GENETIC ASPECTS OF DEVELOPMENTAL PATHOLOGY

RECENT TITLES PUBLISHED BY ALAN R. LISS, INC.
FOR MARCH OF DIMES BIRTH DEFECTS FOUNDATION

Birth Defects Compendium, Second Edition, Daniel Bergsma, *Editor*

BIRTH DEFECTS: ORIGINAL ARTICLE SERIES

1982 — Volume 18

No. 1 **Craniofacial Anomalies: New Perspectives,** Carlos F. Salinas, *Editor*
No. 3A **Annual Review of Birth Defects, 1981, Prenatal Diagnosis and Mechanisms of Teratogenesis,** William L. Nyhan and Kenneth Lyons Jones, *Editors*
No. 3B **Annual Review of Birth Defects, 1981, Dysmorphology,** William L. Nyhan and Kenneth Lyons Jones, *Editors*
No. 4 **Children With Sex Chromosome Aneuploidy: Follow-Up Studies,** Donald A. Stewart, *Editor*
No. 5 **Cumulative Index: Birth Defects: Original Article Series Volumes I (1965)–XVI (1980),** Natalie W. Paul, *Editor*
No. 6 **Genetic Eye Diseases: Retinitis Pigmentosa and Other Inherited Eye Disorders,** Edward Cotlier, Irene H. Maumenee, and Elaine R. Berman, *Editors*
No. 7 **Thalassemia: Recent Advances in Detection and Treatment,** Antonio Cao, Ugo Carcassi, and Peter T. Rowley, *Editors*

1983 — Volume 19

No. 1 **Dentition: Genetic Effects,** Ronald J. Jorgenson, *Editor*
No. 3 **Primary Immunodeficiency Diseases,** Ralph J. Wedgwood, Fred S. Rosen, and Natalie W. Paul, *Editors*
No. 4 **Nervous System Regeneration,** Bernard Haber, J. Regino Perez-Polo, George A. Hashim, and Anna Maria Giuffrida Stella, *Editors*
No. 5 **Annual Review of Birth Defects, 1982, Birth Defects: Clinical and Ethical Considerations,** Sara C. Finley, Wayne H. Finley, and Charles E. Flowers, Jr., *Editors*

1984 — Volume 20

No. 1 **CMV: Pathogenesis and Prevention of Human Infection,** Stanley A. Plotkin, Susan Michelson, Joseph S. Pagano, and Fred Rapp, *Editors*
No. 3 **Craniofacial Mesenchyme in Morphogenesis and Malformation,** Kenneth S. Brown and Carlos F. Salinas, *Editors*

1985 — Volume 21

No. 2 **Diagnostic Accuracy: Effect on Treatment Planning,** Robert J. Shprintzen and Natalie W. Paul, *Editors*
No. 5 **The Patient Within the Patient: Problems in Perinatal Medicine,** Bruce K. Young, *Editor*

1986 — Volume 22

No. 1 **Bone Marrow Transplantation for Treatment of Lysosomal Storage Diseases,** William Krivit and Natalie W. Paul, *Editors*
No. 3 **Prospective Studies on Children With Sex Chromosome Aneuploidy,** Shirley G. Ratcliffe and Natalie W. Paul, *Editors*

Please contact the publisher for information about previous titles in this series published by Alan R. Liss, Inc.

March of Dimes Birth Defects Foundation
Birth Defects: Original Article Series, Volume 23, Number 1, 1987

GENETIC ASPECTS OF DEVELOPMENTAL PATHOLOGY

Solicited Papers and Proceedings of a Symposium Held September 26–28, 1985, in Madison, Wisconsin, as Part of the Interim Meeting of the Society for Pediatric Pathology and Sponsored by the University of Wisconsin-Madison and the March of Dimes Birth Defects Foundation

Editors

Enid F. Gilbert, MD
Departments of Pathology
and Pediatrics
University of Wisconsin
Madison, Wisconsin

John M. Opitz, MD, DSci, hc
Genetic and Birth Defects Unit
Shodair Children's Hospital
Helena, Montana

Associate Editor
Natalie W. Paul
March of Dimes
Birth Defects Foundation
White Plains, New York

Assistant Editor
Melanie Matson
Shodair Children's Hospital
Helena, Montana

ALAN R. LISS, INC., NEW YORK

To enhance medical communication in the birth defects field, the March of Dimes Birth Defects Foundation publishes the *Birth Defects Compendium (2nd Edition)*, an *Original Article Series*, a *Reprint Series*, *Nursing Staff Development Modules*, *Genetics in Practice* (a quarterly newsletter), and provides a series of films and related brochures.

Further information can be obtained from:

Professional Education Department
March of Dimes Birth Defects Foundation
1275 Mamaroneck Avenue
White Plains, New York 10605

Published by:
Alan R. Liss, Inc.
41 East 11th Street
New York, New York 10003

Views expressed in articles published are the authors', and are not to be attributed to the March of Dimes Birth Defects Foundation or its editors unless expressly so stated.

Library of Congress Cataloging-in-Publication Data

Genetic aspects of developmental pathology.

(Birth defects, original article series ; v. 23, no. 1)
Includes index.
1. Fetus—Abnormalities—Genetic aspects—Congresses. 2. Fetus—Abnormalities—Diagnosis—Congresses. I. Gilbert, Enid F., 1927– . II. Opitz, John M. III. Society for Pediatric Pathology (U.S.) IV. University of Wisconsin–Madison. V. March of Dimes Birth Defects Foundation. VI. Series: Birth defects original article series ; v. 23, no. 1. [DNLM: 1. Abnormalities—familial & genetic—congresses. 2. Abnormalities—pathology—congresses. 3. Genetic Screening—congresses. 4. Hereditary Diseases—prevention & control—congresses. W1 BI966 v.23 no.1 / QZ 45 G328 1985]
RG626.B63 vol. 23, no. 1 616'.043 s 86-15299
ISBN 0-8451-1063-2 [618.3'2]

The March of Dimes Birth Defects Foundation is dedicated to the goals of preventing birth defects and ameliorating their consequences for patients, families, and society.

As part of our efforts to achieve these goals, we sponsor, or participate in, a variety of scientific meetings where all questions relating to birth defects are freely discussed. Through our professional education program we speed the dissemination of information by publishing the proceedings of these and other meetings. From time to time, we also reprint pertinent journal articles to help achieve our goals. Now and then, in the course of these articles or discussions, individual viewpoints may be expressed which go beyond the purely scientific and into controversial matters. It should be noted, therefore, that personal viewpoints about such matters will not be censored but this does not constitute an endorsement of them by the **March of Dimes Birth Defects Foundation**.

Dedication

Dedicated to the
Immortal Memory of

JAMES CHRISTIAN GILBERT

(born 3 January 1960, died 11 July 1983)

. . . who realized early that "The earth
is full of things that permit
man a partnership with God . . . "
and that "Man's inner liberation
is God's justification."

Contents

Contributors

Razia Ahmad, MD, Department of Pathology, The Children's Hospital, Denver, CO 80218 **[103]**

Sunita Arya, MD, Departments of Pathology and Laboratory Medicine, The University of Wisconsin Medical School, Madison, WI 53792 **[169,191,293,333,433]**

Daniel R. Beckman, MD, Department of Pathology, University of Wisconsin, Madison, WI 53792 **[47]**

J.A. Bell, DIP MED TECH, Department of Cytogenetics, State Health Laboratory, Brisbane, Queensland, Australia 4000 **[307]**

J.R. Bell, MD, Department of Pathology, Mater Public Hospitals, Brisbane, Queensland, Australia 4000 **[307]**

Stanley Berlow, MD, Department of Pediatrics, University of Wisconsin, Madison, WI 53792 **[47,65]**

Jay Bernstein, MD, Department of Anatomic Pathology, William Beaumont Hospital, Royal Oak, MI 48072 **[115]**

Edward T. Bersu, PhD, Department of Anatomy, University of Wisconsin, Madison, WI 53706 **[315]**

Leslie E. Biesecker, Department of Pediatrics, University of Wisconsin, Madison, WI 53706 **[385]**

Harold J. Bruyere, Jr., PhD, Departments of Pathology and Laboratory Medicine, The University of Wisconsin Medical School, Madison, WI 53792 **[169,443,449,453,459]**

Sherrie Caldwell, MD, Department of Pathology, The Children's Hospital, Denver, CO 80218 **[103]**

James R. Colwill, MD, Departments of Obstetrics and Gynecology, Victoria General Hospital, Victoria, British Columbia, Canada V8Z 6R5 **[179]**

Ernest Cutz, MD, Department of Pathology, Hospital for Sick Children, Toronto, Ontario, Canada M5G 1X8 **[75]**

D.J. deSa, MD, DPHIL, FRC PATH, Department of Pathology, University of Manitoba, Winnipeg, Manitoba, Canada R3E 0W1; present address: Department of Pathology, McMaster University Medical Center, Hamilton, Ontario, Canada L8N 3Z5 **[367]**

M. Renate Dische, MD, PhD, Department of Pathology, The Mount Sinai School of Medicine, New York, NY 10029 **[75]**

William B. Dobyns, MD, Department of Neurology, Medical College of Wisconsin, Milwaukee, WI 53201 **[225]**

Tzann-Tarn Fang, MD, Departments of Pathology and Laboratory Medicine, University of Wisconsin, Madison, WI 53792; present address: 12723 Dairy Brook, Houston, TX 77099 **[449]**

Joan M. FitzGerald, MS, Genetic and Birth Defects Unit, Shodair Children's Hospital, Helena, MT 59604 **[169]**

Frank Frerman, PhD, Department of Pediatrics, University of Colorado, Denver, CO 80262 **[65]**

The numbers in brackets are the opening page numbers of the contributors' articles.

Richard O. Friday, Jr., Department of Radiology, University of Wisconsin, Madison, WI 53706 **[385]**

Enid F. Gilbert, MD, Departments of Pathology and Pediatrics, University of Wisconsin, Madison, WI 53792 **[xv, 47,65,169,191,293,333,385,411,433, 443,449,453,459]**

Jennifer E. Gilbert, Departments of Pathology and Laboratory Medicine, University of Wisconsin, Madison, WI 53792 **[443]**

Stephen Goodman, MD, Department of Pediatrics, University of Colorado, Denver, CO 80262 **[65]**

Bruce A. Gordon, MD, Departments of Biochemistry and Paediatrics, The University of Western Ontario, London, Ontario, Canada N6A 5C1, and Director of Biochemistry, The Children's Psychiatric Research Institute, London, Ontario, Canada N6A 4G6 **[17]**

Dorothy K. Grange, MD, Department of Pathology, University of Wisconsin, Madison, WI 53792; present address: National Institute of Child Health and Human Development, Bethesda, MD 20892 **[191]**

Randi J. Hagerman, MD, Department of Child Development, The Children's Hospital, Denver, CO 80218 **[103]**

M. Daria Haust, MD, Departments of Pathology and Paediatrics, The University of Western Ontario, London, Ontario, Canada N6A 5B7, and Director of Pathology, The Children's Psychiatric Research Institute, London, Ontario, Canada N6A 4G6 **[17]**

M. Heneghan, MD, Department of Radiology, SUNY Stony Brook, Stony Brook, NY 11794 **[401]**

Jorge Las Heras, MD, PhD, Instituto de Investigaciones Clinicas, University of Chile, Hospital Paula Jaraquemada, Casilla 5370-Correo 3, Chile **[421]**

Jürgen Herrmann, MD, Department of Medical Genetics, Great Lakes Genetics, S.C. Wauwatosa, WI 53226 **[191]**

Klaus Heyne, MD, Department of Pediatrics, Medizinische Universität zu Lübeck, D-2400 Lübeck, Federal Republic of Germany **[131]**

George Hoganson, MD, Departments of Pediatrics and Genetics, University of Wisconsin, Madison, WI 53792 **[47,65]**

Hart Isaacs, MD, Department of Pathology, Children's Hospital of Los Angeles, Los Angeles, CA 90024 **[421]**

Dagmar K. Kalousek, MD, Department of Pathology, Children's Hospital and University of British Columbia, Vancouver, British Columbia, Canada V6H 3V4 **[153]**

Cynthia Kaplan, MD, Department of Pathology, SUNY Stony Brook, Stony Brook, NY 11794 **[401]**

A.S. Knisely, MD, Department of Pathology, Cornell Medical Center/The New York Hospital, New York, NY 10021; present address: Departments of Pathology and Laboratory Medicine, Women and Infants Hospital of Rhode Island, Providence, RI 02905 **[75]**

Larry Konick, MD, Department of Pathology, University of Wisconsin, Madison, WI 53706 **[411]**

Steven Kornguth, Departments of Neurology and Physiological Chemistry, University of Wisconsin, Madison, WI 53706 **[341]**

Joan S. Kozel, BS, Department of Educational Resources, The University of Wisconsin Medical School, Madison, WI 53792 **[169]**

Natalie Krassikoff, MD, Departments of Pediatrics and Medical Genetics, University of Wisconsin, Madison, WI 53706 **[385,411]**

I. Lange, MD, FRCS(C), Departments of Obstetrics and Gynecology, University of Manitoba, Winnipeg, Manitoba, Canada R3E 0W1 **[367]**

Renata Laxova, MD, Departments of Pediatrics and Medical Genetics, University of Wisconsin, Madison, WI 53792 **[191,293,385]**

Susan O. Lewin, MB, BCh, FRCP(C), Genetic and Birth Defects Unit, Shodair Children's Hospital, Helena, MT 59604 **[169,277]**

Mario Lituania, MD, Department of Obstetrics, Istituto G. Gaslini, Genova-Quarto 16148, Italy **[131]**

Ronald R. Louie, MD, Departments of Pathology and Pediatrics, University of Wisconsin, Madison, WI 53706; present address: University of Chicago Hospitals and Clinics, Chicago, IL 60637 **[333]**

E. Lyons, MD, FRCP(C), Departments of Ultrasound and Radiology, University of Manitoba, Winnipeg, Manitoba, Canada R3E 0W1 **[367]**

Geoffrey Allan Machin, MD, PhD, Department of Laboratory Medicine, Victoria General Hospital, Victoria, British Columbia, Canada V8Z 6R5 **[179,243,351]**

Margret S. Magid, MD, Department of Pathology, Cornell Medical Center/The New York Hospital, New York, NY 10021 **[75]**

F. Manning, MD, FRSC(C), Departments of Obstetrics and Gynecology, University of Manitoba, Winnipeg, Manitoba, Canada R3E 0W1 **[367]**

Rumiko Matsuoka, MD, Departments of Pathology and Laboratory Medicine, University of Wisconsin, Madison, WI 53792; present address: The Heart Institute of Japan, Tokyo Women's Medical College, Tokyo 162, Japan **[449,453]**

J. McGuire, MB, BS, Departments of Obstetrics and Gynecology, University of Manitoba, Winnipeg, Manitoba, Canada R3E 0W1 **[367]**

Lorraine F. Meisner, PhD, Department of Preventive Medicine, University of Wisconsin, State Laboratory of Hygiene, University of Wisconsin, Madison, WI 53706 **[333]**

Gary Mierau, PhD, Department of Pathology, The Children's Hospital, Denver, CO 80218 **[103]**

Stuart F. Nicholson, MD, Department of Radiology, Foothills Hospital, Calgary, Alberta, Canada T2N 2T9 **[351]**

Carl A. Nimrod, MD, Department of Obstetrics and Gynecology, Foothills Hospital, Calgary, Alberta, Canada T2N 2T9 **[351]**

Makoto Nishibatake, MD, Departments of Pathology and Laboratory Medicine, University of Wisconsin, Madison, WI 53792 **[433]**

Toshio Nishikawa, MD, Departments of Pathology and Laboratory Medicine, University of Wisconsin, Madison, WI 53792; present address: Department of Pathology, Tokyo Women's Medical College, Tokyo 162, Japan **[443,449,453,459]**

Ronald W. Olson, MD, Department of Obstetrics and Gynecology, University of Wisconsin, Madison, WI 53706 **[385,433]**

John M. Opitz, MD, Genetic and Birth Defects Unit, Shodair Children's Hospital, Helena, MT 59604 **[xv,169,191,277,293,449]**

J.H. Pearn, MD, Department of Child Health, Royal Children's Hospital, Brisbane, Queensland, Australia 4000 **[307]**

James C. Pettersen, PhD, Department of Anatomy, University of Wisconsin, Madison, WI 53706 **[315]**

James S. Popkin, MD, Department of Pediatrics, Victoria General Hospital, Victoria, British Columbia, Canada V8Z 6R5 **[179]**

Helga Rehder, MD, Department of Human Genetics, Medizinische Universität zu Lübeck, D-2400 Lübeck, Federal Republic of Germany **[131]**

James F. Reynolds, Jr., MD, Genetic and Birth Defects Unit, Shodair Children's Hospital, Helena, MT 59604 **[169]**

B. Rochelson, MD, Department of Obstetrics and Gynecology, SUNY Stony Brook, Stony Brook, NY 11794 **[401]**

Lucy Balian Rorke, MD, Department of Pathology, The Children's Hospital of Philadelphia, Philadelphia, PA 19104 **[215]**

Leslie Schweitzer, MD, New York Medical School, Psychoanalytic Institute, New York, NY 10003 **[65]**

Glen Snyder, Department of Pediatrics, University of Wisconsin, Madison, WI 53706 **[385]**

Geoffrey H. Sperber, PhD, Department of Oral Biology, Faculty of Dentistry, University of Alberta, Edmonton, Alberta, Canada T6G 2N8 **[243]**

Jürgen Spranger, Department of Pediatrics, University Hospitals, D-6500 Mainz, Federal Republic of Germany **[1]**

Salma M. Styles, PhD, Department of Laboratory Medicine, Victoria General Hospital, Victoria, British Columbia, Canada V8Z 6R5 **[179]**

Yasuo Takagi, MD, Department of Pathology and Laboratory Medicine, University of Wisconsin, Madison, WI 53792; present address: Department of Pediatrics, Showa University, Tokyo, Japan **[453,459]**

Stephen N. Thibodeau, PhD, Department of Pathology, The Children's Hospital, Denver, CO 80218 **[103]**

C. Trunca, PhD, Department of Obstetrics and Gynecology, SUNY Stony Brook, Stony Brook, NY 11794 **[401]**

Hideo Uno, MD, PhD, Wisconsin Regional Primate Research Center, Madison, WI 53706 **[443]**

Gail Waldstein, MD, Department of Pathology, The Children's Hospital, Denver, CO 80218 **[103]**

Michael Weber, MD, Department of Pathology, Medizinische Universität zu Lübeck, D-2400 Lübeck, Federal Republic of Germany **[131]**

Preface

Within recent years, pediatric pathology, as the final point of convergence of all facts, data, and hypotheses concerning the prenatal life, illness, and death of normal, and malformed fetuses and infants, has assumed a previously undreamed of complexity which is well represented by the 33 contributions to this volume.

The papers by Spranger, Bernstein, Rehder, Rorke, and Opitz were presented at a special symposium on genetic aspects of pediatric pathology on Saturday morning, 28 September 1985 at the University of Wisconsin, in conjunction with an interim meeting of the Society for Pediatric Pathology; the other papers are expanded versions of poster demonstrations at the meeting or original investigations especially solicited for this volume.

The fact that pediatric pathology is practiced by physicians (in collaboration with equally valued basic scientists and laboratory staff) means that all common law medico-legal precedents pertain to them as well as to the clinicians who cared for mother/fetus or infant during life with equal liability for failure to identify cause of death and/or malformation, especially of conditions with a substantial recurrence risk. The disappearance of the "locality rule" makes the pediatric pathologist responsible for the diagnosis of *any* previously described condition, regardless of how rare, and, especially, if, the preceding clinicians had missed the diagnosis.

This paragon scholar/scientist then must be clinical, anatomical, and a laboratory pathologist, electron microscoper and histochemist, "developmental" pathologist, cytogeneticist, and biochemist with a more than passing interest in teratology and the "recombinant DNA" aspects of molecular biology, for here is the last chance to collect DNA from cells cultured from fascia lata, amnion, or other tissues, if indicated.

Thus, obstetrician notes small fetus and finds evidence of a severe form of fetal dwarfism on the basis of roentgenograms and ultrasonography at 32 weeks. Mother goes into spontaneous labor soon afterwards and delivers an infant with short bowed limbs, soft skull, numerous fractures, characteristic facial appearance, and roentgenographic evidence of osteogenesis imperfecta, a presumed lethal type II. It is Friday afternoon, and from the delivery room the infant and placenta immediately go to the pathology morgue to be studied on Monday morning when growth of fibroblasts from the infant and placenta may be severely impaired. Yet, as Spranger points out in his review in this volume, in precisely such a case recombinant DNA studies may make it possible to determine if the infant's condition was due to a new mutation (with negligible recurrence risks) or represents the homozygous state of a defect present in both parents (with 25% recurrence risk). To determine linkage phase of DNA probe and disease locus (especially of autosomal dominant conditions such as Huntington chorea), it will be important for the pathologist to study not only the brain or other tissue(s) of the dead person entrusted to him/her for final care, but also to obtain cells from the patient for the preparation of DNA samples.

It seems paradoxical to demand all that expertise (and more if it were up to the insurance "industry") from one person with finite strength and time to read, work and with the very best judgment, training, experience, and ethical sensitivity when in large parts of the United States, e.g. Montana, there are no pediatric pathologists at all and few general pathologists who make fetal/genetic and developmental pathology an area of even passing interest.

Yet some two-thirds of mankind never make it to the end of the first year of life, with most in this group dying in early stages of pregnancy and with the stillbirth rate of 7 or 8/1000 appearing as some sort of irreducible biological constant. More than half of spontaneously aborted embryos and stillborn fetuses have gross developmental abnormalities, and in over 60% of aborted embryos a chromosome abnormality is found. Thus, genetic disorders are the commonest cause of "morbidity" and mortality in humans.

And parents do indeed care, they care desperately about the how and why of their infant's anomaly and/or death, and they want the facts and explanations and genetic and grief counseling. This is documented not only on the basis of our clinical practice involving by now hundreds of cases studied in Madison and/or Helena, but also by a rapidly increasing genre of literature for lay persons in pamphlet, booklet, or book form on pregnancy loss, stillbirth, and infant death.*

The obvious answer is for pathologists to collaborate with many colleagues, including radiologists (especially those with expertise in skeletal radiology); cytogeneticists, clinical, biochemical, and molecular geneticists; anatomists and embryologists (a highly endangered species of academic scientist); and teratologists. Above all, it will be important for the (pediatric) pathologist with an interest in fetal genetic/developmental pathology to cultivate the good will of their MEDLINE operators and librarians for expert literature searches on a given subject. These searches are not free anymore, but compared with the cost of losing a lawsuit over a missed diagnosis, say

*A sampling of the latest publications of this type received in Helena over the last month: "Comfort Us, Lord—Our Baby Died," "Empty Arms: A Guide to Help Parents and Loved Ones Cope With a Miscarriage," "Empty Arms: Emotional Support for Those Who Have Suffered Miscarriage," "Miscarriage," "Newborn Death," "She was Born. She Died," and "Empty Arms and Miscarriage: A Shattered Dream."

of the autosomal recessive Bartsocas-Pappas syndrome, they are very reasonable indeed.

Thus, we have reached an era of sophistication in our knowledge and the application of research and diagnostic techniques as to have catapulted the pediatric pathologist involved in developmental pathology to the forefront of investigations into developmental biology. Think only of the revolutionary advances in peroxisomopathies alone, with X-linked dominant chondrodysplasia calcificans punctata being only the most recent entity added to a rapidly increasing list which began with the Zellweger syndrome only a few years ago!

The papers in this volume were ordered into nine groups according to subject matter, the first dealing with metabolic and connective tissue disorders. In his authoritative review of the developmental pathology of *collagen*, Spranger demonstrates the extraordinary molecular heterogeneity that has been identified as the basis of the lethal forms of *osteogenesis imperfecta*, a subject that should be of deep interest to pathologists since so many lethal disorders of prenatal development are associated with skeletal abnormalities. Waldstein and her coworkers document histologically apparent *elastin* abnormalities of skin of patients with the *fragile X* [fra(X)] or *Martin-Bell syndrome* (MBS) as possible explanation for the evident connective tissue dysplasia in children with that condition.

We are most grateful to Drs. Haust and Gordon for summarizing their elegant ultrastructural studies in the HHH (*hyperornithinemia*, *hyperammonemia*, and *homocitrullinuria*) syndrome. Beckman et al and Hoganson et al from the University of Wisconsin describe, respectively, the pathological findings observed in patients with *5,10-methylene tetrahydrofolate reductase deficiency* and in *glutaric acidemia type II*, the former now considered the commonest hereditary defect in the metabolism of folic acid, and the latter being of exceptional interest since it is one of a growing group of metabolic disorders that are associated with structural defects of differentiation. Knisely and his coworkers from New York present exceptionally well-documented clinical and genetic reports of four new cases of *neonatal hemochromatosis* with pathological findings, results of quantitative iron studies in one case, and a thorough review of the previous literature on the subject of neonatal hemochromatosis.

In a magisterial paper that stands in a class by itself, Bernstein reviews and documents the *hepatic involvement* in a considerable number of *genetic renal syndromes* suggestive either of pleiotropy, or perhaps more likely a common tissue determinant shared by liver and kidney during histogenesis and similarly mutant in both organs in the given disorder, e.g. autosomal recessive infantile polycystic disease.

The five papers in the next section address a broader, more general, and heterogeneous set of topics. Rehder and her coworkers report on selected experiences in a group of exceptionally interesting cases from one of the great world centers of fetal pathology working in closest association with clinical geneticists and experts in prenatal diagnosis, cytogeneticists and pediatricians in Lübeck. Here Rehder et al confirm again that the SC-pseudothalidomide and Roberts syndrome are mild and severe variants of the same disorder because of observation of both forms in the same sibship with the same chromosome abnormality—i.e. paracentromeric heterochromatic puffing as a function of premature sister-chromatid separation.

Dagmar Kalousek has now established an extremely important center for the anatomical and genetic study of embryos and fetuses at the University of British Columbia, one of very few in Canada. Her paper documents a 7-year-experience with early abortion specimens which usually got short shrift in most general pathology labs with almost invariable report of "products of conception." Kalousek's report on almost 1,800 specimens deserves careful reading not only for its high methodologic standards in "routine" studies (still possible in a socialized medicine system), but also for the renewed demonstration of the high rate of chromosome abnormalities (approximately 60%) in the 460 specimens successfully cultured, and even higher (93.3%!) rate in embryos with localized defects.

Bruyere et al summarize the experience (mostly on a methodological basis) of the combined Madison-Helena fetal genetic pathology study groups and demonstrate the immense value of such studies in suggesting teratogenic cause and in the discovery of new genetic entities.

Colwill, working with the distinguished reproductive geneticist and pathologist Geoffrey Machin now of Victoria, B.C., and his collaborators summarize in a valuable paper the observed associations between acute second trimester EPH (edema/proteinuria/hypertension) "gestosis" and fetal anomalies, including sacro-coccygeal teratoma with hydrops fetalis, trisomy 13, and triploidy.

Grange and her coworkers from Madison and Helena document the remarkable pathogenetic heterogeneity of short umbilical cords which fall into at least six more or less distinct groups including ADAM sequence, presumed early amnion rupture ("cyllo/pleurosomus"), acephalus-acardia, presumed primary defect of umbilical cord formation, schisis-association, and presumed fetal hypokinesia.

The section on CNS malformations contains two important papers—a superb general approach to abnormalities of brain differentiation by Lucy Rorke of Philadelphia, and one on the lissencephalies by Bill Dobyns (now of the Milwaukee Children's Hospital) who has made very substantial contributions to the subject of the syndromal and chromosomal and non-syndromal forms of various forms of lissencephaly.

In the section on developmental mechanisms, Sperber and Machin give what is probably the finest available anatomo-histological analysis of the janiceps form of conjoined twinning as an important commentary on the developmental instability of the human midline. The broader aspects of developmental fields are discussed by Opitz and Lewin in the second paper in this section.

The cytogenetic abnormalities of human dysmorphogenesis are so important that a group of five papers on that subject was collected into a special section in the proceedings. Gilbert et al give a brief review of the fetal and placental abnormalities seen in human aneuploidy and polyploidy based on poster exhibits at the meeting. Judy Bell and her coworkers give results of an 8-year survey of chromosome abnormalities in live-born children from Queensland, Australia, showing that nearly half of all chromosome disorders diagnosed up to age 14 are detected in the first week of life, and that in such material there tends to be a substantial underascertainment of the gonosomal aneuploidies 47,XXX, 47,XXY, and 47,XYY.

Pettersen and Bersu of the University of Wisconsin summarize their lovely work on the anatomical/developmental effects of aneuploidy and polyploidy (triploidy) in humans and of trisomy 1, 16, and 19 in the mouse. The work of these two collaborators is virtually unique in the world, one supposes because gross anatomy in general has become a bit unfashionable, to the great detriment of the rest of medicine and biology. Almost 20 years ago Beverly Barash dissected the first 18-trisomy infant at the University of Wisconsin in collaboration with zoologist, anthropologist, and pediatric clinical geneticist; the possibility that she might have discoverd truly atavistic structures in the Darwinian sense filled all but one of the collaborators with deepest apprehension. This was the humble beginning of the anatomical genetics program at the University of Wisconsin which is now leading the world in the field and has done much to support the Waddington-Shapiro hypothesis.

Meisner and coworkers from the University of Wisconsin give an instructive analysis of a fetus with 70,XXYY chromosome constitution with partial hydatidiform degeneration and *female* external genitalia in the presence of abdominal testes.

Kornguth of the University of Wisconsin has joined the team of investigators working on mouse trisomy 16 (homology with human trisomy 21) and has contributed a beautiful paper on the development of the CNS in the trisomy 16 mouse.

Prenatal diagnosis is where a collaborative team of obstetrician, clinical geneticist, ultrasonographer and others frequently arrive at conclusions influencing decisions which may provide the pediatric (genetic) pathologists with a plethora of abnormal fetuses. Machin and his former coworkers from Calgary illustrate and document the operation of such a multidisciplinary team in prenatal diagnosis and management of fetuses with congenital anomalies.

McGuire et al from Winnipeg report on their methods and findings in studying skeletal dysplasias prenatally with ultrasound—an important topic because of the commonness of skeletal involvement in congenital defect. Their material includes thanatophoric dysplasia, hypophosphatasia, achondrogenesis II, and a fascinating new skeletal dysplasia in a pair of sibs.

Laxova et al from the University of Wisconsin report on the ultrasonographic (prenatal?) diagnosis of renal cystic disease.

A section on the clinical and diagnostic aspects of congenital anomalies and tumors includes a somewhat heterogeneous group of papers of exceptional interest.

Kaplan et al from SUNY-Stony Brook report on the use of the femoral cylinder index in the diagnosis of the Ullrich-Turner syndrome. Krassikoff et al from the University of Wisconsin report only the second infant with classical hydrolethalus syndrome born to non-Finnish parents. Las Heras and Isaacs document their extensive experience with congenital tumors at the Children's Hospital of Los Angeles. And Olson, with his collaborators from Madison, returns most instructively to the ever more important subject of nonimmunologic hydrops fetalis, in this case due to intrauterine closure of the foramen ovale.

The last section of the Symposium includes a series of papers by Bruyere and coworkers from the University of Wisconsin on the teratological production of congenital anomalies—mostly of the cardiovascular system of the chick and caused in diverse ways. One of these was a direct outgrowth of a clinical case studied in Helena and Madison of an embryo with truncus arteriosus whose mother had taken four tablets of Tedral® (theophylline, ephedrine, and phenobarbital) at a critical phase of organogenesis.

We are convinced that this group of papers can be considered evidence that the field of pediatric pathology, in its fusion with genetics, has reached a level of sophistication previously undreamed of and is now capable of challenging even the most brilliant minds in medicine and general biology. This is the ideal time in the history of the specialty for a young professional to enter it and to pursue any one of the half-dozen or so areas of subspecialization and research discussed by the authorities represented in this volume. With a good mentor, a critical mind, high enthusiasm, and a modest investment of effort in morgue and in laboratory, such a beginner will attain mature wisdom with daily satisfaction and highest intellectual pleasure.

We want to thank all of our collaborators at the University of Wisconsin for making this meeting such a success, all contributors to this volume for taking the time and making the effort to produce this important group of papers, and the Office of Postgraduate Medical Education (Dr. Thomas C. Meyer, Dean, and Mrs. Sarah Aslakson) of the University of Wisconsin and the March of Dimes Birth Defects Foundation for financial support. We give special thanks to George and Steven Kargas for their untiring efforts during the meeting to ensure that the entire program ran smoothly.

This volume is dedicated in sorrow and gratitude to the beloved memory of our son and friend James Christian Gilbert who died too young but lived in the firm belief that "Man is the language of God."

Enid F. Gilbert
John M. Opitz

The Developmental Pathology of Collagen in Humans

J. Spranger

Children's Hospital, University of Mainz, Federal Republic of Germany

To understand the developmental pathology of collagen a certain knowledge of normal collagen synthesis and structure is required. There are excellent reviews on this subject [1–4] and only a few basic facts will be repeated here.

PHYSIOLOGIC ASPECTS

Collagen is the most abundant mammalian protein. This tough fibrous material is a major constituent of all mesenchymal tissues, most notably of skin, bone, tendons, ligaments, and blood vessels. It provides strength and integrity, transmits force, protects and compartmentalizes the body and its organs.

Over 8 different kinds of collagen have been detected which differ from each other by the sequence of amino acids. Five of them are listed in Table I.

The various collagens have the same basic molecular structure. Each collagen molecule consists of 3 polypeptide chains that are twisted around each other in a right-handed helix. Each chain is twisted in a left-handed helix. Every third amino acid in this chain is glycine, which is essential for correct helix packing. Hence, the typical collagen sequence is Gly-X-Y in which X and Y may be any amino acid except tryptophane, cysteine, and tyrosine. The chains are rich in proline, lysine, and hydroxylysine.

Nine nonallelic collagen genes are presumed to code for the 9 different alpha chains of the 5 major collagens [5]. The $\alpha 1(I)$ collagen gene is located

Birth Defects: Original Article Series, Volume 23, Number 1, pages 1–16

TABLE 1. Collagen Types

Type	Chain composition	Tissue distribution
I	$[\alpha 1\ (I)]_2\ \alpha 2$	Skin, bone, tendons, fasciae, blood vessels
II	$\alpha 1\ (II)_3$	Cartilage
III	$\alpha 1\ (III)_3$	Skin, tendons, fasciae, blood vessels
IV	$\alpha 1\ (IV)_3$	Basement membranes, lens capsule
V	$(\alpha B)_3$ $(\alpha B)_2\ \alpha A$	Fetal membranes, blood vessels; minor components in bone and cartilage

on chromosome 17 and contains about 18 kilobase pairs (kbp) of DNA [6,7]. Intervening sequences divide the gene into a larger number of exons [4]. The $\alpha 2$(I) gene is located on the long arm of chromosome 7 [7] and encompasses about 38 kbp of DNA. About 50 introns divide the gene into short exons of 54 bp [8]. Most exons studied so far in different collagens are 54 bp long. Shorter exons occur whose lengths are in multiples of 9 base pairs, ie, the unit encoding the basic glycine-X-Y triplet.

The gene transcription product, procollagen messenger RNA, is about 8-fold shorter than the parent gene. It is thought that extensive splicing favors recombinations and deletions [9]. In addition, the highly repetitive base sequences GGN-CCN-CCN coding for glycine - proline - hydroxyproline in the alpha chain domains may predispose the genes to unequal cross-over mutations during meiosis [8]. These 2 factors partly explain the great diversity of mutations that have been found.

The ratio of $\alpha 1$(I) and $\alpha 2$(I) species in cytoplasm is about 2:1 and so is the ratio of $\alpha 1$(I):$\alpha 2$(I) propeptide chains (Fig. 1). Since the mRNAs are translated at about equal rates, and since there appears to exist only 1 gene for pro $\alpha 1$(I) and one for pro $\alpha 2$(I) per haploid genome, there must be differences between the 2 mRNAs in their rates of transcription, processing, or metabolic turnover [10]. The mRNA molecules are transported to the cytoplasm and are translated on ribosomes attached to membranes in the rough endoplasmic reticulum.

Procollagen chains are synthesized in the rough endoplasmic reticulum. They consist of a helical domain, a COOH-terminal and a NH_2-terminal propeptide extension. These nonhelical extensions are necessary for chain alignment, formation and stabilization of the triple helix, for prevention of intracellular fibrogenesis, and transport. In the course of chain synthesis and elongation, most prolyl residues in the Y-position of the Gly-X-Y triplet are

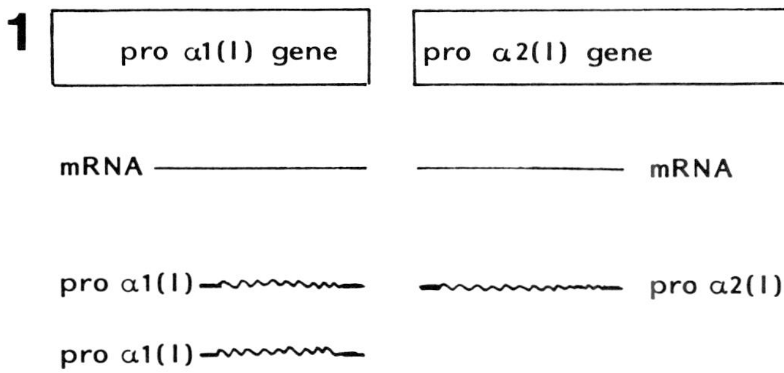

Fig. 1. One gene codes for pro α1(I) and a second one for about half the amount of pro α2(I). The different production rates are probably caused by differences in the rates of transcription, processing, or turnover of mRNA.

hydroxylated by the enzyme prolyl-4-hydroxylase. Hydroxylated prolyl residues stabilize the triple helix. A small proportion of lysyl residues in Y-position is also hydroxylated creating potential sites for O-linked glycosylation. Once synthesis of the chain is complete, it is released from the ribosome and starts to associate with other chains through a domain located within the C-terminal propeptide extension. The triple helix propagates rapidly from the COOH-terminus to the NH_2-terminus of the molecule. It is important to note that modification of the chain, ie hydroxylation and glycosylation, stops once the helix is formed. Interference with, and hence slowing of, the helix formation leads to excessive hydroxylation and glycosylation, ie, overmodification.

After its formation, the intact procollagen molecule is transported to the Golgi apparatus, packaged into Golgi-derived vesicles, moved to the cell surface and secreted. Synthesis, modification, and triple helix formation in the rough endoplasmic reticulum take about 7 minutes, transport and secretion about 20.

Once outside the cell, procollagen molecules aggregate and form fibril precursors. The nonhelical extensions at both ends of the procollagen are cleaved by 2 different proteases. The fibrils are then stabilized by the formation of covalent bonds. This occurs by the oxidative deamination of lysyl or hydrosylysyl residues to the corresponding aldehydes—allysine or hydroxyallysine. The aldehydes react with themselves or with lysine or hydroxylysine and form aldol or aldimine products linking the chains.

GENETIC DISORDERS OF COLLAGEN METABOLISM

The complexity of collagen synthesis and structure explains the large number of known and the much greater number of expected genetic defects

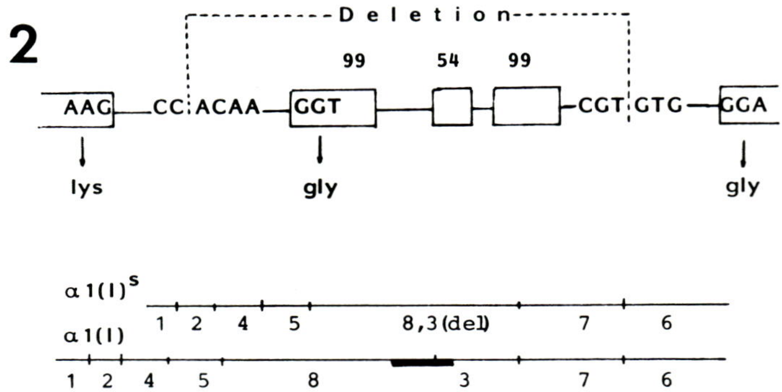

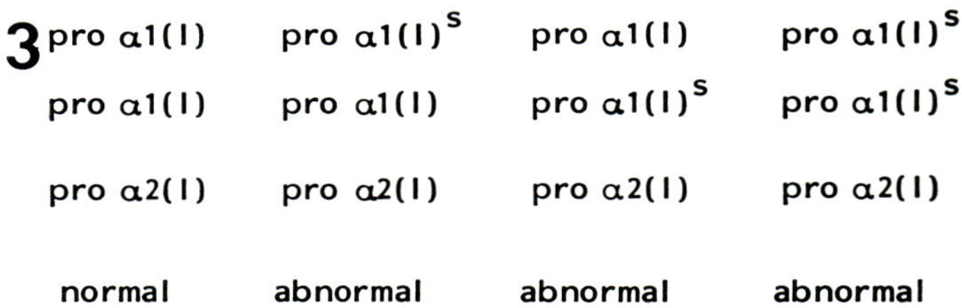

Fig. 2. Scheme of the CB 1262 deletion. It consists of about 650 base pairs, leaves the sequence lys→gly intact and results in a shortened $\alpha1$(I) chain. The numbers refer to the pro $\alpha1$(I) CB fragments. [Adapted from 14 and 15].

Fig. 3. In the CB 1262 deletion (as in any heterozygous mutation affecting the structure of pro $\alpha1$(I) chains) 3 of 4 procollagen trimers contain 1 or 2 abnormal chains (here marked pro $\alpha1(I)^{s}$).

of collagen metabolism. Best studied are defects of type I collagen [11]. A few examples will be presented. Clinically, they lead to abnormalities mainly of bone, skin, and ligaments and clinically to 2 groups of disorders: osteogenesis imperfecta and the Ehlers-Danlos "syndrome." Few firm data are available on patients with the Marfan syndrome.

1)*The CRL 1262 Deletion

In 1975, cells were derived from the skin of a dismembered stillborn infant [12]. They were cultured and stored in the American Type Culture Collec-

*The numbers correspond to those in Figure 8.

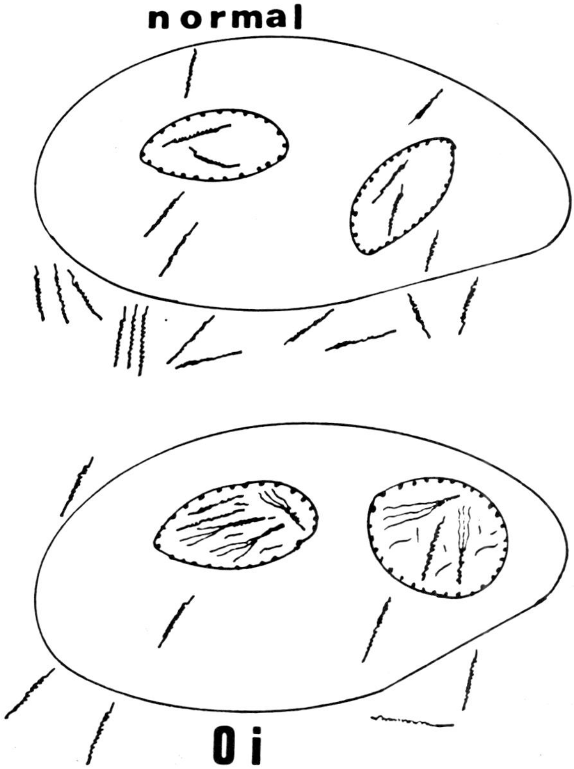

Fig. 4. Protein suicide. Type I procollagen containing abnormal chains cannot be assembled properly or secreted from the endoplasmic reticulum. The endoplasmic reticulum is dilated by excessive amounts of defective procollagen molecules which are degraded. Too little procollagen becomes available to the extracellular space.

tion, Rockville, Md. The study of this cell line, which received the number CRL 1262 by various groups of investigators, has led to important results.

Part of the mutant gene from cell strain CRL 1262 has been cloned and sequenced [13–15]. It was found that the mutation consisted of a deletion of about 650 base pairs. The deletion extended between 2 introns and contained 3 exons coding for 84 amino acids. The loss of these amino acids led to a pro $\alpha 1(I)$ chain that was 84 amino acids shorter than the normal chain (Fig. 2). Since the deletion left the coding sequence in register, the structure of the shortened chain beyond the deletion was normal and it associated with normal $\alpha 1(I)$ and $\alpha 2(I)$ chains. Three out of 4 procollagen molecules contained 1 or

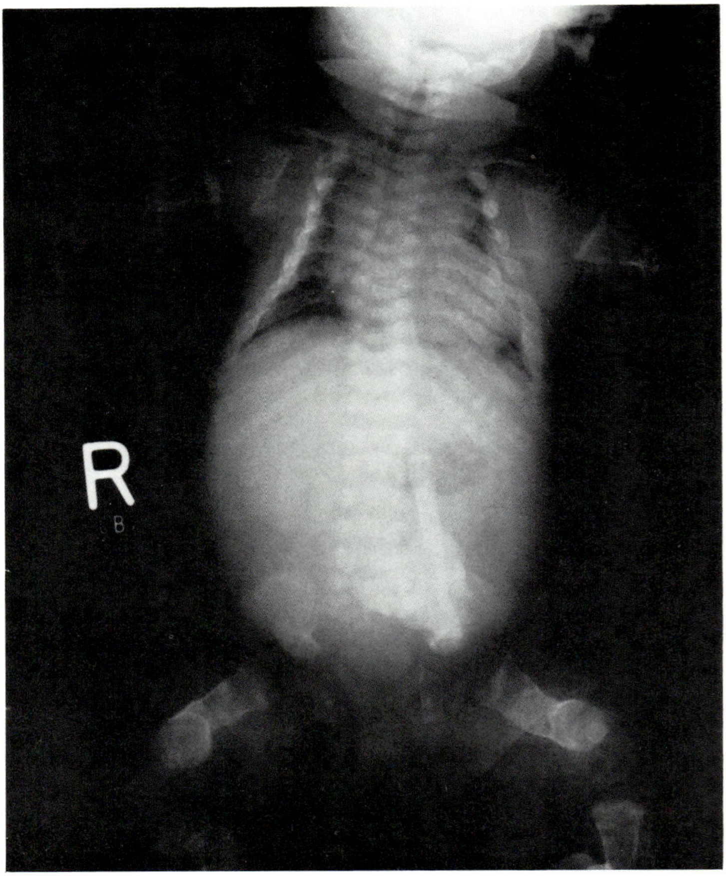

Fig. 5. Osteogenesis imperfecta type II-A. The long bones and ribs are short and broad due to innumerable compression fractures.

2 of these shortened $\alpha 1$(I) chains (Fig. 3). The shortening apparently interfered with helix formation, and procollagen molecules that contained 1 or 2 shortened chains were not folded into a stable triple helix [16]. They were not effectively secreted but remained in the rough endoplasmic reticulum, underwent increased posttranslational modification, and were degraded. Too little type I procollagen was secreted from the cell [17] and too little type I collagen became available to the extracellular tissue [18] (Fig. 4). This led to a number of secondary effects including an increased production of type III procollagen [15]. The clinical result was a lethal bone dysplasia with radiographic characteristics of osteogenesis imperfecta type II-A [12] (Fig. 5).

6

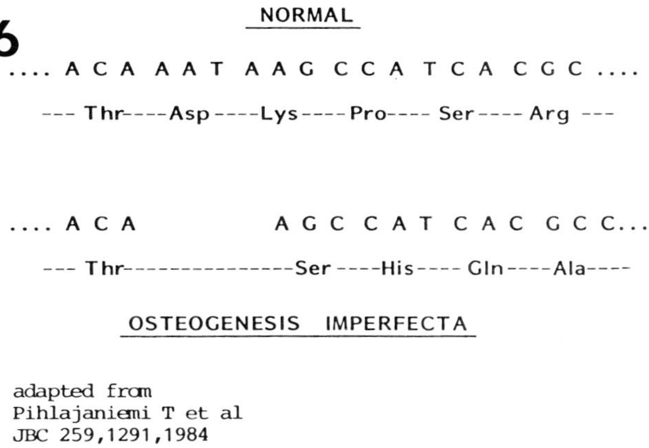

7

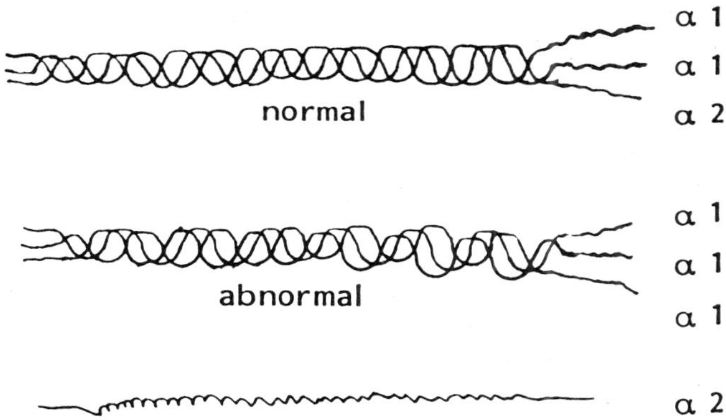

Fig. 6. Frameshift mutation in a patient with osteogenesis imperfecta observed in Göttingen. The deletion of 4 bases AATA (or ATAA or AAAT) changed the sequence of base triplets from ACA-AAT to ACA-AGC and of the corresponding amino acids from threonine-asparagine to threonine-serine.

Fig. 7. Due to the abnormal amino acid sequence in the C-terminal propeptide extension of the $\alpha 2$(I) chains of the patient with the Göttingen mutation, $\alpha 2$(I) chains do not associate with $\alpha 1$(I) chains. Only $\alpha 1$(I) trimers are formed.

The production of a protein that cannot be properly used but instead is degraded after its synthesis has been called "protein suicide" [8,11].

2) The "Göttingen Deletion"

A 2-year-old patient was observed at the University of Göttingen with a severe form of osteogenesis imperfecta [19, 20]. At age 7 weeks, 19 fractures were present and the future course of the disorder was consistent with type

III osteogenesis imperfecta with marked shortness and deformation of the long bones. The parents were consanguineous.

Type I collagen extracted from the patient's skin had no $\alpha 2(I)$ chains and consisted of $\alpha 1(I)$ trimers. Similarly, cultured fibroblasts synthesized and secreted only $\alpha 1(I)$ trimers [19]. The basic defect in this disorder was a deletion of 4 nucleotides in the terminal DNA region that codes for the C-propeptide of the pro $\alpha 2(I)$ chain [21,22]. The deletion of 4 nucleotides out of an AAATAA sequence led to a frameshift changing the last 33 amino acids of COOH-propeptide of the $\alpha 2(I)$ chain (Fig. 6). The changed amino acid sequence prevented the association of $\alpha 2(I)$ with $\alpha 1(I)$ chains. Consequently, only $\alpha 1(I)$ chains associated with each other and only $\alpha 1(I)$ trimers were formed (Fig. 7).

Fibroblasts of both parents, who did not have osteogenesis imperfecta, secreted both $\alpha 1(I)$ trimers and normal type I procollagen composed of two $\alpha 1(I)$ and one $\alpha 2(I)$ chains. Thus, the parents were clinically unaffected heterozygotes for the deletion.

Other Deletions

3) De Wet et al [23] reported observations on fibroblasts from a proband with a lethal form of osteogenesis imperfecta. The cells produced shortened pro $\alpha 2(I)$ chains. The shortening was caused by the deletion of about 20 amino acids from the cyanogen bromide (CB) 3,5 fragment of the chain which contains amino acid residues 361-775 (Fig. 8). The pro $\alpha 2(I)$ chains produced by both parents were normal. Independently, the patient's cells and those of his father produced about half the normal amount of pro $\alpha 2(I)$ chains. The patient apparently had 2 separate mutations at the $\alpha 2(I)$ gene locus: a clinically silent null allele for $\alpha 2(I)$ inherited from the father and a deletion of the functioning gene which probably resulted from a *de novo* mutation.

4) A deletion of about 30 amino acids from the CB 4 fragment of the $\alpha 2(I)$ chain was observed in cultured fibroblasts from a 5-year-old boy with a mild form of dominantly inherited osteogenesis imperfecta [24]. A peculiar clinical manifestation was marked joint laxity. The patient's mother had blue sclerae and was only 134 cm tall. Blue sclerae, dislocated hips, and multiple fractures were present in other maternal relatives. In accord with the dominant inheritance, only one of the two pro $\alpha 2(I)$ genes was mutated and the patient's cells produced equal amounts of normal and of shortened pro $\alpha 2(I)$ chains.

A similar mutation that altered the structure of the N-terminal region of the pro $\alpha 2(I)$ chain produced a clinical disorder that has been classified as

Ehlers-Danlos syndrome type VII or arthrochalasis multiplex congenita [25,26]. Both this and the above-mentioned mutation led to a decreased thermal stability and to a resistance of the procollagen molecule to cleavage by procollagen N-protease.

5) In the same pro $\alpha2(I)$ CB 4 fragment, another deletion of 15–20 amino acids was detected in cultured fibroblasts from a 56-year-old woman with a clinical disorder that could be classified as osteogenesis imperfecta type I [27]. Collagen fibrils in bone and skin were smaller in diameter than normal and those in bone were disorganized.

6) A large deletion of about 100 amino acids from the central portion of the $\alpha2(I)$ chain was found in another patient with type II osteogenesis imperfecta [28]. Since both parents produced normal amounts of structurally normal type I procollagen the disease must have resulted from a new mutation at the $\alpha2(I)$ locus.

7) The CB6 Gly→ Cyst Mutation

Cultured fibroblasts from a patient with type II-A osteogenesis imperfecta produced about equal amounts of normal and abnormal pro $\alpha1(I)$ chains. Extensive studies by Steinmann et al [29] traced the abnormality to the exchange of a single amino acid in the pro $\alpha1(I)$ chain. In its COOH-terminal cyanogen bromide CB6 peptide, 27 amino acids from the terminus, cysteine had been substituted for glycine. This was caused by a single base substitution in a glycine codon [cited by Cohen P, 30]. As a result of this single amino acid substitution, triple helical formation, which proceeds from the COOH- to the NH_2-terminus, was transiently disrupted. This led to the same consequences as in the CRL 1262 deletion: collagen molecules that contained 1 or 2 abnormal chains were overmodified so that the content of hydroxylysine and glycosylated hydroxylysine was more than twice normal. Helix stability was decreased as reflected by a decreased melting temperature. Part of the abnormal material accumulated in the cell and was degraded; cellular secretion was diminished with a reduction of the amount of collagen in the extracellular tissue compartment. The observations of Steinmann and his coworkers provide evidence that a single amino acid substitution can have the same disastrous effects as large deletions, namely "protein suicide" and a lethal clinical disorder.

8) Subtle Structural Alterations

Based on Steinmann's observation [29] that overmodification of the pro α-chains occurred NH_2-terminal to the mutation point, Bonadio and Byers [30] proposed that "overmodification" is a general sign of delayed triple helix

8

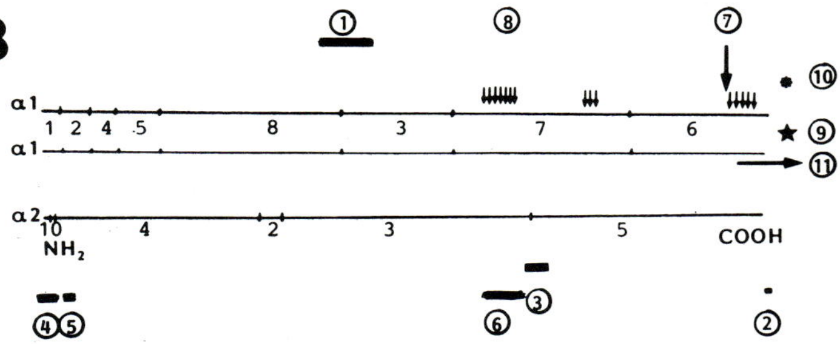

Fig. 8. Structural changes of pro α1(I) and pro α2(I) chains in patients with osteogenesis imperfecta. The numbers refer to those in the text. (1) Deletion of 84 amino acids in one α1(I) allele product. OI type II [12-18]. (2) 4 base deletion leading to changes of the terminal amino acids of the COOH propeptide of the α2(I) chain. OI type III [19–22]. (3) Compound heterozygosity: deletion of 20 amino acids in 1 α2(I) chain and nonfunctional α2(I) gene. Lethal OI [23]. (4) Deletion of about 30 amino acids near NH_2-terminus with ensuing resistence to procollagen-N-proteinase. Dominant OI with marked joint laxity [24]. (5) Small deletion from α2(I) CB 4 propeptide. Mild OI with blue sclerae [27]. (6) Deletion of about 100 amino acids in 1 α1(I) chain. Lethal OI [28]. (7) Amino acid substitution (gly---cys) in α1(I) fragment of one α1(I) allele product. OI type II-A [29] (thick arrow) (8) Presumed single amino acid exchanges with overmodification in NH_2-terminal part of 1 pro α1(I) chain. All patients had OI II-A phenotype [30]. (thin arrows). (9) One allele for pro α1(I) not transcribed into mRNa. Lethal OI [10]. (10) Increased mannose content of COOH-propeptide extension. OI type III [35]. (11) Lengthened pro α1(I) chain. Lethal OI [36].

formation and can be used to locate the mutation site. Helix formation begins at the COOH-terminus of the molecule and propagates toward the NH_2-terminus. It proceeds normally until the mutation site is reached. Thereafter the rate of formation of a stable helix is delayed and the unassembled molecules are available to the modifying enzymes longer than normal. Overmodification results (Fig. 9). The starting point of the overmodification is the mutation site. If it is determined, gene or messenger RNA studies can be directed to it.

Studying cultured cells from 15 patients with osteogenesis imperfecta type II-A according to Sillence [31], Bonadio and Byers located the probable mutation sites to 3 major areas: (a) N-terminal to the collagenase cleaving site with the 1(I) CB7 peptide (7 cases); (b) a region close to the cleavage site (3 cases); and (c) toward the COOH-terminus (5 cases) (Fig. 8). Since all patients secreted normal and abnormal pro α1(I) chains at about equal rates, it can be assumed that they were heterozygotes for a gene coding for the abnormal pro α1(I) chain, ie, that they were carriers of a dominant mutation. This is consistent with the observation that most patients with lethal

9

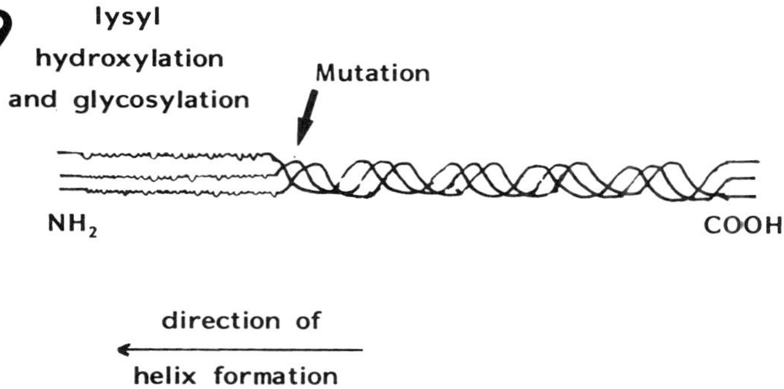

Fig. 9. Scheme depicting the Bonadio and Byers hypothesis [30]. Helix formation proceeds from COOH- to NH_2-terminus and is delayed from the mutation point. Overmodification results in the slow-assembling NH_2-terminal portion of the procollagen molecule. Determination of the overmodified portion allows to locate the mutation site.

osteogenesis imperfecta are isolated, ie probably the result of new dominant mutations.

Apparently, mutations that result in single amino acid substitution are much more common than large deletions [30,32]. They invariably lead to the formation of procollagen with an unstable helix, intracellular accumulation, increased degradation, and decreased secretion of collagen by the cell (Fig. 4). The collagen secreted by osteogenesis imperfecta fibroblasts is sparse, less well oriented, and thinner than normal collagen fibers [33], an observation that has also been made in bone [34].

Other Observations

Preliminary data on some less extensively studied cases suggest additional mechanisms that may lead to abnormal collagen gene products:

9) In 1 patient with lethal osteogenesis imperfecta (IMR 2328), the ratio of newly synthesized pro $\alpha1(I)$ to pro $\alpha2(1)$ chains was 2.45 instead of 2 [10]. This was interpreted as an indication that 1 pro $\alpha2(I)$ gene was not expressed. The significance of this is not known since the clinically unaffected father of another patient (IMR 2629) also had a nonfunctioning pro $\alpha2(I)$ gene [23].

10) In a patient with moderately severe osteogenesis imperfecta, the COOH-propeptide extension contained an increased amount of mannose [35]. This was associated with a type I procollagen that aggregated more readily than normal. How this alteration occurred is unknown.

11) Uitto et al [36] reported on 2 patients with lethal osteogenesis imperfecta who possibly synthesized lengthened pro $\alpha 1(I)$ chains suggesting abnormalities of the stop codon. This has not been fully substantiated.

12) The decreased production of structurally normal type I collagen that has been found in a number of patients [37, 38] has been explained by lowered levels of mRNA [4]. The molecular mechanisms that could reduce the amount of mRNA are unknown.

13) Lysyl Hydroxylase Deficiency

Lysyl hydroxylase catalyzes the transformation of lysine to hydroxylysine. Hydroxylysine is required for cross-link formation. A deficiency of the enzyme alters the formation and structure of cross-links and leads to a clinical disorder with hypermobile joints, hyperextensible skin, and, in some patients, with ocular fragility and keratoconus [39–41].

It is important to note that in the observed cases only type I and III collagen were insufficiently hydroxylated, whereas other collagens were normal [42]. The basis for this is not clear nor why the defect leads to abnormalities of skin and ligaments but not of bone.

CONCLUSIONS AND OUTLOOK

Diversity and complexity of collagen explain the large number of errors of collagen metabolism that have been defined in the last years. A much greater number is to be expected in the future. The number of patients with osteogenesis imperfecta and the Ehlers-Danlos syndrome in whom the defect has been defined is extremely small in comparison to the number of patients in whom the pathogenesis of their disorder is unknown. Up to now, no 2 patients with osteogenesis imperfecta have had the same biochemical defect.

The clinician's tendency to nosologically lump patients into a few categories such as osteogenesis imperfecta, Ehlers-Danlos syndrome, Marfan syndrome, is understandable and clinically useful to a certain degree. On the other hand, it gives a false sense of security and may be dangerous if it results in a firm prognosis and genetic counsel. Even if the subclassification of Sillence [31] is used, it is almost impossible to provide reliable genetic counsel to the patient with osteogenesis imperfecta or his/her family–unless, of course, vertical transmission of the defect has been proven. As to prognosis, a purely empiric approach seems sometimes preferable to a classification-based prognostication [43].

Genetic counseling will become easier with the increasing availability of biochemical tests. For instance, the finding of 2 types of type I procollagen in fibroblast cultures from a patient with osteogenesis imperfecta will point to a disorder which is clinically manifest in the heterozygous state, ie dominant, even if the molecular basis for the abnormal type I procollagen is unknown. Once the methods are speedy enough, such a finding will also provide the means for prenatal diagnosis.

Most studies have been directed toward type I and type III collagen. There is no reason to rule out similar defects in other types of collagen. Abnormalities of type II collagen have been detected in patients with achondrogenesis II [44] and diastrophic dysplasia [45].The close involvement in collagen metabolism of other substances such as copper, iron, ascorbic acid, or α-ketoglutarate and the close relationship of collagen with other connective tissue proteins lead to clinical disorders that closely resemble those caused by primary defects of collagen metabolism. Known examples are the Menkes syndrome, type IX Ehlers-Danlos syndrome (probably a disorder of intracellular copper metabolism) [45,46], or type X Ehlers-Danlos syndrome [47]. Other disorders, such as the Marfan syndrome, Larsen syndromes and Desbucquois syndrome [48], are prominent candidates for further collagen studies, as are patients with idiopathic osteoporosis or patients with unnamed disorders showing loose skin, loose joints, and brittle bones.

REFERENCES

1. Prockop DJ, Kivirikko KI, Tuderman L, Gutman NA: The biosynthesis of collagen and its disorders. N Engl J Med 301:77–85, 1979.
2. Bornstein P, Byers PH: Disorders of collagen metabolism. In Bondy PK, Rosenberg LD (eds): "Metabolic Control and Disease," 8th ed. Philadelphia: W.B. Saunders, 1980, pp 1089–1153.
3. Bornstein P, Sage H: Structurally distinct collagen types. Ann Rev Biochem 49:957–1004, 1980.
4. Byers PH, Bonadio JF: The molecular basis of clinical heterogeneity in osteogenesis imperfecta. Butterworth International Medical Reviews Pediatrics 5: Metabolic and Genetic Disease, J Lloyd, CR Scriver eds. London: Butterworth, In Press.
5. Tolstoshev P, Solomon E: Collagen genes. Nature 300:581–582, 1982.
6. Chu ML, Myers JC, Bernard MP, Ding JF, Ramirez F: Cloning and characterization of five overlapping cDNAs specific for the human pro alpha 1(I) collagen chain. Nucl Acids Res 10:5925–5934, 1982.
7. Huerre C, Junien C, Weil D, Chu ML, Morabito M, Cong NV, Myers JC, Foubert C, Gross MS, Prockop DJ, Boué A, Kaplan JC, de la Chapelle A, Ramirez F: Human type I procollagen genes are located on different chromosomes. Proc Natl Acad Sci USA 79:6627–6630, 1982.
8. Prockop DJ:Osteogenesis imperfecta: Phenotypic heterogeneity, protein suicide, short and long collagen. Am J Hum Genet 36:499–505, 1984.
9. Shapiro JR, Rowe DW: Collagen genes and brittle bones. Ann Intern Med 99:700–704, 1983.

10. de Wet WJ, Chu ML, Prockop DJ: The mRNAs for the pro-alpha 1(I) and pro alpha 2(I) chains of type I procollagen are translated at the same rate in normal human fibroblasts and in fibroblasts from two variants of osteogenesis imperfecta with altered steady state ratios of the mRNAs. J Biol Chem 258:14385–14389, 1983.
11. Prockop DJ, Kivirikko KI: Heritable diseases of collagen. N Engl J Med 311:376–386, 1984.
12. Heller RH, Winn KJ, Heller RM: The prenatal diagnosis of osteogenesis imperfecta congenita. Am J Obstet Gynecol 121:572–573, 1975.
13. Chu ML, Williams CJ, Pepe G, Hirsch JL, Prockop DJ, Ramirez F: Internal deletion in a collagen gene in a perinatal lethal form of osteogenesis imperfecta. Nature 304:78–80, 1983.
14. Barsh GS, Roush CL, Bonadio J, Byer PH, Gelinas RE: Intron-mediated recombination may cause a deletion in an alpha 1 type I collagen chain in a lethal form of osteogenesis imperfecta. Proc Natl Acad Sci USA 82:2870–2874, 1985.
15. Chu ML, Gariulo V, Williams CJ, Ramirez F: Multiexon deletion in an osteogenesis imperfecta variant with increased type III collagen mRNA. J Biol Chem 260:691–694, 1985.
16. Williams CJ, Prockop DJ: Synthesis and processing of a type I procollagen containing shortened pro-alpha1(I) chains by fibroblasts from a patient with osteogenesis imperfecta. J Biol Chem 258:5915–5921, 1983.
17. Barsh GS, Byers PH: Reduced secretion of structurally abnormal type I procollagen in a form of osteogenesis imperfecta. Proc Natl Acad Sci USA 78:5142–5146, 1981.
18. Penttinen RP, Lichtenstein JR, Martin GR, McKusick VA: Abnormal collagen metabolism in cultured cells in osteogenesis imperfecta. Proc Natl Acad Sci USA 72:586–589, 1975.
19. Nicholls AC, Pope FM, Schloon H: Biochemical heterogeneity of osteogenesis imperfecta: New variant. Lancet I: 1193, 1979.
20. Schloon H: personal communication.
21. Dickson LA, Pihlajaniemi T, Deak S, Pope FM, Nichols, A, Prockop DJ, Myers JC: Nuclease S1 mapping of a homozygous mutation in the carboxyl-propeptide-coding region of the pro alpha 2(I) collagen gene in a patient with osteogenesis imperfecta. Proc Natl Acad Sci USA 81:4524–4528, 1984.
22. Pihlajaniemi T, Dickson LA, Pope FM, Korhonen VR, Nicholls A, Prockop DJ, Myers MC: Osteogenesis imperfecta: Cloning of a pro alpha 2(I) collagen gene with a frameshift mutation. J Biol Chem 259:12941–12944, 1984.
23. de Wet W, Pihlajaniemi T, Myers J, Kelly TE, Prockop DJ: Synthesis of a shortened pro-alpha 2(I) chain and decreased synthesis of pro-alpha 2(I) chains in a proband with osteogenesis imperfecta. J Biol Chem 258:7721–7728, 1983.
24. Sippola M, Kaffe S, Prockop DJ: A heterozygous defect for structurally altered pro-alpha 2 chain of type I procollagen in a mild variant of osteogenesis imperfecta. J Biol Chem 259:14094–14100, 1984.
25. Lichtenstein JR, Martin GR, Kohn L, Byers PH, McKusick VA: A defect in the conversion of procollagen to collagen in a form of the Ehlers-Danlos syndrome. Science 182:298–300, 1973.
26. Steinmann B, Tuderman L, Peltonen L, Martin GR, McKusick VA, Prockop DJ: Evidence for a structural mutation of procollagen type I in a patient with the Ehlers-Danlos syndrome type VII. J Biol Chem 255:8887–8893, 1980.

27. Byers PH, Shapiro JR, Rowe DW, David KE, Holbrook KA: Abnormal alpha2-chain in type I collagen from a patient with a form of osteogenesis imperfecta. J Clin Invest 71:689–697, 1983.
28. Byers PH, Bonadio JF, Steinmann B, Barsh GS, Holbrook KA, Greenberg C, Rowe DW, Gelinas R: Molecular heterogeneity in perinatal lethal osteogenesis imperfecta (OI type II). Am J Hum Genet 35:39A, 1983.
29. Steinmann B, Rao VH, Vogel A, Bruckner P, Gitzelmann R, Byers PH: Cysteine in the triple-helical domain of one allelic product of the alpha 1(I) gene of type I collagen produces a lethal form of osteogenesis imperfecta. J Biol Chem 259:11129–11138, 1984.
30. Bonadio J, Byers PH: Subtle structural alterations in the chains of type I procollagen produce osteogenesis imperfecta type II. Nature 316:363–366, 1985.
31. Sillence DO, Barlow KK, Garber AP, Hall JG, Rimoin DL: Osteogenesis imperfecta type II: Delineation of the phenotype with reference to genetic heterogeneity. Am J Med Genet 17:407–424, 1984.
32. Bateman JF, Mascara T, Chan D, Cole WG: Abnormal type I collagen metabolism by cultured fibroblasts in lethal perinatal osteogenesis imperfecta. Biochem J 217:103–115, 1984.
33. Bonadio J, Holbrook KA, Gelinas RE, Jacob J, Byers PH: Altered triple helical structure of type I procollagen in lethal perinatal osteogenesis imperfecta. J Biol Chem 260:1734–1742, 1985.
34. Stöss H, Pesch JH: Structural changes of collagen fibrils in skeletal dysplasias. Virchows Arch Pathol Anat 405:341–364, 1985.
35. Peltonen L, Palotie A, Prockop DJ: A defect in the structure of type I collagen in a patient who had osteogenesis imperfecta: Excess mannose in the COOH-terminal propeptide. Proc Natl Acad Sci USA 77:6179–6183, 1980.
36. Uitto J, Tan E, Müller P, Krieg T, Prockop DJ: Synthesis of lengthened pro alpha 1(I) chains of type I procollagen by skin fibroblasts from two patients with lethal osteogenesis imperfecta. Clin Res 31:468A, 1983.
37. Barsh GS, David KE, Byers PH: Type I osteogenesis imperfecta: A non-functional allele for pro-alpha 1(I) chains of type I procollagen. Proc Natl Acad Sci 79:3838–3842, 1982.
38. Fraser J, Lancaster GA, Scriver CR: Secreted collagen ratios in normal human and osteogenesis imperfecta skin fibroblasts. Conn Tiss Res 11:57–67, 1983.
39. Pinnell SR, Krane SM, Kenzora JE, Glimcher MH: A heritable disorder of connective tissue: Hydroxylysine-deficient collagen disease. N Engl J Med 266:1013–1020, 1972.
40. Sussman M, Lichtenstein JR, Nigra TP, Martin GR, McKusick VA: Hydroxylysine-deficient collagen in a patient with a form of the Ehlers-Danlos syndrome. J Bone Jt Surg 56A:1228–1234, 1974.
41. Steinmann B, Gitzelmann R, Vogel A, Grant ME, Harwood R, Sear CHJ: Ehlers-Danlos syndrome in two siblings with deficient lysyl hydroxylase activity in cultured skin fibroblasts but only mild hydroxylysine deficiency in skin. Helv Paediatr Acta 30:255–275, 1975.
42. Ihme A, Krieg T, Nerlich A, Feldmann U, Rauterberg J, Glanville RW, Edel G, Müller PK: Ehlers-Danlos syndrome type VI: Collagen type specificity of defective lysyl hydroxylation in various tissues. J Invest Dermatol 83:161–165, 1984.
43. Spranger J, Cremin B, Beighton P: Osteogenesis imperfecta congenita. Features and prognosis of a heterogenous condition. Pediatr Radiol 12:21–27, 1982.
44. Horton WA, Machado MA, Chou JW, Eyre DR: Abnormal cartilage collagens in achondrogenesis II. Pediatr Res 19, 248A, 1985.

45. Stanescu V, Stanescu R, Maroteaux P: Pathogenic mechanisms in osteochondrodysplasias. J Bone Jt Surg 66A:817–836, 1984.
46. Kuivaneimi H, Peltonen L, Palotie A, Kaitila K, Kivirikko KI: Abnormal copper metabolism and deficient lysyl oxidase activity in a heritable connective tissue disorder. J Clin Invest 69:730–733, 1982.
47. Holbrook KA, Byers PH: Structural abnormalities in dermal collagen and elastic matrix from the skin of patients with inherited connective tissue disorders. J Invest Dermatol 79:7s–16s, 1982.
48. Desbuquois G, Grenier B, Michel J, Rossignol C: Nanisme chondrodystrophique avec ossification anarchique et polymalformations chez deux soeurs. Arch Franç Pédiatr 23:573–587, 1966.

Possible Pathogenetic Mechanism in Hyperornithinemia, Hyperammonemia, and Homocitrullinuria Syndrome*

M. Daria Haust, MD, and B.A. Gordon, MD

Departments of Pathology (MDH), Paediatrics (MDH, BAG), and Biochemistry (BAG), Children's Psychiatric Research Institute, and The University of Western Ontario, London, Ontario, Canada

INTRODUCTION

The syndrome of hyperornithinemia, hyperammonemia, and homocitrullinuria (HHH syndrome) was first delineated by Shih et al [1] in 1969. These authors reported on a patient with high concentrations of blood ammonia who could be differentiated from the group of inherited hyperammonemias by accompanying high levels of blood ornithine and urinary homocitrulline. The report in 1973 by Wright and Pollitt [2] on a second such patient was followed in 1975 by that of Gatfield et al [3] on a group of 6 related subjects; to date, 11 patients with the HHH syndrome have been reported [1–6].

Clinically, the HHH syndrome is characterized by episodic motor impairment, seizures, intellectual deficits, protein intolerance, and feeding problems in infancy; in some, a bleeding tendency is observed early in life [3]. The clinical manifestations vary considerably from one subject to another. Pedigree analysis indicates that this is an autosomal recessive trait [3].

*Supported by a grant-in-aid Nr. 712 from the Ontario Mental Health Foundation, Toronto, Ontario, Canada.

Birth Defects: Original Article Series, Volume 23, Number 1, pages 17–45

To date the basic metabolic error in the HHH syndrome has not been identified unequivocally, nor can the homocitrullinuria be explained on the basis of any proposed "operating" mechanisms.

Our previous morphologic and biochemical studies [3,7,8], and the results of clinical supplement trials [3,9], all supported the concept that the basic defect in the HHH syndrome resides at the level of the transmembranous transport of ornithine into the hepatic mitochondria for the purpose of "conversion" to citrulline.

The purpose of this presentation is to (1) summarize and illustrate the hepatic ultrastructural abnormalities; (2) report morphologic findings of the peripheral lymphocytes before and after long-term oral ornithine supplements; (3) record some preliminary observations on mitochondrial ultrastructure of cultured dermal fibroblasts in a patient with the HHH syndrome; and (4) discuss these data in the context of possible pathogenetic mechanisms underlying this syndrome.

MATERIAL AND METHODS

Clinical Notes

The patient, who was originally seen at age 7 years and has been followed ever since, is at present an almost 20-year-old, severely retarded young man. He was included as case 1 in a group of 6 HHH patients reported previously [3]. Since that report of over a decade ago, the patient has shown little developmental progress, is of short stature, and, despite carefully controlled and adequate anticonvulsive treatment, continues to have myoclonic and grand mal seizures.

Biochemical Data

Details of the original findings in serum, urine, peripheral WBCs, and liver (and pertaining to the values of either one or the other of the following: ammonia, amino acids, and enzymes); the results of oral "loading" with ornithine, citrulline, and lysine; and the "response" of various biochemical parameters to different amounts of protein intake, were included in the original report [3].

Subsequently, studies were undertaken to test again the effect of oral ornithine "loading," and to assess the therapeutic effects of ornithine administered over a period of 2 years. Fibroblasts, cultured from the patient's skin, were used to study also the oxidation of ornithine and glutamate. Methods employed in all of these procedures will be detailed in another report [10].

Morphologic Studies

Liver. The tissue obtained by needle biopsy was processed for light and electron microscopy as described previously [3,8].

Peripheral lymphocytes. Blood samples were obtained from the patient just before and twice (at a short interval) after the long-term treatment with ornithine supplements (see above).

The pelleted buffy coats of each sample were processed (with appropriate controls) for electron microscopy by the now well-established routine techniques.

Fibroblasts. From the skin of the patient and of 3 appropriate control subjects fibroblasts were grown to confluency in 75 cm^2 Falcon flasks in MEM-media containing 10% fetal calf serum.

For electron microscopy the confluent layers were fixed *in situ* and embedded in plastic (Epon-812) by routine procedures. Thin sections were cut in planes both parallel and perpendicular to the cellular layer. Cutting, mounting and staining, and examination of thin sections proceeded as for hepatic tissue [8].

RESULTS

Biochemical Studies

Some results of these studies were reported briefly [11], and a detailed account will be provided elsewhere [10].

For the purpose of this communication, and in particular the discussion, it suffices to summarize the pertinent findings as follows: (1) While markedly elevating the ornithine level, ornithine supplements decreased the concentration of ammonia in blood; (2) when ornithine was taken with meals over a period of many weeks, postprandial blood ammonia was reduced to an almost normal concentration even with increased protein intake; and (3) there was a considerable reduction of oxidation by cultured dermal fibroblasts of the ornithine-5-^{14}C to $^{14}Co_2$ in the presence of normal oxidation of glutamate-U-^{14}C.

Morphological Studies

Liver. Brief [3,7] and more detailed [8] accounts on the ultrastructural characteristics of this patient's hepatocytes were reported previously. Of these observations, findings considered pertinent to the ensuing discussion are illustrated herein.

Some hepatocytes were structurally unremarkable (Fig. 1); the chromatin distribution in the nucleus and the complement of cytoplasmic organelles

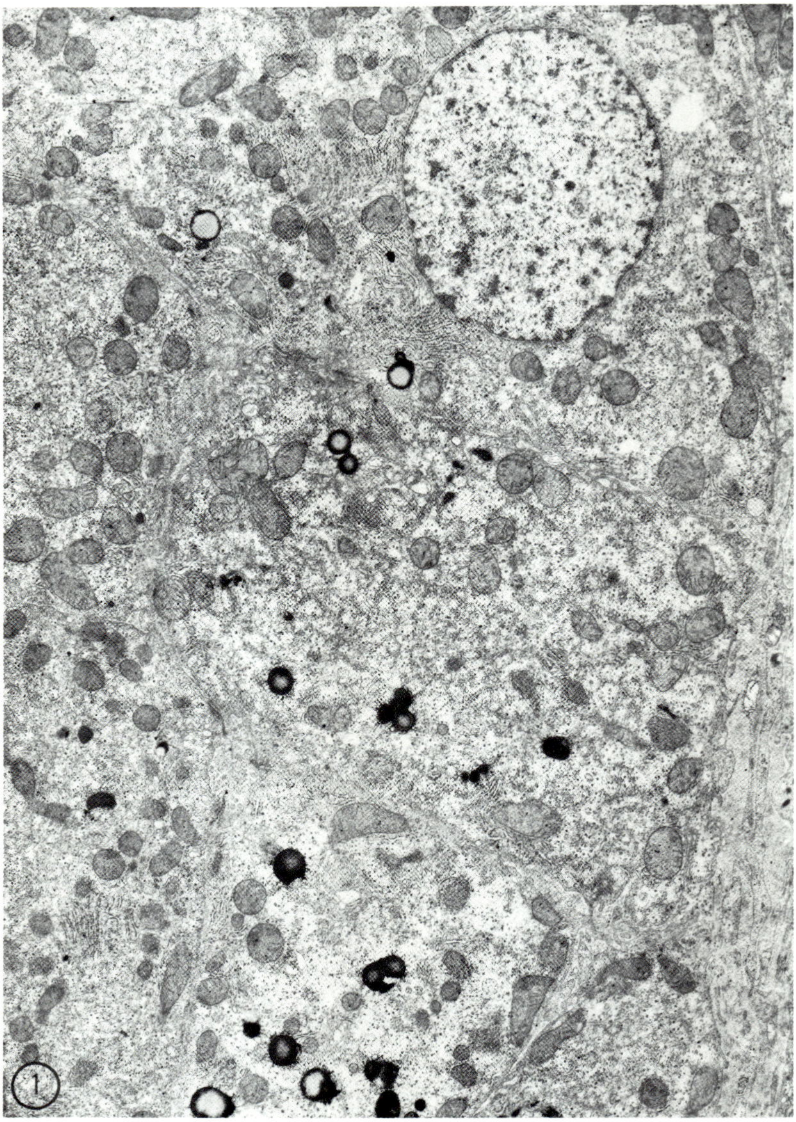

Fig. 1. An area of liver with normal-appearing hepatocytes. The electron-opaque (some with a lucent core) cytoplasmic inclusions are considered to represent lipo-pigment complexes. Magnification × 5,200.

appeared to be normal. A few small, electron-opaque cytoplasmic inclusions, at times with a lucent core (Fig. 1), were interpreted as lipo-pigment complexes.

Other hepatocytes had an altered appearance, which was associated largely with glycogen accumulation. Nonmembrane bound glycogen aggregates were present in the nuclei (Fig. 2) and/or cytoplasm (Fig. 3). In the latter they were "contained" between increased numbers and dilated profiles of smooth surface endoplasmic reticulum (Fig. 3). In these glycogen-rich cells, the mitochondria and other cytoplasmic structures and complexes were usually decreased in number, but not necessarily altered in appearance.

However, most hepatocytes contained distinctly abnormal mitochondria (Figs. 4–8). Generally, in such cells, the number of these organelles was markedly increased, and they tended to concentrate in the perinuclear zone (Fig. 4). Their size and shape varied considerably (Figs. 4–8). Whereas the dimensions of many were comparable with those of normal mitochondria (Fig. 4), bizarre-shaped, very long and giant forms were prominent (Figs. 4–8). Sections parallel to the longitudinal axis of the very long mitochondria (Fig. 4), displayed an unusual internal structure: a thick sievelike or periodic membrane was closely applied to the inner mitochondrial membrane and interposed between it and the matrix (Figs. 4–6). However, at times, both mitochondrial membranes bulged outward, showing the now "naked" sievelike structure (Figs. 4, 6, 7). Its periodic nature was best visualized in tangential sections (Figs. 5–7). The mitochondrial matrix of the "bulge" contained cristae (or their fragments?) only on a rare occasion. The "bulges" varied in size and position on the long or bizarre-shaped mitochondria. They were particularly prominent at points of angulation and at the ends, and here formed bulbous terminations (Fig. 6). In addition, the long mitochondria showed the presence of "tubules." These were usually limited by slightly wavy, ill-delineated membranes, and also ran parallel to the longitudinal axis (Figs. 4–6).

Cross-sections of the abnormal mitochondria at the level of the "bulges" conveyed the impression of a "mitochondrion within a mitochondrion" (Figs. 7,8), as if reflecting an internal budding process. However, on close inspection and higher magnification, the true nature of these images was easily determined; the internal or "budding" mitochondrion lacked both (outer and inner) mitochondrial membranes and was limited by the "naked" sievelike structure (Fig. 8). Cross-sections of the longitudinal tubules showed their peripheral arrangement and triangular shape (Figs. 4, 8).

Peripheral lymphocytes. (1) Before the long-term treatment with ornithine supplement most lymphocytes were of the intermediate or large

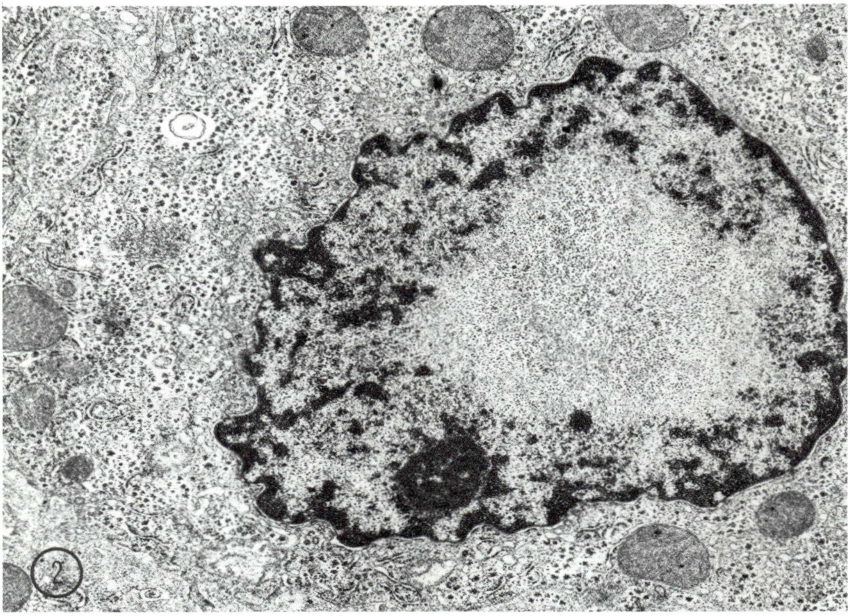
2

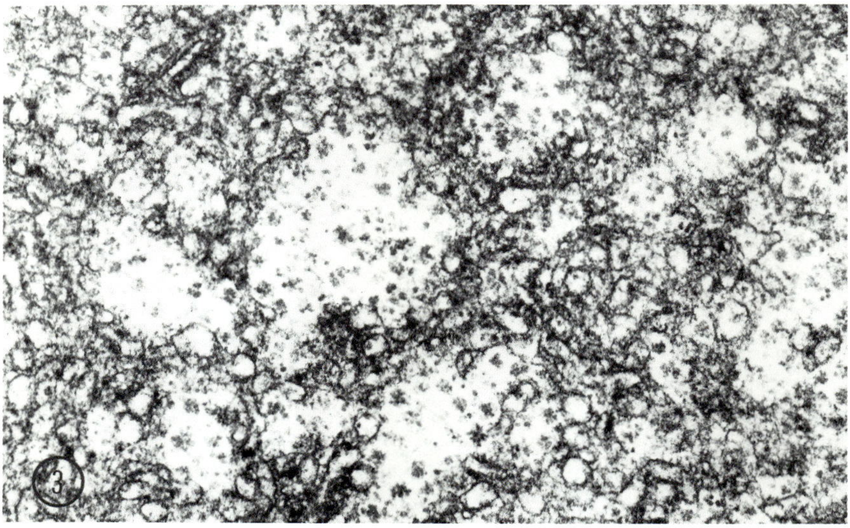
3

variety (Figs. 9–14). Electron microscopic examination showed the presence of cytoplasmic "inclusions" of variable composition and configuration (Figs. 9–14). Some of these were round or oblong, had a homogeneous electron-opaque appearance, and were limited by a unit membrane. Their size was variable but usually approximated that of mitochondria (Figs. 9, 13A), but some were of much smaller dimension (Figs. 12, 13C, 14C). These uniformly appearing structures were compatible with azurophilic granules. At the other end of the spectrum were "inclusions" entirely devoid of a limiting membrane and in direct contact with the hyaloplasm; they consisted of tubular arrays. The size of these approximated those of the above granules, but the shapes were often irregular and angular (Figs. 11–14). Structures with mixed characteristics were common (Figs. 11, 12, 13C, 13D, 14A, 14B). One could trace in electron micrographs the "evolution" of the entirely tubular, nonmembrane bound inclusions from the homogeneous membrane-limited variety (Figs. 13A–D, 14A–D). Almost the entire population of lymphocytes contained the cytoplasmic inclusions, but their number varied from a few to many (Figs. 9 and 12 vs Figs. 11 and 11A). (2) After treatment most lymphocytes were of the small, more mature variety (Figs. 15,16). The number of inclusion-containing cells, and the number of inclusions present in a given cell, were considerably reduced as compared with those before treatment, but these inclusions largely resembled those of tubular arrays (Fig. 17) with or without the limiting membrane.

Cultured fibroblasts. Preliminary assessment of mitochondria by electron microscopy indicated that mitochondrial structure was considerably altered when compared with that of control cells. In most cells, these organelles were extremely long, tortuous, and branching (Figs. 18,19), with bulbous projections often extending from their surface (Fig. 18) and terminal segments (Fig. 19). Whereas the internal structure has yet to be studied in detail, the overall impression was that the organelles commonly displayed unduly regressive changes (Fig. 20), and increased electron-opacity (Figs. 18–20), both types of abnormalities not observed (Fig. 21) even in degenerating (Fig. 22) control fibroblasts.

Fig. 2. Intranuclear accumulation of glycogen that is also increased but dispersed in the cytoplasm of a hepatocyte from another area than that illustrated in Figure 1. The organelles appear normal. Magnification × 11,400.

Fig. 3. "Islets" of glycogen pools are surrounded by numerous dilated smooth-surfaced endoplasmic reticulum in a hepatocyte different than those illustrated in Figures 1 and 2. Magnification × 40,000.

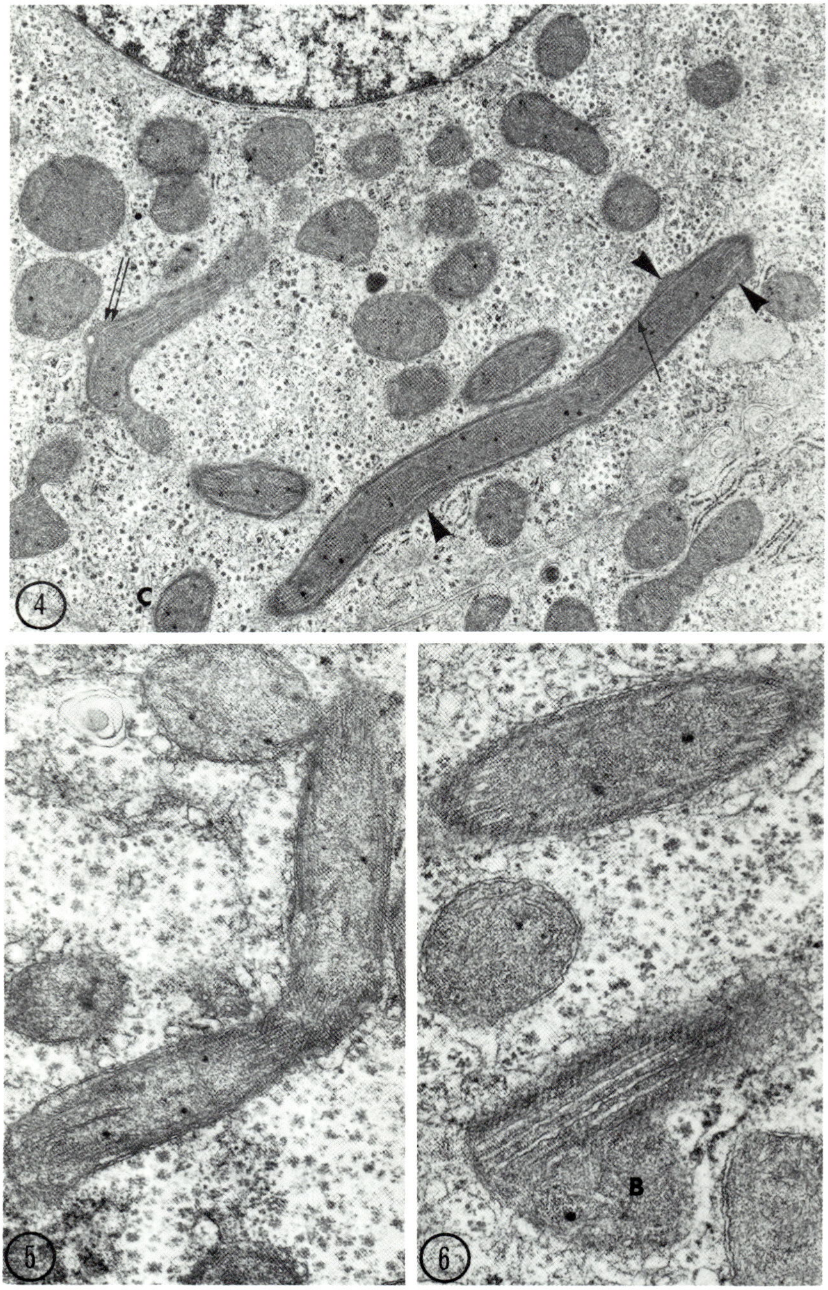
4
C
5
6
B

In only a few cells of 1 normal control subject examined, a small number of mitochondria were reminiscent of some aspects of the patient's organelles, ie, they were increased in length, and occasionally showed branching and terminal bulbous projections (Fig. 22). However, these mitochondria neither displayed the intense electron-opacity, nor the contorted images characterizing the organelles of the patient's fibroblasts. The work on the assessment of these mitochondria (resolution of their internal structure; ratios of normal to abnormal forms; number per cell, and other) continues.

DISCUSSION

The reluctance to accept one of the proposed theories (see below) as the metabolic basis of the HHH syndrome is understandable in view of the failure of each to explain all of the observed changes in this disease.

Hyperammonemia, a component of the HHH syndrome, occurs in genetically determined diseases [12] not only in deficiencies of the urea cycle enzymes, but also may accompany several other metabolic disorders, eg, the organic acidemias (methylmalonic and propionic acidemias, and α-methylacetoacetyl CoA β-ketothiolase deficiency), familial protein intolerance with aberrant transport of dibasic amino acids, and lysine dehydrogenase deficiency [13–15]. However, none of these is associated with other characteristics of the HHH syndrome.

Homocitrullinuria, also present in the HHH syndrome, is associated with citrullinemia [16] in arginino-succinate synthetase (ASS)-deficiency, a disorder not characterized by hyperornithinemia.

Hyperornithinemia [17], a prominent manifestation of the HHH syndrome, could arise as a consequence of alterations in any of the reactions in

---

Fig. 4. Increased number of mitochondria in perinuclear region of a hepatocyte display altered forms and length. The long forms show tubules running parallel to the longitudinal axis, a thick structure applied to the inner mitochondrial membrane (arrow) with sievelike appearance on slightly tangential cut (double arrow), and several small bulges protruding from surface (arrowheads). Note the peripheral arrangement of the tubules on cross-sections (C). Magnification × 15,000.

Fig. 5. Higher magnification of a mitochondrion similar to that illustrated in the left half of Figure 4. The periodicity of the sievelike structure is clearly visible at the angulation and at the end-segments of the mitochondrion. Magnification × 35,000.

Fig. 6. Bulbous projection at the end of a bizarrely shaped mitochondrion (B). The periodicity of the thick membrane is clearly seen also in the mitochondrion at the top of the photograph. Magnification × 35,500.

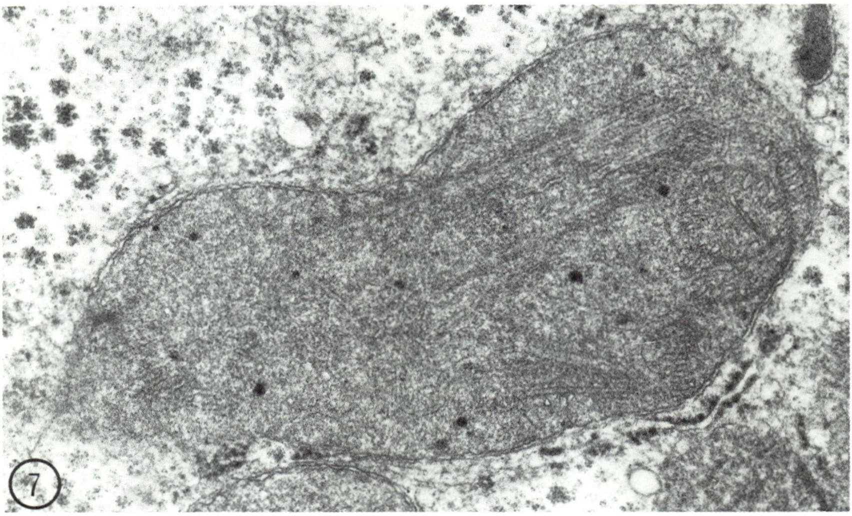
7

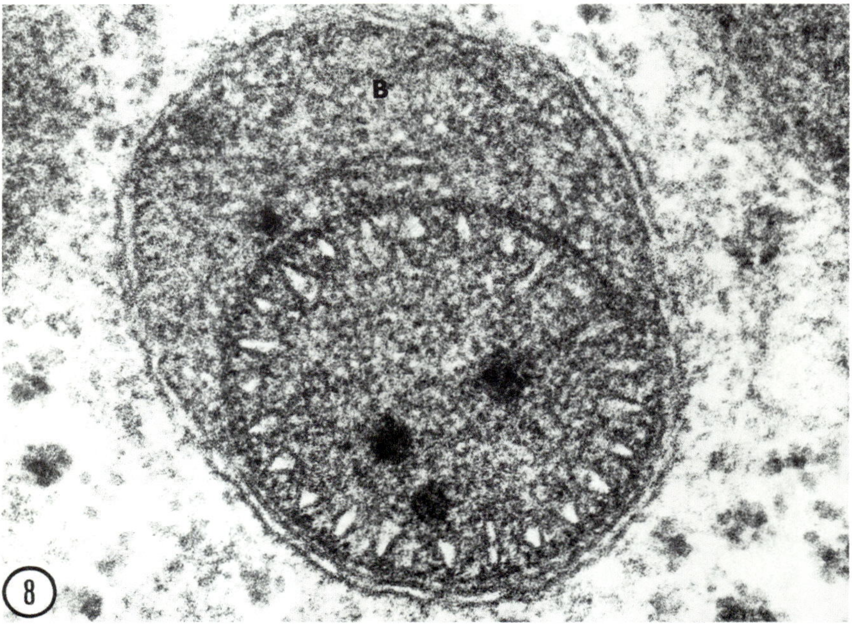
B
8

which ornithine is involved, either directly or indirectly. To date, hyperornithinemia, characterizing an inherited metabolic disease, has been linked conclusively to only one enzymatic "aberration," ie, the defective ornithine-ketoacid transaminase. The disorder was first described in Finland in 1973 by Simell and Takki [18]. The affected adult patients with progressive visual impairment had a gyrate atrophy of the choroid and retina, and 10- to 20-fold increase of serum ornithine levels in the absence of hyperammonemia. Subsequent reports of similar patients, who were natives of other countries [19–23], established that this disorder is not confined to the Finnish people. Data indicate that in this disease the abnormality of the ornithine-ketoacid transaminase activity is the underlying defect [24–26].

Actually, a disorder associated with deficiency of ornithine-ketoacid transaminase was described 5 years earlier by Bickel et al [27]. The disease became manifest in early childhood with prolonged neonatal jaundice, impairment of mental development, certain electroencephalographic changes, an approximately 3-fold elevation of blood ornithine levels, and absent to mild hyperammonemia. The variable hyperammonemia in this condition was underscored in a subsequent report [28]. Thus, in a child with hyperkinesis, psychomotor retardation, refractory seizures, and intermittent ataxia, the levels of blood ammonia were up to 3 times the normal value. Enzyme studies, utilizing ornithine as a substrate, indicated that the activity of the ornithine-ketoacid transaminase in the liver of the 2 first reported patients was less than 20%, and in cultured dermal fibroblasts of the third chiid [27–29] was approximately 10% of normal mean values [30]. However, the results of a more recent study [31] of a patient with mild hyperornithinemia and other changes similar to those of the patients of Bickel et al, question the existence of this entity. In this patient the dermal fibroblasts showed normal ornithine-ketoacid transaminase activity and normal rates of incorporation of the ornithine carbon skeleton into protein [31]. Whether this childhood

---

Fig. 7. This bizarrely shaped giant mitochondrion appears to represent a "mitochondrion within mitochondrion": some having a longitudinal, others a cross-cut appearance. Note that all these "inside" mitochondria lack both mitochondrial limiting membranes; the image represents a cut through several bulges and angulations much more "contorted" than those seen in Figures 4–6. Magnification × 46,500.

Fig. 8. A high-power magnification of a section through a bulge shows the periodic nature of the thick sievelike membrane that at a lower circumference is closely applied to the inner mitochondrial membrane. The tubules, on longitudinal sections (Fig. 4) parallel to the long mitochondrial axis, are on cross-section triangular and closely applied to the periodic membrane. B = bulge. Magnification × 134,000.

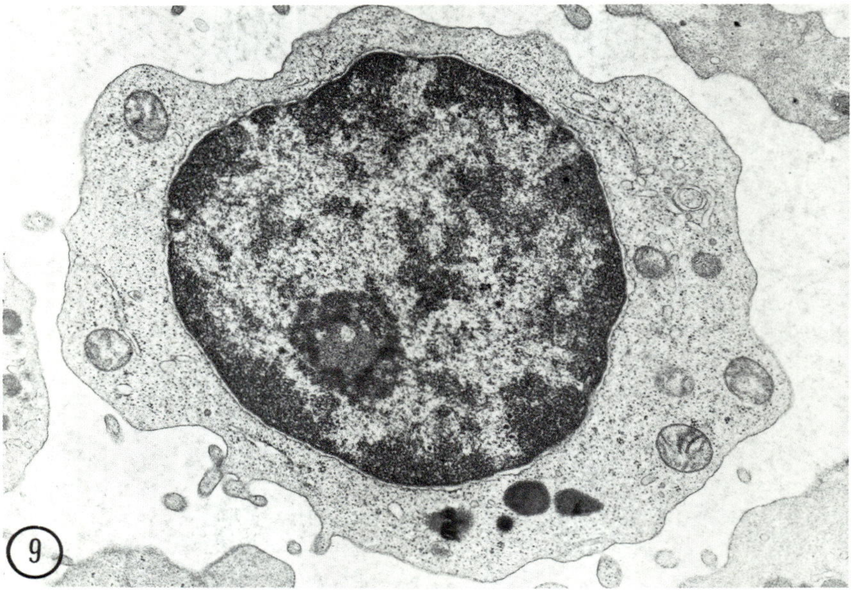
9

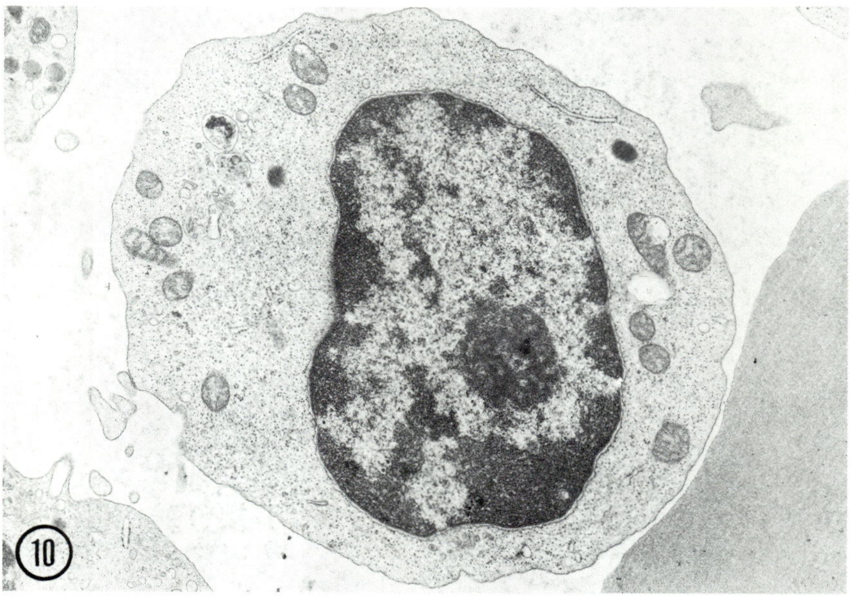
10

disease represents the effects of a primary ornithine-ketoacid transaminase defect or a deficiency secondary to a hepatocellular damage remains uncertain.

There are a few other inborn errors of metabolism that theoretically could affect the level of blood ornithine. Thus, interference with ornithine turnover may involve defects at steps beyond the ornithine-ketoacid transaminase, for example, type II hyperprolinemia is characterized by deficient activity of $\triangle^1$pyrroline-5-carboxylic acid dehydrogenase [32]. However, hyperornithinemia usually, does not accompany this order. Similarly, abnormalities in either of the 2 first enzymes of the urea cycle, ie, carbamyl phosphate synthetase I and ornithine transcarbamylase, theoretically may lead to an elevation of blood ornithine. However, in numerous reported instances in which the primary deficiency was that of either the above 2 enzymes, hyperornithinemia was not a manifestation (see in [3]).

In the HHH syndrome, the activities of both the ornithine transcarbamylase (OTC) and the ornithine-ketoacid transaminase (OKT) are essentially normal [3], and the aberration of either metabolism or transport of ornithine had to be explained on another basis. In an attempt at identifying the site of that defect, Shih et al [1,33] studied the metabolism of dermal fibroblasts obtained from 2 patients with the HHH syndrome, and demonstrated that the activity of the ornithine decarboxylase was considerably reduced. These findings suggested to these investigators that the synthesis of polyamines was disturbed, since this enzyme is involved in the initial step of their metabolic pathway. However, this is not a major pathway in ornithine metabolism, and a defect in this cytoplasmic enzyme cannot readily explain either all of the biochemical or morphologic findings in the HHH syndrome.

On the basis of our original biochemical data and observations on the ultrastructure of hepatic mitochondria, we have postulated that the defect in the HHH syndrome lies in the inability of ornithine to be transported into mitochondria because of the interference by a thick sievelike structure (Figs. 4–8) interposed between the inner membrane and the interior [3, p. 494].

Figures 9–14. Represent lymphocytes obtained from peripheral blood before treatment.

Fig. 9. A large lymphocyte containing 4 electron-opaque granules (bottom). The 2 on the right are clearly membrane-limited. The larger granules approximate the size of mitochondria. Magnification × 9,000.

Fig. 10. Cells as in Figure 9. In addition to 2 smaller electron-opaque granules, there are 2 small aggregates of nondescript and partially electron-dense material (upper left) that is also membrane bound. Magnification × 5,000.

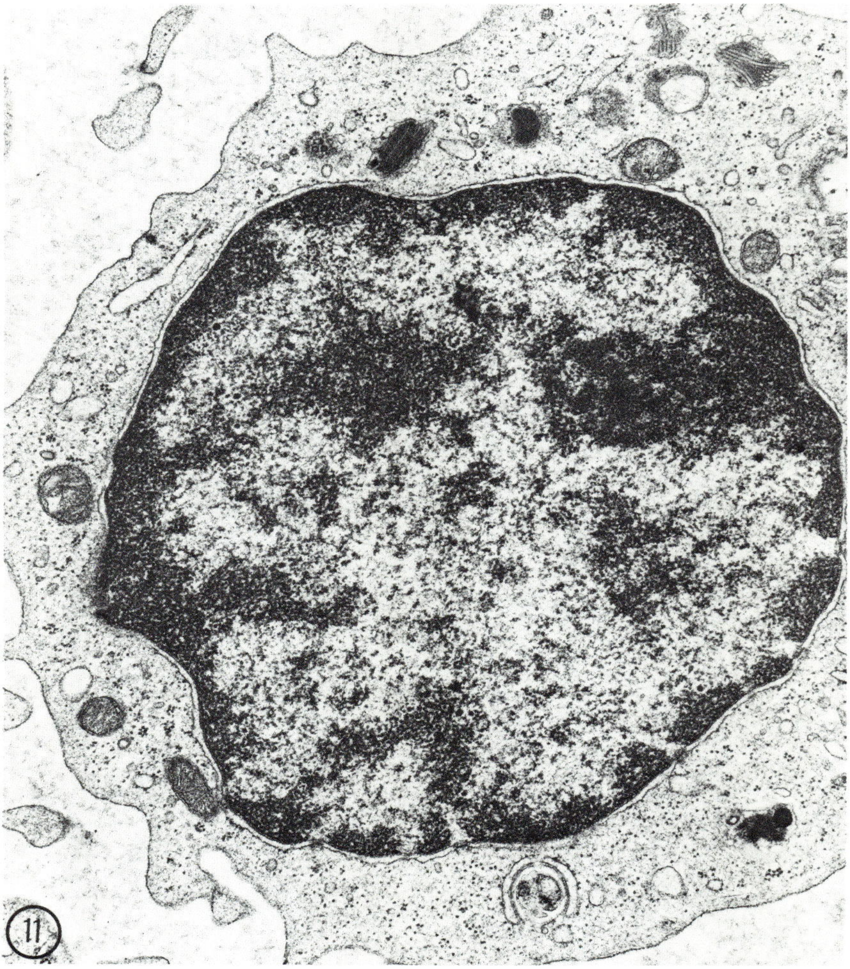

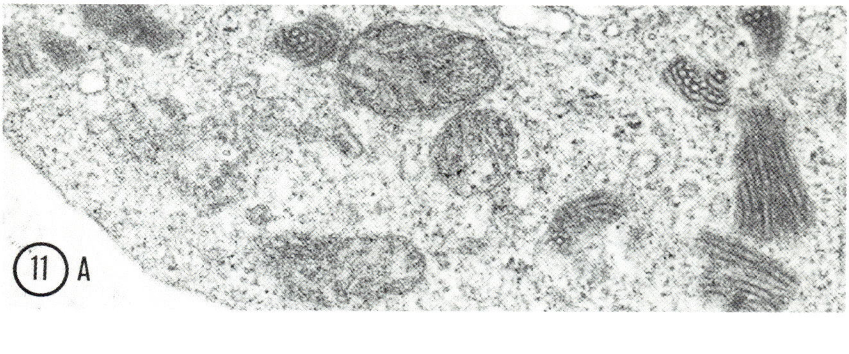

This concept was particularly attractive in the light of the then newly published data of Gamble and Lehninger on the transport of ornithine into mitochondria [34]. They emphasized the fact that the first 2 enzymes of the urea cycle reside in the mitochondrial matrix and thus the operation of the full cycle requires ornithine to enter into, and citrulline to exit from the mitochondria. Their studies indicated that ornithine transport is unidirectional, dependent on respiration and permeant anion, and stereospecific. They proposed that a specific, electrogenic uniport carrier exists for ornithine transport.

Thus, the available information suggested that the ornithine carrier that regulates the transmembranous transport of ornithine into the mitochondria of the HHH-cell had a reduced affinity for this amino acid.

Data from other studies lend support to the concept of "impaired entry" of ornithine into mitochondria, some inferring that it is even possible to overcome this block in transmembranous transport by increasing considerably the blood ornithine level. Clinical trials by Wright and Pollitt [2] and Gatfield et al [3] indicated that acute loads with monitoring of blood ammonia in the post-load period or continuing supplementation with oral ornithine at mealtime and longer term monitoring lead to a reduction in blood ammonia concentration in the HHH patients so treated. Similar results were obtained in the present study; furthermore, when ornithine was administered with meals over a period of many weeks, postprandial blood ammonia concentration was almost normalized, even when the protein intake was increased [10,11]. However, recent data from another center showed that ornithine loading did not prevent induced hyperammonemia in 1 patient with the HHH syndrome [6]. Clarification of this clinically important point must await further studies.

The concept of a block in the entry of ornithine into mitochondria is also supported by data derived from several tissue culture studies using dermal fibroblasts and/or lymphocytes of patients with the HHH syndrome. These suggest that transmembranous transport was diminished [4], and there was a reduced affinity in uptake [31] and catabolism [35] of ornithine by the patient's mitochondria.

Fig. 11. Several tubular aggregates, some completely or partially membrane-limited, are seen in upper and right cytoplasmic region. In the right lower corner a similar inclusion has a small round electron-opaque component. Magnification × 16,000. (A) None of the many tubular structures or arrays are membrane limited. Some are cross-, others longitudinally-cut. Magnification × 45,000.

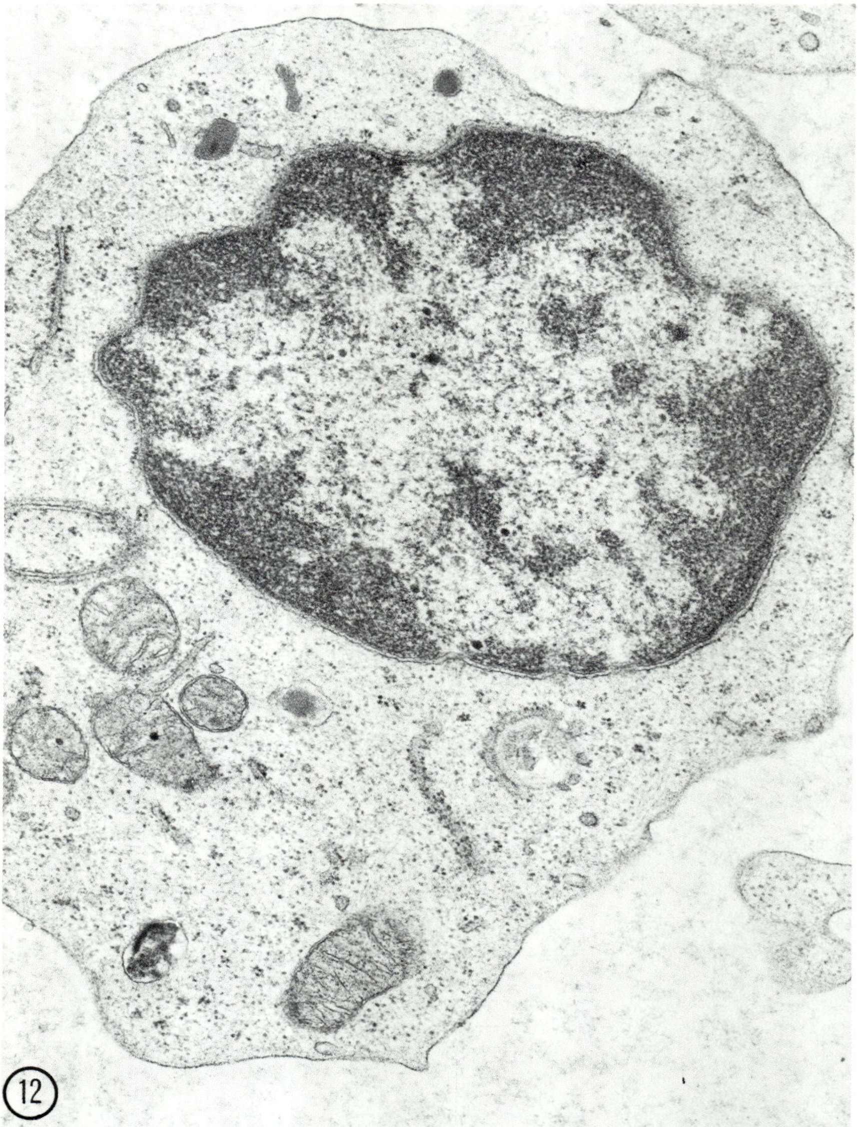

Fig. 12. A large lymphocyte contains 4 membrane bound inclusions; the 2 in upper area are electron-opaque and homogeneous, the 2 in the lower cytoplasm show "loosening" or "degeneration." Magnification × 28,000.

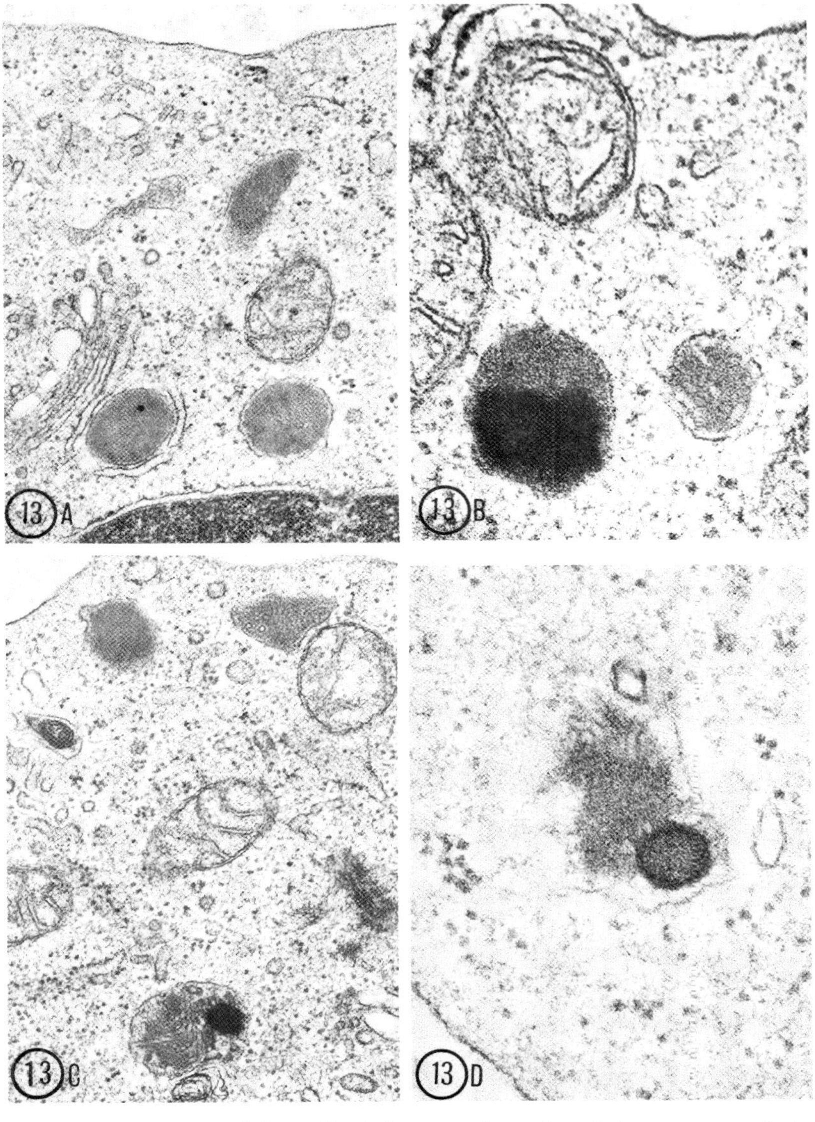

Fig. 13. Various stages of "transition" from membrane bound, homogeneous electron-opaque inclusions (A) to membrane bound mixed (tubular arrays and homogeneous; B-D), and entirely tubular (C; top) structures; Magnifications: A = × 40,000; B = × 75,000; C = x 40,000; D = × 62,000.

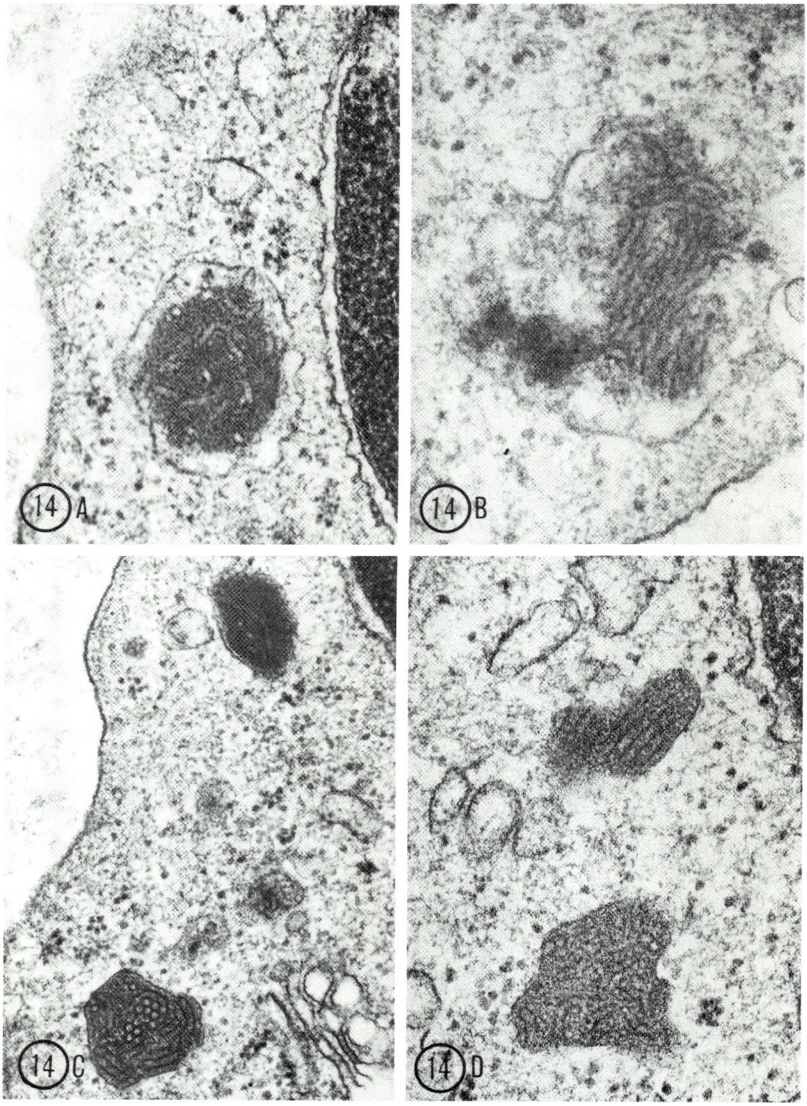

Fig. 14. Various stages of "transition" from membrane bound largely tubular arrays (A, B, C-top) to membrane-free, tubular, angular structures in intimate contact with cytoplasm (C - bottom, D). Magnifications: A = × 60,000; B = × 90,000; C = × 45,000; D = × 50,000.

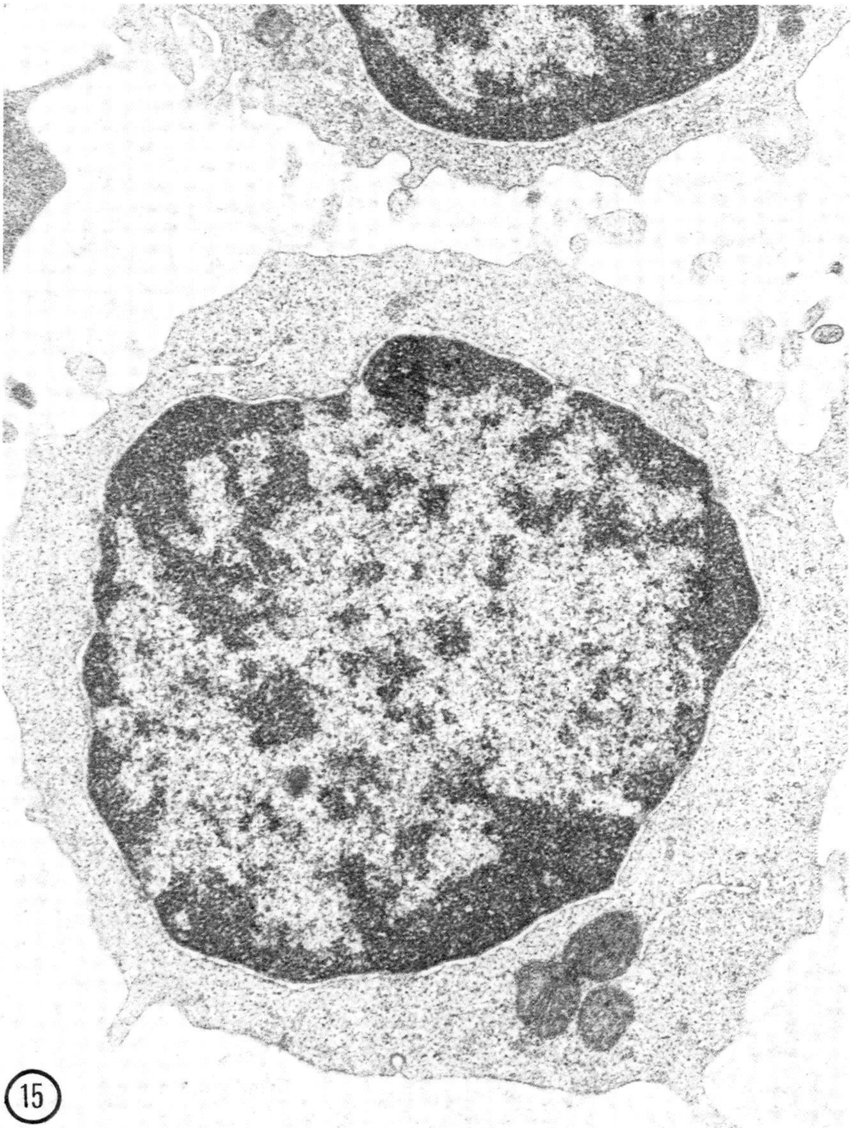

15

Figs. 15–17 represent lymphocytes obtained from peripheral blood after long-term treatment (see text).

Fig. 15. The lymphocyte is free of cytoplasmic inclusions. Magnification × 25,000.

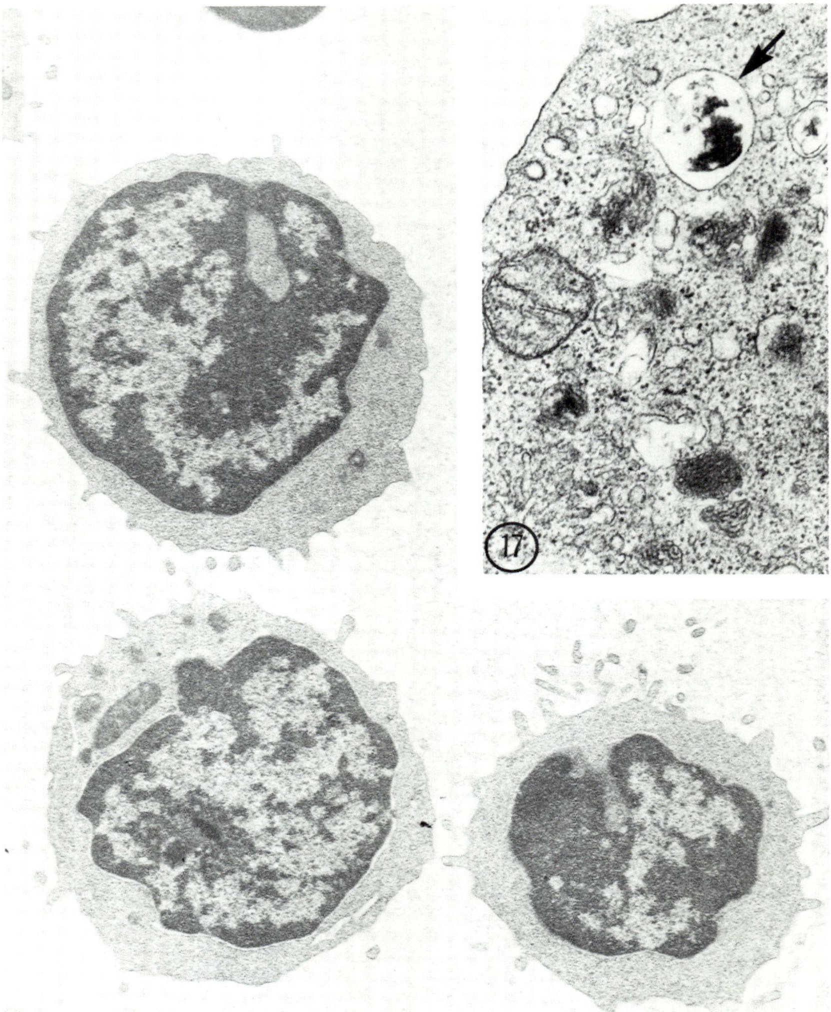
17
16

The work using lymphocytes that is cited above [35] is of some interest in view of our observations on the ultrastructure of peripheral lymphocytes (Figs. 9–17).

The comparison of lymphocytes before and after long-term therapy may be summarized as follows: (1) the number of lymphocytic inclusions (azurophilic granules, tubular conglomerates, and mixture of both) decreased following treatment, with most cells free of these cytoplasmic structures; (2) the tubular transformation is considered to represent changes of azurophilic granules; and (3) the peripheral lymphocytes appeared to be of a smaller, more mature variety during the treatment phase than previously (compare Figs. 9–12 with Figs. 15 and 16).

It is difficult to interpret these findings without resorting to some speculation, since so little is known regarding the nature and role of the lymphocytic "inclusions," their relation to the azurophilic granules seen on light microscopy [36–38], and the precise life span of the lymphocytes [39,40]. Only 10% of peripheral lymphocytes contain a few azurophilic granules [36]. Therefore, it appears that in a disease such as the HHH syndrome, there is an a priori increase in the number of the azurophilic granules that ultimately change to the "tubular" forms. Presumably, with some restoration of integrity of ornithine metabolism, the lymphocytes in the peripheral blood show less degeneration. The tubular aggregates, still observed in the lymphocytes after treatment could represent markers of the former status of a cell that survived for over 2 years. Indeed, some reported data suggest that certain lymphocytes may have a long life span [36,39].

The tubular structures observed in the lymphocytes are not pathognomonic for the HHH syndrome, as similar if not identical structures have been observed in apparently normal subjects and in several conditions (for review, see: Brunning and Parkin [41]). Of interest to the present studies is the report that following administration of dexamethasone to 10 healthy volunteers, the percentage of lymphocytes containing these tubular arrays increased during lymphopenia induced by steroid administration, but that no change occurred

---

Fig. 16. This low-power electron micrograph illustrates that most cells are free of cytoplasmic inclusions. Magnification × 11,000.

Fig. 17. Numerous small, ill-defined, cytoplasmic tubular arrays, similar to those depicted in Figures 13C,D, and 14A–D, are not membrane bound; the contents of the 1 membrane-limited "vesicle" (arrow) are also ill defined and reminiscent of dense curved tubules. These aspects were observed singly or in combination in a small number of mature lymphocytes. Magnification × 25,000.

in the size or number of these arrays in individual cells. The authors interpreted these findings as an indication that a morphologically defined population of lymphocytes from normal peripheral circulation had been linked to a specific response, ie, steroid resistance [42]. Our studies indicate that, at least in the HHH syndrome, the tubular arrays may be derived from the azurophilic granules.

It is unlikely that the smaller lymphocytes observed during treatment resulted from maturation of the larger, granule-containing forms of the untreated patient, since the granules are not known to be discharged from the lymphocytes [36,37]. On that basis one has to conclude that the small, granule-free cells represent *de novo* populations of lymphocytes.

Examination of the peripheral blood from the treated and untreated patients with the HHH syndrome will be required to confirm the above morphologic observations, and their possible significance as a guide to the effectiveness of treatment in our patient.

From our ultrastructural studies of liver, it is uncertain why some hepatocytes contain a normal complement of cytoplasmic organelles (Fig.1), and glycogen and smooth surface endoplasmic reticulum is considerably increased in other cells (Figs. 2, 3). Moreover, it is of interest that not all hepatocytes contained the characteristically altered mitochondria. Such dichotomy in mitochondrial changes occurs in individuals who are heterozygous for OCT-deficiency [43] but not in the liver of homozygous patients of the same disease [43]. This aspect of the HHH syndrome must also await further clarification.

Preliminary observations on the ultrastructure of mitochondria of fibroblasts cultured from the skin of our patient suggest that certain changes are similar to those of hepatic mitochondria [3,8], ie, the increased number, large size, and bizarre forms (compare Figs. 4–8 with Figs. 18 and 19). Thus, our previous proposal [8] relating specificially to the increased number and size of hepatic mitochondria could be extended to those of fibroblasts, ie, that these increases represent attempts at compensation of mitochondrial volume (and function) in the face of metabolic incompetence of these organelles in the HHH syndrome. Data derived from another ultrastructural assessment of similar fibroblasts, while supporting our original findings on the increased volume of hepatic mitochondria [3,8], do not include morphologic evidence of mitochondrial increases in size and number in the fibroblasts [44].

The apparent discrepancies between the other changes of hepatic (Figs. 4–8) and fibroblastic (Figs. 18–20) mitochondria are being explored at present.

In closing, it may be stated that several aspects of the HHH syndrome remain ill understood or controversial; however, on the basis of available

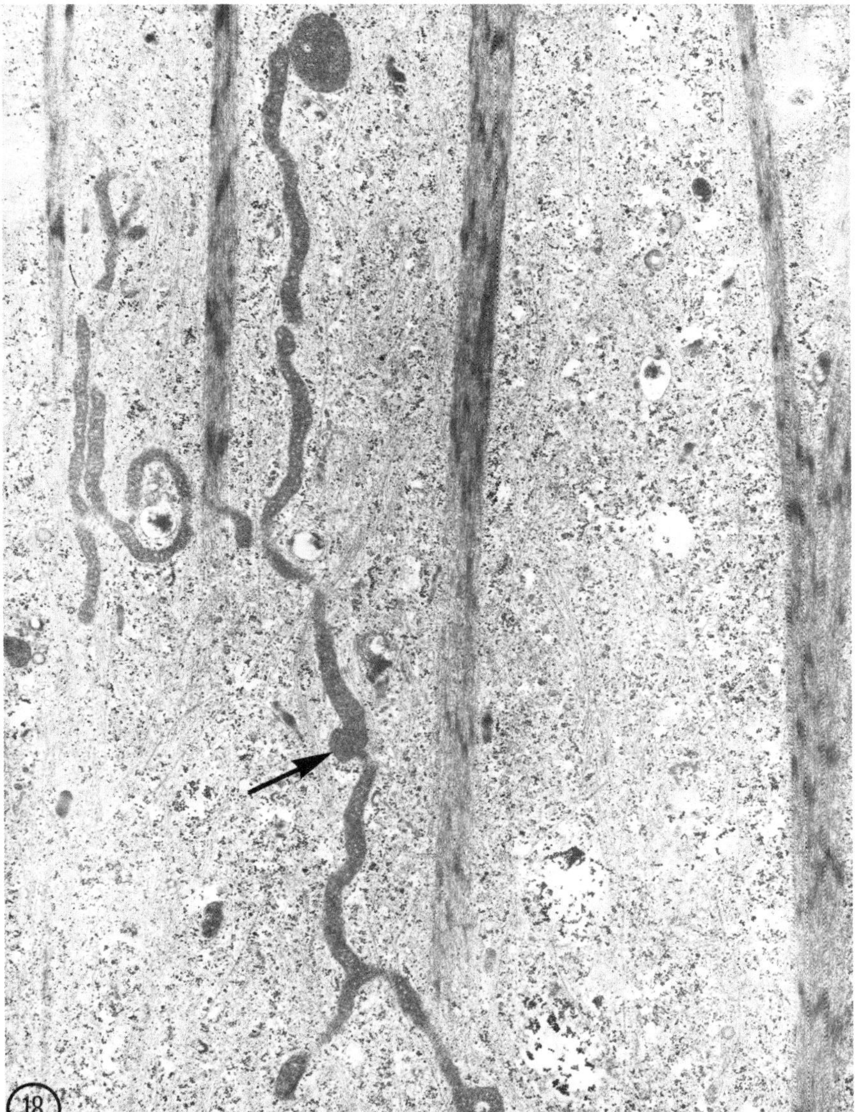

Fig. 18. Fibroblast cultured from patient's skin contains very long, electron-opaque, contorted mitochondria with curling (left, mid-photograph), branching (bottom), and budding (arrow). Magnification × 12,000.

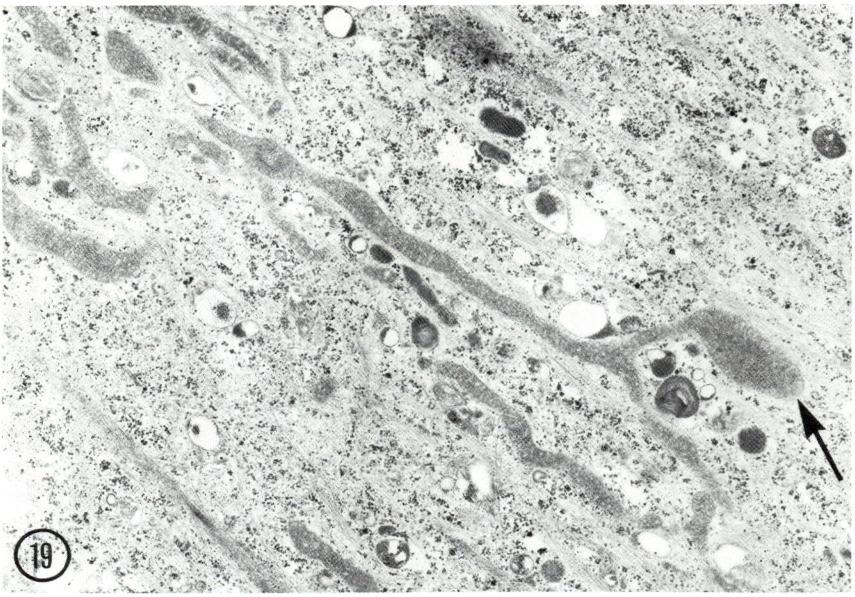
19

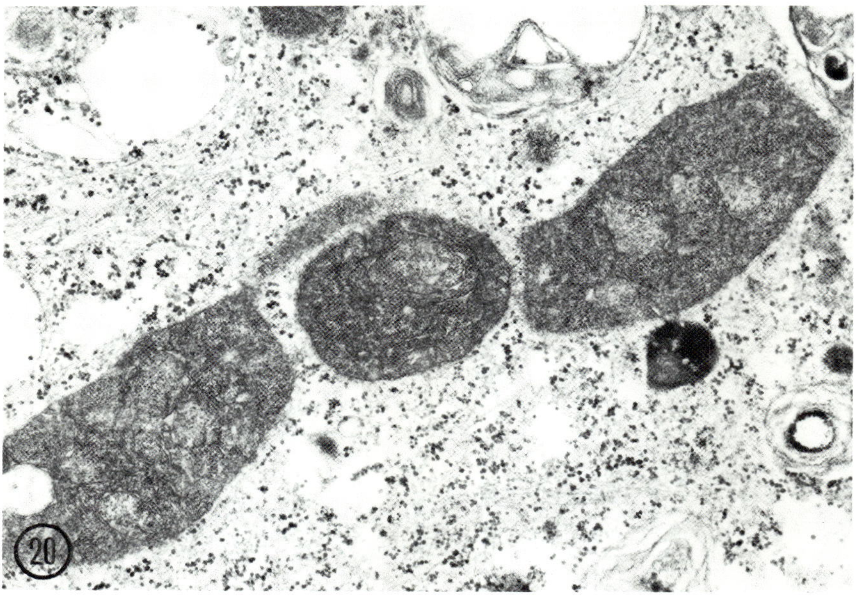
20

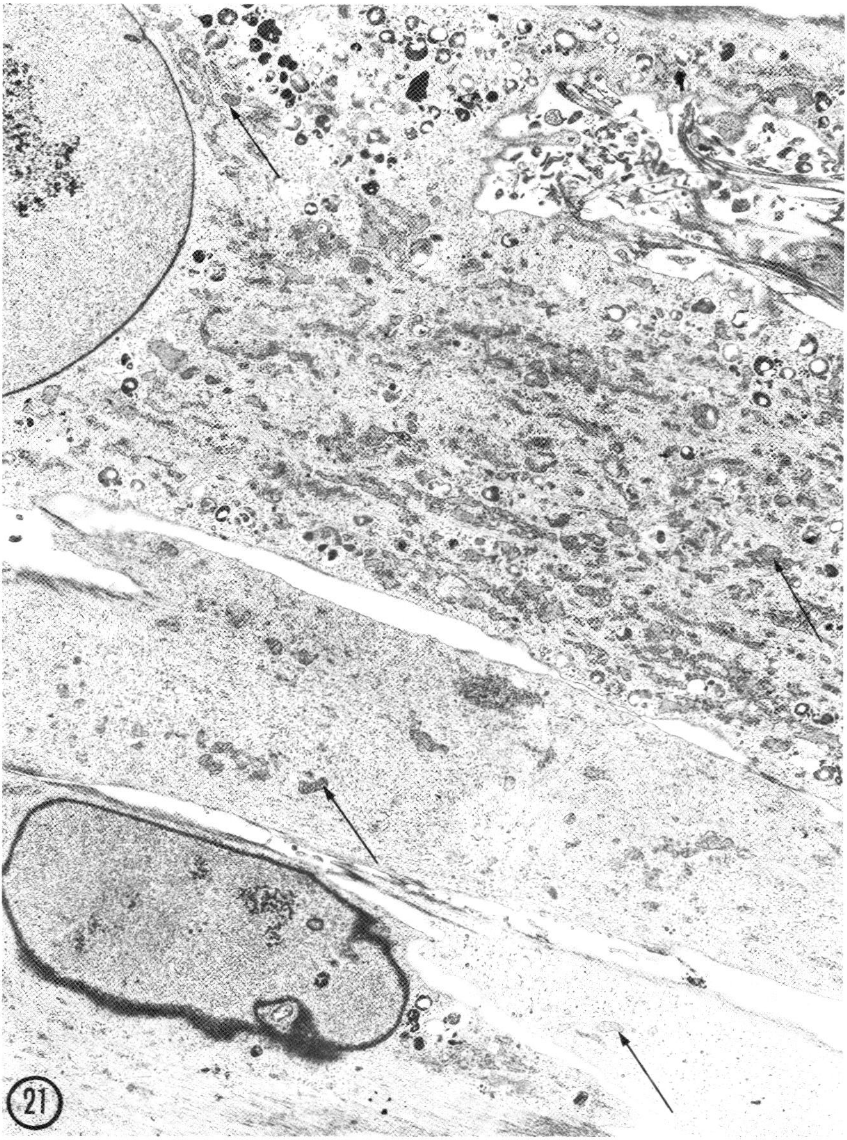

Fig. 21. Fibroblast cultured from skin of a control subject. The mitochondria in all cells depicted are small, few in number, and inconspicuous (arrows). Magnification × 4,000.

Fig. 19. Tissue as in Figure 18, but characteristics of degeneration evident in cytoplasm (round electron-opaque and concentrically membranous "bodies"). One branch of the long mitochondrion terminates in a bulbous projection (arrow). Magnification × 13,000.

Fig. 20. Cell as in Figure 19. The internal structure of the 3 large electron-opaque mitochonia, while difficult to resolve, shows some unusual arrays of cristae in addition to probable degenerative changes. Magnification × 35,000.

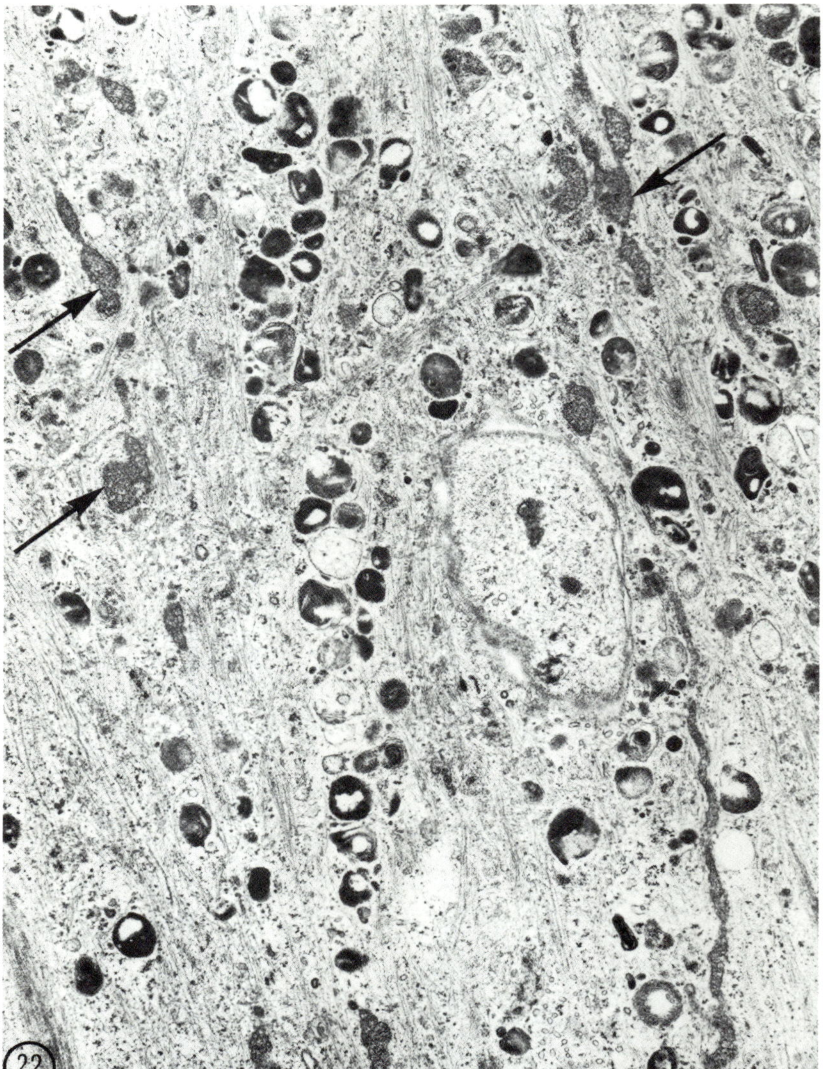

Fig. 22. Tissue as in Figure 21. The fibroblast is in a more advanced degenerative stage than that illustrated in Figure 19. One long mitochondrion (right lower half of illustration) and several oddly shaped or branching, but short, forms are also present (arrows). These changes do not quite approximate those seen in Figures 18–20. Magnification × 6,000.

information it appears reasonable to link the metabolic defect in this disease with the transmembranous transport of ornithine into the mitochondrial matrix.

ACKNOWLEDGMENTS

The authors thank Mr. Roger Dewar, Ms. Irena Wojewodzka, and Mrs. Renate Feulgen for their expert technical assistance, and Mrs. Marion Webster and Mrs. Lya Motesharei for efficient typing of the manuscript.

REFERENCES

1. Shih VE, Efron ML, Moser HW: Hyperornithinemia, hyperammonemia, and homocitrullinuria. A new disorder of amino acid metabolism associated with myoclonic seizures and mental retardation. Am J Dis Child 117:83–92, 1969.
2. Wright T, Pollitt RJ: Psychomotor retardation, epileptic and stuporous attacks, irritability and ataxia associated with ammonia intoxication, high blood ornithine levels, and increased homocitrulline in the urine. Proc R Soc Med 66:221, 1973.
3. Gatfield PD, Taller E, Wolfe DM, Haust MD: Hyperornithinemia, hyperammonemia, and homocitrullinuria associated with decreased carbamyl phosphate synthetase I activity. Pediatr Res 9:488–497, 1975.
4. Hommes FA, Ho CK, Roesel RA, Coryell ME, Gordon BA: Decreased transport of ornithine across the inner mitochondrial membrane as a cause of hyperornithinaemia. J Inher Metab Dis 5:41–47, 1982.
5. Oyanagi K, Tsuchiyama A, Itakura Y, Sogawa H, Wagatsuma K, Nakao T: The mechanism of hyperammonaemia and hyperornithinaemia in the syndrome of hyperornithinaemia, hyperammonaemia and homocitrullinuria. J Inher Metab Dis 6:133–134, 1983.
6. Simell O, MacKenzie S, Clow CL, Scriver CR: Ornithine loading did not prevent induced hyperammonemia in a patient with the HHH syndrome. Pediatr Res 19:1283–1287, 1985.
7. Haust MD, Gatfield PD: Hepatic ultrastructure in a child with carbamyl phosphate synthetase deficiency, hyperornithinaemia, hyperammonaemia and homocitrullinuria. Arch Dis Child 50:663, 1975 (Abs).
8. Haust MD, Gatfield PD, Gordon BA: Ultrastructure of hepatic mitochondria in a child with hyperornithinemia, hyperammonemia, and homocitrullinuria. Hum Pathol 12:212–223, 1981.
9. Fell V, Pollitt RJ, Sampson GA, Wright T: Ornithinemia, hyperammonemia and homocitrullinuria: A disease associated with mental retardation and possibly caused by defective mitochondrial transport. Am J Dis Child 127: 752–756, 1974.
10. Gordon BA, Gatfield PD, Haust MD: The hyperornithinemia, hyperammonemia, homocitrullinuria syndrome: An ornithine transport defect remediable with ornithine supplements. Submitted for publication.
11. Gordon BA, Gatfield PD, Wolfe MD: Studies on the metabolic defect in patients with hyperammonemia, hyperornithinemia and homocitrullinuria. Clin Res 24: 668 A, 1976.
12. Shih VE: Congenital hyperammonemic syndromes. Clin Perinatol 3: 3–14, 1976.
13. Mahoney MJ: Organic acidemias. Clin Perinatol 3: 61–78, 1977.

14. Kekomäki M, Visakorpi JK, Perheentupa J, Saxén J: Familial protein intolerance with deficient transport of basic amino acids. An analysis of 10 patients. Acat Paediatr Scand 56:617–630, 1967.
15. Burgi W, Richterich R, Colombo JP: L-lysine dehydrogenase deficiency in a patient with congenital lysine intolerance. Nature 211:854–855, 1966.
16. Levin B, Oberholzer VG, Palmer T: Citrullinemia and alternative urea cycle. Pediatr Res 7:728, 1973.
17. Valle D, Simell O: The hyperornithinemias. In Stanbury JB, Wyngaarden JB, Frederickson DS, Goldstein JL, Brown MS (eds): "The Metabolic Basis of Inherited Disease," 5th Ed New York: McGraw-Hill Book Company, 1983, pp 382–401.
18. Simell O, Takki K: Raised plasma-ornithine and gyrate atrophy of the choroid and retina. Lancet 1: 1031–1033, 1973.
19. McCulloch C, Marliss EB: Gyrate atrophy of the choroid and retina: Clinical, ophthalmologic and biochemical considerations. Trans Am Ophthalmol Soc 73: 153–171, 1976.
20. Berson EL, Schmidt SY, Rabin AR: Plasma amino-acids in hereditary retinal disease. Ornithine, lysine and taurine. Br J Ophthalmol 60: 142–147, 1976.
21. Sengers RCA, Trijbels JMF, Brussart JH, Deutman AF: Gyrate atrophy of the choroid and retina and ornithine ketoacid transaminase deficiency. Pediatr Res 10: 894, 1976 (Abs).
22. Kennaway NG, Weleber RG, Buist NRM: Gyrate atrophy of choroid and retina: Deficient activity in ornithine ketoacid aminotransferase in cultured fibroblasts. [Letter]. N Engl J Med 297: 1180, 1977.
23. Valle D, Brusilow SW, Walser M, Kaiser-Kupfer MI: Hypoammonemia in gyrate atrophy of choroid and retina. Pediatr Res 12: 513, 1978 (Abs).
24. Valle D, Kaiser-Kupfer MI, Del Valle LA: Gyrate atrophy of the choroid and retina: Deficiency of ornithine aminotransferase in transformed lymphocytes. Proc Natl Acad Sci USA 74: 5159–5161, 1977.
25. Shih VE, Berson EL, Mandell R, Schmidt SY: Ornithine ketoacid transaminase deficiency in gyrate atrophy of the choroid and retina. Am J Hum Genet 30: 174–179, 1978.
26. O'Donnell JJ, Sandman RP, Martin RG: Gyrate atrophy of the retina: Inborn error of L-ornithine-2-oxoacid aminotransferase. Science 200: 200–201, 1978.
27. Bickel H, Feist D, Müller H, Quadbec G: Ornithinämie, eine weitere Aminosäurenstoffwechselstörung mit Hirnschädigung. Dtsch med Wscher 93: 2247–2251, 1968.
28. Garnica AD, Rennert OM, Chan WY: Ornithine ketoacid transaminase deficiency associated with hyperammonemia, hyperornithinemia. Pediatr Res 10: 365, 1976 (Abs).
29. Kekomäki MP, Räihä NCR, Bickel H: Ornithine-ketoacid aminotransferase in human liver with reference to patients with hyperornithinemia and familial protein intolerance. Clin Chim Acta 23: 203–208, 1969.
30. Shih VE, Shulman JH: Ornithine-ketoacid transaminase activity in human skin and amniotic fluid in cell culture. Clin Chim Acta 27: 73–75, 1970.
31. Shih VE, Mandell R, Herzfeld A: Defective ornithine metabolism in cultured skin fibroblasts from patients with the syndrome of hyperornithinemia, hyperammonemia and homocitrullinuria. Clin Chim Acta 118: 149–157, 1982.
32. Valle D, Goodman S, Applegarth D, Shih VE, Phang JM: Type II hyperprolinemia $\triangle^1$-pyrroline-5-carboxylic acid dehydrogenase deficiency in cultured skin fibroblasts and circulating lymphocytes. J Clin Invest 58: 598–603, 1976.
33. Shih VE, Mandell R: Metabolic defect in hyperornithinemia. [Letter] Lancet 2: 1522–1523, 1974.

34. Gamble JG, Lehninger AL: Transport of ornithine and citrulline across the mitochondrial membrane. J Biol Chem 248: 610–618, 1973.
35. Gray RGF, Hill SE, Pollit RJ: Reduced ornithine catabolism in cultured fibroblasts and phytohaemagglutinin-stimulated lymphocytes from a patient with hyperornithinemia, hyperammonemia and homocitrullinuria. Clin Chim Acta 118: 141–148, 1982.
36. Rhodin JAG: "Histology. A Text and Atlas."London, Toronto: Oxford University Press, 1974.
37. Ackerman GA: Structural studies of the lymphocyte and lymphocyte development. In Gordon AS (ed): "Regulation and Hematopoiesis," Vol 2. New York: Appleton-Century-Crofts, 1970, pp 1297–1338.
38. Tanaka Y, Goodman JR: "Electron Microscopy of Human Blood Cells." New York: Harper & Row, 1972.
39. Gowans JL: Life-span, recirculation and transformation of lymphocytes. Int Rev Exp Pathol 5: 1–24, 1966.
40. Zucker-Franklin D: The ultrastructure of lymphocytes. Semin Hematol 6: 4–27, 1969.
41. Brunning RD, Parkin J: Ultrastructural studies of parallel tubular arrays in human lymphocytes. Am J Pathol 78: 59–70, 1975.
42. Payne CM, Glasser L: The effect of steroids on peripheral blood lymphocytes containing parallel tubular arrays. Am J Pathol 92: 611–618, 1978.
43. Haust MD, Gatfield PD, Gordon BA: Ultrastucture of liver in homo- and heterozygous subjects for OCT-deficiency. Unpublished observations.
44. Metoki K, Hommes FA, Dyken P, Kelloes C, Trefz J: Ultrastructural changes in fibroblast mitochondria of a patient with HHH-syndrome. J Inher Metab Dis 7: 147–150, 1984.

Pathological Findings in 5,10-Methylene Tetrahydrofolate Reductase Deficiency

Daniel R. Beckman, MD, George Hoganson, MD, Stanley Berlow, MD, and Enid F. Gilbert, MD

Departments of Pathology, Pediatrics and Genetics, University of Wisconsin Hospitals, Madison, Wisconsin 53792

INTRODUCTION

Vivian Shih first described 5,10-methylene tetrahydrofolate reductase (MTHFR) deficiency in 1972 [1,2] and since then about 25 patients have been reported with what is now considered the commonest hereditary defect in the metabolism of folic acid. Even in this small sample, and like most autosomal recessive hereditary metabolic diseases, there is clinical and biochemical heterogeneity [3]. The most frequent form of the condition begins in infancy with lethargy and hypotonia. A severe convulsive disorder soon follows. The infant is developmentally delayed and the child is severely retarded. Microcephaly is almost always present. Death can occur during an episode of apnea, or may follow respiratory problems. Few children with the infantile form of MTHFR deficiency live beyond the first decade. Therapy with folinic or folic acid, vitamins B_6 and B_{12}, methionine supplements, and betaine, in various combinations has helped a few patients [4–8]. A report on prenatal diagnosis appeared recently [9].

The diagnosis is generally first suspected when on metabolic screening urinary nitroprusside reaction is obtained. Quantitative amino acid analyses demonstrate homocystine in urine and blood. However, the levels are usually lower than in classic homocystinuria secondary to cystathionine synthase (CS) deficiency [10]. Plasma methionine levels generally are low. Methyl-

Birth Defects: Original Article Series, Volume 23, Number 1, pages 47–64

malonic aciduria and megaloblastic anemia are *not* present; 5-methyl tetrahydrofolate levels in blood and CSF are reduced. Low CSF neurotransmitter metabolite levels (5-hydroxyindoleacetic acid, 3-methoxy-4-hydroxy-phenylglycol and homovanillic acid (5HIAA, MHPG and HVA)) were first reported in 1980 [8,11]. Presently the diagnosis is confirmed by enzymatic assays performed on lymphocytes or skin fibroblasts.

In the differential diagnosis of homocystinuria, other conditions must be considered. Nutritional deficiency or defective absorption of vitamin B_{12} and hereditary metabolic defects in the cellular metabolism of cobalamin [12–14], aka cobalamin mutants, can cause homocystinuria. CS deficiency is the commonest inborn error of metabolism associated with elevated plasma and urinary homocystine levels. In this disease [15], the vascular manifestations of arteriosclerosis and thromboses cause devastating CNS complications.* Similar findings have been reported in MTHFR deficiency [18,19] and in patients with cobalamin defects and homocystinuria [20,21] (Fig. 1) We concur with others who have reported that the homocystinemia is responsible for the vascular lesions. However, our emphasis is on the origin in MTHFR deficiency of the astrogliosis and demyelination that may reflect the adverse combination of CNS folate deficiency, inadequate neurotransmitter production, and chronic hypomethioninemia on the developing brain.

Despite numerous biochemical and clinical reports, we have been able to locate only 4 pathologic reports of this disease since the original description by Kanwar [18] in 1976. The purpose of this report is to describe the pathologic findings in 2 autopsied patients.

HISTORY

Patient 1. B.D. 7/25/74

Symptoms of lethargy, poor feeding, and apneic spells with cyanosis were the cause of this male infant's first hospitalization at age 2 1/2 weeks. Except for an EEG that was reported as "grade I bitemporal dysrhythmia," results

*Neuropathologic findings in a male patient with homocystinuria and hypermethioninemia were reported from this institution in 1965 [16]. Cystathionine was not present in his cerebrum [17]. No enzyme studies were reported. The method of sample preparation for blood amino acid analysis, at that time, may explain the failure to find homocystine in plasma. After an unusual course for cystathionine synthase deficiency—severe failure to thrive, spastic quadriplegia, zonular cataracts—the patient died at age 1 year. At autopsy, spongy degeneration and demyelination in the white matter, cerebellum, basal ganglia, brain stem, and spinal cord were found, but have not been reported in other patients with CS deficiency.

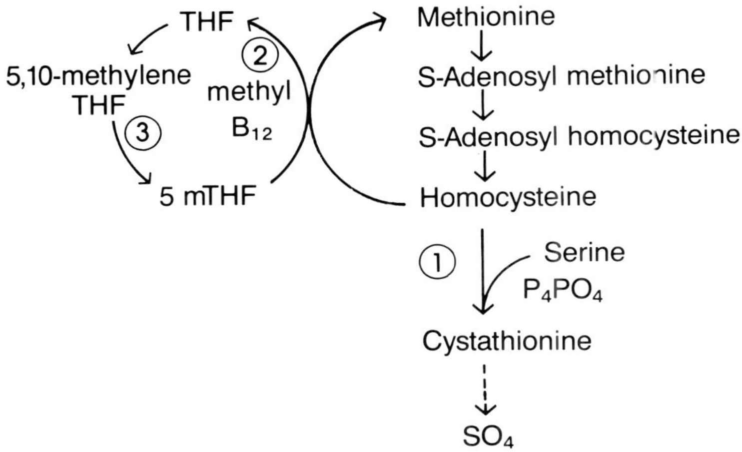

1 Cystathionine Synthase
2 methyl THF homocysteine methyl transferase
3 5,10-methylene THF reductase

Fig. 1. Metabolic pathways of methionine in brain.

of other laboratory studies (including a urinary amino acid paper chromatography screen and the nitroprusside test) were unremarkable. By age 3 months, he was below the 3rd centile in length, weight, and head circumference. At 6 months, no response to visual stimuli was noted. Normal responses were obtained on the electroretinogram (ERG) and visual evoked response (VER). When a diagnosis of seizure disorder was made at 10 months on clinical and EEG evidence, phenobarbital and dilantin treatment was begun. He was profoundly hypotonic and retarded at age 17 months when another comprehensive diagnostic evaluation was performed. At that time, the urine nitroprusside test was reactive; quantitative urine amino acid analyses showed homocystinuria. Plasma methionine was 0.1 mg/dl (nl$=0.4\pm0.1$) and homocystine 0.3 mg/dl (nl$=0$). Serum folate levels determined by radioimmunoassay (RIA) were 2.2 and 3.3 ng/ml (nl$=$5-19 ng/ml). Dr. Paul Wong reported 10% MTHFR activity in the patient's lymphocytes (see Table I); the levels in the parents were reduced to approximately 50% of normal. Folic acid (20 mg/day) was administered orally for 6 weeks with no change in plasma methionine, homocystine levels, or his clinical condition.

TABLE I. Biochemical Findings in MTHFR Deficiency

	Patient No. 1	Patient No. 2	Normal values
5,10 mTHFr activity:			
Lymphocytes	1.46*		11.37 + 3.77
Fibroblasts		0.8*	5.04 + 1.36
Plasma amino acids: mg/dl			
Methionine	0.1–0.16	tr.–0.16	0.4 + 0.1
Homocystine	0.3–0.6	0.6–1.0	0
Cystine	0.2–0.7	0.4–0.6	0.5+0.2
Folic acid: ng/ml			
Serum	2.3–3.6	3.5	5–19
CSF	—	26	10.6–85
CSF Neurotransmitter metabolites: ng/ml			
5HIAA	—	20.1	42.7+6.2
HVA	—	28	120.3 + 12.6
MHPG	—	11.9	14.2 + 1.7

*nmol formaldehyde produced/hour/mg protein

During the last 6 months of his life, he had myoclonic seizures that were refractory to treatment. He required gavage feedings, was rarely awake, and had little voluntary movement.

At age 27 months, he was readmitted to the hospital because of respiratory distress and a temperature of 97°. *Haemophilus influenza* and *Staphylococcus aureus* were grown from blood cultures. Despite intravenous ampicillin and penicillin treatment, he had a sudden respiratory arrest 5 days after admission and died.

Patient 2. B.D. 7/31/83

This male infant was considered to be healthy with normal development until age 3 months when a mass was noted in his left calf. Biopsy showed an infantile fibrosarcoma [22,23]. No metastases were found on investigation, and the tumor was excised under 50% nitrous oxide (N_2O) anesthesia, 4 hours in duration. Two weeks after the operation he had an apneic spell during feeding. On hospital admission, developmental regression was documented; he was markedly hypotonic and had no head control. His head circumference, which at birth was 36 cm, was then 39 cm. His EEG was grossly abnormal and he was treated with phenobarbital 5 mg/kg/day. A CT scan was reported as showing generalized cortical atrophy. Ophthalmologic examination showed no fixation, nor did he follow objects. ERG was normal but no VER was elicited. A nitroprusside reaction occurred on urine metabolic screening. Quantitative urinary amino acid analyses demonstrated homocystine but methionine was *not* detected in the urine. Plasma amino acid determinations were homocystine 0.61 mg/dl and methionine 0.06 mg/dl. Serum folate levels (RIA) were 3.8 and 3.5 ng/ml. CSF folate (RIA) was 26 ng/ml (n=10.6-85). 5-methyl THF levels performed by Dr. David Rosenblatt, Montreal, using a bacterial assay were serum 2.1 ng/ml and CSF 1.3 ng/ml. Both values and the ratio were reduced. The latter test is considered to give a more accurate measure of 5-methyl THF levels (David Rosenblatt, Montreal).

Neurotransmitter metabolites in CSF (William Seifert, Houston, TX) were:

		ng/ml
	Patient	Normal (mean ± SEM)
5HIAA	20.1	42.7 ± 6.2
HVA	28	120.3 ± 12.6
MHPG	11.9	14 ± 1.1

Fibroblast MTHFR activity, assayed by Dr. Paul Wong, Chicago, IL, was 0.8 nmol formaldehyde produced/hour/mg protein (nl 5.04±1.36).

The patient was given intravenous *Leukovorin* (folinic acid) 10 mg/day without biochemical or clinical improvement. Administration of betaine, 250 mg/kg/day, p.o., cleared homocystine from urine and plasma but did not increase plasma methionine. He also received vitamins B_{12} and B_6 and a methionine supplement for only 1 day before his acute, sudden death in an apneic spell at age 4 1/2 months.

GROSS PATHOLOGY

Both children appeared grossly normal with normal body height, weight and circumferential measurements. The cardiovascular systems were grossly normal except in patient 1 where small lipid atheromatous plaques were present in the ascending aorta, proximal left coronary artery, and ventricular surfaces of the mitral valve leaflets. The lungs in patient 1 showed dark red hemorrhagic areas but no thromboemboli could be identified. In patient 2, pulmonary congestion was present. Hepatosplenomegaly was seen in patient 2; the liver weighed 260 g (normal 160 g) and the spleen 34 g (normal 16 g). The kidneys were also slightly enlarged in patient 2.

The brains in both cases were abnormal with significant cerebral atrophy; that of patient 1 weighed 640 g (normal 1064 g), that of patient 2 weighed

410 g (normal 540 g) (Fig. 2). Varying degrees of polymicrogyri (Fig. 3) were present in both brains but no evidence of thrombosis was noted. Asymmetry and demyelination were present (Fig. 4) with a generalized decrease in the amount of white matter. Hypoplasia of the corpus callosum was seen in patient 1. No hemorrhage or necrosis was present and no significant changes were seen in the midbrain, pons, medulla, cerebellum, or spinal cord.

MICROSCOPIC PATHOLOGY

In patient 1 sections through the coronary arteries showed intimal thickening and subintimal fibrosis. Both patients showed fragmentation and disruption of the elastic lamellae within the aorta (Fig. 5). No medial necrosis or thrombosis was present. Foci of pulmonary hemorrhage without throm-

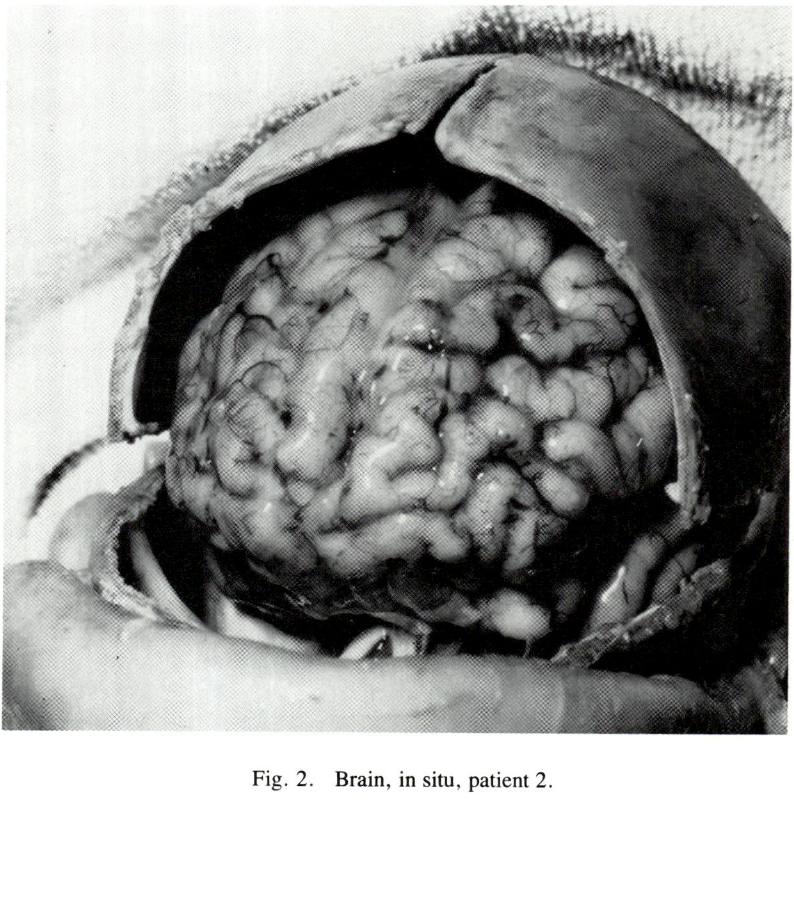

Fig. 2. Brain, in situ, patient 2.

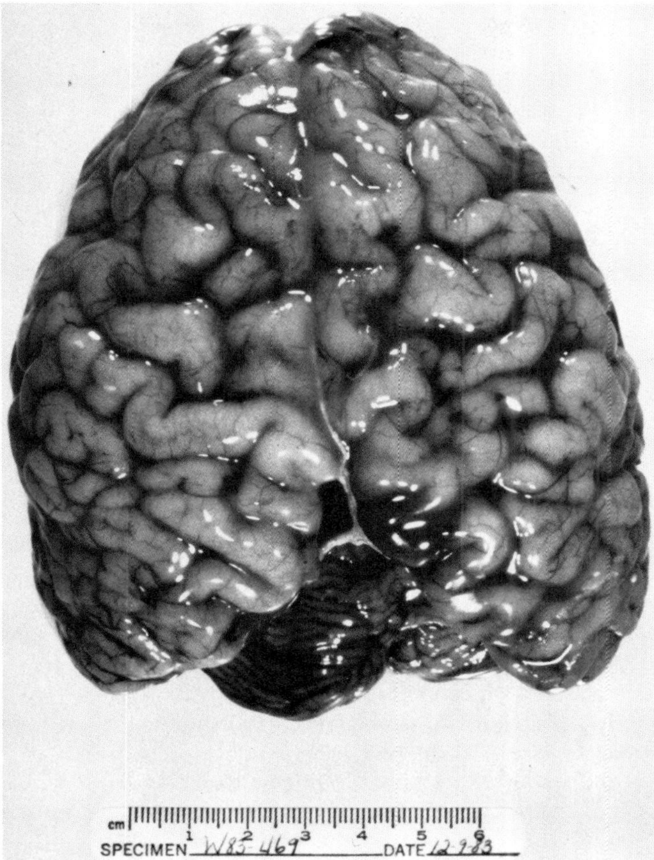

Fig. 3. Brain, polymicrogyria, patient 2.

bosis consistent with early infarction were present in patient 1, but patient 2 showed only pulmonary congestion. Hepatic changes consisted of mild fatty metamorphosis with some congestion of the central veins and sinusoids. No necrosis or inflammation was present. No evidence of recurrent or metastatic fibrosarcoma was seen in patient 2.

Several microscopic changes were present in the brain, especially in patient 1. The cortical gray matter showed changes of fibrillary astrogliosis of the molecular layer while in the white matter there was reduced myelina-

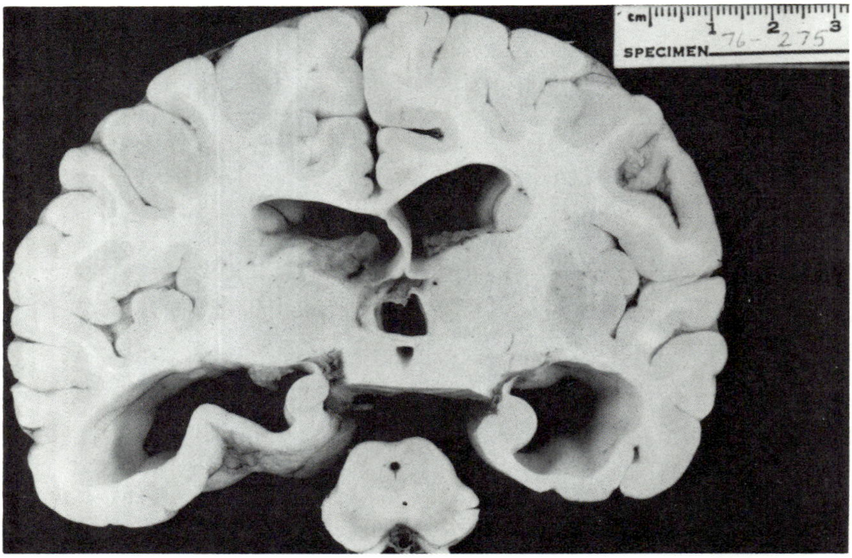

Fig. 4. Brain, asymmetry, patient 2.

tion. This was quite marked and disproportionately severe in patient 2 despite the fact that death occurred at an early age (4 months). This suggests that another pathophysiologic mechanism may be contributing to demyelination. Perivascular spaces contained loose connective tissue with occasional lymphocytes (Fig. 6). The oligodendroglial cells appeared to be numerically reduced. No significant changes were seen in the basal ganglia or thalami. Similar changes were also present in the midbrain, medulla, and cerebellum with demyelination, astrogliosis, and depletion of oligodendroglial cells. Neurons in the cerebellar cortex appeared intact. Sections of the upper cervical spinal cord were not available in patient 2, but those in patient 1 showed ovoid-shaped areas of demyelination, especially in the posterior columns, very similar to the changes seen in subacute combined degeneration (vitamin B_{12} deficiency). Demyelination was also present in the optic chiasm in patient 1, but changes in the optic nerves were not as significant. Lipid-filled macrophages were conspicuous in the choroid plexus of patient 1 (Figs. 7,8), but these cells were not as prominent in patient 2. No significant thromboemboli were seen in either brain.

ELECTRON MICROSCOPY

Tissue sections from the aorta, liver, skeletal muscle, and brain were processed for electron microscopy. Hepatocytes had round to oval nuclei

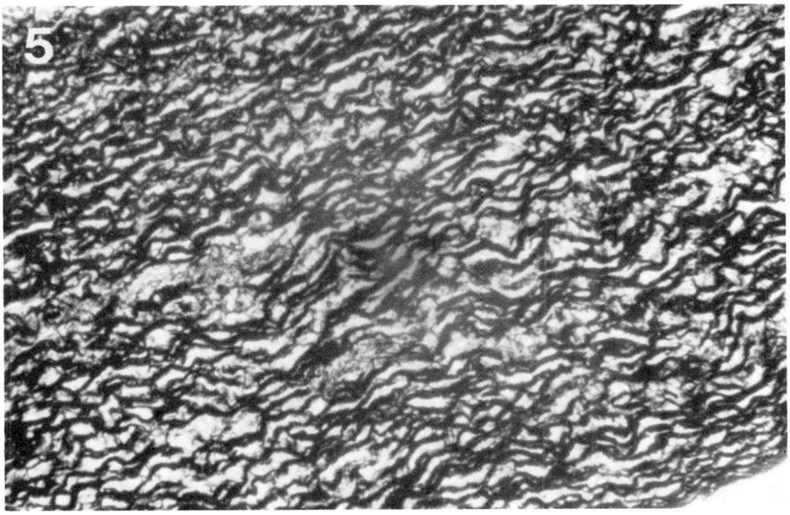

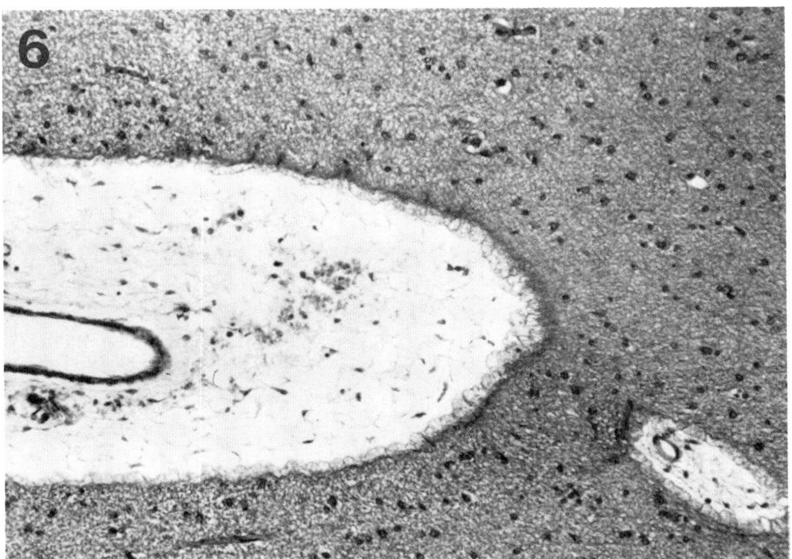

Fig. 5. Aorta, disruption of elastic lamellae (x250).

Fig. 6. Brain, widening of perivascular space (x250).

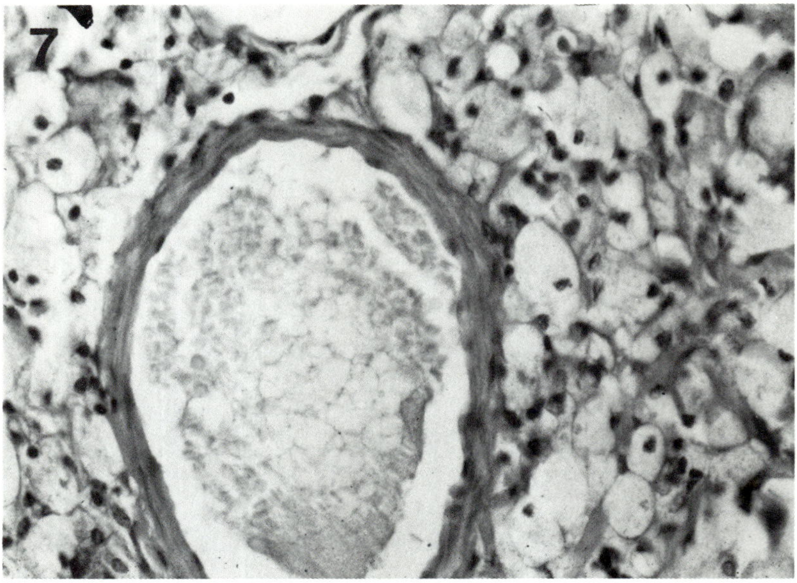

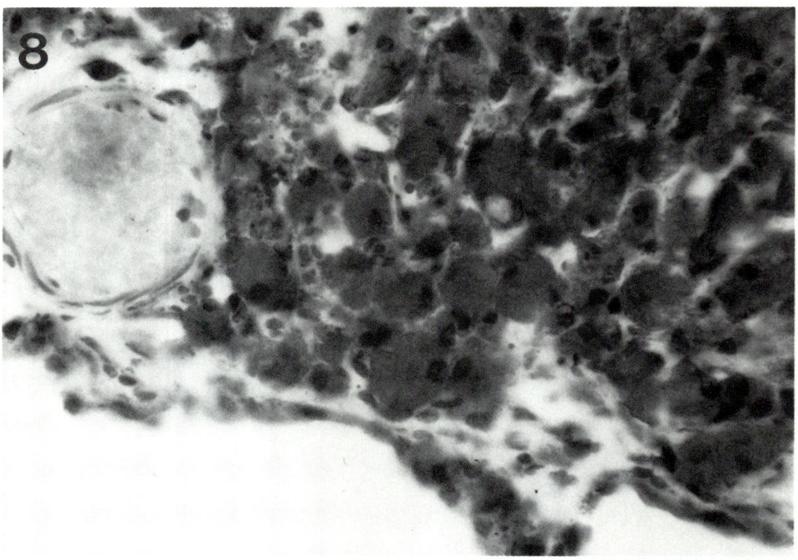

Fig. 7. Choroid plexus, lipid-filled macrophages (x250).

Fig. 8. See Figure 7 (x400).

with some peripheral condensation of nuclear chromatin. Frequently observed in the cytoplasm were lipid droplets and occasional multivesicular bodies in close approximation to lysosomes. Occasional electron-dense lipofuscin deposits were noted. Some mitochondria were of giant size and lobulated with peripheral projections. Glycogen was prominent; rough endoplasmic reticulum was arranged in parallel arrays. Bile canaliculi and Kupffer cells appeared normal.

The aorta showed prominent endothelial cells with a considerable increase in subendothelial collagen. In the media there was fragmentation and disruption of the elastic lamellae; interlamellar spaces were wide and contained flocculent material (Fig. 9). Smooth muscle cells of the media showed early degenerative changes with some loss of myofilaments. Similar ultrastructural changes were also seen in the coronary and mesenteric vessels in patient 1.

In the brain, neurons showed loss of Nissl bodies. Some astrocytes had reactive changes with increased intracytoplasmic fibrils. Severe degenerative changes were noted in the myelin sheaths with separation of the layers and formation of large cystic spaces which connected to the degenerating adjacent nerve fibers (Fig. 10). Axon cylinder degeneration, presumably due to

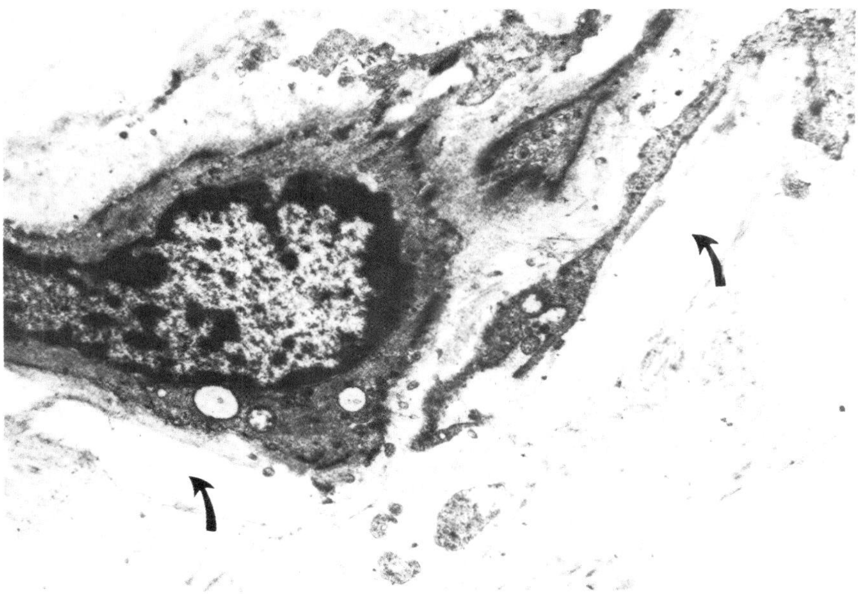

Fig. 9. Aorta, showing fragmentation and disruption of the elastic lamellae with interlamellar spaces containing flocculent material (arrows). Magnification, x16,000.

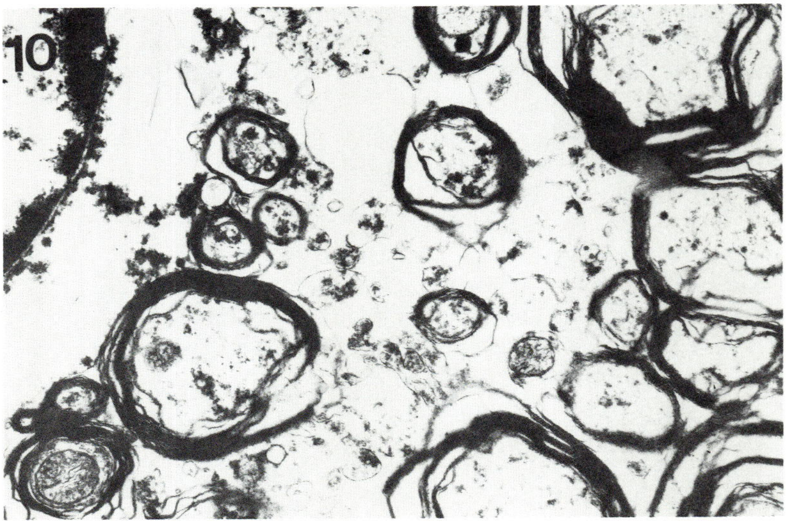

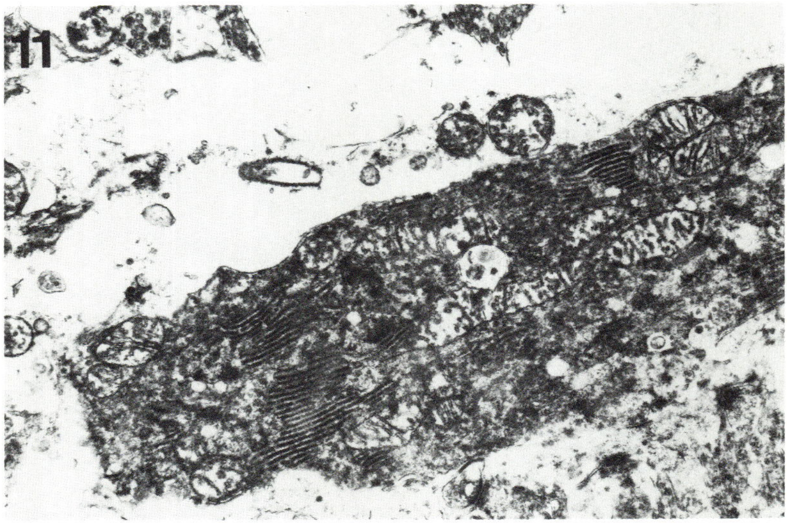

Fig. 10. Myelin sheath showing separation of myelin leaflets forming cystic spaces. Magnification, x22,000.

Fig. 11. Purkinje cell of cerebellar cortex showing parallel arrays of endoplasmic reticulum within the cytoplasm. Mitochondria are numerous and contain parallel and sometimes disrupted and twisted cristae. Magnification, x22,000.

compression by spongy swelling of myelin sheaths, was also prominent. Sections of a dendrite of a Purkinje cell showed parallel arrays of endoplasmic reticulum also present in the cell body (Fig. 11). Focal irregular areas of dense amorphous material were also present in the cellular matrix. The mitochondria were enlarged and contained parallel but sometimes disrupted and twisted cristae. In patient 1, sections were also taken of the internal capsule, which showed degenerative cystic myelin and axonal changes similar to those seen in the cortex.

Sections of striated muscle were also examined in patient 1. These showed focal areas of irregularity of the myofibers with disrupted Z bands and disorganization of the myofilaments (Fig. 12). Mitochondria were enlarged with irregular cristae. Some atypical cytoplasmic bodies, consisting of dense, coarsely granular material, were also present surrounded by myofilaments.

DISCUSSION

Most of the descriptions of the pathologic changes in homocystinuria have focused on the vascular anomalies [20,24,25], and the lesions have been

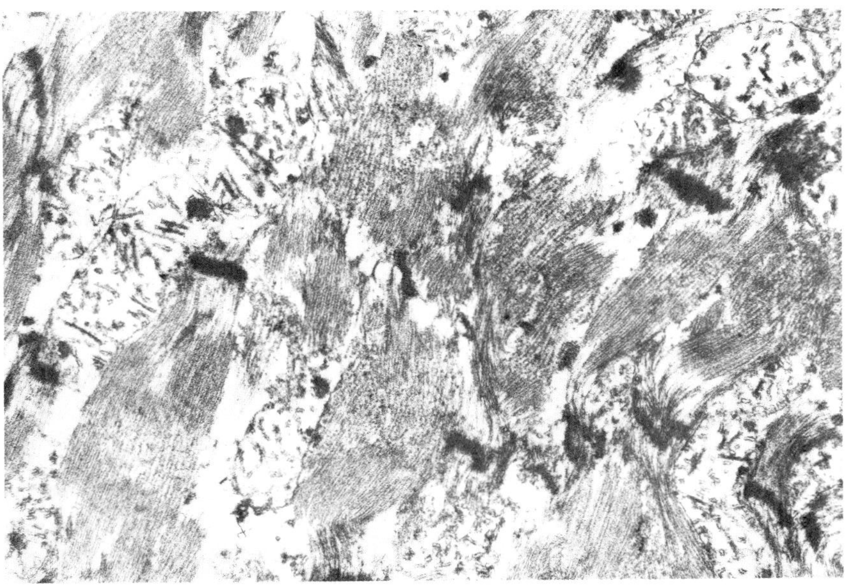

Fig. 12. Skeletal muscle fiber showing disrupted Z bands and disorganization of myofilaments. Uranyl acetate and lead citrate. Magnification, x24,000.

attributed to the vasculo-toxic effects of elevated levels of homocystine. The original description of the pathologic changes of MTHFR deficiency by Kanwar et al is no exception [18]; they emphasized the gross, microscopic, and ultrastructural changes with complete descriptions of the liver, brain, aorta, skeletal muscles, and kidneys. The other reports of the pathologic changes of MTHFR deficiency are not as detailed, but the cases can be compared to the present patients. Narisawa [26] described a young girl who died at 9 months with the usual clinical manifestations. She was diagnosed at 6 months. The postmortem description was limited to the brain, which showed cortical atrophy (weight 610 g [normal 810 g]), marked dilatation of the ventricular system, and fresh thrombosis of the superior sagittal sinus. Also noted was atrophy of the cerebellum, brain stem, and basal ganglia. Microscopic changes included neuronal loss, cellular degeneration in gray matter, and defective myelination.

Baumgartner and Wick [19] described a patient who died at 3 1/2 years after a minor respiratory infection. The child had had progressive hypotonia, microcephaly, and seizures leading to a diagnosis at 18 months. The pathologic description included widespread vascular lesions consisting of focal intimal proliferation with destruction of the internal elastic lamella most prominent in the coronary and the external iliac arteries. The brain was atrophic (weight 710 g) and vascular lesions were noted in small intracerebral vessels. Multiple foci of perivascular demyelination and gliosis were present but these were not described as diffuse. The authors commented that these lesions were similar to the cerebral lesions previously described in pernicious anemia (PA) and speculated that "elevated plasma homocysteine might play an important role in the pathogenesis of the neurological abnormalities of PA."

Haan et al [27] described a boy who died at 7 1/2 years. The autopsy showed bronchopneumonia and marked cerebral atrophy with a brain weight of 690 g (normal 1260 g). Extensive gliosis and demyelination were prominent, but intravascular thrombosis and thickening of cerebral vessel walls were not seen despite his relatively long survival. No other pathologic abnormality was described.

In reviewing the pathologic changes in the different forms of homocystinuria (CS deficiency, cobalamin mutants, and MTHFR deficiency), we are struck by many similarities, which suggest that high levels of homocystine are responsible for the vascular lesions that are the one common denominator in all 3 forms. Although most cases described have vascular changes, the degree of thrombosis is quite variable. Kanwar et al [18] concluded that the thrombosis was secondary to the arterial changes because vascular abnormalities were observed without thrombosis. He also speculated whether the initial vascular event was endothelial damage or connective tissue injury; abnormal proteoglycans seemed to support the latter possibility.

As we have discussed previously, the neuropathologic vascular abnormalities of MTHFR deficiency are similar to those described in CS deficiency [24,25]. There is abundant evidence that links homocyst(e)ine to endothelial injury [28] and arteriosclerosis [29], although questions have been raised about the experimental models that have been employed in the laboratory [30,31].

However, in MTHFR deficiency, it is also necessary to explain the additional findings of demyelination, astrogliosis, and lipid-filled macrophages that are associated in many infants with an apparently progressive course of seizures, microcephaly, and severe psychomotor retardation.

Erbe [32] has emphasized the generally consistent findings in the infantile form of the disease, ie, low plasma methionine, low plasma and CSF folate with normal cobalamin levels, and the absence of megaloblastic anemia. He has suggested that the "CNS seems particularly vulnerable to the biochemical abnormalities" and indicts methionine deficiency as the major cause of the neuropathology. We certainly agree and can point to the undetectable methionine in the CSF of our patient 2 (Table I) as further evidence of severe methionine deprivation.

In addition, this paper adds a second example, our patient 1, to a previous report [33] of subacute combined degeneration (SCD) in MTHFR deficiency. SCD is a well-recognized complication of PA, but the mechanism whereby cobalamin deficiency causes SCD has not been precisely defined. However, recently, N_2O exposure has been employed as a model for PA, since cobalamin is inactivated by it [34] and N_2O anesthesia produces a neuropathy in monkeys that pathologically is similar to SCD [35]. N_2O oxidizes cobalamin I to inert cobalamin III thereby inactivating methionine synthetase (Fig. 1) and producing methionine deficiency. The brain does not have an alternate route (as liver uses betaine: homocysteine methyltransferase) for the *de novo* synthesis of methionine [34]. Thus, when brain methionine synthesis is blocked, the CNS becomes completely dependent on circulating, and mainly dietary, methionine.

How methionine deficiency specifically causes demyelination—by interfering with methylation, by formate starvation, or by some other mechanism—is not known [34]. In any case, such a pathologic process would be expected to be more severe in the infantile brain and to produce lipid-filled macrophages.

The significance of these observations and conclusions is multifaceted. First, it should now be obvious that in MTHFR deficiency we are dealing with a disease that primarily affects the CNS. Treatment must be directed at the brain and the efficacy of treatment measured by brain function and CSF levels of metabolites. Treatment should be begun early, preferably before onset of symptoms. Second, this group of hereditary metabolic defects involving methionine synthetase must be studied not only for themselves but in the context of their relationship to the "methylfolate trap" hypothesis [36], to PA and the pathogenesis of SCD. Especially significant are the interrelationships among methionine, folate, B_{12}, and neurotransmitter production in the CNS. Although we have emphasized the low methionine levels, we recognize that lowered CSF folate and decreased levels of neurotransmitter probably play a significant role in the CNS changes. In patient 2, it is possible that N_2O exposure further compromised reduced levels of methionine synthetase activity and contributed to the progression of his disease.

Last, we must consider the significance of the fibrosarcoma in patient 2. To our knowledge, this is the first report of a neoplasm in the approximately 25 patients who have been reported with MTHFR deficiency. Speculation about the relationship of hypomethylation to carcinogenesis in humans must await further research or additional reports in MTHFR deficiency.

ACKNOWLEDGMENTS

We thank Drs. Robert F. Schilling, Robert Steele, and N.L. Benevenga for their discussions of these patients and their helpful suggestions. Mr. Robert Colwell performed the amino acid analyses.

REFERENCES

1. Shih VE, Salam MZ, Mudd SH, Uhlendorf BW, Adams RD: A new form of homocystinuria due to $N^{5,10}$methylenetetrahydrofolate reductase deficiency (Abstract). Pediatr Res 6:135, 1972.
2. Mudd SH, Uhlendorf BW, Freeman JM, Finkelstein JD, Shih VE: Homocystinuria associated with decreased methylene tetrahydrofolate reductase activity. Biochem Biophys Res Comm 46:905–912, 1972.
3. Rowe PB: Inherited disorders of folate metabolism. In Stanbury JB, Wyngaarden JB, Fredrickson DS, Goldstein JL, Brown MS (eds): "The Metabolic Basis of Inherited Disease." New York: McGraw-Hill, 1983, pp 516.
4. Harpey JP, Rosenblatt DS, Cooper BA, LeMoel G, Roy C, Lafourcade J: Homocystinuria caused by 5,10 methylentetrahydrofolate reductase deficiency: A case in an infant responding to methionine, folinic acid, pyridoxine and vitamin B12 therapy. J Pediatr 98:275–278, 1983.
5. Allen RJ, Wong P, Rothenberg SP, DiMauro S, Headington JT. Progressive neonatal leukoencephalomyopathy due to absent methylenetetrahydrofolate reductase, responsive to treatment. (Abstract) Ann Neurol 8:211, 1980.

6. Wendel U, Bremer HJ: Betaine in the treatment of homocystinuria due to 5,10 methylene THF reductase deficiency. Eur J Pediatr 142:147–150, 1984.
7. Freeman JM, Finkelstein JD, Mudd SH: Folate-responsive homocystinuria and "schizophrenia." N Engl J Med 292:491–496, 1975.
8. Harpey JP, Moel GL, Zittoun J: Follow-up in a child with 5,10-methylene tetrahydrofolate reductase deficiency. J Pediatr 103:1007, 1983.
9. Christensen E, Brandt NJ: Prenatal diagnosis of 5,10-methelenetetrahydrofolate reductase deficiency (letter to the editor). N Engl J Med 313:50–51, 1985.
10. Wong PWK, Justice P, Hruby M, Weiss EB, Diamond E: Folic acid nonresponsive homocystinuria due to methylenetetrahydrofolate reductase deficiency. Pediatrics 59:749–756, 1977.
11. Singer HS, Butler I, Rothenberg S, Valle D, Freeman J: Interrelationships among serum folate, CSF folate, neurotransmitters and neuropsychiatric symptoms. Neurology 30:419, 1980.
12. Rosenberg L: Disorders of propionate and methylmalonate metabolism. In Stanbury JB, Wyngaarden JB, Fredrickson DS, Goldstein JL, Brown MS (eds): "The Metabolic Basis of Inherited Disease." New York: McGraw-Hill, 1983, pp. 491–494.
13. Schuh S, Rosenblatt DS, Copper BA, Schroeder ML, Bishop AJ, Seargent LE, Haworth JC: Homocystinuria and megaloblastic anemia responsive to vitamin B12 therapy. N Engl J Med 310:666–690, 1984.
14. Baumgartner R, Wick H, Maurer R, Egli N, Steinmann B: Congenital defect in intracellular cobalamin metabolism resulting in homocytinuria and methylmalonic aciduria. Helv Paediatr Acta 34:465–482, 1979.
15. Mudd SH, Levy HL: Disorders of transulfuration. In Stanbury JB, Wyngaarden JB, Fredrickson DS, Goldstein JL, Brown MS (eds): "The Metabolic Basis of Inherited Disease." New York: McGraw-Hill, 1983, pp. 522–559.
16. Chou S, Waisman HA: Spongy degeneration of the central nervous system: Case of homocystinuria. Arch Pathol 79:357–363, 1965.
17. Gerritsen T, Waisman HA: Homocystinuria: Absence of cystathionine in the brain. Science 145:588, 1964.
18. Kanwar YS, Manaligod TR, Wong PWK: Morphologic studies in a patient with homocystinuria due to 5,10-methylenetetrahydrofolate reductase deficiency. Pediatr Res 10:598–609, 1976.
19. Baumgartner R, Wick, H, Ohnacher, H, Probst, A, Maurer, R: Vascular lesions in two patients with congenital homocystinuria due to different defects of remethylation. J Inher Metab Dis 3:101–103, 1980.
20. McCully KS: Vascular pathology of homocystinemia: Implications for the pathogenesis of arteriosclerosis. Am J Pathol 56:111–128, 1969.
21. Dayan AD, Ramsey RB: An inborn error of B12 metabolism associated with cellular deficiency in coenzyme forms of the vitamin. J Neurol Sci 23:117–120, 1974.
22. Soule E, Pritchard DJ: Fibrosarcoma in infants and children. Cancer 40:1711–1721, 1977.
23. Chung EB, Enzinger FM: Infantile fibrosarcoma. Cancer 38:729–739, 1976.
24. Gibson JB, Carson NA, Neill AW: Pathological findings in homocystinuria. J Clin Pathol 17:427–437, 1964.
25. Carson NAJ, Dent CE, Field CMB, Gaull GE: Homocystinuria. J Pediatr 66:565–583, 1965.
26. Narisawa K: Brain damage in the infantile type of 5,10-methylene tetrahydrofolate reductase deficiency. In MI Bates, EH Reynolds (eds): "Folic Acid in Neurology, Psychiatry and Internal Medicine." New York: Raven Press, 1979, pp. 391–400.

27. Haan EA, Rogers JG, Lewis GP, Rowe PB: 5,10-methylene tetrahydrofolate reductase deficiency. Clinical and biochemical features of a further case. J Inher Metab Dis 8:53–57, 1985.
28. Wall RT, Harlan JM, Harker LA, Striker GE: Homocysteine-induced endothelial cell injury *in vitro*: A model for the study of vascular injury. Thromb Res 18:113–121, 1980.
29. Harker LA, Ross R, Slichter J, Scott CR: Homocystine-induced arteriosclerosis. JCI 58:731–741, 1976.
30. Reddy CSR, Wilcken DEL: Experimental homocystinemia in pigs: Comparison with studies in sixteen homocystinuric patients. Metabolism 31:778–783, 1982.
31. Dudman NPB, Wilcken DEL: Homocysteine thiolactone and experimental homocystinuria. Biochem Med 27:244–253, 1982.
32. Erbe RW: Congenital defects in folate metabolism. Adv Hum Genet 9:293–354, 1979.
33. Smith I, Hyland K, Kendall B, Leeming R: Clinical role of pteridine therapy in tetrahydrobiopterin deficiency. J Inher Metab Dis 8 Suppl 1:39–45, 1985.
34. Chandrin I, Deacon R, Lumb M, Muir M, Perry J: Cobalamin-folate interrelations: A critcial review. Blood 66:479–489, 1985.
35. Scott JM, Weir DG: The methyl folate trap. Lancet 2:337–340, 1981.
36. Baumgartner ER, Stokstad ELR, Wick H, Watson JE, Kusano G: Comparison of folic acid coenzyme distribution patterns in patients with methylenetetrahydrofolate reductase and methionine synthetase deficiencies. Pediatr Res 19:1288–1292, 1985.

Glutaric Acidemia Type II and Flavin-Dependent Enzymes in Morphogenesis

George Hoganson, MD, Stanley Berlow, MD, Enid F. Gilbert, MD, Frank Frerman, PhD, Stephen Goodman, MD, and Leslie Schweitzer, MD

University of Illinois at Chicago-Health Sciences Center, Department of Pediatrics, m/c 586 Chicago, Illinois 60612 (GH), University of Wisconsin, Departments of Pediatrics and Pathology, Madison, Wisconsin 53706 (SB, EFG), University of Colorado, Department of Pediatrics, Denver, Colorado 80262 (FF, SG), New York Medical School, Psychoanalytic Institute, New York, New York 10003 (LS)

INTRODUCTION

Glutaric acidemia type II (GA II) is an autosomal recessive disorder characterized clinically by metabolic acidosis, hypoglycemia, and the excretion of a specific group of organic acids in urine [1–7]. GA II is a clinically and biochemically heterogenous disorder; 1 subgroup of patients has been noted to have congenital anomalies neonatally [8–10]. The biochemical disturbances of the disease are secondary to a defect in electron transfer from the acyl coenzyme A dehydrogenases to coenzyme Q in the electron transport chain. Electron transfer flavoprotein (ETF) and ETF dehydrogenase function in this electron transfer [11,12]; thus, patients with neonatal GA II can be separated into 2 groups, namely those with ETF and ETF dehydrogenase deficiency. While the biochemical changes resulting from these 2 biochemical defects are similar, the presence of congenital anomalies has been associated only with ETF dehydrogenase deficiency [12,13]. The finding of multiple congenital anomalies in certain GA II patients indicates that tissue differentiation may be adversely affected in some metabolic disorders, and that this represents a special aspect of this group of disorders. Opitz has referred to the group of metabolic disorders that result in defects of cellular differentia-

Birth Defects: Original Article Series, Volume 23, Number 1, pages 65–74

tions as "prenatal metabolic dysplasias" [14]. Reports of other metabolic diseases with prenatal effects have appeared in association with defects in valine metabolism [15] and in lactic acidosis [16].

The Zellweger (or cerebro-hepato-renal) syndrome appears to be another example of a metabolic dysplasia in which pathologic and morphologic manifestations are similar to those present in GA II patients [17,18]. A pathologic finding common to both disorders is renal cystic dysplasia, ie, changes of abnormal histologic differentiation of glomeruli and tubules. There are other chromosome and multiple malformation syndromes in which renal cystic dysplasia occurs [19]. Thus, different developmental insults, including hereditary metabolic defects, can adversely affect tissue differentiation in a similar pattern.

We report on the pathologic findings in 2 patients with GA II. Because of the presence of similar biochemical findings and the known teratogenic effect of riboflavin deficiency in fetal rats, kidneys from riboflavin-deficient fetal rats were also examined. Our results suggest that certain flavin-dependent protein(s) and/or metabolites of these proteins may play an important role in normal tissue development and impairment of these proteins can adversely affect development.

CLINICAL REPORTS

Patient 1

Clinical manifestations of patient 1 were previously reported [9]. A 1786 g male infant was born to consanguineous parents. Intrauterine growth retardation had been diagnosed during pregnancy. At birth, the infant had Apgar scores of 1 and 4 at 1 and 5 minutes, respectively. Shortly after birth the infant developed acidosis, hypoglycemia, hyperammonemia, and *Escherichia coli* sepsis. The infant died at 3½ days. Large increases in lactic, hexanoic, ethylmalonic, glutaric, adipic, and 4-hydroxyphenyllactic acids were present in serum and urine. 2-hydroxyisolvaleric, suberic, octenedioic, and 2-hydroxyglutaric acids were also present in the urine. Plasma and urine proline levels were increased. The pattern of organic acids present suggested the diagnosis of glutaric acidemia type II.

The head circumference (OFC) was 32 cm (40th centile for gestation). The skull was dolichocephalic and the anterior fontanelle was enlarged. Craniotabes was present. The ears appeared low-set and the palate was highly arched. An irregular mass was palpable in the right upper quadrant of the abdomen. Valgus deformity of the feet was present. Third-degree hypospadias and bilateral cryptorchidism were present.

The kidneys together weighed 50 g (normal 10 g each). Cortical and medullary surfaces of the kidneys were studded with cysts that measured up to 1 cm in diameter and were most numerous in the cortex. Sections of the kidneys demonstrated that the cysts were both tubular and glomerular (Fig. 1). Some cysts were frequently associated with pericystic fibrosis; others resembled persistent metanephric ducts and were marginated by fibrocollagenous collars. The appearance was consistent with renal cystic dysplasia. The liver was slightly enlarged and congested. A mild degree of fatty change of the parenchymal cells was present. A considerable amount of iron was demonstrated by Perls Prussian blue reaction. No biliary dysgenesis or changes of cirrhosis were present. The brain weighed 310 g (normal 290 g) and the gross appearance was normal. Hemorrhage into the central nervous system was noted. Sections of the brain showed some evidence of disordered neuronal migration with lack of clear delineation of the cerebral cortical neuronal layers.

Patient 2

A 2.22 kg male infant was delivered at 35 weeks gestation to a 34-year-old mother by elective cesarean section. An increased OFC was identified by ultrasonography before delivery. Apgar scores were 6 and 8 and the infant was hypotonic at birth. The infant was similar in appearance to patient 1 and developed acidosis, hypoglycemia, hypoxemia, and died on the third day of life. He was the ninth child of nonconsanguineous parents; 5 previous children were similarly affected; 4 male infants had findings including macrocephaly, enlarged anterior fontanelle, hypospadias, hydroureter, and hydronephrosis. One previous affected female infant had macrocephaly and enlarged kidneys. The other children in the family, 2 males and 1 female, are alive and well.

On examination, the infant's OFC was 36.5 cm (> 90th centile for gestational age). The anterior fontanelle measured 6 × 7 cm and the cranial sutures were widely separated. Facial appearance was abnormal: the infant had a high forehead, flat nasal bridge, and prominent infraorbital skin folds. Hepatomegaly and enlarged kidneys were present.

Diagnosis of glutaric acidemia type II was based on the urinary organic acid pattern. The head CT scan showed numerous small areas of intracranial calcifications.

On postmortem examination the kidneys contained numerous cysts similar to those described in patient 1. Fatty changes and iron storage were present within the hepatic parenchymal cells. Cerebral sections revealed disordered neuronal migration.

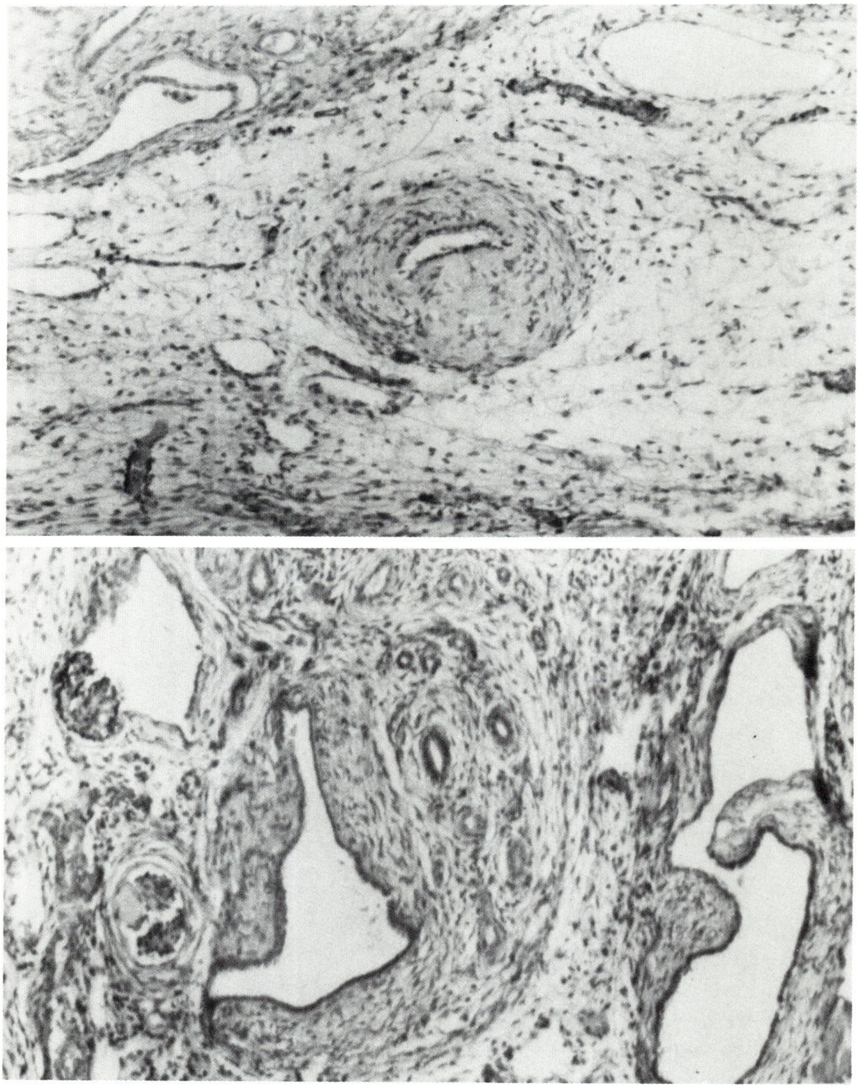

Fig. 1. Renal cystic dysplasia present in GA II patient (patient 1).

Riboflavin-Deficient Rats

Rat embryos were kindly supplied by Thomas Shepard, Central Laboratory of Human Embryology, University of Washington, Seattle.

Riboflavin deficiency was produced by restricting riboflavin intake and feeding galactoflavin, a riboflavin antagonist [20]. Kidneys from eight 20-day gestation fetal rats, 4 riboflavin-deficient, and 4 control animals were examined by light microscopy. Control animal findings revealed normal renal architecture and development of glomerular and collecting system (Fig. 2). All kidneys from riboflavin-deficient animals showed localized areas of fibrosis and cyst formation (Fig. 2). Similar changes were not present in the control animal kidneys. Other malformations present in the riboflavin-treated animals have been reported [20].

DISCUSSION

The 2 infants with GA II were noted to have multiple congenital anomalies and tissue dysplasia. The renal cystic dysplasia and cerebral dysgenesis are similar to that noted in sibs with GA II reported by Bohm et al [8]. These authors describe the cerebral dysgenesis in their patients as "warty" due to the presence of localized areas of marked cerebral dysplasia which resulted in a wartlike surface of the cerebral cortex. While the infants reported here did not exhibit such gross cerebral dysplastic changes, evidence of abnormal tissue differentiation was present on a cellular level. Presumably the differences reflect a varying degree to which cerebral tissue differentiation was perturbed in these cases. Sweetman et al [4] noted cystic kidneys, reactive gliosis of the CNS, and minor anomalies in another case of GA II. Similar findings were also present in a male and a female case reported in 1984 [10]. Additional histologic findings common to these cases include fatty degeneration and iron storage in the liver. Absent in the present report were the pancreatic and biliary duct dysplastic changes that have been noted previously [8]. The common abnormalities noted in these patients appear to be associated with the presence of the metabolic defect. The morphologic and pathologic manifestations of 7 cases of GA II are summarized in Table I.

Postmortem studies have not been reported in all patients with GA II, so the frequency of morphologic abnormalities in this disorder is unknown. Renal abnormalities in a 7-week-old female were limited to mild fatty infiltration of the renal tubular epithelium, suggesting that the developmental abnormalities are not present in all individuals with neonatal GA II [5]. Characterization of the specific defect(s) that cause GA II in conjunction with pathologic examination of affected cases should be helpful in determining if

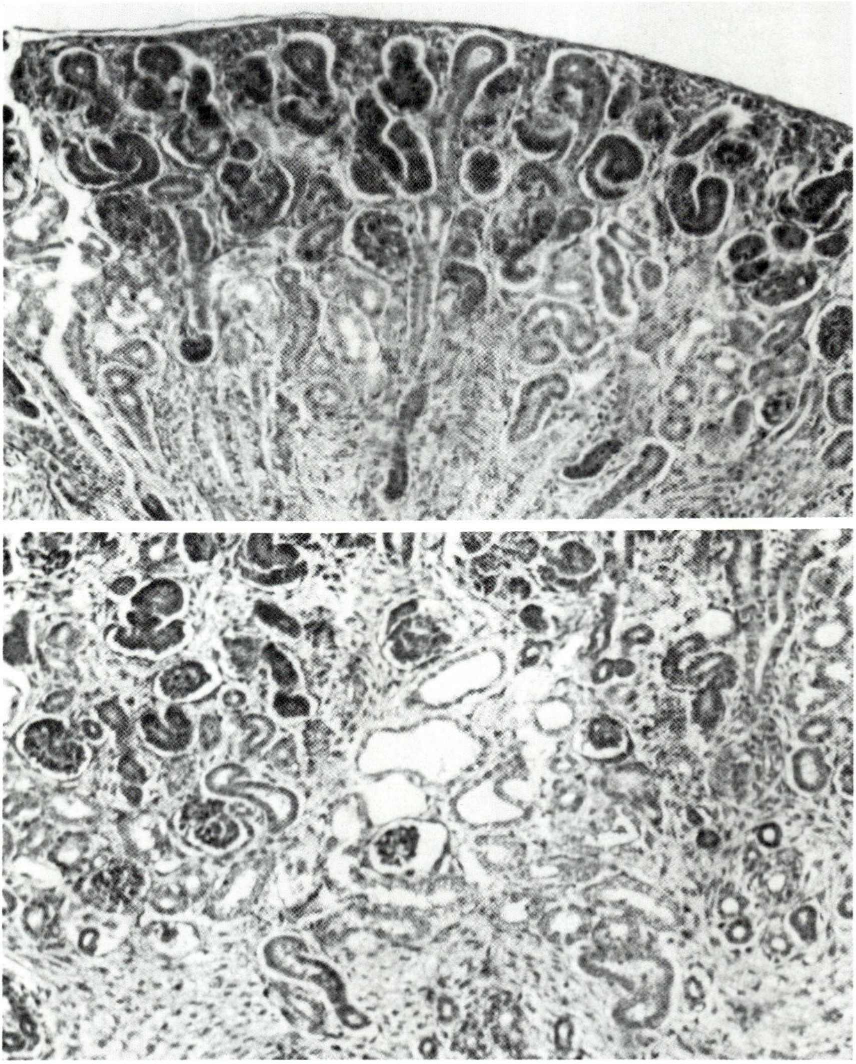

Fig. 2. Histology of fetal rat kidney from 20-day gestation riboflavin-deficient and galactoflavin-treated maternal rat. Normal histology (top) and riboflavin-deficient (bottom) showing normal structure and an area of multiple cysts respectively.

TABLE I. Morphologic and Pathologic Findings in GA II Patients

General	Hepatomegaly (7/7)
Prematurity (3/7)	Fatty degeneration
Breech delivery (2/7)	Iron storage
Hypotonia (6/7)	Biliary duct dysplasia
Skull	Pancreatic duct and acini dysplasia
Macrocephaly	Renal enlargement (7/7)
Dolichocephaly	Multiple cysts
Enlarged fontanelle	Cystic renal dysplasia
Facial anomalies	Genital anomalies (4/6)
Hypertelorism	Hypospadias
Small palpebral fissures	Cryptorchidism
Ear anomalies	CNS (3/7)
Flattened nasal bridge	Gyral abnormalities
High-arched palate	Cerebral cortex dysgenesis ranging from symmetric warty dysplasia to poorly demarcated neuronal layers
Micrognathia	
Congenital heart disease	
Ventricular septal defect	Other
Patent ductus arteriosus	Equinovarus deformity of the feet (3/5)

a specific mutation is associated with the presence of developmental abnormalities. Biochemical studies have identified ETF dehydrogenase deficiency in 3 patients with congenital anomalies [12,13]. However, congenital anomalies were absent in cases of ETF deficiency and some cases of ETF dehydrogenase deficiency, suggesting that the biochemical abnormalities of GA II (ie, organic acid profile) are not specifically associated with the development of congenital anomalies. Absence of ETF dehydrogenase cross-reacting material is 1 characteristic common to 3 cases of GA II with congenital anomalies evaluated [12,13]. Further experience is needed to determine if a mutation that results in the absence of ETF dehydrogenase protein leads to development of congenital anomalies.

Pathologic findings in the patients with GA II are remarkably similar to those present in the Zellweger syndrome, and anomalies shared in common are listed in Table II. Renal cystic dysplasia and cerebral dysgenesis are present in both disorders. Hepatic iron storage and fatty infiltration are also present but represent nonspecific findings. The underlying metabolic defects in the GA II and the Zellweger syndrome appear to be different. GA II results from the defective electron transfer from acyl CoA dehydrogenases to coenzyme Q in the electron transport chain [11,12]. While the defect underlying Zellweger syndrome is unknown, defects in bilirubin, pipecolic acid, and long chain fatty acid metabolism, mitochondrial oxidation, cytochrome defects, and the absence of peroxisomes have been noted [21–25]. The authors (unpublished) have found normal urine organic acid profile in 2

TABLE II. Anomalies Common to GA II and Zellweger Syndrome

Craniofacial	Equinovarus deformity
Cranial shape	Genital
Enlarged fontanelles	Hypospadias
Epicanthal folds	Cryptorchidism
Skin folds under eyes	CNS
High forehead	Gyral abnormality
Flattened nasal bridge	Cerebral dysgenesis
Micrognathia	Renal cystic dysplasia

patients with the Zellweger syndrome. These findings suggest that the phenotypic overlap noted results from a common tissue response to the defects present in these disorders. Possible explanations of how a metabolic defect could give rise to abnormal morphogenesis include the production of a toxic substance(s) or deficiencies of intermediates or proteins that are important at certain developmental stages.

Riboflavin deficiency in rats produces an organic aciduria similar to that present in glutaric acidemia [26]. The effects of riboflavin deficiency on the developing rat fetus have been studied previously; offspring of pregnant rats made riboflavin deficient by dietary restriction of riboflavin and the administration of galactoflavin, a riboflavin antagonist, showed craniofacial and skeletal malformations [20]. Miscellaneous other malformations including hydronephrosis and cardiac defects were less frequently noted. These malformations presumably resulted from flavin deficiency and its effect on flavin-dependent enzymes [27]. Kidneys from riboflavin-deficient, 20-day rat embryos showed the presence of small tubular cysts (Fig. 2) similar to those present in renal cystic dysplasia. Activity levels of certain flavin-dependent enzymes were found to be decreased in the riboflavin-deficient rat [27], however, no information is available on ETF and ETF dehydrogenase levels. A common pathogenetic mechanism, if present, that results in congenital malformation in both GA II and riboflavin deficiency in the rats remains to be determined.

In conclusion, it appears that in 1 form of GA II, in the Zellweger syndrome, and in riboflavin deficiency a metabolic defect adversely affects tissue differentiation and results in the phenotypes described. The common finding of renal cystic changes in these disorders would appear to justify closer pathologic examination of patients with related metabolic disorders. Metabolic studies should be performed in multiple malformation syndromes having similar pathologic findings. Pathologic examination of infants with other metabolic disorders may identify other conditions in which embryonic development is affected. In addition, these results suggest that riboflavin-dependent proteins and/or the metabolites of these proteins may play a role in normal morphogenesis. Functional abnormalities of these proteins secondary to a genetically determined defect or cofactor deficiency may interfere with normal tissue differentiation.

REFERENCES

1. Przyrembel H, Wendel U, Becker K, Bremer HL, Bruinvis L, Ketting D, Wadman SK: Glutaric aciduria type II: Report on a previously undescribed metabolic disorder. Clin Chim Acta 66:227, 1976.
2. Goodman SI, McCabe ERB, Fennessey PV, Mace JW: Multiple acyl-CoA dehydrogenase deficiency (glutaric aciduria type II) with transient hypersarcosinemia and sarcosinuria: Possible inherited deficiency of an electron transfer flavoprotein. Pediatr Res 14:12, 1980.
3. Gregersen N, Kolvraa S, Rasmussen K, Christensen E, Brandt NJ, Ebbesen F, Hansen FH: Biochemical studies in a patient with defects in the metabolism of acyl-CoA and sarcosine: Another possible case of glutaric aciduria type II. J Inherited Metab Dis 3:67, 1980.
4. Sweetman L, Nyhan WL, Trauner DA, Merritt TA, Singh M: Glutaric aciduria type II. J Pediatr 96:1020, 1980.
5. Goodman SI, Stene DO, McCabe ERB, Norenberg MD, Shikes RH, Stumpf DA, Blackburn GK: Glutaric acidemia type II: Clinical, biochemical and morphologic considerations. J Pediatr 100:946, 1982.
6. Coude FX, Ogier H, Charpentier C, Thomassin G, Checoury A, Amedee-Mansme O, Saudubray JM, Frezal J: Neonatal glutaric aciduria type II: An X-linked recessive inherited disorder. Hum Genet 59:263, 1981.
7. Lehnert W, Wendel V, Lindenmeier S, Böhm N: Multiple acyl-CoA dehydrogenation deficiency (glutaric aciduria type II), congenital polycystic kidneys, and symmetric warty dysplasia of the cerebral cortex in two brothers. I. Clinical, metabolic, and biochemical findings. Eur J Pediatr 132:56, 1982.
8. Bohm N, Uy J, Kiebling M, Lehnert W: Multiple acyl-CoA dehydrogenation deficiency (glutaric aciduria type II), congenital polycystic kidneys, and symmetric warty dysplasia of the cerebral cortex in two newborn brothers. II. Morphology and pathogenesis. Eur J Pediatr 139:60, 1982.
9. Goodman SI, Reale M, Berlow S: Glutaric acidemia type II: A form with deleterious intrauterine effects. J Pediatr 102:411–413, 1983.
10. Bove J, Chalmers RA, Tracey B, Watson D, Gray R, Keeling J, King G, Pett TB, Lindenbaum R, Rocchiccioli F, Saudubray J: Prenatal diagnosis of dysmorphic neonatal-lethal type II glutaric aciduria. Lancet 1:846–847, 1984.
11. Rhead W, Amendt B: Electron transferring flavoprotein deficiency in the multiple acyl-CoA dehydrogenation disorders, glutaric aciduria type II and ethylmalonic-adipic aciduria. J Inherited Metab Dis 7 (Suppl 2):99–101, 1984.
12. Frerman FE, Goodman SI: Deficiency of electron transfer flavoprotein or electron transfer flavoprotein: Ubiquinone oxidoreductase in glutaric acidemia type II fibroblasts. Proc Natl Acad Sci USA 82:4517–4520, 1985.

13. Goodman SI, Frerman FE: Glutaric acidaemia type II (multiple acyl-CoA dehydrogenation deficiency). J Inherited Metab Dis 7 (Suppl 1):33–39, 1984.
14. Friedman A, Bethzhold J, Hong R, Gilbert EF, Viseskul C, Opitz JM: Clinicopathologic conference: A three-month-old infant with failure to thrive, hepatomegaly, and neurological impairment. Am J Med Genet 7:171–186, 1980.
15. Brown GK, Hunt SM, Scholen R, Fowler K, Grimes A, Mercer JF, Truscott RM, Cotton RG: β-hydroxyisobutyryl coenzyme A deacylase deficiency: A defect in valine metabolism associated with physical malformations. Pediatrics 70:532, 1982.
16. Sherwood G, Robinson BH: Dysmorphism in congenital lactic acidosis. Pediatr Res 18:300A, 1984.
17. Gilchrist KW, Gilbert EF, Goldfarb S, Goll U, Spranger JW, Opitz JM: Studies of malformation syndromes of Man XIB: The cerebro-hepato-renal syndrome of Zellweger: Comparative pathology. Eur J Pediatr 121:99–118, 1976.
18. Opitz JM, ZuRhein GM, Vitale L, Shahidi NT, Howe JJ, Chou SM, Shanklin DR, Sybers HD, Dood AR, Gerritsen T: The Zellweger syndrome (cerebro-hepato-renal syndrome). March of Dimes—Birth Defects Foundation BD:OAS V(2):144–158, 1969.
19. Gilbert EF, Opitz JM: Renal abnormalities in malformation syndromes. In Edelman CM, Berstein J (eds): "Pediatric Kidney Disease." Boston: Little, Brown and Company, in Press.
20. Shepard TH, Lemire RJ, Aksu O, Mackler B: Studies of the development of congenital anomalies in embryos of riboflavin-deficient, galactoflavin fed rats. I. Growth and embryologic pathology. Teratology 1:75–92, 1968.
21. Monnens L, Bakkeren J, Parmentier G, Janssen G, van Haelst U, Trijbels F, Eyssen H: Disturbances in bile acid metabolism of infants with the Zellweger (cerebro-hepato-renal) syndrome. Eur J Pediatr 133:31–35, 1980.
22. Trijbels JMF, Monnens LAH, Bakkeren JAJM, Van Raay-Selten AHJ, Corstiaensen JMB: Biochemical studies in the cerebro-hepato-renal syndrome of Zellweger: A disturbance in the metabolism of pipecolic acid. J Inherited Metab Dis 2 (Suppl 2):39–42, 1980.
23. Goldfischer S, Moore CL, Johnson AB, Spiro AG, Valsamis MP, Wisniewski HK, Ritch RH, Norton WT, Rapin I, Gartner LM: Peroxisomal and mitochondrial defects in the cerebro-hepato-renal syndrome. Science 182:62–64, 1973.
24. Moser AE, Singh I, Brown FR III, Solish GI, Kelley RI, Benke PJ, Moser HW: The cerebrohepatorenal (Zellweger) syndrome. Increased levels and impaired degradation of very-long-chain fatty acids and their use in prenatal diagnosis. N Engl J Med 18:1141–1146, 1984.
25. Datta NS, Wilson GN, Hajra AK: Deficiency of enzymes catalyzing the biosynthesis of glycerol-ether lipids in Zellweger syndrome. A new category of metabolic disease involving the absence of peroxisomes. N Engl J Med 17:1080–1083, 1984.
26. Goodman SI: unpublished observation.
27. Aksu O, Mackler B, Shepard TH, Lemire RJ: Studies of the development of congenital anomalies in embyros of riboflavin-deficient, galactoflavin fed rats. II. Role of the terminal electron transport systems. Teratology 1:93–102, 1968.

Neonatal Hemochromatosis

A.S. Knisely, MD, Margret S. Magid, MD, M. Renate Dische, MD, PhD, and Ernest Cutz, MD

Departments of Pathology, Cornell Medical Center/The New York Hospital, New York, New York 10021 (ASK, MSM), Mt. Sinai School of Medicine, New York, New York 10029 (MRD), and University of Toronto, Toronto, Ontario, Canada (EC)

INTRODUCTION

Idiopathic hemochromatosis is an inherited disorder of iron metabolism in which various tissues contain excessive amounts of iron in association with cellular injury and reactive fibrosis [1]. The reticuloendothelial system is relatively unaffected [2,3]. The disease typically manifests itself in midlife as hypogonadism, diabetes, arthritis, or cardiac or liver disease [2], although some cases have presented as early as adolescence [4]. The iron enters the body by excess intestinal absorption over years [5]. Neonatal hemochromatosis is a rare disorder of the newborn, characterized clinically by signs of hepatic insufficiency that in many cases includes a prominent hemorrhagic diathesis. Histopathologically, there are hepatic fibrosis and cirrhosis with cholestasis and giant-cell transformation, concentrations of stainable iron in the liver higher than those in normal newborn infants [6], and marked siderosis of extrahepatic tissues that spares the reticuloendothelial system. Here we present our findings in 4 new cases of neonatal hemochromatosis, with family and quantitative tissue iron studies in 1 case, and review previous reports. Our observations indicate autosomal recessive or codominant inheritance as possible in this disorder and suggest that antenatal diagnosis may be feasible. They do not support the hypothesis that the primary pathogenesis is excess transplacental uptake of iron analogous to the intestinal hyperabsorption seen in adult hemochromatosis.

Birth Defects: Original Article Series, Volume 23, Number 1, pages 75–102

CASE HISTORIES

Patient 1

A 2780 g white female infant was born at term to a 29-year-old G3P2 woman. Two sibs were alive and well. Pregnancy was uncomplicated but oligohydramnios was noted at delivery. On the first day of life, the infant developed cyanosis, lower limb edema, anuria, and seizures. The mother's blood type was O+; screening found no unusual antibodies. The infant's blood type was A+; direct and indirect antiglobulin (Coombs) testing was unreactive. The hemoglobin was 14.7 g/dl, albumin 2.1 g/dl, calcium 7.4 mg/dl, and glucose 35 mg/dl. Blood cultures grew *Klebsiella* and a course of antibiotics was administered. Radiologic studies and cystoscopy for persistent anuria failed to identify urinary tract abnormalities. One day before death, a nasogastric aspirate and the urine became grossly bloody and hemoglobin dropped to 10.3 g/dl; blood transfusions were given. Massive hematochezia and epistaxis developed, and the infant died at age 5 days. An autopsy was performed.

Patient 2

A 2990 g white female infant was born after 38 weeks of gestation to a 25-year-old primigravida. Lethargy and hypothermia were noted shortly after birth; antibiotics were given. There was no evidence of isoimmune hemolytic disease. The infant was anuric and bled from the nose and mouth, and the hemoglobin fell from 15.7 g/dl at birth to 8.8 g/dl on the second day. The prothrombin time and partial thromboplastin time were prolonged; fibrin split products were not present, and the platelet count was 133K/mm^3. Hypoglycemia and hypocalcemia were noted. Abnormal values were partly corrected by exchange transfusion, but frank hematemesis and hematochezia persisted, convulsions developed, and the patient died at age 9 days. An autopsy was performed.

Patient 3

A white male infant was born at term to a G2P1 25-year-old woman after an uneventful pregnancy. An older sib was well. Although the infant was apparently healthy at birth, at 30 hours of age apneic episodes not related to feeding were noted. At age 3 days, the infant was cyanotic with moderate respiratory distress, jittery, and hyperreflexic. The ears were apparently low-set. Both liver and spleen extended 2.5 cm below the costal margin. There was no evidence of isoimmune hemolytic disease. Hypoglycemia, hypocalcemia, and slight jaundice were present. Intermittent generalized seizure activity developed. Bleeding from the umbilical stump, blood in the nasogastric aspirate, and gross hematuria appeared and were not corrected by exchange transfusions and administration of two units of platelets. Additional problems included oliguria unresponsive to diuretics and congestive heart failure with pulmonary edema. The infant died at 7 days after an episode of bradycardia and respiratory arrest. An autopsy was performed.

Patient 4

The sister of patient 3, a 2300 g white female infant, was born at 38 weeks of gestation by dates. Pregnancy was unremarkable. At birth, the infant was dusky, areflexic, and without spontaneous respirations. She refused feedings and intermittently assumed an opisthotonic posture. There was no evidence of isoimmune hemolytic disease. The hemoglobin was 15.8 g/dl, a platelet count was 74K/mm^3, serum glucose was 18 mg/dl, and serum calcium was 6.8 mg/dl. Her hospital course was marked by unrelenting acidosis, a diffuse hemorrhagic diathesis, tonic seizures, oliguria, and persistent hypoglycemia, hyperkalemia, and hypocalcemia. Plasma and urine levels of a variety of amino acids were abnormally elevated; levels of amino acids in a sample of maternal plasma were normal. Her chromosomes, prepared using circulating lymphocytes, were normal. Death occurred at age 4 days. An autopsy was performed.

SELECTED AUTOPSY FINDINGS

Tissues from all patients were fixed in either Zenker's formol or formalin and embedded in paraffin. No placentas were available for study. Sections were stained with hematoxylin and eosin, Gömöri's iron stain [7], and Masson's trichrome connective tissue stain. All normal weights are taken from Schultz et al [8].

Patient 1

The body was edematous and jaundiced with widespread petechial hemorrhages and ecchymoses, pulmonary and gastrointestinal hemorrhages, and a hemorrhagic renal infarct. The liver was small (49 g; normal, 131 g), firm, and finely nodular; the extrahepatic biliary tree was patent. The spleen weighted 18.6 g (normal, 11 g) and there were esophageal varices. Microscopy of the liver (Figs. 1, 2) disclosed micronodular cirrhosis with diffuse fibrosis, giant-cell transformation of hepatocytes, neocholangiole formation, and intracanalicular bile stasis. Granules of hemosiderin crowded the cytoplasm of the hepatocytes but were less conspicuous in Kupffer cells. No inflammatory reaction and no infectious agents were identified. Abundant

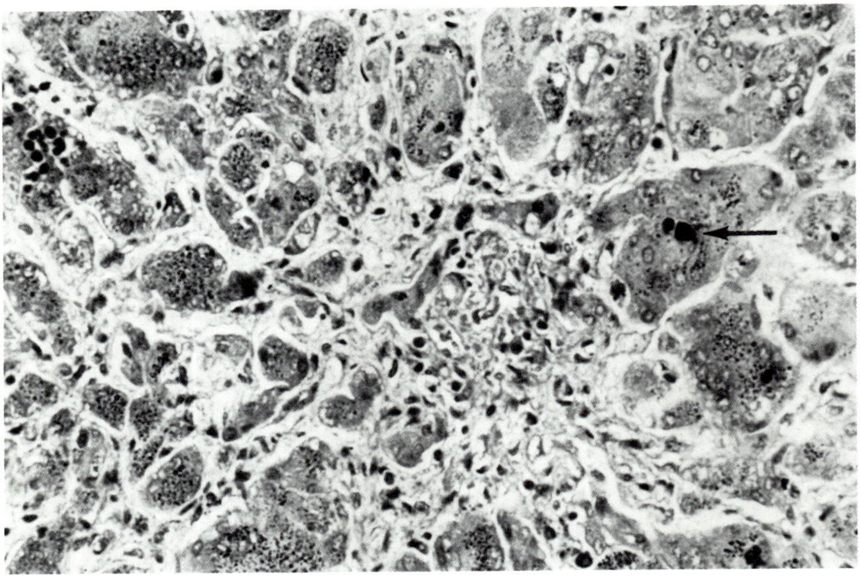

Fig. 1. Liver, patient 1. Nearly all hepatocytes contain finely granular material that stains positively for iron (Fig. 2). Inspissated bile (arrow), giant-cell change, and diffuse fibrosis are present. Hematoxylin and eosin, ×300.

extramedullary hematopoiesis was present. The islets of Langerhans were hypertrophied and hyperplastic. There were iron deposits (Table IIIC) in many epithelia, including the renal distal convoluted tubules (Fig. 3) and endometrial and endocervical lining (Fig. 4), the parenchyma of various organs, and the myocardium (Fig. 5). Only scanty amounts of iron, in rare scattered macrophages, were present in the spleen, lymph nodes, and bone marrow.

Patient 2

The body was edematous and jaundiced, with widespread ecchymoses and pulmonary and gastrointestinal hemorrhages. The finely granular liver weighed 58 g (normal, 131 g). The extrahepatic biliary tract was patent. The spleen weighed 18 g (normal, 11 g). Microscopy of the liver showed changes resembling those of patient 1 but with steatosis of hepatocytes and diffuse fibrosis rather than cirrhosis. Esophageal varices were present and the islets of Langerhans were hypertrophied and hyperplastic. Sections of the brain showed periventricular leukomalacia and hemorrhage. Abundant iron was

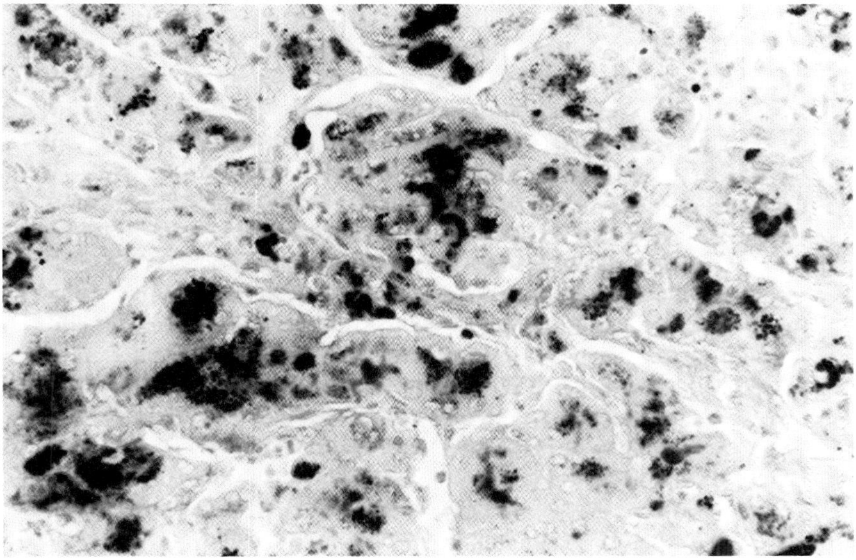

Fig. 2. Liver, patient 1. Abundant stainable iron is evident. Gömöri iron stain with eosin counterstain, ×300.

present in many tissues (Table IIIC). The spleen, lymph nodes, and bone marrow contained stainable iron similar in distribution and quantity to that in patient 1.

Patient 3

The body was jaundiced and edematous. Extensive pulmonary and retroperitoneal hemorrhages were present. The liver was coarsely nodular and weighed 47 g (normal, 129 g). The extrahepatic biliary tract was patent. The spleen weighed 16 g (normal, 11 g). Microscopic findings in the liver closely resembled those in patient 2. Esophageal varices and hypertrophy and hyperplasia of the islets of Langerhans were present. Sections of the brain showed changes consistent with anoxic encephalopathy. Table IIIC gives the location of iron deposits; the spleen, lymph nodes, and bone marrow contained only scanty amounts in occasional macrophages.

Patient 4

No description of gross findings at autopsy is available. Microscopy found abnormalities closely resembling those in patient 1, with pulmonary hemor-

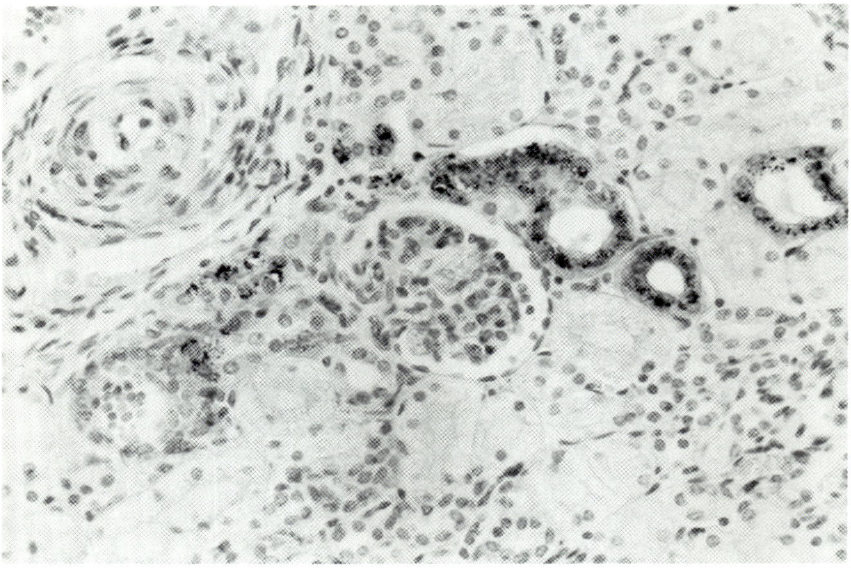

Fig. 3. Renal cortex, patient 1. Epithelial cells of the distal convoluted tubules contain abundant stainable iron. Gömöri iron stain with eosin counterstain, ×190.

rhages and hemorrhagic renal infarcts, marked giant-cell change, cholestasis, cirrhosis, and diffuse fibrosis in the liver, esophageal varices with congestion and fibrosis of the spleen, and hyperplasia and hypertrophy of the islets of Langerhans. Necrotizing enteritis and anoxic-ischemic encephalopathic changes were also present. Iron in the spleen, lymph nodes, and bone marrow was restricted to rare scattered macrophages. The distribution of other iron deposits is given in Table IIIC.

FAMILY AND IRON STUDIES, PATIENT 1

Both parents denied ingestion of medications containing iron and drinking alcohol to excess. The results of complete blood counts, determinations of glucose 6-phosphate dehydrogenase activity, serum protein electrophoreses, and tests of liver function were normal in both parents. Values for levels of serum iron and iron-binding capacity in both parents are given in Table IV.

The iron content of ashed aliquots of the liver and heart of patient 1 was determined by atomic absorption spectrophotometry. The results are given in Table V.

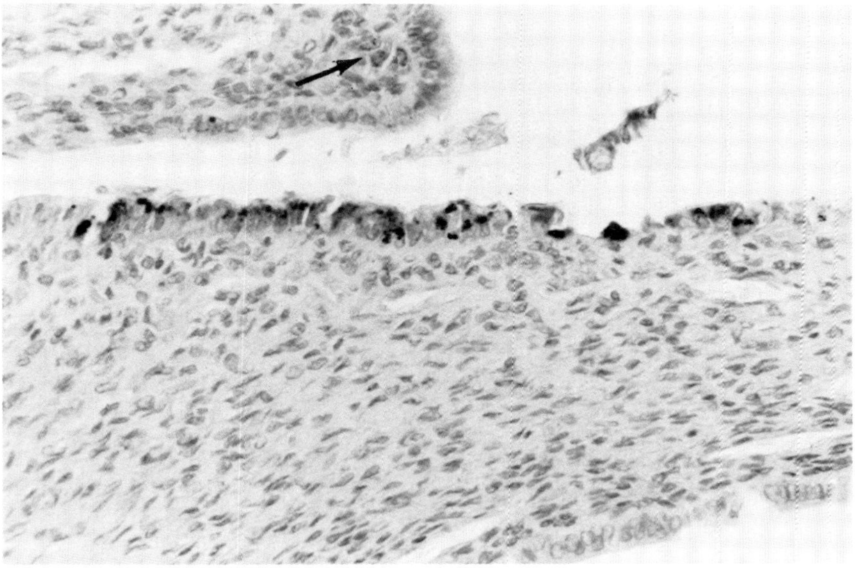

Fig. 4. Endocervix and endometrium, patient 1. There are focally heavy deposits of stainable iron in endometrial epithelium; lesser amounts are present in a submucosal endocervical gland (arrow). Gömöri iron stain with eosin counterstain, ×300.

REVIEW OF THE LITERATURE

Hemosiderosis in infants was reported as early as 1914 [9]. It was later observed in a wide range of diseases of the newborn infant, particularly erythroblastosis fetalis [10–12]. Differentiation among various disorders that lead to hemosiderosis became possible only with the discovery of blood-group incompatibility and its relationship to hemolytic disease. In some cases of severe isoimmune disease, hepatic fibrosis and cirrhosis at birth were described [13–15]. Further work established that a wide range of insults, including infections and metabolic disorders, lead to intrauterine damage to the liver, and that a characteristic but nonspecific response of the liver to injury is giant-cell hepatitis [16,17].

The Swiss worker Cottier was the first to identify a distinct form of neonatal cirrhosis with giant cell transformation that was characterized by tissue deposition of excessive amounts of iron in a pattern of distribution different from that seen in isoimmune hemolytic disease. Because the pattern paralleled that of adult hemochromatosis in which excess enteric absorption

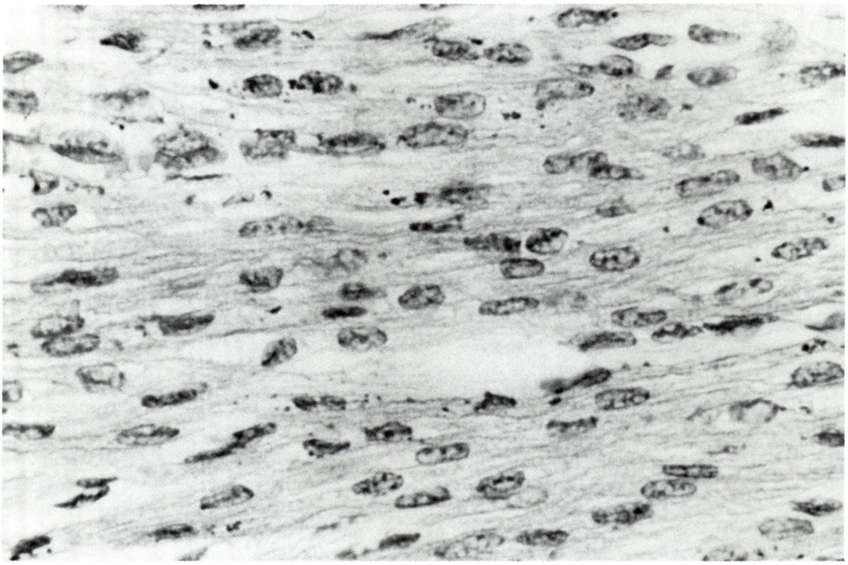

Fig. 5. Ventricular myocardium, patient 1. There are granules of stainable iron within cardiac myocytes. Gömöri iron stain with eosin counterstain, ×450.

of iron occurs, he ascribed the new entity to excessive placental uptake of iron and called it "hemochromatosis in the newborn" [18].

Shortly thereafter a similar case was observed in Czechoslovakia [19]. American workers independently attributed the disease to defects in the mobilization of iron from ferritin [20,21]. There have been 3 more reports of cases that meet rigorous criteria for the diagnosis of neonatal hemochromatosis [22–24], and some cases earlier attributed to immune hemolytic disease [25] or neonatal hepatitis [26–28] can also, with varying degrees of confidence, be considered examples of neonatal hemochromatosis. Other cases in the literature may represent variants of the disease, but they are difficult to evaluate because of coexistent *Cytomegalovirus* infection (Dible et al [26], case 2) or unusually long survival with histories of repeated transfusion (Nezelof et al [29]; Greco et al [30]; Goldfischer et al [22], case 2); some also lack extrahepatic iron [29]. These cases have not been considered in this review. Only 21 previously reported cases fit strict requirements that we define as:

1. A rapidly progressive clinical course with death *in utero* or in the early neonatal period;

2. Increased tissue iron deposition in multiple organs, particularly in the liver, pancreas, heart, and endocrine glands, with the extrahepatic reticuloendothelial system relatively unaffected; and

3. No evidence for hemolytic disease, syndromes associated with hemosiderosis, or exogenous iron overload from transfusions.

CLINICAL MANIFESTATIONS

Clinical data for the present 4 cases are reported above. Selected clinical findings for the 25 identified cases of neonatal hemochromatosis are summarized in Table I.

Blood grouping or alloantibody studies are reported for 19 cases. Specific reports that the maternal serum was free of alloantibodies, or that red blood cells of the infant were nonreactive on direct antiglobulin (Coombs) testing, are available in 15 cases. No reactive Coombs test or other evidence of maternal immunization was identified in any case. Only 2 mothers were known to be Rh-negative; 2 of their 4 affected children were specifically reported to be Coombs-nonreactive, and in a third case the maternal serum was antibody-free.

Gestational age at birth is known in 22 cases. All 22 were delivered at or later than 32 weeks, but 9 were born before 37 weeks, giving a 40.9% incidence of prematurity. Only one infant was stillborn. Five of 20 cases, or 25%, were small for gestational age [8].

Maternal age, where known, ranged from 17 [24] to 34 [22,24] years, with a mean of 26. All parents were clinically well, although 3 mothers [18,19,27] had histories of varying degrees of hepatic dysfunction.

The 25 cases include 5 pairs of full sibs [18,20,21,27] other than the present patients 3 and 4 and one pair of half-sibs [43]. There was one set of 3 full sibs; a fourth child in this family died at age 3 days with "bleeding from the mouth and intestines" [26]. Sex is not recorded in 2 infants. In the other cases, the male to female ratio is 12 to 11. None of these cases is known to have been black or Asian.

Abbreviated clinical histories for previously reported cases are presented in Table II. Presenting signs in all 25 cases were nonspecific and generally reflected multi-system failure. The disease was always fatal. Survival ranged from minutes after birth to 9 days, with a mean of 2.7 days. Due to the rapidly progressive nature of the disorder, extensive laboratory evaluations were not possible. Biochemical data are reported for a small number of

TABLE I. Selected Clinical Findings in Cases of Neonatal Hemochromatosis

Authors	Case No.	Sex	Birth weight (g)	Gestational age*	Blood group studies†
Reiffenstuhl [25]		F	1,900	Term	Mo O+; In A+, no anti-A in cord serum
Dible et al [26]	1		2,735	Term	Mo A+
	3	F	3,100	36 w	Mo O+; In O+, Coombs −
	4	M	3,730	38 w	Mo O+, nonimmunized; In O+, Coombs −
	5				
Ehrlich and Ratner [27]	1	M	2,180	35 w	Mo A+; In A+, Coombs −
	2	F	3,080	Term	
Cottier [18]	1	F			
	2	M	"Under-weight"		Mo "not immunized against paternal cells"
Tomik [19]	1	M	2,800	Term	Mo Rh+; In O+
Fienberg [20]	A1	M	1,927	Term	Mo A+
	A2	M	1,593	8 m	Mo A+
	B1	M	2,300	Term	Mo A−; In A+, Coombs −
	B2	M	1,818	8 m	Mo A−; In Rh+, Coombs −
Laurendeau et al [21]	1	F	2,330	37 w	Mo B−, nonimmunized
	2	F	2,830	38 w	Mo B−, nonimmunized; In Coombs−
Goldfischer et al [22]	1	M	1,390	34 w	
Jacknow et al [23]	1	F		36 w	
	3	M		35 w	
Blisard and Barton [24]	1	F	1,740	34 w	Mo nonimmunized
	2	M	3,860	35 w	Mo nonimmunized
Present	1	F	2,780	Term	Mo O+, nonimmunized; In A+, Coombs −
	2	F	2,990	38 w	No evidence of isoimmune hemolytic disease
	3	M		Term	No evidence of isoimmune hemolytic disease
	4	F	2,300	38 w	No evidence of isoimmune hemolytic disease

*w = weeks; m = months.
†Mo = mother; In = infant.

TABLE II. Abbreviated Clinical Histories of Previously Reported Cases of Neonatal Hemochromatosis

Authors	Case No.	Clinical course	Age at death
Reiffenstuhl [25]		Cyanosis and seizures; progression of cyanosis and death	20 h
Dible et al [26]	1	Cyanosis at birth; "black material" vomited at 24 h; no icterus	6 h
	3	Cyanosis and generalized edema at birth; no icterus; serum albumin 0.53 g/dl	10 h
	4	Cyanosis of hands and feet at birth; death following 2 episodes of generalized and more severe cyanosis	36 h
	5	Stillborn	
Ehrlich and Ratner [27]	1	Hematemesis, icterus, and thigh ecchymosis at 17 h; hematochezia at 1 d; hemoglobin (Hb) 12 g/dl, platelet count normal; persistent hematemesis and hematochezia; cyanosis, seizures, cerebral cry, and death	45 h
	2	Perioral cyanosis at birth with progressive worsening refractory to oxygen	6½ h
Cottier [18]	1	Death immediately after birth	
	2	Persistent vomiting and circulatory collapse	48 h
Tomik [19]	1	Cyanosis at birth; development of petechiae on skin and conjunctivae, icterus, oozing at venipuncture sites; nasogastric aspirate bloody; dyspnea, persistent cyanosis, apnea and bradycardia, and death	24 h
Fienberg [20]	A1	Vomiting at 12 h; cyanotic episode, convulsions, icterus immediately antemortem	27 h
	A2	Vomiting of coffee-ground material; apnea	50 h
	B1	Icterus at birth; recurrent episodes of cyanosis and apnea	3 d
	B2	Abnormal respiratory pattern, cyanosis, flaccidity	20 h
Laurendeau et al [21]	1		25 h
	2	Generalized edema at birth with abdominal distension; peripheral progressing to generalized cyanosis; dark brown vomitus on several occasions	47 h
Goldfischer et al [22]	1	Apgar 8; anuric for 25 h with blood urea nitrogen 8, creatinine 2.2 mg/dl; Hb 12.3 g/dl, platelet count normal; apneic episodes	2 d
Jacknow et al [23]	1	Death in delivery room	
	3	"Died . . . of liver failure"	4 d

(continued)

TABLE II. Abbreviated Clinical Histories of Previously Reported Cases of Neonatal Hemochromatosis (continued)

Authors	Case No.	Clinical course	Age at death
Blisard and Barton [24]	1	Hypotonic at birth; Apgar scores 3 and 6; cord blood hematocrit (hct) 26% and glucose 27 mg/dl; hypoxemia, renal failure, acidosis, hyperbilirubinemia, coagulopathy, elevated liver enzymes; serum albumin 1.5 g/dl; hemoptysis and bradycardia terminally	7 d
	2	Cyanotic, hydropic, and lethargic at birth; Apgar scores 1 and 3; hct 33% and liver function studies abnormal; persistent bradycardia and respiratory failure	24 h

cases; in these, hypoglycemia, hypoalbuminemia, and hypocalcemia were found. Levels of hepatocellular enzymes were measured in only 2 infants and were elevated in both. A bleeding diathesis was described in 10 of the 22 infants who survived for more than a few minutes.

PATHOLOGY

Table III presents a summary of selected aspects of gross pathology and histopathology in the 25 identified cases of neonatal hemochromatosis.

In all cases, there was severe damage to the liver *in utero* (Table IIIA). The livers were fibrotic or cirrhotic, usually shrunken, and often bile-stained. The extrahepatic biliary tract was patent in every instance. Congestive splenomegaly and esophageal varices were found in the present 4 cases, and splenomegaly was often reported without mention of varices [18,19,21,25–27]. There was significant hemorrhage in 14 infants at various sites (Table IIIB).

Microscopy disclosed striking deposition of hemosiderin in hepatocytes with smaller amounts in biliary epithelium and Kupffer cells. There was diffuse fibrosis with variable regenerative activity, and frank cirrhosis was frequently present. Giant-cell transformation of hepatocytes was found in 23 cases. Hepatocellular necrosis was frequently noted, but inflammation was insignificant. Cholestasis was present in nearly all cases and often was accompanied by steatosis and bile-duct proliferation. Hypertrophy and hyperplasia of the islets of Langerhans were present in 15 cases (Table IIIA).

The distribution of iron showed a distinctive pattern (Table IIIC). In all cases, the absence of any but the most trivial iron deposition in the spleen,

TABLE III A. Selected Aspects of Pathology—Histopathology of Liver and Pancreas

Authors	Case No.	Liver*: Fibrosis (F) Cirrhosis (C) Necrosis (N)	Liver*: Giant-cell change (G) Steatosis (S) Cholestasis (C)	Pancreas (Islet-cell hypertrophy and hyperplasia)
Reiffenstuhl [25]		C	G, C	
Dible et al [26]	1	F, C	G, C	
	3	F, C	G, C	
	4	F, C	G, S, C	
	5	F	Autolyzed	
Ehrlich and Ratner [27]	1	F, N	G, S, C	+
	2	F, N	G, S, C	+
Cottier [18]	1	F, N	G, S	
	2	F, N	G, S	+
Tomik [19]		F, C, N	G, C	+
Fienberg [20]	A1	F, N	G, C	+
	A2	F	G	+
	B1	F	G	+
	B2	F	G, S, C	+
Laurendeau et al [21]	1	F	G	
	2	F, C	G, S, C	+
Goldfischer et al [22]	1	F		
Jacknow et al [23]	1	C, N	G	
	3	C, N	G	
Blisard and Barton [24]	1	F	G, C	+
	2	F	G, C	+
Present	1	C	G, C	+
	2	F	G, S, C	+
	3	C	G, S, C	+
	4	F, C	G, C	+

*All livers contained heavy deposits of iron.

lymph nodes, and bone marrow was striking. The reticuloendothelial system contained significant amounts of iron only in the liver. Because detailed studies of iron distribution were not given in all cases, the frequency with which individual organs are involved can only be outlined. Stains for iron generally showed large quantities within (in addition to the liver) pancreatic exocrine acinar cells, renal tubular epithelium, the myocardium, parenchymal cells in the definitive adrenal cortex, thyroid follicular epithelium, and the islets of Langerhans. Other tissues that were less frequently reported as sites of iron deposition included choroid plexus epithelium, the adenohypo-

TABLE IIIB. Selected Aspects of Pathology—Placental Findings and Complications

Authors	Case No.	Placental findings	Complications
Dible et al [26]	3	Enlarged	
	4	Enlarged	
Ehrlich and Ratner [27]	1	Normal size; iron in basement membrane of villi	Kernicterus; multifocal gastrointestinal hemorrhage
	2		Intracranial hemorrhage
Cottier [18]	2		Kernicterus; pulmonary and intracranial hemorrhage
Tomik [19]			Pulmonary and gastrointestinal hemorrhage
Fienberg [20]	A2	Iron in basement membrane of villi	Intracranial hemorrhage and periventricular leukomalacia
Laurendeau et al [21]	1		Gastrointestinal hemorrhage
	2	Enlarged; iron in chorionic villi and decidua	
Goldfischer et al [22]	1	"Minimal iron"	Pulmonary hemorrhage
Blisard and Barton [24]	1		Pulmonary hemorrhage
	2	Enlarged; iron in trophoblast	Nonimmune hydrops fetalis
Present	1		Portal hypertension and hemorrhagic diathesis with pulmonary, gastrointestinal, and renal hemorrhages
	2		Portal hypertension and hemorrhagic diathesis with pulmonary and gastrointestinal hemorrhages; periventricular leukomalacia and hemorrhage
	3		Portal hypertension and hemorrhagic diathesis with pulmonary hemorrhage; anoxic encephalopathy
	4		Portal hypertension and hemorrhagic diathesis with pulmonary hemorrhage and hemorrhagic renal infarcts; anoxic encephalopathy; necrotizing enteritis

TABLE IIIC. Selected Aspects of Pathology—Extrahepatic Iron Distribution*

Authors	Case No.	Pancreas: Acini	Pancreas: Islets	Heart	Kidney	Adrenal	Thyroid	Miscellaneous
Reiffenstuhl [25]		+	−		+			
Dible et al [26]	3							
	4							
Ehrlich and Ratner [27]	1	+	−	+	+	−	−	
	2	+	−					
Cottier [18]	2	+	+	+	+			Pituitary, choroid plexus, salivary gland acini, sweat gland and gastric crypt epithelium, and Brunner glands
Tomik [19]		+	+	+	+	+	−	Salivary gland acini
Fienberg [20]	A1	+	+	+	+	+		Respiratory submucous glands
	A2	+	+	+	+	+		Respiratory submucous glands
	B1	+	+	+	+	+		Respiratory submucous glands
	B2	+	+	+	+	+		Respiratory submucous glands
Laurendeau et al [21]	1	−	−					
	2	+	+	+	+			
Goldfischer et al [22]	1	+		+				
Jacknow et al [23]	1				+			
	3		+ (site unspecified)				+	
Blisard and Barton [24]	1	+	+	+	+	+	+	Pituitary, gastric crypt, and endometrial epithelium
	2	+		+	+	−	+	Colonic epithelium
Present	1	+	+	+	+	+	+	Choroid plexus, respiratory submucous glands, gastric crypt, endometrial, and endocervical epithelium
	2	+	+	+	+	+	+	Pituitary, choroid plexus
	3	+	−	+	+	−	+	
	4	+	+	+	+	−	+	

*No spleen was described as containing more than traces of stainable iron.

physis, salivary gland acinar cells, gastric crypt epithelium, endometrial and endocervical glands, submucosal glands in the respiratory tract, sweat gland epithelium, Brunner glands, and colonic epithelium.

Only 7 placentas were examined (Table IIIB). Four were enlarged, 1 in association with fetal hydrops. None contained markedly abnormal quantities of stainable iron.

SERUM IRON STUDIES IN RELATIVES

Studies of relatives of index cases of adult hemochromatosis can identify abnormalities in iron metabolism that both enable the diagnosis of adult hemochromatosis to be made before clinical signs and symptoms appear [31] and allow the differentiation of varieties of adult hemochromatosis [32]. Among the studies used both in index cases and relatives are measurements of serum levels of iron, transferrin, and ferritin [31], computerized roentgenographic [33] and nuclear magnetic resonance [34] tomography of the liver, and human leukocyte antigen (HLA) typing [35]. No such studies have been performed on any index case of neonatal hemochromatosis. Levels of serum iron, iron-binding capacity, transferrin, or ferritin have been measured in 1 or both parents in 5 matings that have produced 1 or more previously reported index cases of neonatal hemochromatosis [18,20–23], in a single sib of an index case [23], and in both parents of the present patient 1. These data are shown in Table IV.

TISSUE IRON STUDIES

The diagnosis of adult hemochromatosis is most definitively made by finding excessive amounts of iron in a liver biopsy. Concentrations in untreated patients have averaged 40 times normal levels [2]. Quantitative studies of tissue iron in neonatal hemochromatosis have been made in only 5 instances [18,21,26,27] other than the present patient 1. The data in the literature and from patient 1 are shown in Table V, together with available control values. The only attempt at evaluation of levels of iron-binding proteins in tissues was made by Jacknow et al [23], who in their case 3 found "markedly increased hepatocellular ferritin" by immunofluorescence. Biopsy specimens of liver from 2 mothers with histories of varying degrees of hepatic dysfunction were interpreted as showing mild hepatocellular injury, but no excess of iron was found in either [18,27].

DISCUSSION

Review of the 25 identified cases of neonatal hemochromatosis shows that, in addition to producing a syndrome of hepatic insufficiency at birth,

TABLE IV. Serum Iron Studies in Relatives

	Serum iron, mcg %	Total iron-binding capacity, mg %	Saturation in %	Transferrin, ng/ml	Ferritin, mcg/ml
Cottier [18]					
Mother	85	—	—	—	—
Fienberg [20]					
Pair A					
Mother	98	292	34	—	—
Father	98	279	34	—	—
Laurendeau et al [21]					
Mother	190 (90–160)*	228 (248–422)*	83.2	—	—
Goldfischer et al [22]					
Case 1					
Mother	—	—	—	210 (176–385)	27 (10–300)
Father	—	—	—	290 (176–385)	89 (10–300)
Jacknow et al [23]					
Mother	"Low"	—	—	"Increased"	"Undetectable"
Sib	"Low"	—	—	"Increased"	"Undetectable"
Present Case 1					
Mother	160 (50–150)	410 (235–450)	39 (15–45)	—	—
Father	201 (50–150)	401 (235–450)	50 (15–45)	—	—

*( ) = normal ranges.

the disease shows a strong association with premature birth (40.9%) and intrauterine growth retardation (25%), possibly as a consequence of hepatic injury. Risk is not related to sex or advanced maternal age. Occurrence in sibs is frequent; parents have been clinically well.

Cases of neonatal hemochromatosis are distributed in a pattern consistent with either disease mediated by maternal antibodies against a fetal antigen or an error in metabolism inherited as an autosomal codominant or recessive trait. The former hypothesis is weakened by the existence of 3 cases born to primiparas (Fienberg, case A1 [20]; Blisard and Barton, case 2 [24]; present patient 2), but maternal immunization against paternal antigens can occur before a first pregnancy. Second or third cases in a sibship have not been more severe than index cases. Evidence for abnormal iron metabolism in first-degree relatives of index cases, which might support the latter etiology, is inconclusive. Liver biopsy specimens from 2 mothers did not contain

TABLE V. Tissue Iron Quantitation

Organ	Author/Case No.	Organ weight, g (normal) [8]	Mg iron/100 g tissue (weight)	
			Wet	Dry
Liver*	Dible et al [26]			
	Case 3	37 (131)	—	300
	Case 4	116 (129)	—	130
	Ehrlich and Ratner [27]			
	Case 1	40 (131)	—	729
	Cottier [18]			
	Case 2	50 (130)	1,290	3,820
	Present patient 1	49 (131)	228	615
Heart†	Present patient 1	21 (21)	58	190
Kidneys‡	Ehrlich and Ratner [27]			
	Case 1	24 (29)	—	141
Placenta**	Laurendeau et al [21]			
	Case 2	—	—	83

Normal Values–Tissue Iron

*Liver: mg iron/100 g tissue wet weight: 270 (water-soluble iron), 108 (water-insoluble iron), 378 (total non-heme iron) [36]; Mg iron/100 g tissue dry weight: 177 (total "non-haemin" iron) [37], 250 ("total iron" including blood) [38].

†Heart: Mg iron/100 g tissue dry weight: 16.6 (heme iron), 22.8 (non-heme iron), 40.5 (total iron) [39].

‡Kidneys: Mg iron/100 g tissue dry weight: 20.5 (total "non-haemin" iron) [37].

**Placenta: Mg iron/100 g tissue wet weight: 2.51 [40], 7.7 [41], 9.08 [42] (all total iron); mg iron/100 g tissue dry weight: 4.2 to 12 (water-insoluble non-heme iron) [43].

excessive amounts of iron [18,27], and serum levels of iron and iron-binding proteins were normal in 3 mothers and 2 fathers. Abnormal values were present in 5 first-degree relatives of index cases. The mother of the infants reported by Laurendeau et al had high levels of serum iron, low total iron-binding capacity, and high saturation, but she was taking oral iron supplements at the time she was studied [21]. The mother of the cases reported by Jacknow et al and her child who survived infancy (case 2) had low serum iron levels without anemia, increased serum levels of transferrin, and undetectable serum levels of ferritin. Concentrations of ferritin in the liver of her third child (case 3) were assessed by immunofluorescent staining as increased. Since her 1st and 3rd children were half-sibs, it was concluded that "mutant ferritin," transmitted as a dominant trait and resulting in iron sequestration within the liver, was responsible for neonatal hemochromatosis in that kindred [23], but codominant inheritance or abnormalities in ferritin metabolism, rather than of ferritin itself, are possible. Both the mother and the father of the present patient 1 had high levels of serum iron and total iron-binding capacity, and saturation in the father also was high, suggesting autosomal codominant inheritance of an error in iron metabolism. Neonatal hemochromatosis, like adult idiopathic hemochromatosis [32], may prove to be genetically heterogeneous.

The histopathologic response in infants with hemochromatosis differs in several respects from that in adults. Giant-cell change of hepatocytes and pancreatic islet-cell hypertrophy and hyperplasia are nonspecific responses to injury and stress in the fetus and neonate. These are common in neonatal hemochromatosis and are not seen in the adult disease. Although the liver of infants shows reactive fibrosis and cirrhosis, other organs as a rule do not; minimal fibrosis was seen in the pancreas in only 3 cases (Reiffenstuhl [25]; Dible et al, case 3 [26]; Laurendeau et al, patient 2 [21]), while it is a constant finding in chronic iron overloading [44,45]. This may be related to the duration of exposure to iron, which is necessarily much briefer in infants. Evidence of portal hypertension is frequent. The hemorrhagic diathesis, hypoalbuminemia, and low total serum calcium seen in many patients probably reflect liver disease. Other findings in infants who survived several days are common in severely ill newborn infants and are nonspecific.

Normal maternofetal transfer of iron is incompletely understood. It is a one-way process [46,47] in which maternal transferrin binds to receptors on placental trophoblast [48] whose concentration is proportional to rates of iron transfer [49]. The bound transferrin is internalized by the trophoblast [50] and iron is released to fetal apotransferrin [51]. Hepatic endothelial cells then bind and desialate transferrin and present it to hepatocytes [52,53]. Fetal iron accumulates against a concentration gradient [41,54] even in maternal iron deficiency [40], and most of it is found in the liver [55].

Abnormal numbers or function of placental transferrin receptors could lead to primary excessive placental uptake of maternal iron. Similar abnormalities in hepatic endothelium or hepatocytes, or failure to mobilize hepatic iron from ferritin [20,21,23], could cause deposition of excessive amounts of iron in the liver while lowering circulating fetal iron levels and leading to compensatory placental hyperabsorption of iron. Antibodies to autologous transferrin can cause compensatory hypersiderinemia, with tissue siderosis and injury that mimic idiopathic hemochromatosis [56]; maternal immunization against a fetal iron-binding compound might give a similar picture. Disorders affecting the poorly understood class of low-molecular-weight iron-binding compounds [57,58] also might, through "signal error," lead to excessive maternofetal iron transfer.

Siderosis may also nonspecifically accompany liver damage caused by various agents [59]. In liver damage, serum levels of ferritin rise [60], and the capacity to manufacture apotransferrin [61] may decline. Placental uptake of maternal iron is to some extent independent of fetal status [46,49]; if maternofetal transfer of iron continues unabated in the presence of fetal liver damage, the proportional saturation of fetal iron-binding capacity will rise. Since cells take up disaturated transferrin more readily than monosaturated transferrin [62], hepatic dysfunction per se may increase uptake of iron by extrahepatic tissues. The nonspecific siderosis associated with liver damage does not spare reticuloendothelial cells, while in neonatal hemochromatosis the macrophage system is largely free of iron pigment. This sparing is not absolute; as in adult hemochromatosis [3], iron pigment is present in some macrophages, indicating that they are able to accept iron in some form. It may be that iron encountered in normal phagocytic activity is internalized while the uptake of iron as transferrin is abnormal. Although some alteration in macrophage function is present in neonatal hemochromatosis, its nature and relationship to hepatic damage and extrahepatic siderosis are unclear.

It has not yet been shown that excess iron *in utero* leads to neonatal hepatic fibrosis and cirrhosis. In 2 infants stillborn to mothers given iron dextran at or after the 29th week of gestation, concentrations of hepatic ferritin and hemosiderin were higher than those in control individuals, but no abnormalities in hepatic histology were present [38]. Similar treatment during late gestation in rabbits and rats produced increased concentrations of iron in the kidneys and livers of the pups, without tissue damage [63]. If excess iron acts as a hepatotoxin in the fetus, greater amounts, or more chronic or earlier exposure, may be required to produce its effects; the hepatic isoferritin present at birth differs from that found at 20 weeks of gestation [64], and there may be age-related differences in handling of and susceptibility to iron.

Nor has it yet been established that infants with neonatal hemochromatosis have an absolute, quantitative excess of body iron. Although tissue concentrations of iron in these infants are elevated (Table V), there are difficulties in interpreting these data that extend beyond variation in methods used for iron assays and failures to distinguish among heme, transferrin/ferritin, and hemosiderin iron. The liver of infants with neonatal hemochromatosis often is small and fibrotic. In consequence, total hepatic iron content may be normal despite greatly elevated liver iron concentration. To investigate this possibility, hepatic iron concentrations were recalculated in terms of standard liver weights [9] when feasible (Table VI). Unfortunately, standard weights for dried organs of fetuses and infants are not available, and many data in case reports of neonatal hemochromatosis are expressed only as weight of iron per unit weight of dried tissue. Attempts to extrapolate such data to give iron concentrations in wet tissue were not made, since the dry weight/wet

TABLE VI. Adjusted Concentrations of Liver Iron

	Body length (cm)	Body weight (g)	Liver weight (g)	Fe, mg/100 g wet weight	Total Fe content (mg)
Cottier [18]					
Case 2	49	2,770	50	1,290	645
Present patient No. 1	52	2,750	49	228	112

	Liver weight (g) appropriate for body length [8]	Adjusted Fe, mg/100 g wet weight	Liver weight (g) appropriate for body weight [8]	Adjusted Fe, mg/100 g wet weight	Normal hepatic iron levels
Cottier [18]					
Case 2	130	496	89	724	270 mg water-soluble iron, 108 mg water-insoluble iron, 387 mg total non-heme iron per 100 g liver, wet weight [36]
Present patient No. 1	131	85	96	105	

weight ratio of 1 to 5 reported for normal livers [55] may not hold for fibrotic ones.

These calculations show that the adjusted hepatic iron concentration is elevated only in case 2 of Cottier. In our patient 1, the adjusted hepatic iron concentration is actually lower than normal. It can be inferred that the same is true for adjusted hepatic iron concentrations in the cases reported by Dible et al [26], Ehrlich and Ratner [27], and Laurendeau et al [21]. The data suggest a shift of normal iron stores from a small liver to extrahepatic sites, although an increase in total body iron has not been ruled out. The immunofluorescence data of Jacknow et al [23], showing an increase in hepatocytic ferritin, are consistent with either interpretation.

Placental iron content has been measured in only 1 case of neonatal hemochromatosis. While a sample of the placenta of case 2 of Laurendeau et al [21] contained elevated concentrations of iron, the histology of that sample was not examined, and varying degrees of focal hemosiderin deposition in the placenta are normal [65]. The mother was also receiving oral iron supplementation. High placental iron concentrations here may reflect an underlying abnormality in iron metabolism, sampling variation, or increased maternal iron intake.

The differential diagnosis of neonatal hemosiderosis in association with hepatic fibrosis and cirrhosis includes isoimmune hemolytic disease as well as several rare congenital syndromes. In isoimmune hemolytic disease severe hepatic damage and hemosiderosis may coexist, and iron deposition in extrahepatic sites may be marked [14]. Unlike neonatal hemochromatosis, clinical evidence of fetomaternal incompatibility with maternal alloimmunization and extensive iron deposition in macrophages of the extrahepatic reticuloendothelial system are present. The pattern of iron distribution in hereditary dyserythropoietic anemia type II (hereditary erythroblastic multinuclearity with positive acidified serum test, or HEMPAS), resembles that of isoimmune hemolytic disease [66]. Hepatic injury in the neonate has not been reported in HEMPAS. Other intrinsic erythrocytic or erythropoietic disorders that lead to hemolysis may show similar patterns.

Other disorders in which neonatal siderosis and hepatic lesions may be associated include the cerebrohepatorenal syndrome of Zellweger [67,68] and its variants [69], "hypermethionemia" [70], now considered a member of the group of aminoacidemias called hepatorenal tyrosinemia [71,72], and leprechaunism [73–79]. These entities are readily separable, clinically and pathologically, from neonatal hemochromatosis. The hypotonia and characteristic cerebral, renal, and skeletal abnormalities of infants with Zellweger syndrome are distinctive. Antemortem laboratory studies in these infants can identify diagnostic defects in peroxisomal long-chain fatty acid metabolism [80,81]. Hepatorenal tyrosinemia can be distinguished clinically by the "fishy" or "cabbagelike" odor of patients and by abnormal amino acid levels in plasma and urine. Extrahepatic siderosis is absent. The phenotypic anomalies of leprechaunism are pathognomonic. Although extrahepatic parenchymal siderosis occurs, widespread iron deposition in tissue macrophages is also present [78]. The latter is not seen in neonatal hemochromatosis.

FUTURE STUDIES

Because neonatal hemochromatosis is both fulminant and rare, it is unlikely that an index case in a particular kindred will be recognized antemortem; all reported cases have been diagnosed at autopsy. The diagnosis should be entertained when overwhelming hepatic failure is seen in a newborn infant. The studies used in diagnosis and differentiation of adult hemochromatosis have not been applied to neonatal hemochromatosis, and their results would be of interest. Since renal tubular epithelial cells in these infants commonly contain iron, a Rous test for hemosiderin in the urine [82] may be a simple initial screen. Abnormal levels of iron, transferrin, and ferritin in the serum may help make the diagnosis. Examination of a liver biopsy specimen should be valuable, if a biopsy is not precluded by hypocoagulability. Noninvasive imaging may be useful in demonstrating iron overload. Studies of iron metabolism in relatives of an index case would be of particular value in defining the inheritance of the disorder.

Since neonatal hemochromatosis has frequently occurred in sibs, pregnancies in matings that have previously produced an index case should be monitored. A Rous test of the amniotic fluid may be diagnostic. Concentrations of iron and iron-transport compounds in the amniotic fluid [83–85] may also indicate abnormalities in iron metabolism. The hepatic architecture of isoimmune hydrops fetalis is distinctive on ultrasonography of the fetus [86], and it may also be possible to identify *in utero* the hepatic fibrosis associated with neonatal hemochromatosis.

If excess transplacental transport of iron contributes to the liver damage seen in neonatal hemochromatosis, it may advisable to consider early induction of labor to end third-trimester iron loading [87]. Although hepatic injury has been extensive in all reported cases, iron-depletion therapy, which has led to regression of cirrhosis in some cases of adult hemochromatosis [88], may be of value. Liver transplantation probably offers the best hope of survival [89].

Quantitative studies of tissue iron that distinguish among heme iron, iron in the forms of transferrin and ferritin, and iron in hemosiderin have not been done for either normal infants and fetuses or infants with neonatal hemochromatosis, and should be undertaken. The available data suggest that the increase in histochemically demonstrable iron in the liver of infants with neonatal hemochromatosis reflects an increase in hepatic iron concentration but not in total hepatic iron content, while both iron concentration and iron content are elevated in the heart and kidneys. These findings suggest that extrahepatic siderosis in neonatal hemochromatosis may result from shunting of iron away from an injured liver.

We conclude that 2, and possibly 3, abnormalities in iron handling are present in neonatal hemochromatosis. The absence of iron deposits within macrophages indicates an abnormality in reticuloendothelial function. High concentrations of stainable iron in the liver suggest that hepatic iron metabolism is disordered. The absorption of more iron than the fetal liver can store may reflect a primary abnormality in placental iron handling; alternatively, liver damage may disrupt the mechanisms that link hepatic and placental iron metabolism, or iron absorption may be an autonomous process. At present it is not clear which of these is the primary disorder, but the available data argue against the hypothesis that neonatal hemochromatosis is caused by primary placental hyperabsorption of iron.

REFERENCES

1. Weir MP, Gibson JF, Peters TJ: Haemosiderin and tissue damage. Cell Bioch Funct 2:186–194, 1984.
2. Sheldon J: Haemochromatosis. London: Oxford University Press, 1935.
3. Herring WG, Gay RM: Absence of stainable bone marrow iron in hemochromatosis. South Med J 74:1088–1094, 1981.
4. Cazzola M, Ascari E, Barosi G, Claudiani G, Daccó M, Kaltwasser JP, Panaiotopoulos N, Schalk KP, Werner EE: Juvenile idiopathic haemochromatosis: A life-threatening disorder presenting as hypogonadotrophic hypogonadism. Hum Genet 65:149–154, 1983.
5. Björn-Rasmussen E: Iron absorption: Present knowledge and controversies. Lancet 1:914–916, 1983.
6. Langley FA: Haemopoiesis and siderosis in the foetus and newborn. Arch Dis Child 26:64–75, 1951.
7. Gömöri G: Microtechnical demonstration of iron. A criticism of its methods. Am J Pathol 12:655–663, 1936.
8. Schultz DM, Giordano DA, Schulz DH: Weights of organs of fetuses and infants. Arch Pathol 74:244–250, 1962.
9. Sträter R: Beiträge zur Lehre von der Hämochromatose und ihren Beziehungen zur allgemeinen Hämosiderose. Virchows Arch 218:1–30, 1914.
10. Gilmour JR: Erythroblastosis foetalis. Part I. Arch Dis Child 19:1–11, 1944.
11. Gilmour JR: Erythroblastosis foetalis. Part II. Arch Dis Child 19:12–20, 1944.
12. Gilmour JR: Erythroblastosis foetalis. Part III. Arch Dis Child 19:21–25, 1944.

13. Zollinger HU: Pathologische Anatomie und Pathogenese des familiären Morbus haemolyticus neonatorum (Erythroblastose, Hydrops congenitus, Icterus gravis neonat. usw.). Helv Paediatr Acta 1 [Suppl II]:127–160, 1946.
14. Zeitlhofer J, Speiser P: Diffuse intraacinäre Lebercirrhose und Hydrops congenitus bei Rh.-Incompatibilität. Oest Z Kinderheilk 5:217–232, 1950.
15. Craig JM: Sequences in the development of cirrhosis of the liver in cases of erythroblastosis fetalis. Arch Pathol 49:665–686, 1950.
16. Craig JM, Landing BH: Form of hepatitis in neonatal period simulating biliary atresia. Arch Pathol 54:321–333, 1952.
17. Peace R: Fatal hepatitis and cirrhosis in infancy. A critical analysis of thirty-two cases studied at necropsy. Arch Pathol 61:107–119, 1956.
18. Cottier H: Ueber ein der Hämochromatose vergleichbares Krankheitsbild bei Neugeborenen. Schweiz Med Wochenschr 37:39–43, 1957.
19. Tomik F: Leberzirrhose bei einem Neugeborenen mit gigantozellulärer Transformation der Leberzellen. Zentralbl Allg Pathol 100:447–452, 1960.
20. Fienberg R: Perinatal idiopathic hemochromatosis: Giant cell hepatitis interpreted as an inborn error of metabolism. Am J Clin Pathol 33:480–491, 1960.
21. Laurendeau T, Hill JE, Manning GB: Idiopathic neonatal hemochromatosis in siblings. An inborn error of metabolism. Arch Pathol 72:410–423, 1961.
22. Goldfischer S, Grotsky HW, Chang C-H, Berman EL, Richert RR, Karmarkar SD, Roskamp JO, Morecki R: Idiopathic neonatal iron storage involving the liver, pancreas, heart, and endocrine and exocrine glands. Hepatology 1:58–64, 1981.
23. Jacknow G, Johnson D, Freese D, Smith C, Burke B: Idiopathic neonatal iron storage disease. Lab Invest 48:7P, 1983.
24. Blisard KS, Bartow SA: Neonatal hemochromatosis. Hum Pathol 17:376–383, 1986.
25. Reiffenstuhl G: Infantile Lebercirrhose und ABO-Inkompatibilität. Schweiz Zeit Allg Pathol 16:197–209, 1953.
26. Dible JH, Hunt WE, Pugh VW, Steingold L, Wood JHF: Foetal and neonatal hepatitis and its sequelae. J Pathol Bact 67:195–206, 1954.
27. Ehrlich JC, Ratner IM: Congenital cirrhosis of the liver with kernicterus. Report of two cases in siblings with a discussion of the relationship to so-called neonatal hepatitis and to iso-immunization disease. Am J Pathol 31:1013–1047, 1955.
28. Krainin P, Lapan B: Neonatal hepatitis in siblings. Report of two cases with giant multinucleated liver cells and fatal termination. JAMA 160:937–940, 1956.
29. Nezelof C, Watchi J-M, Gauter P, Brault A: Cirrhose infantile pigmentaire familiale. À propos d'une observation. Presse Med 75:451–456, 1967.
30. Greco MA, Richards HMS, Finegold MJ: Parenchymal cell siderosis in infancy. Lab Invest 38:387, 1978.
31. Bassett ML, Halliday JW, Ferris RA, Powell LW: Diagnosis of hemochromatosis in young subjects: Predictive accuracy of biochemical screening tests. Gastroenterology 87:628–633, 1984.
32. Muir WA, McLaren GD, Braun W, Askari A: Evidence for heterogeneity in hereditary hemochromatosis. Evaluation of 174 persons in nine families. Am J Med 76:806–814, 1984.
33. Howard JM, Ghent CN, Carey LS, Flanagan PR, Valberg LS: Diagnostic efficacy of hepatic computed tomography in the detection of body iron overload. Gastroenterology 84:209–215, 1983.
34. Leung AW-L, Steiner RE, Young IR: NMR imaging of the liver in two cases of iron overload. J Comput Assist Tomogr 8:446–449, 1984.

35. Simon M, Alexandre J-L, Fauchet R, Genetet B, Bourel M: The genetics of hemochromatosis. In Steinberg AG, Bearn AG, Motulsky AG, Childs B (eds): Progress in Medical Genetics, New Series, Vol 4. "Genetics of Gastrointestinal Disease." Philadelphia: W.B. Saunders, 1980, pp 135–168.
36. Bauminger BB, Walters G: Increased hepatic iron stores in the human fetus after maternal total dose infusion of iron dextran. Ann Clin Biochem 19:238–240, 1982.
37. Brückmann G, Zondek SG: Iron, copper and manganese in human organs at various ages. Biochem J 33:1845–1857, 1939.
38. Ramage H, Sheldon JH, Sheldon W: A spectrographic investigation of the metallic content of the liver in childhood. Proc R Soc Lond Ser B 113:308–327, 1933.
39. Kooyman JC: Investigations on serum- and tissue-iron. Acta Med Scand 134:205–220, 1949.
40. Singla PN, Chand S, Agarwal KN: Cord serum and placental tissue iron status in maternal hypoferremia. Am J Clin Nutr 32:1462–1465, 1979.
41. Tsuchiya H, Mitani K, Kodama K, Nakata T: Placental transfer of heavy metals in normal pregnant Japanese women. Arch Environ Health 39:11–17, 1984.
42. Apte SV, Iyengar L, Nagarajan V: Effect of antenatal iron supplementation on placental iron. Am J Obstet Gynecol 110:350–351, 1971.
43. Bauminger BB, Walters G, Whicher JT, Duke AB: Effect of total dose infusion of iron dextran on the storage iron content of the human placenta. J Clin Pathol 35:502–506, 1982.
44. Ellis JT, Schulman I, Smith CH: Generalized siderosis with fibrosis of liver and pancreas in Cooley's (Mediterranean) anemia with observations on the pathogenesis of siderosis and fibrosis. Am J Pathol 30:287–309, 1954.
45. Suda K: Hemosiderin deposition in the pancreas. Arch Pathol Lab Med 109:996–999, 1985.
46. Bothwell TH, Pribilla WF, Mebust W, Finch CA: Iron metabolism in the pregnant rabbit. Iron transfer across the placenta. Am J Physiol 193:615–622, 1958.
47. Orlic D, Lev R: Fetal monkey absorption of ^{55}Fe from amniotic fluid. Am J Anat 142:457–470, 1975.
48. Galbraith GMP, Galbraith RM, Temple A, Faulk WP: Demonstration of transferrin receptors on human placental trophoblasts. Blood 55:240–242, 1980.
49. McArdle HJ, Morgan EH: Transferrin and iron movements in the rat conceptus during gestation. J Reprod Fertil 66:529–536, 1982.
50. Galbraith GMP, Galbraith RM, Faulk WP: Immunological studies of transferrin and transferrin receptors of human placental trophoblast. Placenta 1:33–46, 1980.
51. Fletcher J, Suter PEN: The transport of iron by the human placenta. Clin Sci 36:209–220, 1969.
52. Soda R, Tavassoli M: Liver endothelium and not hepatocytes or Kupffer cells have transferrin receptors. Blood 63:270–276, 1984.
53. Tavassoli M, Soda R, Kataoka M, Kishimoto T, Harjes K: Endothelial processing of iron-transferrin (Fe-TF) complexes in the liver. Blood 64:43a, 1984.
54. Okuyama T, Tawada T, Furuya H, Villee CA: The role of transferrin and ferritin in the fetal-maternal-placental unit. Am J Obstet Gyncol 152:344–350, 1985.
55. Iob V, Swanson WW: A study of fetal iron. J Biol Chem 124:263–268, 1938.
56. Westerhausen M, Meuret G: Transferrin-immune complex disease. Acta Haematol 57:96–101, 1977.
57. Jacobs A: Low molecular weight intracellular iron transport compounds. Blood 50:433–439, 1977.

58. Jones RL, Grady RW, Sorette MP, Cerami A: Host-associated iron transfer factor in normal humans and patients with transfusion siderosis. J Lab Clin Med 107:431–438, 1986.
59. Ruebner BH, Miyai K: The pathology of neonatal hepatitis and biliary atresia with particular reference to hemopoiesis and hemosiderin deposition. Ann NY Acad Sci 111:375–291, 1963.
60. Prieto J, Barry M, Sherlock S: Serum ferritin in patients with iron overload and with acute and chronic liver diseases. Gastroenterology 68:525–533, 1975.
61. Thorbecke GJ, Liem HH, Knight S, Cox K, Muller-Eberhard U: Sites of formation of the serum proteins transferrin and hemopexin. J Clin Invest 52:725–731, 1973.
62. Huebers HA, Finch CA: Transferrin: Physiologic behavior and clinical implications. Blood 64:763–767, 1984.
63. Beliles RP, Palmer AK: The effect of massive transplacental iron loading. Toxicology 5:147–158, 1975.
64. Alpert E, Coston RL, Drysdale JW: Carcino-foetal human liver ferritins. Nature 242:194–196, 1973.
65. McKay DG, Hertig AT, Adams EC, Richardson MV: Histochemical observations on the human placenta. Obstet Gynecol 12:1–36, 1958.
66. Vargas PL, Pino Preira R, García Urrutia H, Vela Cobo H, González R: Anemia diseritropoyética congénita tipo II con intensa hemosiderosis hepática en un lactante de un mes. Bol Med Hosp Infant Mex 36:611–620, 1979.
67. Patton RG, Christie DL, Smith DW, Beckwith JB: Cerebro-hepato-renal syndrome of Zellweger. Two patients with islet cell hyperplasia, hypoglycemia, and thymic anomalies, and comments on iron metabolism. Am J Dis Child 124:840–844, 1972.
68. Vitale L, Opitz JM, Shahidi NT: Congenital and familial iron overload. N Engl J Med 280:642–645, 1969.
69. Versmold HT, Bremer HJ, Herzog V, Siegel G, von Bassewitz DB, Irle U, von Voss H, Lombeck I, Brauser B: A metabolic disorder similar to Zellweger syndrome with hepatic acatalasia and absence of peroxisomes, altered content and redox state of cytochromes, and infantile cirrhosis with hemosiderosis. Eur J Pediatr 124:261–275, 1977.
70. Perry TL, Hardwick DF, Dixon GH, Dolman CL, Hansen S: Hypermethionemia: A metabolic disorder associated with cirrhosis, islet cell hyperplasia, and renal tubular degeneration. Pediatrics 36:236–250, 1965.
71. Perry TL: Tyrosinemia associated with hypermethioninemia and islet cell hyperplasia. Can Med Assoc J 97:1067–1072, 1967.
72. Gaull GE, Rassin DK, Solomon GE, Harris RC, Sturman JA: Biochemical observations on so-called hereditary tyrosinemia. Pediatr Res 4:337–344, 1970.
73. Donohue WL, Uchida I: Leprechaunism. A euphemism for a rare familial disorder. J Pediatr 45:505–519, 1954.
74. Kálló A, Lakatos I, Szijártó L: Leprechaunism (Donohue's syndrome). J Pediatr 66:372–379, 1965.
75. Rogers DR: Leprechaunism (Donohue's syndrome). A possible case, with emphasis on changes in the adenohypophysis. Am J Clin Pathol 45:614–619, 1966.
76. Ordway NK, Stout LC: Intrauterine growth retardation, jaundice, and hypoglycemia in a neonate. J Pediatr 83:867–874, 1973.
77. Hartdegen RG, Dogliotti M, Rabinowitz L, Bartlett RG: Leprechaunism. Case report in a black African child. Br J Dermatol 93:587–591, 1975.
78. Adams JM, Gordon LP, Dutton RV, Rosenberg HS, Rudolph AJ: Leprechaunism (Donohue's syndrome) in a low birth weight infant. South Med J 70:998–1001, 1977.

79. D'Ercole AJ, Underwood LE, Groelke J, Plet A: Leprechaunism: Studies of the relationship among hyperinsulinism, insulin resistance, and growth retardation. J Clin Endocrinol Metab 48:495–502, 1979.
80. Datta NS, Wilson GN, Hajra AK: Deficiency of enzymes catalyzing the biosynthesis of glycerol-ether lipids in Zellweger syndrome. A new category of metabolic disease involving the absence of peroxisomes. N Engl J Med 311:1080–1083, 1984.
81. Moser AE, Singh I, Brown FR, Solish GI, Kelley RI, Benke PJ, Moser HW: The cerebrohepatorenal (Zellweger) syndrome. Increased levels and impaired degradation of very-long-chain fatty acids and their use in prenatal diagnosis. N Engl J Med 310:1141–1146, 1984.
82. Rous P: Urinary siderosis. Hemosiderin granules in the urine as an aid in the diagnosis of pernicious anemia, hemochromatosis, and other diseases causing hemosiderosis of the kidney. J Exp Med 28:645–658, 1918.
83. Galask RP, Snyder IS: Antimicrobial factors in amniotic fluid. Am J Obstet Gynecol 106:59–65, 1970.
84. Nusbaum MJ, Zettner A: The content of calcium, magnesium, copper, iron, sodium, and potassium in amniotic fluid from eleven to nineteen weeks' gestation. Am J Obstet Gynecol 115:219–226, 1973.
85. Thadepalli H, Gangopadhyay PK, Maidman JE: Amniotic fluid analysis for antimicrobial factors. Int J Gynaecol Obstet 20:65–72, 1982.
86. Weiss PAM: Typische Ultraschallbilder bei schwerer fetaler Rhesus-Erkrankung. Geburtshilfe Fraunheilkd 34:640–644, 1974.
87. Pribilia W, Bothwell TH, Finch CA: Iron transport to the fetus in man. In Wallerstein RO, Mettier SR (eds): "Iron in Clinical Medicine." Berkeley: University of California Press, 1958, pp 58–64.
88. Powell LW, Kerr JFR: Reversal of "cirrhosis" in idiopathic haemochromatosis following long-term intensive venesection therapy. Aust Ann Med 1:54–57, 1970.
89. Starzl TE, Zitelli BJ, Shaw BW, Iwatsuki S, Gartner JC, Gordon RD, Malatack JJ, Fox IJ, Urbach AH, Van Thiel DH: Changing concepts: Liver replacement for hereditary tyrosinemia and hepatoma. J Pediatr 106:604–606, 1985.

Since submission of this manuscript five further communications concerning neonatal hemochromatosis have appeared [90–94].

90. Kurnetz R, Yang SS, Holmes R, Harrison DD: Neonatal jaundice and coagulopathy. J Pediatr 107:982–987, 1985.
91. Witzleben C, Uri A: "Infantile hemochromatosis"—pathogenetic entity or non-specific response? Lab Invest 54:70A, 1986.
92. Silver MM: Perinuclear vesicles in five cases of perinatal hemochromatosis. Lab Invest 54:9P, 1986.
93. Silver MM, Valberg LS: Tissue iron quantitation in five cases of perinatal hemochromatosis. Lab Invest 54:9P, 1986.
94. Glista BA, Bautista A, Prudencio M, Desposito F: Neonatal iron storage disease. Pediatr Res 20:410A, 1986.

Fragile X Syndrome: Skin Elastin Abnormalities

Gail Waldstein, MD, Gary Mierau, PhD, Razia Ahmad, MD, Stephen N. Thibodeau, PhD, Randi J. Hagerman, MD, and Sherrie Caldwell, MD

Departments of Pathology (GW, GM, RA, SNT, SC), and Child Development (RJH), The Children's Hospital, Denver, Colorado 80218

INTRODUCTION

The fra(X) or Martin Bell (MB) syndrome is a common form of X-linked mental retardation (XLMR) characterized by distinct clinical manifestations in the affected males. They have a large forehead, prominent long ears, some prognathism and macroorchidism post-puberty. In addition, many patients have conditions compatible with a clinical connective tissue disorder. These include hyperextensibility of finger joints, flat feet, increased stretchability of skin, highly arched palate, mitral valve prolapse, and aortic dilatation [1,2]. The cytogenetic laboratory evaluation for this sydrome is the recognition of a fragile site at Xq27.3 when the lymphocytes are cultured in folic acid-deficient media. The karyotype is then identified as 46,XY,fra(Xq27.3) [3] and the percentage of fragile site-bearing cells is noted.

The connective tissue abnormalities are clinically reminiscent of cutis laxa and the Ehlers-Danlos syndromes (Table I). These manifestations suggest underlying abnormalities in collagen or elastin, although a specific biochemical defect has not been identified in fra(X) patients.

We undertook a preliminary study of biopsies in mentally retarded fra(X) males with connective tissue dysfunction. We attempted to analyze fibroblast cultures for lysyl oxidase, a critical enzyme in covalent collagen construction and a key component in the structural integrity of elastin. To date, these analyses have had technical difficulties, precluding interpretation. Half of

Birth Defects: Original Article Series, Volume 23, Number 1, pages 103–114

TABLE I. Comparison of Syndromes With Connective Tissue Disorders

	Cutis laxa	Fragile X	Ehlers-Danlos
Inheritance	Autosomal recessive (rare X-linked form)	X-linked	AD:types I, II, III, VIII AR:types IV, VI, VII, IX XLR: type V
Dominant clinical findings	Pulmonary emphysema, GI, GU diverticula, hernias	Mental retardation macroorchidism, large ears	Excess skin stretch-ability, joint laxity, GI diverticula, vascular aneurysms
Hyperextensible joints	− (+ X-linked)	+	++
Collagen	Normal	Normal	Some quantitative decrease, structurally normal
Elastic fibers	Decreased in number, variable diameter, fragmented or granular	Fewer; lack arborization, fragmented and curled	Relative increase, normal structure
Acid mucopoly-saccharides	Increased	Decreased	Increased

each biopsy was submitted for light and electron microscopy with the hope of identifying structural correlates for the observed clinical abnormalities in the fra(X) patients.

METHODS AND RESULTS

Five males with XLMR were chosen for this pilot study because they had cytogenetically documented fra(X) syndrome. Their percentages of fra(X) bearing cells varied from 18 to 42%. Their age ranged from 16 to 42 years. All had macroorchidism and prominence of ears and forehead. These patients also manifested a variety of mild to moderate connective tissue dysfunction, including hyperextensibility of finger joints, excessively stretchable skin, flat feet, highly arched palate, and mitral valve prolapse documented by ultrasonography.

Two normal males were used as control subjects. Neither showed the fra(X) chromosome in 100 lymphocytes appropriately cultured. These men were 33 and 38 years old with no evidence of mental impairment and had no physical stigmata of fra(X) syndrome or of a connective tissue disorder.

A 6 mm punch biopsy of the skin of the flexor surface of the forearm was obtained after cleansing with betadine and anesthetizing with 1.0 cc of 1% Xylocaine. Appropriate consent was obtained and sterile technique was employed. The biopsy was immediately hemisected with a sterile blade and half was submitted for fibroblast culture; the other half was subdivided for light and electron microscopy. Approximately 2/3 of this half biopsy was promptly placed in B_5 fixative for 2–4 hours, postfixed in formalin, and routinely processed for light microscopy. 4μ sections were subsequently stained with hematoxylin and eosin, Masson trichrome, Verhoeff-Van Gieson elastin stain, orcein elastin stain, and the Hale colloidal iron method for acid mucopolysaccharides. The remaining portion was fixed in 2.5% gluteraldehyde, postfixed in 2% osmium tetroxide, and processed for electron microscopy in customary fashion. Sections were stained with uranyl acetate and lead citrate for routine study. The tannic acid method of Kajikawa et al [4] was employed to study the quantity and distribution of elastin within elastic fibers.

The biopsy material was examined by light microscopy on 2 separate occasions by one observer and on 2 separate occasions by a second observer before breaking the code regarding controls and patients. Generally, agreement between observers was good with the exception of minor variations in interpretation of the Hale stain for acid mucopolysaccharide. Three regions of the dermis were evaluated with each of the stains in terms of deposition of mucopolysaccharides, orientation and distribution of collagen fibers, and organization, configuration, and quantity of elastin fibrils.

The *results* are summarized in Table II. The areas studied included superficial or papillary dermis, deep or reticular dermis, and their junction. Acid mucopolysaccharide was prominent in the papillary dermis of both control males (Fig. 1) but was sparse to inapparent in all the fra(X) patients (Fig. 2) except 1 teenage boy. It surrounded skin appendages in the reticular dermis equally in both controls and patients.

Study of collagen in the papillary dermis by light microscopy suggested thicker fibers with some crowding in the specimens from patients with fra(X) except 1 teenager whose collagen fibrils had a delicate composition. One control male evidenced thick collagen fibers and the other had delicate collagen in the papillary dermis. Both control males had collagen orientation in the superficial region parallel to the surface. Four fra(X) males had fibers that were oriented primarily perpendicularly to the surface. One had fibers which were oriented both in parallel and perpendicular planes. The reticular dermal collagen was generally thick and had a haphazard orientation with respect to the surface, both in control and fra(X) syndrome biopsies. Consid-

TABLE II. Comparison of Fragile X Syndrome and Control Males*

Case No.	Clinical findings	Age (yrs)	Fra (X) Cells (%)	Elastin (papillary dermis)	Elastin (juncture)	Elastin (reticular dermis)
1	Hyperextensible jts.; mitral valve prolapse; highly arched palate	32	18	Curled	Long fibers	Thick > > thin; fragmented; blunt ends
2	Loose, stretchable skin; hyperextensible jts.; flat feet	42	34	Curled	Haphazard	Thick> > thin; fragmented; blunt ends
3	Hyperextensible jts.; loose stretchable skin; flat feet	16	42	Partial arborization	Sparse; long fibers	Thick and thin; blunt/tapered ends
4	Mitral valve prolapse; flat feet	17	24	Wisps	Tangential	Thin > > thick; blunt/tapered ends
5	Mitral valve prolapse; pectus excavatum; flat feet; hyperextensible jts.	29	18	Partial arborization	Haphazard	Thick fragmented; curled; blunt ends
6	Normal control	38	0	Arborization	Long fibers	Long; thick; blunt/tapered ends
7	Normal control	33	0	Arborization	Long fibers	Long; thick; blunt/tapered ends

*All fragile X males had macroorchidism, large ears, and a prominent forehead.

eration of the orientation of skin section with respect to the long axis of the forearm was not incorporated in this study. Abnormalities in collagen fiber size or periodicity were not detected in either the papillary or reticular dermis of patients with the fra(X) syndrome by electron microscopic study.

Examination of the biopsies with both Verhoeff-Van Gieson and orcein stain showed differences in distribution of elastin fibers. The control material had an arborizing or branching pattern with supporting, longitudinally oriented elastin fibers giving rise to perpendicularly oriented extensions, appearing to reach up or to arborize toward the epidermis (Fig. 3). The papillary dermis of the fra(X) males had wisps of delicate fibrils, often oriented perpendicularly and tangentially to the surface, but rarely supported by longitudinal fibers (Fig. 4). There were fewer fibers than in control males,and in some patients the fibers were twisted and clumped. Electron microscopic examination of both patient and control elastic fibers documented an amorphous or gel component intermingled with a microfibrillary component in an irregular fashion (Fig. 5). This normal composition of elastic fibrils in this locale produced the anticipated vacant spots when examined with the tannic acid stain.

The area of junction between the papillary and reticular dermis was distinct in these sections when examined with elastic tissue stains. The control males had abundant, long fibers oriented parallel to the surface (Fig. 6). All fra(X) males had fewer fibers, the majority with tangential to haphazard surface orientation (Fig. 7).

The elastic fibers of the reticular dermis shared some patterns in all the specimens. Most fibrils were longitudinally oriented with respect to surface and lay parallel to each other (Fig. 8). The fra(X) patients tended to have more fragmented portions of elastic fibers or greater fracturing (Fig. 9). All biopsies had fibers that were blunt-ended, whereas control males and 3 younger fra(X) biopsies had many fibers with tapered ends as well. Fiber diameter seemed variable. The control subjects had predominantly thick, long elastic fibers in the reticular dermis although a few thin fibers were identified. Most patients had an admixture of fibers with thick and thin cross-sectional diameters with thick fibers generally dominating. Electron microscopic study revealed the microfibrillary component of the elastic fibers of the deep dermis in both groups to be nearly obscured by the homogeneous deposition of amorphous elastin (Fig. 5). This is recognized as the normal appearance of elastic fibers in this location.

DISCUSSION

In a subset of patients with the fra(X) syndrome there are manifestations of a connective tissue disorder including joint hyperextensibility and some-

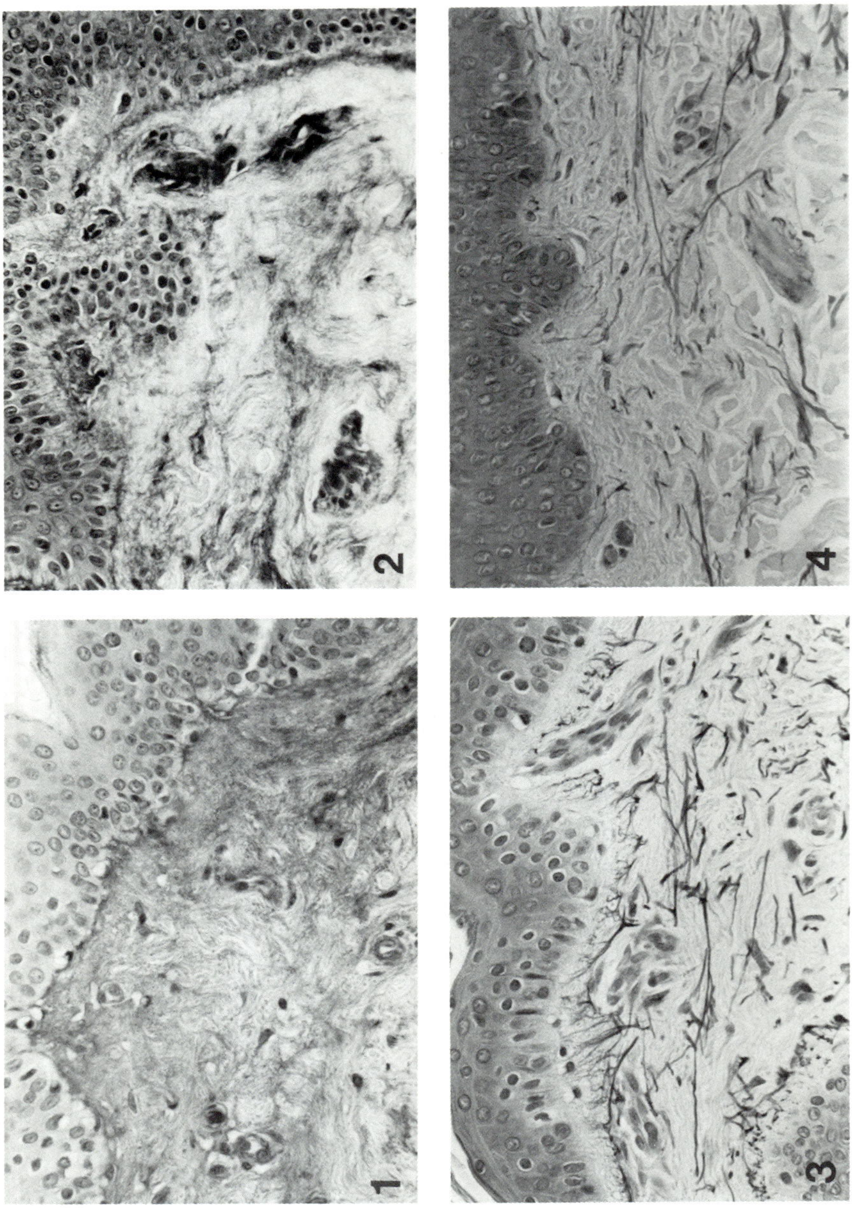
2
4
1
3

what loose, unusually stretchable skin. Other clinical problems in these patients include mitral valve prolapse, flat feet, highly arched palate, and occasional pectus excavatum. These findings presumably also reflect a defect in structural alignment of the underlying connective tissues.

From our pilot study, the abnormalities of elastic fiber morphology is fra(X) patients provides one explanation for many of the connective tissue stigmata observed. The malalignment of elastin, its relative paucity and variable configuration, may affect the tensile qualities of joint capsules, ligaments, and tendons and provide a basis for the looseness and stretchability of skin seen in these men. The long, prominent ears characterizing fra(X) patients may be a further manifestation of elastin network problems. Another classic finding in this syndrome is macroorchidism, which has been related to increase in interstitial volume of the testes [5]. This may also relate to imperfect elastin anatomy in the interstitium, or perhaps to an aberration in the composition of ground substance. The ground substance in the papillary dermis of fra(X) men is decreased as delineated histologically with the acid mucopolysaccharide stain. This material is known to coat the protein core of elastin fibers in normal individuals and has previously been described as disordered in other connective tissue dysplasias [6].

Comparing and contrasting the connective tissue problems in fra(X) patients with those of Ehlers-Danlos syndrome and cutis laxa patients may provide valuable insights into pathophysiologic mechanisms. The intricacies of inheritance, molecular structure of collagen and elastin, their anatomic distribution in connective tissues, the relationship to the acid mucopolysaccharide ground substance, and the ultimate expression in the clinical findings of the patient provide a monumental correlative task, demanding an interdisciplinary approach. A simplistic comparison of clinical findings, microscopic observations, and inheritance is provided in Table II. Clearly, current biochemical methods and more precise clinical descriptions, will permit more

---

Fig. 1. Normal skin; papillary dermis: Densely staining acid mucopolysaccharides. Hale's colloidal iron. Original magnification ×100.

Fig. 2. Fra(X) patient; papillary dermis: Absence of acid mucopolysaccharide. Hale's colloidal iron. Original magnification ×100.

Fig. 3. Normal skin; papillary dermis: A delicate arborizing pattern of elastic fibers supported by longitudinal fibers. Orcein stain. Original magnification ×100.

Fig. 4. Fra(X) patient; papillary dermis: Paucity of elastin with rare tangential fibers. Orcein stain. Original magnification ×100.

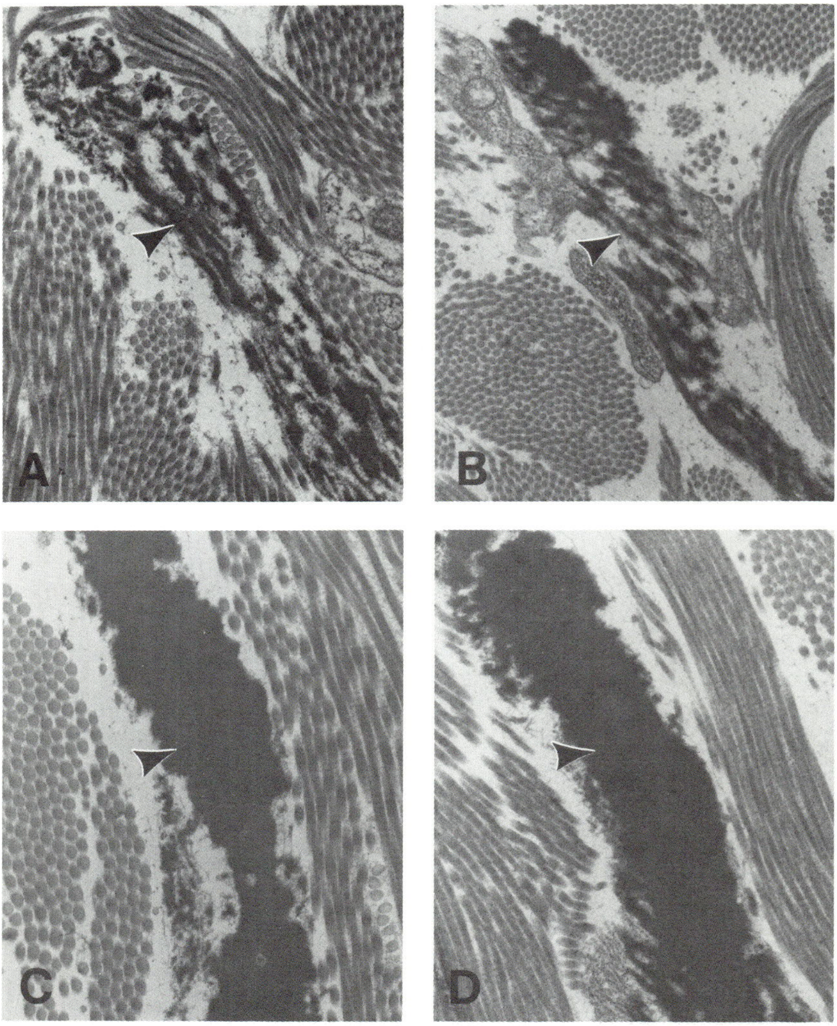

Fig. 5. The quantity and distribution of elastin (arrows) within the elastic fibers of fragile X patients seems not to differ from that of normal controls. (A) Superficial dermis, fragile X patient. (B) Superficial dermis, age-matched control. (C) Deeper dermis, fragile X patient. (D) Deeper dermis, normal control. Tannic acid stain, ×26,400.

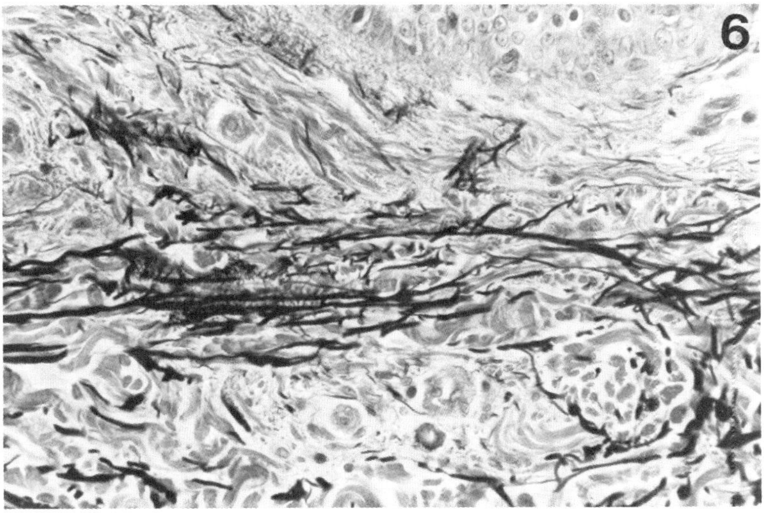

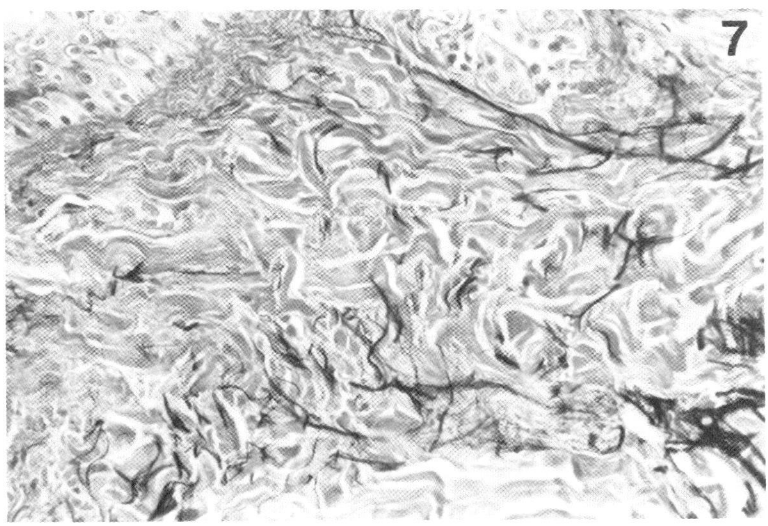

Fig. 6. Normal skin; junction of papillary/reticular dermis: Abundant long fibers oriented parallel to surface epidermis. Verhoeff-Van Gieson stain. Original magnification ×100.

Fig. 7. Fra(X) syndrome; junction of papillary/reticular dermis: Rare fibers haphazardly oriented. Verhoeff-Van Gieson stain. Original magnification ×100.

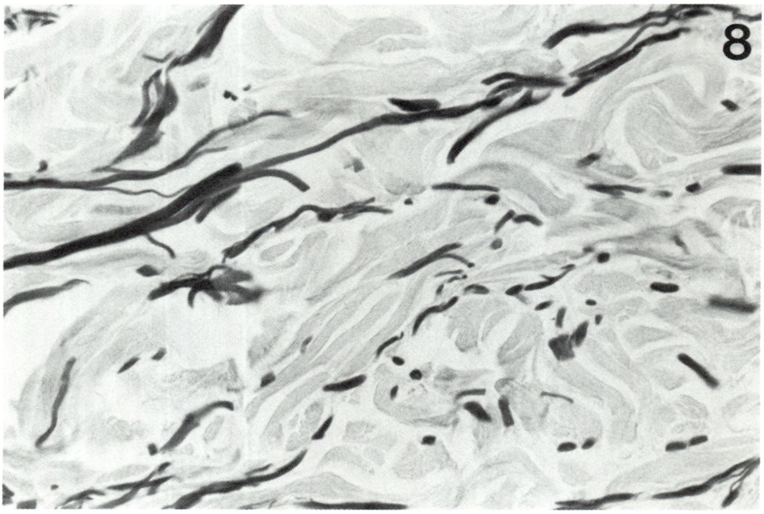

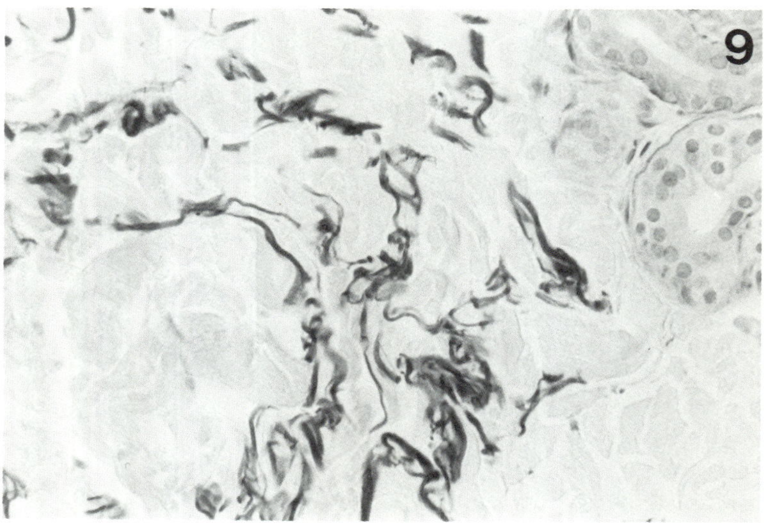

Fig. 8. Normal skin; deep or reticular dermis: Fairly uniform elastic fibers align parallel to the surface. Orcein stain. Original magnification ×100.

Fig. 9. Fra(X) patient; deep dermis: Fragmented, twisted fibers with uneven diameters and irregular surface orientation. Orcein stain. Original magnification ×100.

distinct delineation of the variants of Ehlers-Danlos syndrome and cutis laxa than are summarized in Table II.

However, there is some value in reviewing old conceptual frames when attempting to unravel these interrelationships. The proposal by Jansen of a "defective wickerwork" as an explanation for the dermal findings in Ehlers-Danlos syndrome is still attractive. If the "wickerwork" is indeed unsound because of faulty or maldistributed collagen, there might well be a compensatory elastin proliferation to provide dermis, joints, and vessel walls with appropriate tensile properties for function [7]. An alternate explanation for the collapse of the dermis noted in the Ehlers-Danlos syndrome is destruction of collagen with fewer fibers remaining and an apparent increase in the elastin [8]. The comparison of fra(X) syndrome with changes described in cutis laxa is more compatible in terms of skin histology. The common type of cutis laxa, with pendulous skin of the face and trunk, has fragmented and decreased elastic fibers that often degenerate further with age. Collagen is histologically normal [9]. An explanation for the skin changes of cutis laxa may be a defective elastin "wickerwork." To extrapolate this hypothesis to the skin of fra(X) patients seems logical. There is a rare X-linked variant of cutis laxa that is clinically similar to the connective tissue dysfunction in fra(X) patients. The skin changes in the X-linked variant of cutis laxa are less severe than in the usual autosomal recessive type and these patients often have considerable joint laxity as well. Studies of this variant of cutis laxa have shown a disturbance of collagen rather than of elastin and a deficiency in the lysyl oxidase enzyme [10]. Pathophysiologic considerations have been forwarded linking the lysyl oxidase genetic locus to the X chromosome and suggesting that while the enzyme may relate to the structural integrity of the elastic wickerwork, it may not be as essential to the ultrastructural composition of elastin and/or collagen in this disorder. Electron microscopic abnormalities were not found in the skin of patients with the X-linked variant of cutis laxa [11].

While it is tempting to expound on the possible relationships between these variable connective tissue diseases and patients with fra(X) syndrome, it is important to recall that there are major differences as well. The fra(X) patients present as mentally retarded individuals presumably with no compromise in life span and with a relatively mild connective tissue dysfunction. The histologic observations reported here represent a pilot study suggesting that the underlying abnormalities in the connective tissue of patients with the fra(X) syndrome may indeed relate to elastin abnormalities. Greater numbers of patients and control individuals may corroborate these preliminary data. Biochemical aspects of connective tissue metabolism should be explored.

Finally, the pathogenetic complexities including clinical findings, elastic fibers abnormalities, changes in acid mucopolysaccharides, and possibly the relationship to lysyl oxidase demand definition.

REFERENCES

1. Hagerman RJ, Van Housen K, Smith ACM, McGavran L: Consideration of connective tissue dysfunction in the fragile X syndrome. Am J Med Genet 17: 111–121, 1984.
2. Opitz JM, Westphal JM, Daniel A: Discovery of a connective tissue dysplasia in the Martin-Bell syndrome. Am J Med Genet 17:101–109, 1984.
3. Harrison CJ, Jack EM, Allen TD, Harris R: The fragile X: A scanning electron microscope study. J Med Genet 20: 280–285, 1983.
4. Kajikawa K, Yamaguchi T, Katsudo S, Miwa A: An improved stain for elastic fibers using tannic acid. J Electron Microsc 24:287–289, 1975.
5. Ruvalcaba RHA, Myhre SA, Roosen-Runge EC, Beckwith JB: X-linked mental deficiency megalotestes syndrome. JAMA 238:1646–1650, 1977.
6. Goltz RW, Hult AM: Generalized elastolysis (cutis laxa) and Ehlers-Danlos syndrome (cutis hyperelastica): A comparative clinical and laboratory study. South Med J 58:848–854, 1965.
7. Jansen LH: The structure of the connective tissue, an explanation of the symptoms of the Ehlers-Danlos syndrome. Dermatology 110:108–120, 1955.
8. Goltz RW, Hult AM, Goldfarb M, Gorlin RJ: Cutis laxa. Arch Dermatol 92:373–387, 1965.
9. Mehregan AH, Lee SC, Nabai H: Cutis laxa (generalized elastolysis). J Cutan Pathol 5:116–126, 1978.
10. Byers PH, Narayanan AS, Bornstein P, Hall JG: An X-linked form of cutis laxa due to deficiency of lysyl oxidase. In Bergsma D, Schimke RN (eds): "Cytogenetics, Environment and Malformation Syndromes." New York: Alan R. Liss, Inc. for The National Foundation–March of Dimes. BD:OAS XII (5):293–298, 1976.
11. Byers, PH, Siegel RC, Holbrook KA, Narayanan AS, Bornstein P, Hall JG: X linked cutis laxa. N Engl J Med 303: 61–65, 1980.

Hepatic Involvement in Hereditary Renal Syndromes

Jay Bernstein, MD

Department of Anatomic Pathology, William Beaumont Hospital, Royal Oak, Michigan 48072

INTRODUCTION

Cystic abnormalities of the liver accompany many hereditary renal syndromes, including autosomal recessive ("infantile") polycystic disease (IPCD), hereditary renal dysplasia, and hereditary tubulointerstitial nephritis. The hepatic abnormalities in those conditions are similar, comprising hepatic fibrosis and biliary dysgenesis.

The term *congenital hepatic fibrosis* (CHF) is used to describe portal and perilobular fibrosis with an excess of bile ducts. The term was adopted by Kerr et al [1] from Parker's paper on fibrosis of the liver as a congenital anomaly [2]. Although his was not the initial description of the abnormality, Parker characterized the histopathologic changes of hepatic fibrosis and attributed them to maldevelopment. At least 3 of the patients had IPCD, and 1 had Meckel syndrome; 2 other patients had nonsyndromal hepatic fibrosis without evidence of cystic disease in the kidneys.

Kerr and colleagues used the term CHF to describe a group of young patients who had portal hypertension and hepatic fibrosis with an excess of bile ducts. A similar abnormality appears to have been described by Dustin [3], Grumbach and Bourvillon [4], and possibly by Mozziconacci et al [5]. The occurrence of portal hypertension in 3 sibs with an identical hepatic abnormality and polycystic kidney disease had been reported by Campbell et al [6], and additional cases were reported by Lathrop [7] and Sedacca et al

Birth Defects: Original Article Series, Volume 23, Number 1, pages 115–130

[8]. Following Kerr's example, the term CHF was used by McCarthy et al [9] in describing hepatic fibrosis and bile duct hyperplasia in a group of children and adults, all but 1 of whom had cystic kidneys. The infants in their study had typical IPCD; some of the older patients, both children and adults, had portal hypertension.

Many of the patients described by Kerr et al [1] were subsequently shown by excretory urography to have renal medullary ductal ectasia [10], an abnormality described by Reilly and Neuhauser [11] as characteristic of IPCD, despite its resemblance to medullary sponge kidney [12]. Although congenital hepatic fibrosis is heterogeneous, as will be discussed, most patients have polycystic disease of the kidney [13].

Since Kerr's paper [1], the term CHF has gained wide currency, but it has also gained several meanings both morphologic and clinical [14]. Kerr and his colleagues [1,10], and many since, have used CHF to mean a syndrome of portal hypertension in patients with noncirrhotic hepatic fibrosis and bile duct excess; Bernstein [15] has used it as descriptive of the hepatic abnormality in IPCD; Landing and colleagues [16,17] have used it in a restricted sense for what they interpret as a condition different from hepatic polycystic disease in IPCD.

The hepatic abnormality in CHF consists of enlarged and fibrotic portal areas with an apparent proliferation of bile ducts [2,9,18–20] (Fig. 1). The involved portal areas appear not to contain central bile ducts, and the portal vein branches often appear to be small, sometimes multiple [18,21,22]. Although the portal hypertension is commonly attributed to a presinusoidal block [1], because of the portal fibrosis or the portal vein abnormalities, a postsinusoidal block may be present in the same patients [23]. Fibrosis around central veins is sometimes prominent in CHF, especially in cases of renal dysplasia (Fig. 2), and there may be obstruction of hepatic vein tributaries. The biliary abnormality is a form of biliary maldevelopment, as it seems to be an arrest in the differentiation of bile ducts [18]. We might assume on stereologic grounds alone [24] that the occurrence of elongated biliary profiles in almost every portal area of a random section of liver reflects the presence of sac-like rather than duct-like or tubular biliary structures [20,25–27], a feature already shown by reconstructions of the biliary cysts [16,28,29]. On the basis of his stereologic studies and reconstructions, Jørgensen [18] had concluded that the arrangement of biliary structures must be interpreted as a system of flattened sacs around the margins of the portal tract in its ramifications through the liver, what he termed "the ductal plate malformation." That arrangement was characterized by Landing and colleagues [16] as a doubled-layered sleeve. Such an arrange-

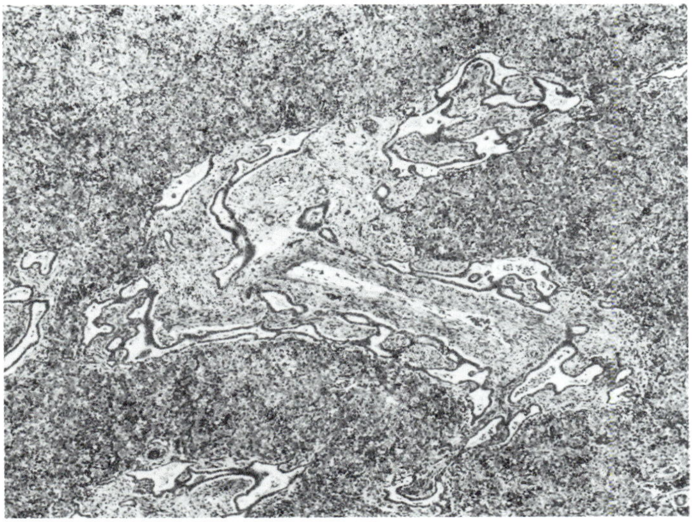

Fig. 1. Congenital hepatic fibrosis in autosomal recessive polycystic disease (IPCD) in a newborn infant: The portal areas are enlarged, appearing to be encircled by elongated, interconnecting, and almost continuous biliary structures that in three-dimensional reconstruction are flattened sacs. A centrally located portal bile duct cannot be identified. Apparently proliferated ductules are present at the limiting plates of the hepatic lobules, and some ductules appear to be situated within the lobules. The portal area appears to contain more than one portal vein branch; the hepatic artery is unaltered. H&E stain, magnification ×42.

ment would account for the appearance of elongated and interconnecting ducts in every plane of section.

Biliary dysgenesis (the term we prefer for the biliary abnormality) in CHF may be accompanied by gross ductal dilatation and sometimes by large intrahepatic cysts [18,20]. The saccular and fusiform ductal dilatations develop without evidence of anatomic obstruction; communicating ectasia of the intrahepatic bile ducts is known as Caroli disease [30,31]. The diagnosis is usually demonstrated by cholangiography, which establishes its nonobstructive nature and differentiates it from other cystic abnormalities. Although Caroli disease may occur without other abnormalities, it occurs most often in association with renal cystic disease and medullary ductal ectasia [32].

AUTOSOMAL RECESSIVE INFANTILE POLYCYSTIC DISEASE

The prototype of biliary dysgenesis (Fig. 1) is found in neonatal IPCD [33–35] (Fig. 3). The portal areas are enlarged, with apparent bile duct

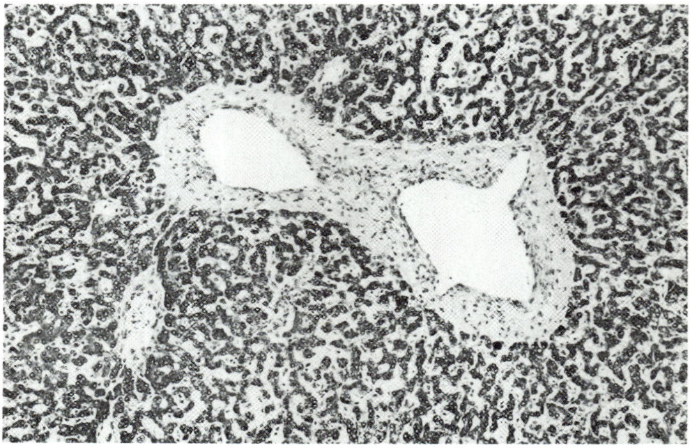

Fig. 2. Congenital hepatic fibrosis with central perivenous fibrosis: Perivenous fibrosis is sometimes prominent in CHF, as in this newborn infant who also had renal dysplasia, phocomelia of the upper limbs, and congenital heart disease. Perivenous fibrosis is a potential cause of postsinusoidal obstruction. H&E stain, magnification ×63.

proliferation, and that "proliferation" reflects a relatively complex arrangement of flattened sacs or cisterns [18]. The biliary structures in histologic sections are often disposed in almost continuous, irregularly interrupted rings around centrally placed blood vessels, but the arrangement is often much more complex, with tributaries residing within the hepatic lobules. The biliary spaces are elongated in the two-dimensional profiles, with rounded contours and local constrictions. The abnormality in young infants occasionally includes ductular proliferation next to the limiting plates of the hepatic lobules, and bile stasis and inspissation are seldom present.

Even in newborn infants the biliary sacs may be dilated [36] and grossly cystic [27]. Large spaces are trabeculated, so that sections of the cysts seem to contain epithelialized islands or inclusions. Biliary dilatation apparently occurs without anatomic obstruction.

Older children seem to have more fibrosis and the biliary sacs have a more variable, pinched appearance and haphazard arrangement (Fig. 4). The liver has increased sonographic echogenicity, partly because of fibrosis and partly because of cysts [37,38]. We have thought the abnormality to evolve with progressive fibrosis [12,18], perhaps as an inherent characteristic of the disease [39,40], but Landing and colleagues [16] have subdivided the hepatic abnormality according to the relative severity of fibrosis and found the division not to be age-related. They have, in showing an increased proportion

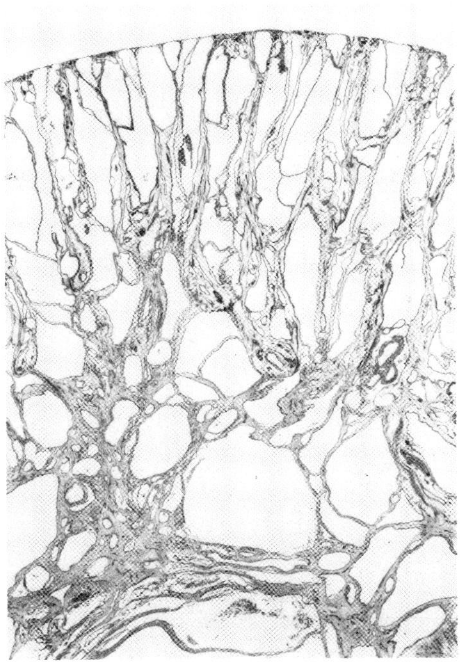

Fig. 3. Autosomal recessive polycystic disease (IPCD) in a newborn infant: The typical renal abnormality consists of dilated collecting ducts that form fusiform or sac-like cysts extending through the cortex from more dilated and rounded collecting ducts within the medulla. Although the typical cortical architecture of alternating medullary rays and cortical labyrinths is obscured by the dilated ducts, nephronic induction is said to be normal. Nonetheless, there may appear to be a paucity of nephrons because of renal enlargement by the cysts and because of variable interstitial edema. H&E stain, magnification, ×7.5.

of fibrous tissue in one subgroup of patients, claimed heterogeneity for what we have regarded as one disease. Their morphometric evaluation of the renal abnormality supports their interpretation of the hepatic findings [41], although we have thought the differences they described in the kidneys to be related to the initial severity of expression, modified by the natural evolution of the lesion (Fig. 5).

The evolution in the liver may be influenced by epigenetic factors such as ascending cholangitis [42] and localized ductal obstruction by inspissated bile [19], both of which could lead to accelerated fibrosis and ductular proliferation. Patients with CHF are at high risk of biliary infection [43], either cholangiolitis or suppurative cholangitis. Purulent biliary infection is a partic-

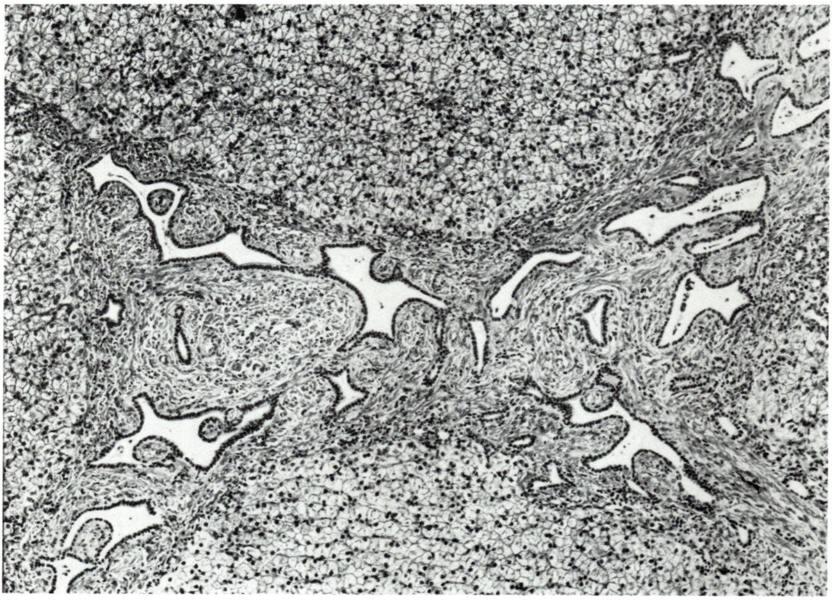

Fig. 4. Congenital hepatic fibrosis in an older child: The hepatic abnormality in a 2-year-old with portal hypertension consists, in comparison with that of a newborn infant (Fig. 1), of relatively more fibrosis, with a pinched and angulated appearance of the biliary structures. Some of the profiles are small and rounded, suggesting a mixture of sac-like and duct-like configurations. H&E stain, magnification ×25.

ular risk in patients with Caroli disease, which predisposes them to stasis and lithiasis. Plugs of inspissated bile are common in older children, although those patients are seldom jaundiced. The development of jaundice usually indicates a complication such as ascending infection or acquired hepatocellular damage. The advancing fibrosis results in perilobular fibrosis that may be barely distinguishable from micronodular cirrhosis.

OTHER HEREDITARY RENAL SYNDROMES

Biliary dysgenesis and an abnormality morphologically indistinguishable from congenital hepatic fibrosis are also seen in association with hereditary renal dysplasia and hereditary tubulointerstitial nephritis. The hepatic abnormalities differ only quantitatively from the hepatic abnormalities in IPCD. Histopathologic examination of the liver in Meckel syndrome (Fig. 6) shows the same pattern of biliary dysgenesis—flattened sacs with variable dilata-

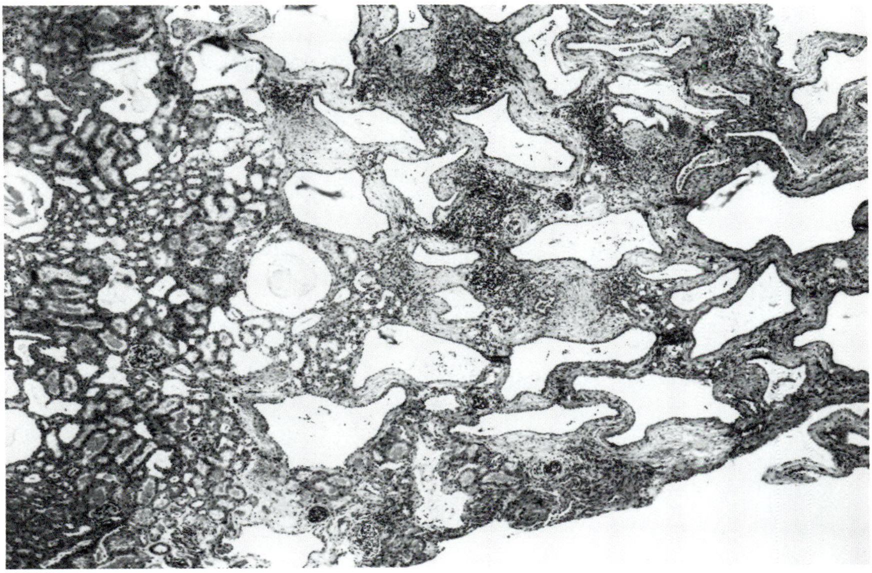

Fig. 5. Autosomal recessive polycystic disease (IPCD) in an older child: The renal abnormality in a 2-year-old with portal hypertension (same case as in Fig. 4) consists of medullary ductal ectasia with focal cortical cysts. There is irregular dilatation of convoluted tubules, and the medulla contains a moderate infiltrate of chronic inflammatory cells. H&E stain, magnification ×12.5.

tion—as demonstrated by anatomic reconstructions [44,45]. Meckel syndrome is perhaps the best known of the hereditary syndromes that include renal cystic dysplasia (Fig. 7), and renal dysplasia is the most consistent anomaly in syndrome [46–48]. The renal abnormality in the other syndromes of hereditary dysplasia (Table I) is histologically the same, and almost all of those syndromes include biliary dysgenesis.

The hepatic abnormality in Meckel syndrome seems more often to be grossly cystic than the similar abnormality in IPCD, and cysts exceeding 10 cm in diameter are relatively common in newborn infants with Meckel syndrome. Landing et al [17] found a higher ratio of portal connective tissue to biliary structures in comparison with the abnormalities of IPCD and CHF, but the differences have not always been apparent. Meckel syndrome has often been taken for polycystic disease [44,45]. Children with Meckel syndrome seldom live long enough to develop portal hypertension and the other complications of biliary dysgenesis, but the potential exists.

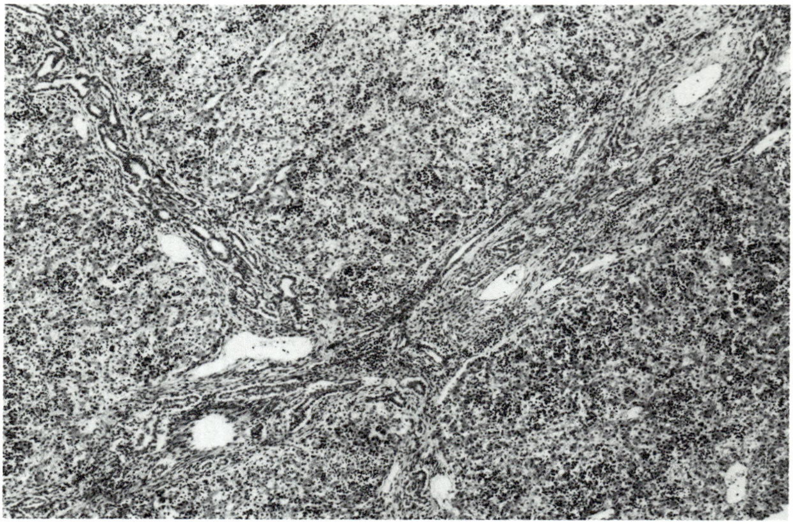

Fig. 6. Congenital hepatic fibrosis in Meckel syndrome: The hepatic abnormality in a newborn infant with Meckel syndrome consists of large portal areas with biliary dysgenesis, strongly resembling other forms of CHF. H&E stain, magnification ×48.

Biliary dysgenesis is a regular manifestation of Jeune and Zellweger syndromes (Figs. 8, 9), but the reports are too few to determine its frequency in the other syndromes of renal cystic dysplasia (Table I). Hepatic involvement is, by definition, a constant component of renal-hepatic-pancreatic dysplasia, sometimes referred to as Ivemark syndrome, in which gross cysts are relatively common [49]. We have also been impressed by the frequency in those cases of hepatic central perivenous fibrosis, which may add an element of postsinusoidal obstruction. However, portal hypertension has not been a characteristic of the condition, as most affected children have died within the first year of life. Although we have not encountered an ascending biliary infection, the possibility cannot be ruled out.

Hepatic fibrosis and biliary dysgenesis have been described in several forms of hereditary tubulointerstitial nephritis, among them juvenile nephronophthisis [50] (Figs. 10, 11), Bardet-Biedl syndrome [51], and Jeune syndrome [52]. (Jeune syndrome has, in its several manifestations, encompassed both renal dysplasia and tubulointerstitial nephritis, phenotypic differences of uncertain genetic implication [53].) Landing et al [17] found in Jeune syndrome without renal dysplasia a relatively small size of portal tract, compared to those of IPCD and CHF, and in nephronophthisis they found

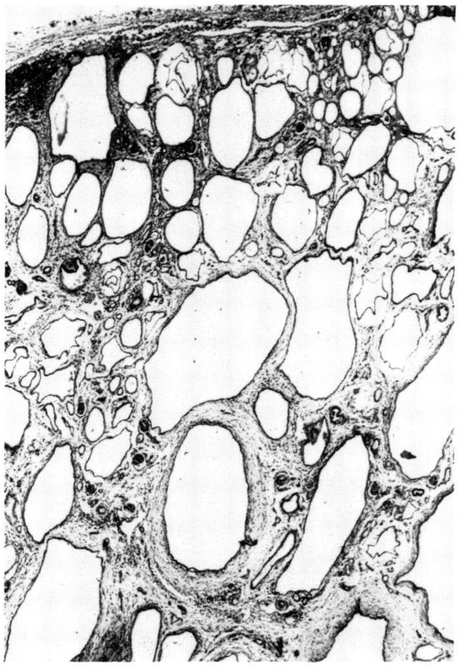

Fig. 7. Renal cystic dysplasia in Meckel syndrome. The typical renal abnormality of Meckel syndrome is abnormal metanephric differentiation with an abundance of cystic collecting ducts and a paucity of nephrons. The abnormal collecting ducts take the form of primitive ducts with fibromuscular collars and linings of undifferentiated columnar or cuboidal epithelium. The lobar development of the kidney is also altered, with poor corticomedullary differentiation and rudimentary medullary development. (Newborn sib of infant whose liver is illustrated in Fig. 6). H&E stain, magnification ×25.

relatively small biliary "ducts." The portal tracts in our own cases of nephronophthisis with hepatic fibrosis have contained a relatively large amount of fibrous tissue that seemed on inspection to increase with age; the biliary sacs at postmortem examination seemed more pinched and more compressed than they had in biopsy specimens during the patient's life (Fig. 10).

SUMMARY

The hepatic abnormality that accompanies IPCD, hereditary renal cystic dysplasia, and hereditary tubulointerstitial nephritis, comprises maldevelop-

TABLE I. Hereditary Syndromes That Include Morphologically Similar Renal Cystic Dysplasia

Meckel syndrome
Zellweger cerebrohepatorenal syndrome
Renal-hepatic-pancreatic dysplasia
Chondrodysplasia syndromes
Majewski and Saldino-Noonan short rib-polydactyly syndromes
Jeune asphyxiating thoracic dysplasia
Ellis-van Creveld chondroectodermal dysplasia
Elejalde acrocephalopolydactylous dysplasia
Trisomy 9 syndrome
Trisomy 13 syndrome
Glutaric aciduria, type II

ment of the intrahepatic bile ducts and portal fibrosis. The biliary abnormality results in flattened sacs that do not differentiate into bile ducts, and the portal areas contain increased amounts of connective tissue with what seems to be hypoplasia of the portal veins. Those abnormalities have been interpreted as the basis of a presinusoidal block that develops into portal hypertension. We find that the portal abnormalities are often accompanied by central perivenous fibrosis, which might contribute to a postsinusoidal block, as suggested by some clinical studies.

The proportions of portal fibrous tissue and biliary structures vary among the different types of hepatic fibrosis, and Landing et al [17] emphasized the difference between typical IPCD and another group with more hepatic fibrosis and less severe renal involvement. While it seems a good bet to predict that genetic heterogeneity underlies some of the variation encountered in IPCD, we have found very few studies of sequential biopsies and very few comparisons between biopsy and autopsy specimens in cases of hepatic fibrosis. Landing et al [17], in studying a few cases morphometrically, were unable to identify age-related changes, but our own evaluations of the hepatic abnormality in hereditary tubulointerstitial nephritis indicate that the abnormality changes with time. We have also seen the development of severe portal and perilobular fibrosis, almost indistinguishable from micronodular cirrhosis, in patients with IPCD, and we think the hepatic abnormality to be modified by epigenetic factors such as ascending infection, portal inflammation, and localized biliary obstruction. In support of an "evolution," both natural and unnatural, are the common observations that complications develop over long periods of time. Hepatic structure is likely to be modified over similar periods of time.

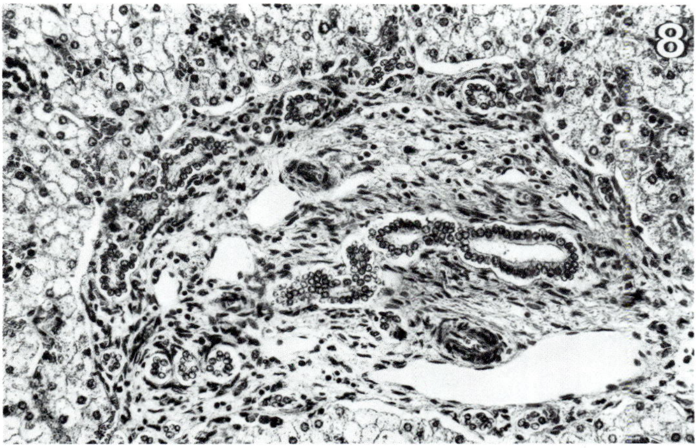

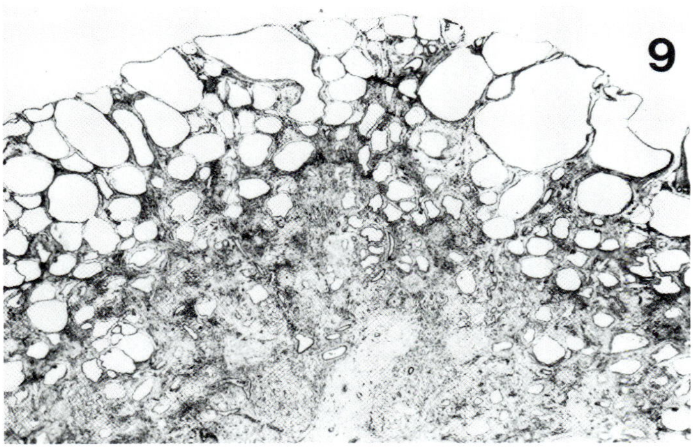

Fig. 8. Congenital hepatic fibrosis in Zellweger syndrome. Although portal enlargement is usually less striking than in IPCD, the same pattern of biliary dysgenesis pertains. Note the multiple small branches of the portal vein. H&E stain, magnification ×160.

Fig. 9. Renal cystic dysplasia in Zellweger syndrome. The renal cortex is cystic, mostly because of dilated collecting ducts. There is moderate nephronic development, and some of the cysts are dilated glomeruli that contain small capillary tufts. There is very poor medullary development, and the specimen bears a striking resemblance to the renal abnormality of Meckel syndrome. H&E stain, magnification ×12.5.

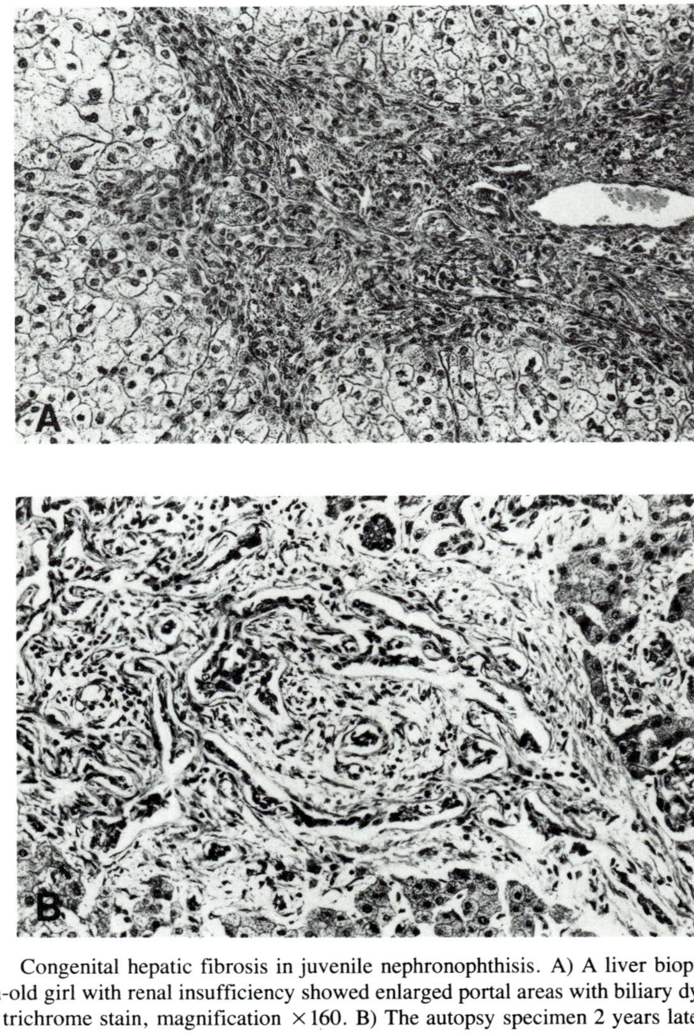

Fig. 10. Congenital hepatic fibrosis in juvenile nephronophthisis. A) A liver biopsy from a 6-month-old girl with renal insufficiency showed enlarged portal areas with biliary dysgenesis. Masson trichrome stain, magnification ×160. B) The autopsy specimen 2 years later showed CHF with a relative increase of portal connective tissue. Masson trichrome stain, magnification ×160.

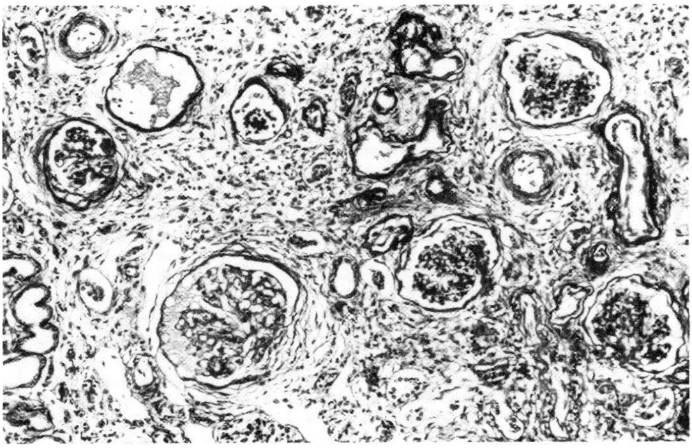

Fig. 11. Tubulointerstitial nephritis. The renal abnormality in the case illustrated in Figure 10 consists of severe tubular atrophy with interstitial fibrosis and secondary glomerular changes. PAS stain, magnification ×100.

REFERENCES

1. Kerr DNS, Harrison CV, Sherlock S, Milnes Walker R: Congenital hepatic fibrosis. QJM 30:91–117. 1961.
2. Parker RGF: Fibrosis of the liver as a congenital anomaly. J Pathol 71:359–368, 1956.
3. Dustin P Jr: Anatomie pathologique du syndrome de Banti. Acta Gastroentérol Belg 15:313–343, 1952.
4. Grumbach R, Bourillon J, Auvert J-P.: Maladie fibro-kystique du foie avec hypertension portale chez l'enfant: Deux observations. Arch Anat Pathol 30:74–77, 1954.
5. Mozziconacci P, Auvert J, Attal C, Girard F, Habib R, Trung P-H: Maladie "fibro-kystique" du foie avec hypertension portale. Arch Franç Pédiatr 15:1269–1278, 1958.
6. Campbell GS, Bick HD, Paulsen EP, Lober PH, Watson CJ, Varco RL: Bleeding esophageal varices with polycystic liver. Report of three cases. N Engl J Med 259:904–910, 1958.
7. Lathrop DB: Cystic disease of the liver and kidney. Pediatrics 24:215–224, 1959.
8. Sedacca CM, Perrin E, Martin L, Schiff L: Polycystic liver: An unusual case of bleeding esophageal varices. Gastroenterology 40:128–137, 1961.
9. McCarthy LJ, Baggenstoss AH, Logan GB: Congenital hepatic fibrosis. Gastroenterology 49:27–36, 1965.
10. Kerr DNS, Warrick CK, Hart-Mercer J: A lesion resembling medullary sponge kidney in patients with congenital hepatic fibrosis. Clin Radiol 13:85–91, 1962.
11. Reilly BJ, Neuhauser EBD: Renal tubular ectasia in cystic disease of the kidneys and liver. AJR 84:546–554, 1960.
12. Bernstein J: Heritable cystic disorders of the kidney. The mythology of polycystic disease. Pediatr Clin North Am 18:435–444, 1971.

13. Murray-Lyon IM, Ockenden BG, Williams R: Congenital hepatic fibrosis—Is it a single entity? Gastroenterology 64:653–656, 1973.
14. Landing BH: Tubulointerstitial and medullary cystic diseases of children—current concepts. Sidney Farber Lecture. Annual Meeting of the Pediatric Pathology Club, San Francisco, California, 10 March 1984.
15. Bernstein J: Polycystic disease. In Edelmann CM Jr (ed): "Pediatric Kidney Disease," Vol II. Boston: Little, Brown & Co, 1978, Chap 40, pp 557–570.
16. Landing BH, Wells TR, Reed GB, Narayan MS: Diseases of the bile ducts in children. In Gall EA, Mostofi FK (eds): "The Liver." International Academy of Pathology Monograph 13. Baltimore: Williams & Wilkins, 1973, Chap 22, pp 480–509.
17. Landing BH, Wells TR, Claireaux AE: Morphometric analysis of liver lesions in cystic diseases of childhood. Hum Pathol 11(Suppl):549–560, 1980.
18. Jørgensen MJ: The ductal plate malformation. Acta Pathol Microbiol Scand A, Suppl 257:1–88, 1977.
19. Nathan M, Batsakis JG: Congenital hepatic fibrosis. Surg Gynecol Obstet 128:1033–1041, 1969.
20. Bernstein J: Hereditary renal disease. In Churg J, Spargo BH, Mostofi FK (eds): "Kidney Disease: Present Status." International Academy of Pathology Monograph. Baltimore: Williams & Wilkins, 1979, Chap 13, pp 295–326.
21. Krainer L: Intrahepatic bile duct malformation associated with portal hypertension. Gastroenterology 33:265, 1957.
22. Hodgson HJF, Davies DR, Thompson RPH: Congenital hepatic fibrosis. J Clin Pathol 29:11–16, 1976.
23. Clermont RJ, Maillard J-N, Benhamou J-P, Fauvert R: Fibrose hépatique congénitale. Can Med Assoc J 97:1272–1278, 1967.
24. Elias H: Three dimensional structure identified from single sections. Science 174:933–1000, 1971.
25. Jørgensen M: A stereological study of intrahepatic bile ducts. 3. Infantile polycystic disease. Acta Pathol Microbiol Scand A 81:670–675, 1973.
26. Jørgensen M: A stereological study of intrahepatic bile ducts. 4. Congenital hepatic fibrosis. Acta Pathol Microbiol Scand A 82:21–29, 1974.
27. Bernstein J: Cystic diseases of the liver in infancy. Presented at an International Workshop on Neonatal Hepatitis and Biliary Atresia, sponsored by the National Institute of Arthritis, Metabolism, and Digestive Diseases and by the John E. Fogarty International Center for Advanced Study in the Health Sciences, March 1977. In Javitt NB (ed): "Neonatal Hepatitis and Biliary Atresia." DHEW Publication No. (NIH) 79-1296, pp 331–338.
28. Norris RF, Tyson RM: The pathogenesis of the polycystic liver. Reconstructions of cystic elements in two cases. Am J Pathol 23:201–215, 1947.
29. Jørgensen M: A case of abnormal intrahepatic bile duct arrangement submitted to three-dimensional reconstruction. Acta Pathol Microbiol Scand A 79:303–306, 1971.
30. Caroli J, Soupault R, Kossakowski J, Plocker L, Paradowska Mme: La dilatation polykystique congénitale des voies biliaires intra-hépatique. Essai de classification. Sem Hôp Paris 34:488–495, 1958.
31. Caroli J, Couinaud C, Soupault R, Porcher R, Etévé J: Une affection nouvelle, sans doute congénitale, des voies biliaires. La dilatation kystique unilobaire des canaux hépatiques. Sem Hôp Paris 34:496–502, 1958.
32. Murray-Lyon IM, Shilkin KB, Laws JW, Illing RC, Williams R: Non-obstructive dilatation of the intrahepatic biliary tree with cholangitis. QJM 41:477–489, 1972.

33. Bunting CH: Congenital cystic kidney and liver with family tendency. J Exp Med 8:271–288, 1906.
34. Potter EL: "Pathology of the Fetus and the Newborn." Chicago: Year Book Medical Publishers, 1952, pp 336–337.
35. Lundin PM, Olow I: Polycystic kidneys in newborns, infants and children. A clinical and pathological study. Acta Paediatr Scand 59:185–200, 1961.
36. Heggö O, Natvig JB: Cystic disease of the kidneys. Autopsy report and family study. Acta Pathol Microbiol Scand 64:459–469, 1965.
37. Rosenfield AT, Siegel NJ, Kappelman NB, Taylor KJW: Gray scale ultrasonography in medullary cystic disease of the kidney and congenital hepatic fibrosis with tubular ectasia: New observations. AJR 129:297–303, 1977.
38. Kelsey JA, Bowie JD: Gray-scale ultrasonography in the diagnosis of polycystic kidney disease. Radiology 122:791–795, 1977.
39. Albukerk J, Duffy JL: Fibrogenesis in congenital hepatic fibrosis. An electron and light microscopic study. Arch Pathol 92:126–135, 1971.
40. Thaler MM, Ogata ES, Goodman JR, Piel CF, Korobkin MT: Congenital fibrosis and polycystic disease of liver and kidneys. Am J Dis Child 126:374–380, 1973.
41. Helczynski L, Wells TR, Landing BH, Lipsey AI: The renal lesion of congenital hepatic fibrosis: Pathologic and morphometric analysis, with comparison to the renal lesion of infantile polycystic disease. Pediatr Pathol 2:441–455, 1984.
42. Alvarez F, Bernard O, Brunelle F, Hadchouel M, Leblanc A, Odiévre M, Alagille D: Congenital hepatic fibrosis in children. J Pediatr 99:370–375, 1981.
43. Stickler GB, Neel IV, Baggenstoss AH, Bernstein J: Polycystic kidney disease in infants. In Brodehl J, Ehrich JHH (eds): "Paediatric Nephrology." Proceedings of the Sixth International Symposium of Paediatric Nephrology, Hannover, Federal Republic of Germany, 29 August–2nd September 1983. Berlin: Springer-Verlag, 1984, pp 363–367.
44. Jørgensen M: Three-dimensional reconstruction of intrahepatic bile ducts in a case of polycystic disease of the liver in an infant. Acta Pathol Microbiol Scand A 80:201–206, 1972.
45. Adams CM, Danks DM, Campbell PE: Comments upon the classification of infantile polycystic diseases of the liver and kidney, based upon three-dimensional reconstruction of the liver. J Med Genet 11:234–243, 1974.
46. Fraser FC, Lytwyn A: Spectrum of anomalies in the Meckel syndrome, or: "Maybe there is a malformation sydrome with at least one constant anomaly." Am J Med Genet 9:67–73, 1981.
47. Moerman Ph, Verbeken E, Fryns JP, Goddeeris P, Lauweryns JM: The Meckel syndrome. Pathological and cytogenetic observations in eight cases. Hum Genet 62:240–245, 1982.
48. Rapola J, Salonen R: Visceral anomalies in the Meckel syndrome. Teratology 31:193–201, 1985.
49. Bernstein J, Chandra M, Kahn E, Creswell J, Daum F, Malouf NN, McVicar M, Weinberg AG, Wybel RE: Renal-hepatic-pancreatic dysplasia: A syndrome reconsidered. Am J Med Genet (in press).
50. Boichis H, Passwell J, David R, Miller H: Congenital hepatic fibrosis and nephronophthisis. A family study. QJM 42:221–333, 1973.
51. Pagon RA, Haas JE, Bunt AH, Rodaway KA: Hepatic involvement in the Bardet-Biedl syndrome. Am J Med Genet 13:373–381, 1982.

52. Turkel SB, Diehl EJ, Richmond JA: Necropsy findings in neonatal asphyxiating thoracic dystrophy. J Med Genet 22:112–118, 1985.
53. Bernstein J, Brough AJ, McAdams AJ: The renal lesion in syndromes of multiple congenital malformations. Cerebrohepatorenal syndrome; Jeune asphyxiating thoracic dystrophy; tuberous sclerosis; Meckel syndrome. In Bergsma D (ed): "Urinary System and Others." Baltimore: Williams & Wilkins, BD:OAS X(4):35–43, 1973.

Fetal Pathology—Nonchromosomal

Helga Rehder, MD, Michael Weber, MD, Klaus Heyne, MD, and Mario Lituania, MD

Institut für Humangenetik (HR), Institut für Pathologie (MW), and Kinderklinik (KH) der Medizinischen Universität zu Lübeck, Federal Republic of Germany, and Servizio di Ostetricia, Istituto G. Gaslini, Genova, Italy (ML)

INTRODUCTION

Thanks to the efforts of an International Working Group, causal and pathogenetic terminology of developmental disorders was subjected to a new classification [1]. In this the term "syndrome," which formerly—in a more general way—applied to any nosologic entity of more or less constantly associated pathologic defects, is now restricted to a recognizable pattern of multiple, pathogenetically related anomalies and is in other respects replaced by terms such as sequence, developmental field defect, association, or deformation.

This new classification is a challenge to every fetal and pediatric pathologist not only to register and to document objectively associated anomalies occurring within a malformation complex, but also to interpret the findings, to differentiate secondary defects occurring as a sequel of a primary defect, to trace common developmental disturbances or precursor lesions, and to address issues of syndromology in order to learn what to look for, since some

Dedicated to Professor H.R. Wiedemann on his 70th birthday.

Birth Defects: Original Article Series, Volume 23, Number 1, pages 131–151

anomalies are more frequently associated than others with certain syndromes. Rash conclusions and overstatements should be avoided. Pathologists may be the only ones to ever see a malformed fetus or stillborn infant, and the outcome of genetic counseling and of subsequent preventive or prenatal diagnostic measures may depend heavily on their findings and conclusions.

The following examples demonstrate the importance and limitations of a developmental morbid anatomy.

HERLITZ SYNDROME

Epidermolysis bullosa atrophicans generalisata gravis Herlitz (R-EBA-GH, also called Herlitz syndrome) is a causally and pathogenetically well-defined monogenic disorder. Among the different types of epidermolysis bullosa classified according to clinical picture, mode of inheritance, site of blister formation within the skin, and the presence or absence of scarring, the Herlitz syndrome represents a lethal type within the group of nonscarring atrophying epidermolyses with an autosomal recessive transmission [2,3]. As a mechano-bullous disorder, it is characterized by generalized traumatic and "spontaneous" blistering with secondary skin atrophy, congenital crusted erosions and ulcerations on the limbs with involvement and "dystrophy" of fingernails. Mucous membranes are also involved. Blister formation is junctional with separation between the plasma membrane of the epidermal basal cells and the basal lamina [4]. As long as the basal lamina remains intact, granulation and scarring do not occur.

The basic defect is an ultrastructural anomaly of basal cells. Electron microscopic investigations have shown that the one gene defect results in reduction and hypoplasia of the hemidesmosomes that are important for a normal dermo-epidermal junctional connection [3,5,6]. This ultrastructural defect is evident only in intact, unseparated skin biopsies. But the pathologist may assume junctional blistering in autopsy material and differentiate it at least from the dermatolytic blisters of other types of epidermolysis bullosa by demonstrating the PAS-positive basal lamina at the blister bottom attached to the dermis and the absence of a reactive granulation or scarring.

Up to now, 16 published cases of epidermolysis bullosa letalis were associated with congenital pyloric atresia [7–16]. We have seen 2 further cases. One concerned a preterm female infant of the 34th gestational week with polyhydramnios. She was the second, but the first affected child of a healthy 23-year-old mother and a 26-year-old father. Epidermolysis bullosa atrophicans gravis Herlitz had already been diagnosed by electron microscopy [17] in a second cousin at Heidelberg. At birth, the proposita had mutilations of the distal limbs, ears, and nose, an ectropion of the right lower eyelid, and severe traumatic blistering and erosions of the skin, involving large areas of the body surface (Fig. 1a), as well as bleeding of the oral, laryngeal, and tracheal mucosa following intubation. She died of aspiration at age 1 day. A segmental, 2 cm long pyloric atresia was found at autopsy

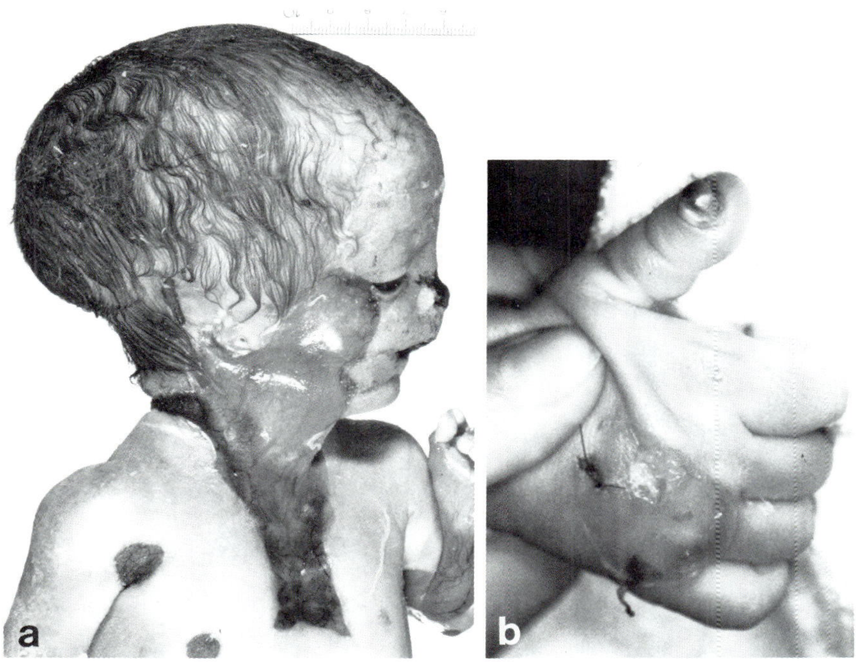

Fig. 1. (a) Preterm infant with severe manifestation of recessive epidermolysis bullosa gravis type Herlitz (R-EBA-GH). (b) Newborn infant with less severe skin alterations in R-EBA-GH displaying blister formation on the back of the hand and nail dystrophy.

(Fig. 2). On paraffin histology (Fig. 3), the skin lesions were consistent with R-EBA-GH; proof by electron microscopy investigations was impossible because of severe autolytic changes (Anton-Lamprecht, Heidelberg).

In the second case, a girl was born to consanguineous parents, a healthy 40-year-old mother and a 40-year-old father, both of Turkish origin. At age 3 days she was operated on because of membranous pyloric atresia. Skin lesions were not as severe as in the first case but were noted shortly after birth as localized erosions on both knees. However, Herlitz syndrome was suspected at age 4 weeks when blister formation became more evident (Fig. 1b). The girl suffered from severe recurrent enteritis and tracheobronchitis, indicating involvement of the gastrointestinal and respiratory mucosa; she died at 20 weeks of marasmus. Autopsy was not performed, but skin biopsies had been taken before death and biopsies from anal and rectal mucosa were taken shortly after death. Paraffin and EM histologic findings were consistent with junctional blistering (Anton-Lamprecht, Heidelberg). The rectal mucosa showed chronic proctitis and the surgical specimen of the pyloric membrane

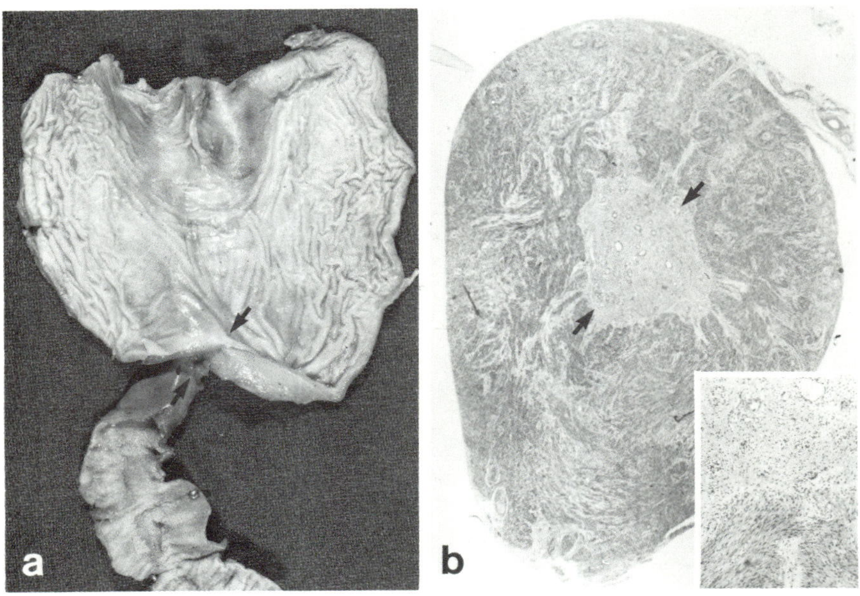

Fig. 2. (a) Dissected stomach and duodenum in R-EBA-GH with segmental atresia of the pylorus (arrow). (b) Histologic cross-section of the atretic pylorus showing defect of mucosa and muscularis mucosae and obliteration of the lumen by granulation and scarring tissue (arrow) HE × 16. (Insert: higher magnification of granulation tissue HE × 48.)

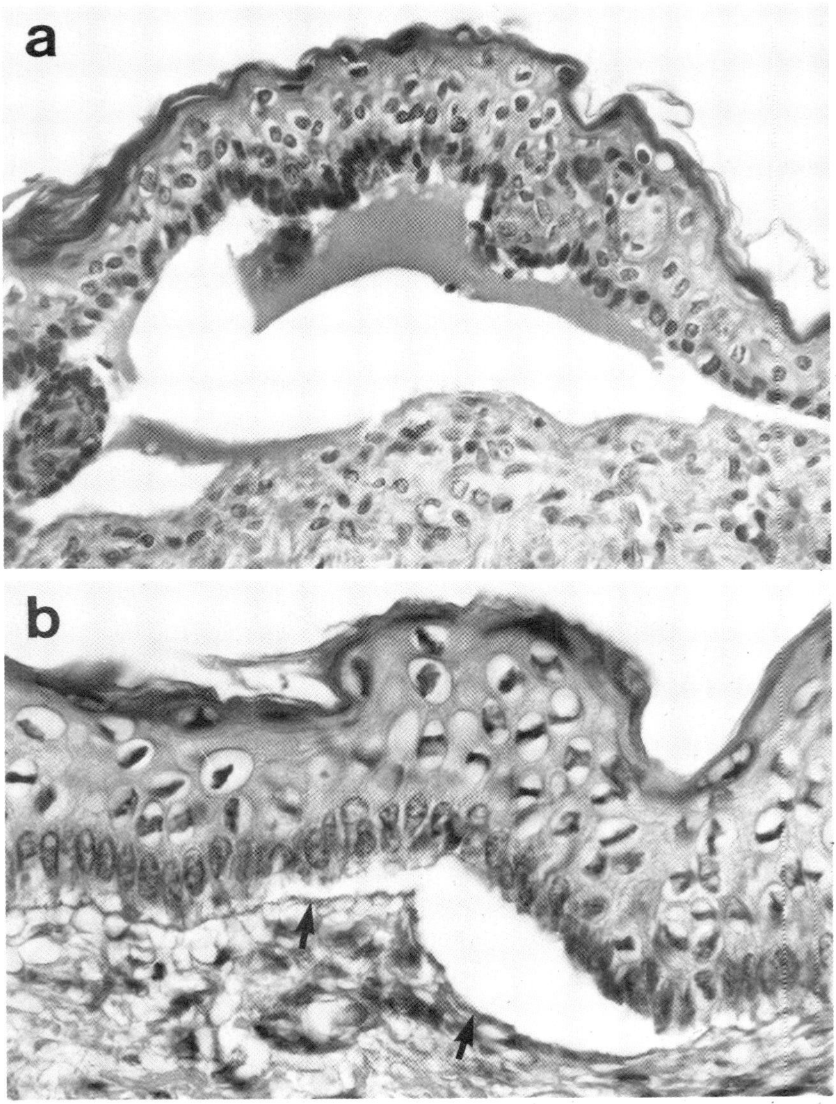

Fig. 3. Histologic section of the skin in R-EBA-GH with junctional blister formation and separation between the epidermal basal cells and the dermis. HE × 400. (a), the basal lamina remaining attached to the dermis (arrow). PAS × 640 (b).

displayed granulation tissue and inflammatory pyloric mucosa (Weber et al, in preparation).

Since autosomal recessive inheritance has also been suggested in some cases of pyloric atresia, the question arose whether the concurrence of EB with pyloric atresia represented a coincidental association of 2 different mutant genes (the frequency of epidermolysis bullosa being 1.9–5.3 per 1,000,000 in Norway [3] and of pyloric atresia 1 per 1,000,000 [18,19]), or whether they reflect linkage or a pleiotropic effect of a single mutant gene [7,10,14].

Pyloric atresia may be segmental or septal in these cases. In the segmental type, a defect of the mucosa, including parts of the muscularis mucosae and submucosa, and an obliteration of the pyloric lumen by granulation and fibrous tissue is found, the histologic picture being identical to that seen in traumatic intestinal obstruction [20]. The muscularis propria is still intact. Adjacent gastric mucosa, and to a different extent esophageal and intestinal mucosa, may show dehiscence between the epithelium and the underlying lamina propria similar to the lesions seen in the epidermis. In the membranous type of atresia, which is more common in the esophagus, larynx and trachea in scarring epidermolysis bullosa dystrophica [21–24], the mucosa is intact but shows an inflammatory and fibrous reaction; atresia is due to web formation following mucosal adhesions.

From these histologic findings we concluded (1) that the pyloric atresia in our patients was a granulomatous and scarring sequel of a preceding mucosal lesion, (2) that the primary mucosal lesion was consistent with the junctional blistering of the epidermis, indicating mucosal involvement in the basic disorder of R-EBA-GH, and (3) that the scarring reaction of the pylorus in a nonscarring type of EB was due to the special mechanical, acidic, and enzymatic injury by gastric contents, leading not only to subepithelial cleavage but also to traumatic lesions of the underlying basal lamina and tunica propria and, thus, to erosions and ulcerations with consecutive inflammatory reaction. Thus, pyloric atresia seems to represent a sequel to EB type Herlitz that may be acquired pre- or postnatally [13,15,16].

It should be mentioned that maceration may simulate junctional blistering, at least in paraffin histology. This led to confusion in a case of a stillborn infant presenting with bullae and denuded areas all over the body surface. Clinically, congenital EB was suspected because of the family history of a chronic skin disease in 2 deceased 70-year-old granduncles. Whereas the obstetrician had stated "perinatal" death, the autopsy findings of severe autolytic changes even in internal organs and of placental infarcts were in favor of prenatal death and, thus, of maceration rather than of epidermolysis bullosa. Anamnestic, clinical, and morphologic data are considered carefully before serious procedures, such as a skin biopsy in a subsequent pregnancy, are performed [17,25].

ROBERTS SYNDROME

Roberts syndrome is a pleiotropic autosomal recessive disorder. It is characterized by growth retardation, symmetrical hypo- and campomelia with reduction anomalies, and by craniofacial abnormalities including bilateral cleft lip and cleft palate, prominent premaxilla, proptosis, lid coloboma, cloudy corneae, facial hemangiomata, and sparse, silvery hair. Penile or clitoral enlargement are often present at birth and persistent branchial arch defects and ear anomalies have been described [26–33]. In severely affected cases, hypomelia may present as tetraphocomelia or even amelia and the palatal cleft may extend into a large median facial cleft with huge fronto-ethmoido-naso-maxillary encephalocele. A similar disorder of autosomal recessive transmission has been delineated as SC-phocomelia [34,35] but is now regarded as a milder manifestation of the same recessive gene [30,36]. Roberts-SC syndrome patients have chromosome abnormalities in the form of premature sister-chromatid separation, most prominently in centromeric and paracentromeric heterochromatic regions (heterochromatic puffing), and reduced cell growth *in vitro* [37–40].

Roberts syndrome patients may have internal anomalies such as renal abnormalities (horseshoe kidneys, cystic kidneys), genital anomalies (cryptorchidisim, bicornuate uterus), or lumbar spina bifida. In 5 cases, cardiovascular malformations have been noted at autopsy, presenting as patent ductus arteriosus in all, as patent foramen ovale in 3, and as crescent-shaped atrial septal defect, secundum type, in 2 cases [29,31,41]. In 1 case of SC-phocomelia, ventricular septal defect was suspected clinically [42]. Since closure of the foramen ovale and the ductus arteriosus in general is not completed until the 18th postnatal day, and since all 5 affected infants died within hours or days after birth, patency of the ductus arteriosus and foramen ovale (and possibly also the incomplete atrial septal defect) cannot be designated as true malformations but may at the most indicate a persisting fetal circulation.

We have seen 3 fetuses with Roberts syndrome after prenatal ultrasound diagnosis of limb anomalies [43]. Two were sibs from a sibship in which a first-born daughter was healthy and the second child, a boy, is living but severely affected by limb deficiency with defects of both radii and ulnae, oligodactyly, bilateral cleft lip and cleft palate, and other characteristics of

Roberts syndrome (Fig. 4a). A ventricular septal defect was diagnosed by ultrasonography while cardioangiography was not performed and vascular anomalies were thus not excluded. Subsequent pregnancies resulted in 2 affected, female and male fetuses. Limb deficiency was of lesser severity and no facial clefts but furrows of lips and philtrum were present in the first, demonstrating that SC phocomelia is a milder manifestation of Roberts syndrome (Figs. 4b, 5). A third case seen by us was a "monster," the first affected child of an Italian couple, a 34-year-old woman and her 36-year-old husband. They had had a normal female before and 3 spontaneous abortions at about the second month of pregnancy. This fetus was aborted in the 30th gestational week because of severe polyhydramnios. It was diagnosed as

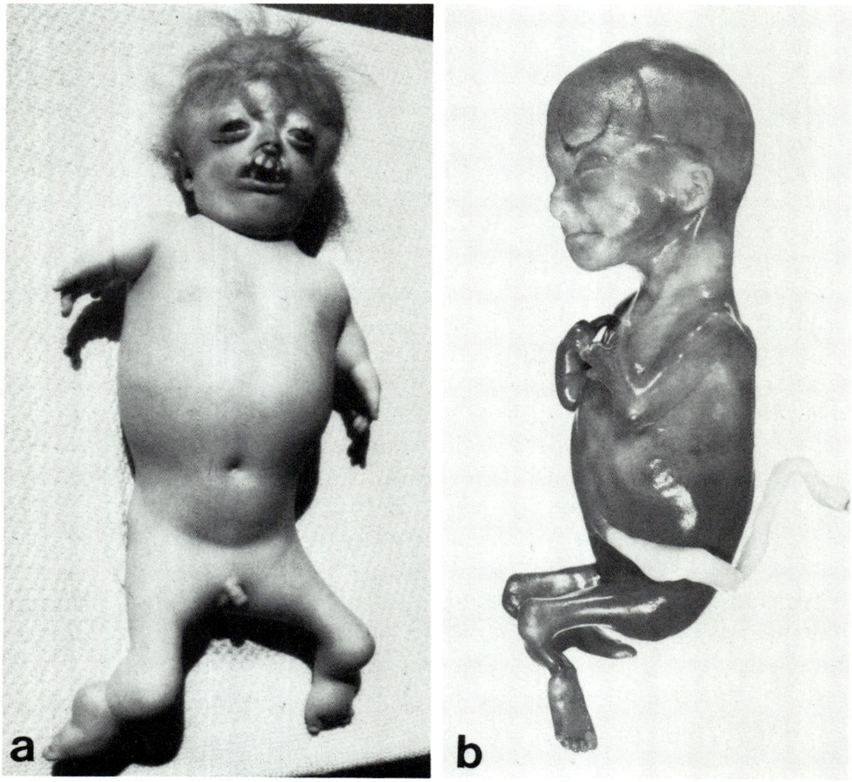

Fig. 4. (a) 3-year-old male infant with severe manifestation of Roberts syndrome (sib of Figs. 4b and 5). (b) Female fetus with milder manifestation of Roberts syndrome (see Fig. 6a).

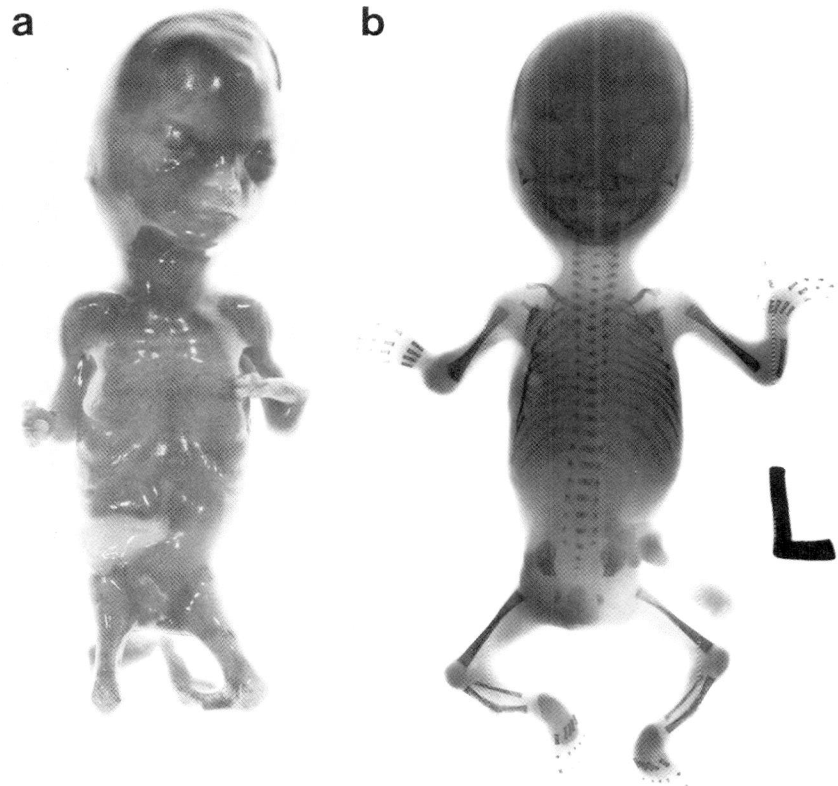

Fig. 5. Male fetus with Roberts syndrome and defects of upper limbs and bowing of lower legs. (a) External aspect. (b) X-ray (sib. of 4a and b).

Roberts syndrome and represented the most severe manifestation of the disorder with amelia, only 1 finger and 2 toes each being attached to the body, with median facial cleft and large fronto-ethmoido-naso-maxillary encephalocele (Fraccaro et al, in preparation).

In 2 of the 3 fetuses, namely in the first aborted fetus of the family with 3 affected sibs and in the monsterlike Italian fetus, cardiovascular malformations were present. They were a small ventricular septal defect and segmental atresia of the left aortic arch, reaching from the origin of the left carotid artery to the junction of the ductus arteriosus with persistence of the right aortic arch and thus formation of an incomplete aortic ring around the trachea and esophagus in 1 fetus (Fig. 6a). In the other fetus an identical atresia of the preductal segment of the left aortic arch with an aorticopulmonary window was found (Fig. 6b).

Roberts syndrome and atresia of the aortic arch are extremely rare conditions. An interrupted aortic arch is found in only 1.3% of children with complex cardiac malformations [45] and in 2 to 3% of aneuploid individuals as, for example, in trisomy 21 or 18 (personal observations). Thus, a chance association of Roberts syndrome and aortic arch anomalies in 2 of 3 investigated fetuses seems to be highly unlikely. Since the aorta and aortic arch derive from the primitive anterior and posterior aorta and the branchial arteries that supply the craniofacial region and branchial pouches, and give rise to the upper limb vessels, and since limbs and head including the branchial arches are mainly involved in the malformation complex of Roberts syndrome, a common pathogenetic pathway, coinciding with a disturbance of the process of obliteration of the branchial arch arteries, could result in the characteristic facial abnormalities and in aortic arch atresia. However, the conclusion that this may represent another example of a developmental

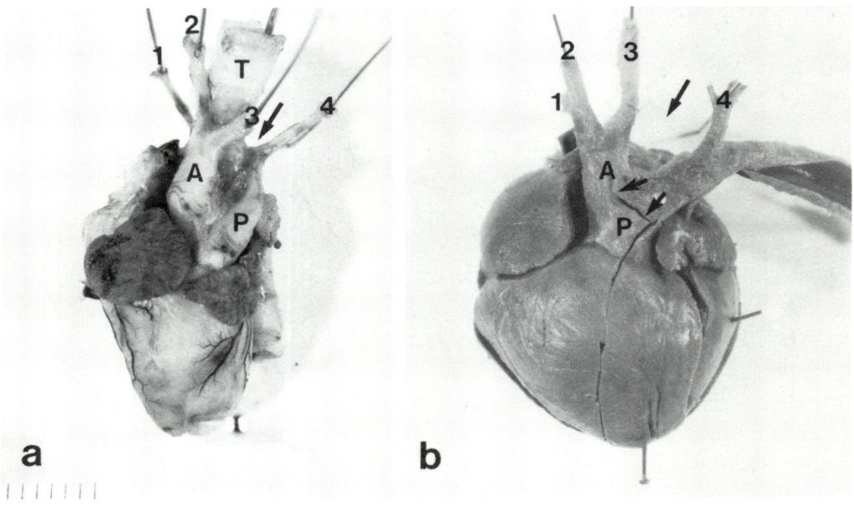

Fig. 6. Frontal aspect of heart and great vessels (a) in a fetus with Roberts syndrome (Fig. 4b) displaying preductal atresia of the left aortic arch (arrow) and persistence of the right aortic arch with incomplete aortic ring around trachea and esophagus; (b) in a monster with severe manifestation of Roberts syndrome showing again interrupted aortic arch (arrow) and additional aorticopulmonary window (arrows). Right subclavian (1) and carotid artery (2), left carotid (3) and subclavian artery (4). T = trachea, A = aorta, P = pulmonary artery and ductus Botalli.

field defect, which, by definition, describes a "dysmorphogenetically reactive unit in different dysmorphogenetic causes" [44], would require similar associations in disorders other than Roberts syndrome, as has been described in the DiGeorge anomaly [45,46]. Aortic arch anomalies may easily be overlooked in small autopsy specimens and should be looked for carefully, especially in cases with severe craniofacial abnormalities.

VATER ASSOCIATION

Different malformations may occur together in varying combinations, but there is a nonrandom tendency for some defects to associate more frequently than others. Thus, ear anomalies have been claimed to be frequently associated with renal anomalies or Wilms tumor or cleft lip and palate with ventricular septal defect of the heart [47]. The VATER association (vertebral anomalies, ventricular septal defect, anal atresia, tracheo-esophageal fistula, esophageal atresia, radial aplasia, and renal malformations) represents another example [48]. It is regarded as "part of a spectrum of congenital anomalies that ranges from the occurrence of any of these defects up to the full set" [49]. The reason that these malformations tend to associate together is not known. A common mesenchymal defect or teratogenetic determination period has been discussed.

Most cases of the VATER association have an unremarkable family or teratogenic history and the recurrence risk is less than 1%. However, some of the above-mentioned abnormalities may concur in etiologically well-defined syndromes such as radial defect, cardiac, renal and ear anomalies, and tracheoesophageal fistula in trisomy 18, radial aplasia and congenital heart defect in autosomal recessive Holt-Oram syndrome; or anal, renal, radial, and ear anomalies in a familial disorder with autosomal dominant transmission [50], in the thalidomide syndrome, or in infants of diabetic mothers [51]. In these conditions the rash diagnosis of a VATER association may lead to faulty recurrence risk counseling.

With respect to the difficulties in interpretation, it was shown that syndromic anal atresia may be associated with numerous malformations but rarely with tracheoesophageal fistula, and vice versa, and that in the presence of both (ie anal atresia and tracheoesophageal fistula), a Mendelian etiology seems to be unlikely [51]. This must alert the pathologist to investigate carefully.

We have seen a male preterm infant, the first child of a 21-year-old mother and a 21-year-old father, with an uneventful family history. It had a full set of VATER anomalies including vertebral anomalies, ventricular septal defect, anal atresia, radial aplasia, unilateral renal agenesis, cleft palate, ear anomalies, and mild hydrocephaly, but with the exception of an esophageal atresia and tracheoesophageal fistula. However, attached to the lower segment of the esophagus, just above the diaphragm, 2 small cysts were found, lined by tracheal mucosa and containing tracheal cartilage within their walls (Fig. 7).

The trachea is formed from the esophagus by longitudinal invagination of mesoderm and septation of the lumen. Disturbance of this developmental process leads to a spectrum of tracheoesophageal malformations of which tracheoesophageal fistula type III (following the classification of Ladd [52]) is the most frequent [53]. This statement accounts for the isolated forms and also for the associated and syndromic TE-fistulas. Other types may occur in any of these conditions.

A bronchogenic cyst attached to the wall of the esophagus may easily escape recognition. It can be interpreted as a mild manifestation of the same developmental disorder that in its severe manifestation presents as tracheo-

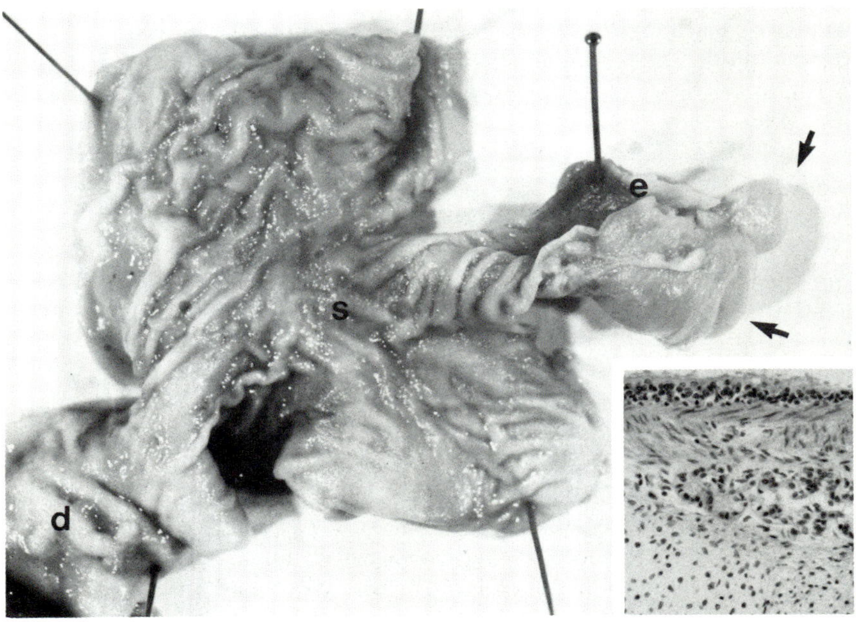

Fig. 7. Dissected stomach (s) with two bronchogenic cysts (arrow) attached to the lower esophagus (e) lined by tracheal mucosa and containing cartilage within the wall (s. insert HE × 160). d = duodenum.

esophageal fistula. In association with anal atresia and other characteristic anomalies it justifies the use of the VATER appellation in the present case.

CONGENITAL TERATOMA

Malformations may not only associate together but also with dysplasias such as tumors. For example Wilms tumor is often found in syndromic or nonsyndromic developmental disorders, as are other dysontogenetic tumors [54]. We have seen neuroblastoma associated with dysraphic malformations, with spina bifida in one case, and with gastroschisis in another.

Congenital teratoma, which in most cases develops at an extragonadal site (mainly the sacrococcygeal area) may be coexistent with various anomalies [55]. Among these, skeletal malformations, especially of the sacrococcygeal bone, predominate and in 1 survey even occurred at a 20% rate [56]. The frequent association with bone defects of the sacrum and coccyx led to the delineation of a familial form of sacrococcygeal teratoma with autosomal dominant transmission. It is characterized by a triad of anorectal malformations, sacral abnormalities, and a presacral tumor, presenting as anterior meningocele, lipoma, hamartoma, dermoid cyst, cystic intestinal duplication, or teratoma [57,58]. It was suggested that when osseous malformations are found in addition to a sacrococcygeal teratoma either in the tumor carrier or in other relatives, they may indicate a genetic etiology [59].

Osseous anomalies in upper segments of the spine have been found coexistent with anterior meningocele and anterior meningoencephalocele, with duplication cysts, namely enterogenic (Fig. 8) and bronchogenic cysts and with pericardial defects [60,61, personal observations], but have not been mentioned in connection with mediastinal or pericardial teratoma.

We have examined a hydropic fetus, the first child of a healthy 26-year-old woman and her 34-year-old husband, that was aborted in the 22nd gestational week with a prenatally diagnosed cardiac tumor. The female fetus had an intrapericardial teratoma that arose at the foot of the aorta, and expanded to the right within the pericardial cavity, compressing the vena cava, heart, and lungs, and thus leading to massive pleural, pericardial, and abdominal effusions and hydrops formation. The teratoma was rather solid with only few cysts and microscopically showed differentiation of acinar, bronchogenic, hepatocellular, neuroectodermal, mesenchymal, and cartilaginous structures. In addition to the intrapericardial teratoma, vertebral anomalies, were present, ie, bifid thoracic vertebrae 8–10 with partial dislocation (Fig. 9). In both parents skeletal abnormalities were excluded.

Intrapericardial teratoma is a rare condition and only 48 cases had been published by 1975 [62,63]. However, since it is characteristically multicystic,

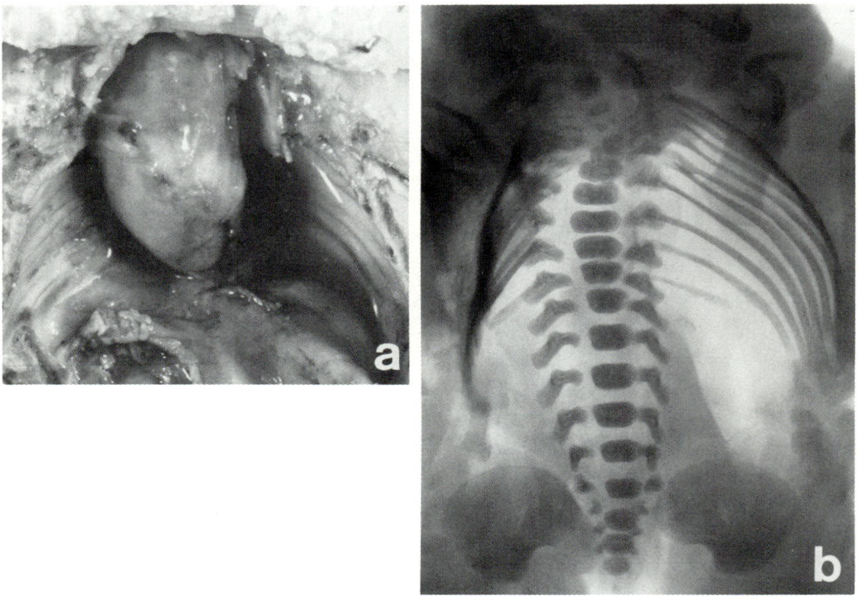

Fig. 8. (a) Enterogenic duplication cyst attached to the thoracic spine. (b) Associated splitting and dislocation of thoracic vertebrae.

some of the cystic tumors diagnosed as bronchogenic cysts are thought to correspond to teratomas.

The question arises whether the development of intrapericardial teratoma of the other above-mentioned conditions and the associated vertebral defects are pathogenetically related, analogous to the triad of anorectal, sacral, and presacral anomalies. Vertebral "splitting" is thought to result in local disturbance in the formation of mesoderm between the neural and enteric tube and, thus, in defective separation of neuroectodermal and entodermal structures [58], whereby the teratoma could arise from persistent pluripotential embryonic cells at this site. This explanation, if applied to the upper spine, would suggest that upper chord splitting may enhance a spectrum of different intrathoracic malformations, including teratomas, and would, thus, extend the scope of the "split notochord syndrome." However, further cases have to be evaluated carefully to exclude coincidental association of vertebral defects of the upper spine, duplication cysts, and intrathoracical teratoma.

MECKEL SYNDROME

Meckel syndrome is a presently well-known autosomal recessive malformation syndrome. In extensive reviews on more than 150 cases, characteristic

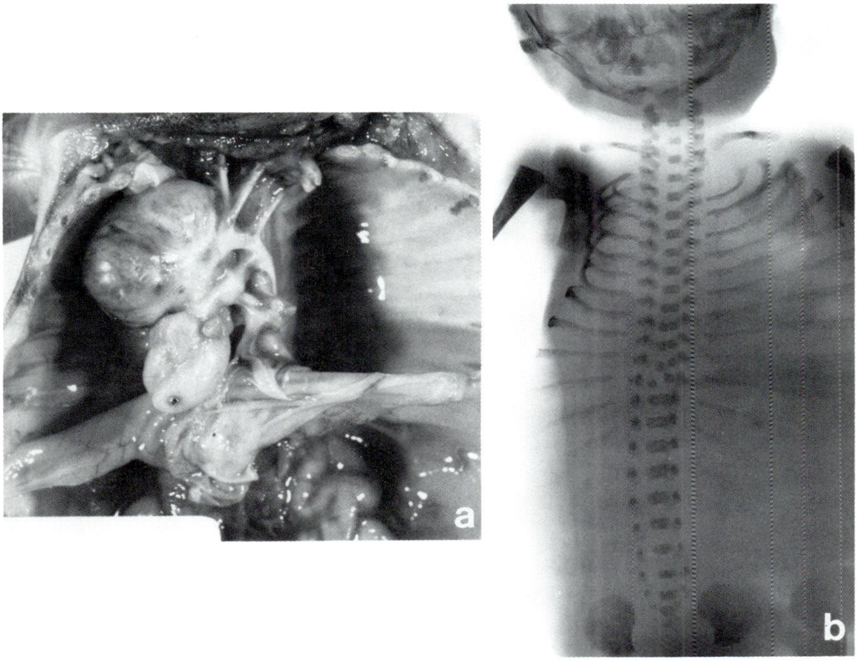

Fig. 9. (a) Intrapericardial teratoma arising from the aortic root. (b) Associated splitting and dislocation of thoracic vertebrae.

anomalies were listed; among these, occipital encephalocele, polydactyly, and polycystic kidneys represent major diagnostic signs, while other more or less frequent findings such as arrhinencephaly, hydrocephaly, anencephaly, cleft lip and/or palate, lobulated tongue, microphthalmia, retinal dysplasia, cardiac, hepatic, urinary tract, and genital anomalies, are thought to be of secondary diagnostic significance [64–69]. We described 5 cases of Meckel syndrome that, in addition to an apical occipital encephalocele, had a second defect of the basal occipital bone with occult cerebellar encephalocele [70].

The finding of an additional lower occipital bone defect with or without meningocele was confirmed in 7 cases of Meckel syndrome by Paetau et al [71], but was definitely excluded in 1 by the same authors, suggesting its frequent, though not consistent, occurrence in this disorder. Meanwhile, we have studied 8 further Meckel syndrome fetuses (Table I) and were able to demonstrate a second basal occipital bone defect of varying size in each of these. In 3 fetuses the defect was rather large, leaving only a small osseous bridge between the 2 occipital gaps and extending onto the first to second

TABLE I. Clinical Manifestations of 8 Fetuses With Meckel Syndrome

Case No.	1	2	3	4	5	6	7	8
Sex	♂	♂	♂	♂	♂	♂	♂	♂
Weight (g)	780	3,000	2,720	700	340	295	2,180	1,300
Crown-rump-/crown-heel-length (cm)	19/29	?/49	33/40	19,5/28,5	16/22,5	16,5/24,5	30/46	24/34,5
Apical occipital encephalocele	+	+	+	+	+	+	+	+
Occipitocervical encephalocele +/bone defect (+)	(+)	+	+	(+)	+	+	+	+
Microcephaly	+	+	+	+	+	−	+	+
Arrhinencephaly +/holoprosencephaly ++	+	++	++	−	−	−	−	+
Sloping forehead	+	+	+	+	−	−	−	+
Hypertelorism	+	+	+	+	+	+	+	+
Macrostomia	+	+	+	+	+	+	+	+
Retro-/microgenia	+	+	+	−	+	+	+	+
Large, apparently low-set ears	+	+	+	+	+	+	+	+
Cleft palate +/cleft uvula (+)	(+)	+	+	+	+	+	−	+
Lobulated tongue	−	+	+	+	+	+	−	+
Polydactyly	6 6 6 6	5 5 5 5	6 5 6 6	6 6 6 6	6 5 6 6	5 6 6 6	5 5 5 5	6 6 6 6
Clubfeet	+	−	+	+	+	−	+	+
Polycystic kidneys	+	+	+	+*	+	+	+	+
Intrahepatic bile duct proliferation	+	+	+	+	Cysts	+	+	+
Pancreatic duct dilatation	−	+	+	+	+	−	+	+
Cystic epididymis	+	+	+	+	+	+	+	+
Hypoplastic genitalia	+	−	+	+	+	+	−	+
Hypoplastic lungs	+	+	+	+	+	+	+	+
Cardiac +/vascular anomaly (+)	(+)	−	−	−	−	−	−	−
Additional minor anomalies	+	+	+	+	+	+	+	+

*Cystic horseshoe kidney.

vertebral arch. Partially hemorrhagic cerebellar and spinal tissue was penetrating through the opening into a herniated meningeal sac, thus forming a subcutaneous occipitocervical meningoencephalocele. In 3 cases the lower bone defect and cerebellar herniation were less extensive, and in the remaining 2 cases there was only an angular extension of an enlarged foramen magnum covered by galeal membrane, preventing meningeal and cerebellar herniation (Fig. 10).

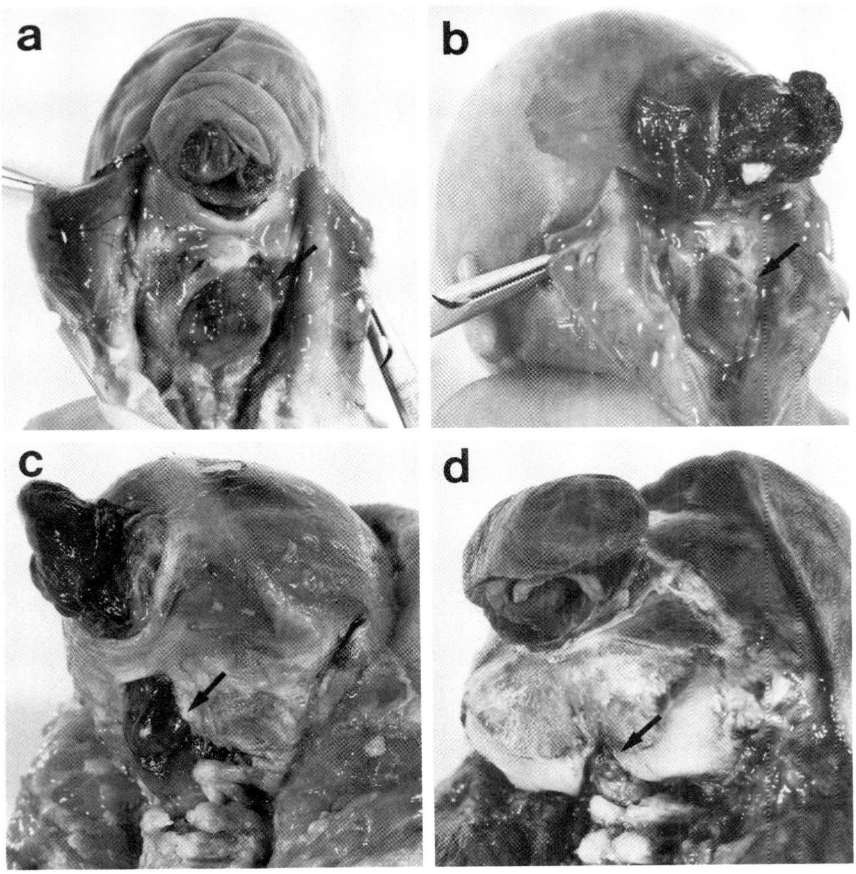

Fig. 10. Meckel syndrome: Occipital encephalocele and associated second bone defect of the basal occiput with (a–c) or without (d) additional occipitocervical encephalocele (arrow) (s. Table I, a = case 6, b = case 5, c = case 2, d = case 1).

The association of 2 cranial clefts in the apical and basal occiput certainly seems unique at first look. Whether this type of dysraphic malformation is characteristic of Meckel syndrome, in which even more extensive cranioschisis and rachischisis have been observed [71], or whether it may also occur in nonsyndromic encephalocele cases, reflecting the complicated sequence of neural tube closure in humans, remains an open question at present, since occult occipitocervical dysraphias are easily missed and thus, may escape recognition.

ACKNOWLEDGMENTS

We are gratefully indebted to Prof. W. Kuhn, Frauenklinik der Universität Göttingen; Prof. F. Lehmann, Städtische Krankenanstalten Bielefeld; Prof. F. Oberheuser, Frauenklinik der Medizinischen Universität zu Lübeck; Prof. R. Rauskolb, Albert-Schweitzer-Krankenhaus Northeim; Dr. E. Schmolling, Knappschafts-Krankenhaus Recklinghausen; Prof. J. Schneider, Frauenklinik der Medizinischen Hochschule Hannover; Prof. H. Schultze-Mosgau, Stadtkrankenhaus Cuxhaven; and Dr. V. Zimmeck, Friederikenstift Hannover, for providing the fetuses and clinical data. Furthermore, we thank Prof. I. Anton-Lamprecht for constructive criticism of the piece on the Herlitz syndrome, and Irene Gausmann, Edith Albinski, and Marianne Kock for their skillful technical and editorial assistance.

This work was supported by a grant of the Deutsche Forschungsgemeinschaft to H.R. (Re 429/5-6).

REFERENCES

1. Opitz JM, Gilbert EF: Pathogenetic analysis of congenital anomalies in humans. Pathobiol Ann 12:301–349, 1982.
2. Gedde-Dahl T: Sixteen types of epidermolysis bullosa. Acta Dermatovener, Suppl 95:74–87, 1981.
3. Gedde-Dahl T, Anton-Lamprecht I: Epidermolysis bullosa. In Emery AEH, Rimoin DL (eds): "Principles and Practice of Medical Genetics." Edinburgh, London, Melbourne, New York: Churchill Livingstone, 1983, pp 672–687.
4. Pearson RW, Potter B, Strauss F: Epidermolysis bullosa hereditaria letalis. Clinical and histological manifestations and course of the disease. Arch Dermatol 109:349–355, 1974.
5. Hashimoto I, Gedde-Dahl T, Schnyder UW, Anton-Lamprecht I: Ultrastructural studies in epidermolysis bullosa hereditaria. IV. Recessive dystrophic types with junctional blistering. Arch Dermatol Res 257:17–32, 1976.
6. Anton-Lamprecht I, Schnyder UW: Zur Ultrastruktur der Epidermolysen mit junktionaler Blasenbildung. Dermatologica 159:377–382, 1979.
7. Korber JS, Glasson MJ: Pyloric atresia associated with epidermolysis bullosa. J Pediatr 90:600–601, 1977.

8. Garcia-Valles MC, Caro AM, Orgaz AH: Atresia del piloro y epidermolysis ampollosa. Una coincidencia? An Esp Pediat 10:745–750, 1977.
9. Pederson PV, Hertel J: Pyloric atresia and epidermolysis bullosa. J Pediatr 91:852–853, 1977.
10. DeGroot WG, Postuma R, Hunter AGW: Familial pyloric atresia associated with epidermolysis bullosa. J Pediatr 92:429–431, 1978.
11. Swinburne LM, Kohler HG, Terrace H: Familial pyloric atresia associated with epidermolysis bullosa. J Pediatr 94:162, 1979.
12. El Shafie M, Stidham GL, Klippel CH, Katzman GH, Weinfeld JJ: Pyloric atresia and epidermolysis bullosa letalis: A lethal combination in two premature newborn siblings. J Pediatr Surg 14:446–449, 1979.
13. Adashi EY, Louis FJ, Vasquez M: An unusual case of epidermolysis bullosa hereditaria letalis with cutaneous scarring and pyloric atresia. J Pediatr 96:443–446, 1980.
14. Peltier FA, Tschen EH, Raimer SS, Kuo TT: Epidermolysis bullosa letalis associated with congenital pyloric atresia. Arch Dermatol 117:728–731, 1981.
15. Honig PJ, Yoder M, Ziegler M: Acquired pyloric obstruction in a patient with epidermolysis bullosa letalis. J Pediatr 102:598–600, 1983.
16. Chang CH, Perrin EV, Bove KE: Pyloric atresia associated with epidermolysis bullosa: Special reference to pathogenesis. Pediatr Pathol 1:449–457, 1983.
17. Anton-Lamprecht I: Prenatal diagnosis of genetic disorders of the skin by means of electron microscopy. Hum Genet 59:392–405, 1981.
18. Parrish RA, Kanavage CB, Wells JA, Moretz WH: Congenital antral membrane. Surg Gynecol Obstet 127:999–1004, 1968.
19. Thompson NW, Parker W, Schwartz S, Holt JF: Congenital pyloric atresia. Arch Surg 97:792–796, 1968.
20. Therkelsen AJ, Rehder H: Intestinal atresia caused by second trimester amniocentesis. Case report. Br J Obstet Gynaecol 88:559–562, 1981.
21. Bergenholtz A, Olsson O, Arwill T, Lundström N-R: Die Epidermolysis bullosa hereditaria dystrophica mit Oesophagusveränderungen. Arch Klin Exper Dermatol 217:518–533, 1963.
22. Katz J, Gryboski JD, Rosenbaum HM, Spiro HM: Dysphagia in children with epidermolysis bullosa. Gastroenterology 52:259–262, 1967.
23. Thompson JW, Ahmed AR, Dudley JP: Epidermolysis bullosa dystrophica of the larynx and trachea. Acute air way obstruction. Ann Otol 89:428–429, 1980.
24. Hillemeier C, Touloukian R, McCallum R, Gryboski J: Esophageal web: A previously unrecognized complication of epidermolysis bullosa. Pediatrics 67:678–682, 1981.
25. Anton-Lamprecht I, Arnold ML, Holbrook KA: Methodology in sampling of fetal skin and pitfalls in the interpretation of fetal skin specimens. Semin Dermatol 3:203–215, 1984.
26. Roberts JB: A child with double cleft of lip and palate, protrusion of the intermaxillary portion of the upper jaw and imperfect development of the bones of the four extremities. Ann Surg 70:252–253, 1919.
27. Appelt H, Gerken H, Lenz W: Tetraphokomelie mit Lippen-Kiefer-Gaumenspalte und Clitorishypertrophie - ein Syndrom. Paediatr Paedol 2:119–124, 1966.
28. Judge C: A sibship with the pseudothalidomide syndrome and an association with Rh incompatibility. Med J Aust 2:280–281, 1973.
29. Freeman MVR, Williams DW, Schimke RN, Temtamy SA, Vachier E, German J: The Roberts syndrome. Clin Genet 5:1–16, 1974.

30. Grosse FR, Pandel C, Wiedemann HR: The tetraphocomelia-cleft palate syndrome. Description of a new case. Humangenetik 28:353–356, 1975.
31. Zergollern L, Hitrec V: Three siblings with Robert's syndrome. Clin Genet 9:433–436, 1976.
32. Zergollern L, Hitrec V: Four siblings with Robert's syndrome. Clin Genet 21:1–6, 1982.
33. Mann NP, Fitzsimmons J, Fitzsimmons E, Cook P: Roberts syndrome: Clinical and cytogenetic aspects. J Med Genet 19:116–119, 1982.
34. Herrmann J, Feingold M, Tuffli A, Opitz JM: A familial dysmorphogenetic syndrome of limb deformities, characteristic facial appearance and associated anomalies: The "pseudothalidomide" or "SC-syndrome." In Bergsma D (ed): "Limb Malformations." March of Dimes Birth Defects Foundation. BD:OAS V(3):81–89, 1969.
35. Hall BD, Greenberg MH: Hypomelia-hypotrichosis-facial hemangioma syndrome (Pseudothalidomide, SC syndrome, SC phocomelia syndrome). Am J Dis Child 123:602–604, 1972.
36. Herrmann J, Opitz JM: The SC phocomelia and the Roberts syndrome: Nosologic aspects. Eur J Pediat 125:117–134, 1977.
37. Tomkins D, Hunter A, Roberts M: Cytogenetic findings in Roberts-SC phocomelia syndrome. Am J Med Genet 4:17–26, 1979.
38. German J: Robert's syndrome. I. Cytological evidence for a disturbance in chromatin pairing. Clin Genet 16:441–447, 1979.
39. Quazi QH, Kassner EG, Masakawa A, Madahar C, Choi SJ: The SC phocomelia syndrome: Report of two cases with cytogenetic abnormality. Am J Med Genet 4:231–238, 1979.
40. Tomkins DJ, Sisken JE: Abnormalities in the cell-division cycle in Roberts syndrome fibroblasts: A cellular basis for the phenotypic characteristics? Am J Hum Genet 36:1332–1340, 1984.
41. Waldenmaier C, Aldenhoff P, Klemm T: The Roberts' syndrome. Hum Genet 40:345–349, 1978.
42. Leonard P, Rendle-Short J, Shardoon L: Roberts'-SC phocomelia syndrome with cytogenetic findings. Hum Genet 60:379–380, 1982.
43. Römke C, Froster-Iskenius U, Heyne K, Hof M, Grzejzcyk G, Rauskolb R, Rehder H, Schwinger E: Roberts syndrome and SC phocomelia. A single genetic entity? Clin Genet submitted.
44. Opitz JM: Editorial Comment: The development field concept. Am J Med Genet 21:1–11, 1985.
45. Freedom RM, Rosen FS, Nadas AS: Congenital cardiovascular disease and anomalies of the third and fourth pharyngeal pouch. Circulation 46:165–172, 1972.
46. Conley ME, Beckwith JB, Mancer KFK, Tenkhoff L: The spectrum of the DiGeorge syndrome. J Pediatr 94:883–890, 1979.
47. Hilson D: Malformation of ears as sign of malformation of genito-urinary tract. Br Med J 2:785–789, 1957.
48. Quan L, Smith DW: The VATER association. J Pediatr 82:104–107, 1973.
49. Barry JE, Auldist AW: The VATER association. One end of a spectrum of anomalies. Am J Dis Child 128:769–771, 1974.
50. Kurnit DM, Steele MW, Pinsky L, Dibbins A: Autosomal dominant transmission of a syndrome of anal, ear, renal, and radial congenital malformations. J Pediatr 93:270–273, 1978.
51. Pinsky L: The syndromology of anorectal malformation (atresia, stenosis, ectopia). Am J Med Genet 1:461–474, 1978.

52. Ladd WE: Surgical treatment of esophageal atresia and tracheoesophageal fistulas. N Engl J Med 230:625–637, 1944.
53. Morison JE (ed): "Foetal and Neonatal Pathology." London: Butterworths, 1963.
54. Mulvihill JJ, Miller RW, Fraumeni JF Jr (eds): "Genetics of Human Cancer." New York, Raven Press, 1977.
55. Altmann RP, Randolph JG, Lilly JR: Sacrococcygeal teratoma: American Academy of Pediatrics Surgical Section Survey - 1973. J Pediatr Surg 9:389–398, 1974.
56. Conklin J, Abell MR: Germ cell neoplasms of the sacrococcygeal region. Cancer 20:2105–2117, 1967.
57. Hunt PT, Davidson KC, Ashcraft KW, Holder TW: Radiography of hereditary presacral teratoma. Radiology 122:187–191, 1977.
58. Currarino G, Coln D, Votteler T: Triad of anorectal, sacral and presacral anomalies. Am J Roentgenol 137:395–398, 1981.
59. Davidson KC: Hereditary presacral teratoma (letter to the editor). JAMA 237:2286–2287, 1977.
60. Haller JA, Mazur DO, Morgan WW: Diagnosis and management of mediastinal mass in children. J Thoracic Cardiovasc Surg 58:385–393, 1969.
61. Vaage S, Knutrud O: Congenital duplications of the alimentary tract with special regard to their embryogenesis. A follow-up study in 16 surgically corrected cases. Prog Pediatr Surg 7:103–123, 1974.
62. Torres-Aybar FG, Basora G, López-Busquets RH, Rodríguez-Estapé HF: Intrapericardial teratoma: A cause of cardiac tamponade in infancy. Bol Assoc Med PR 67:366–368, 1975.
63. Gonzalez-Crussi F (ed): "Extragonadal Teratomas." Washington Armed Forces Inst. Pathol., 1982.
64. Opitz JM, Howe JJ: The Meckel syndrome (Dysencephalia splanchnocystica, the Gruber syndrome). Birth Defects. BD:OAS V/(2):167–179, 1969.
65. Mecke S, Passarge E: Encephalocele, polycystic kidneys and polydactyly as an autosomal recessive trait simulating certain other disorders: The Meckel syndrome. Ann Génét 14:97–103, 1971.
66. Fraser FC, Lytwyn A: Spectrum of anomalies in the Meckel syndrome, or maybe there is a malformation syndrome with at least one constant anomaly. Am J Med Genet 9:67–73, 1981.
67. Moerman P, Verbeken W, Fryns JP, Goddeeris P, Lauweryns JM: The Meckel syndrome. Pathological and cytogenetic observations in eight cases. Hum Genet 62:240–245, 1982.
68. Salonen R, Norio R: The Meckel syndrome in Finland: Epidemiologic and genetic aspects. Am J Med Genet 18:691–698, 1984.
69. Rapola J, Salonen R: Visceral anomalies in the Meckel syndrome. Teratology 31:193–201, 1985.
70. Rehder H, Labbé F: Prenatal morphology in Meckel's syndrome (with special reference to polycystic kidneys and double encephalocele). Prenat Diag 1:161–172, 1981.
71. Paetau A, Salonen R, Haltia M: Brain pathology in the Meckel syndrome: A study of 59 cases. Clin Neuropath 4:56–62, 1985.

Anatomic and Chromosome Anomalies in Specimens of Early Spontaneous Abortion: Seven-Year Experience

Dagmar K. Kalousek, MD

Department of Pathology, B.C. Children's Hospital and University of British Columbia, Vancouver, B.C., Canada

INTRODUCTION

It has been recognized for a long time that spontaneous pregnancy loss in humans represents about 15 to 20% of *clinically recognized* pregnancies [1]. The causes of spontaneous intrauterine death vary greatly with the developmental age of the conceptus. The probability of spontaneous demise of the conceptus is highest in early pregnancy. Nearly half of all embryonic loss is associated with chromosome abnormalities [2]. The incidence of localized and systemic defects in embryonic morphogenesis is reported to be high in spontaneously and therapeutically aborted embryos [3–5]. The effects of various gene(s) defects on early embryonic developments are largely unknown in humans.

There are many reasons for pathologists to study the specimens of early spontaneous abortions. Much more needs to be learned about morphologic abnormalities in embryos to understand their significance and the pathogenesis of common developmental defects detected at birth. At the present time even the distinctions between "normal" and "abnormal" embryonic morphology are often exceedingly difficult to make since we do not yet know, in many instances, how continued growth and development affect the potential disability of conceptuses with borderline embryonic abnormalities such as moderate localized posterior edema. In case of spontaneous pregnancy loss,

Birth Defects: Original Article Series, Volume 23, Number 1, pages 153–168

especially when it is a repeated event, the parents are anxious to know the chance of an embryonic/fetal abnormality recurring in a subsequent pregnancy or the chance of repeated loss. These are very practical questions and pathologists have an essential role to play in supplying the scientific basis for follow-up genetic counseling and prenatal management of future pregnancies.

In this paper the results of detailed morphologic studies on 1794 specimens of early spontaneous abortions supplemented by cytogenetic analysis of 460 specimens are reported and the clinical significance of such studies is discussed.

MATERIALS AND METHODS

During the 7-year period (1978–84) the Embryofetopathology Laboratory at the Children's Hospital (previously Vancouver General Hospital) received and examined 1794 early spontaneous abortion specimens from singleton pregnancies.

An early spontaneous abortion is defined here as the spontaneous loss of a recognized intrauterine pregnancy before 12 completed gestational weeks, or a specimen consisting of a gestational sac with an embryo. An embryo has been defined as a developing human measuring 30 mm or less in crown-rump length (CRL). Well-developed embryos more than 10 mm in length were evaluated developmentally by external characteristics based on Streeter's and O'Rahilly's classifications [6–8]. The actual developmental age of embryos was derived from their CRL and developmental stage [9]. The diagnosis of isolated or combined localized external defects(s) was made after the evaluation of developmental stage. Due to incomplete morphogenesis during the embryonic period, the diagnosis of a specific defect present in an embryo depends heavily on the correct evaluation of the developmental stage. Degenerated and partially fragmented embryos were not evaluated for the presence of localized defects. The term "embryonic growth disorganization" was used as suggested by Poland and Miller [10] with minor modifications [11].

As indicated above, the actual developmental age was derived from the CRL and developmental stage of the embryo. The developmental age was 14 days less than the number of days between the first day of the last menstrual period and the day of abortion (gestational age). The discrepancy between the developmental age derived from morphology of embryos and calculated gestational age reflected the length of time of retention *in utero* after embryonic death and generally correlated with the finding of macerated or severely damaged embryo.

All specimens were examined under the dissecting microscope and histologically. Of the 582 specimens in which gestational sac tissue was set up in tissue culture, a karyotype was obtained in 460 specimens. The specimens selected for tissue culture and cytogenetic analysis originated from pregnancies in which the mothers had previously had one or more spontaneous abortion(s).

Cell cultures for cytogenetic studies were initiated from amnion and chorion whenever possible. The chorionic villi were cleaned from decidual contamination under dissecting microscope. In many specimens of ruptured or fragmented chorionic sac only chorionic villi alone were used for cell culture initiation.

RESULTS

Specimen Morphology

Table I provides general description of 1794 specimens studied. It shows that 11.9% of specimens contained no embryonic/fetal tissue, but consisted of maternal decidua. The largest group was represented by ruptured or fragmented gestational sacs with no embryo proper (38.5%). Some of these sacs were well formed with abundant chorionic villi, amnion, and a portion of cord/body stalk; others were represented only by isolated clusters of chorionic villi. Embryonic growth disorganization was detected in 24% of all specimens and in 48% of complete specimens. A large proportion of these specimens (190) consisted of *intact empty sacs* (Fig. 1). These specimens were designated *GD1*, representing complete or very early failure of devel-

TABLE I. Specimen Morphology

	Total specimens			
Morphology	N	%	N	%
GD1			190	10.6
GD2	430	24.0	128	7.1
GD3			97	5.4
GD4			15	0.8
Normal embryos			187	10.4
Embryos with localized defect(s)	461	25.7	140	7.8
Fragmented/degenerating embryos			134	7.5
Ruptured sacs	690	38.5	282	15.7
Fragmented sacs			408	22.7
Decidua	213	11.9	213	11.9
Total	1,794	100.0	1,794	100.0

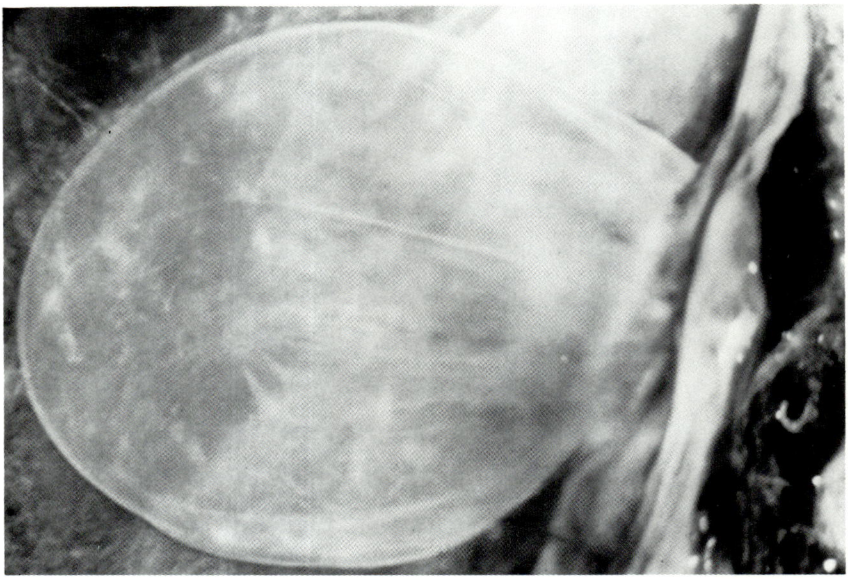

Fig. 1. Empty intact chorionic sac (GD1) with severely reduced chorionic villi development and no indication of the presence of amniotic sac and embryo in it.

opment of the embryo proper. The intact sacs usually contained mucoid fluid with no evidence of an embryo or body stalk. Amnion, if present, was closely applied to the chorion and structurally abnormal. Chorionic villi of these sacs were usually sparse, clubbed, and cystic. Microscopically they were vascular and hydropic with attenuated trophoblast.

GD2 specimens (Fig. 2) consisted of a chorionic sac containing solid embryonic tissue 1–4 mm in length with no recognizable external features and no retinal pigment. This embryonic tissue was either firmly attached to the internal aspect of amnion or a short body stalk could be identified in these specimens. A yolk sac could be easily distinguished from the embryo proper by its position between amnion and chorionic plate. The chorionic villi and amnion showed similar abnormalities as in GD1.

GD3 specimens (Fig. 3) represented elongated smooth embryos up to 10 mm long without any morphologic hallmarks but with retinal pigment identifying a cephalic pole. Sparse, hypoplastic villi showing focal hydropic degeneration were common in these conceptions.

GD4 embryos (Fig. 4) were the least common. They consisted mainly of a recognizable head, trunk, and limb buds characterized by developmental

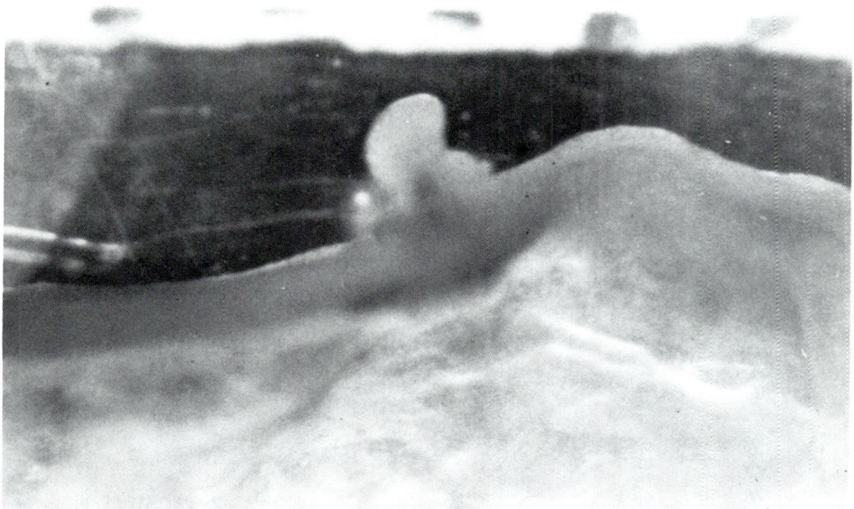

Fig. 2. Typical GD2 specimen showing a globular mass of embryonic tissue 2 mm in diameter without any evidence of internal or external organization. This tissue is attached to the internal aspect of amnion.

inconsistency such as a head too small for developmental age established by embryonic length (usually 10–15 mm) or marked retardation in upper and lower limb development.

Normal embryos (Fig. 5) were classified as such when harmonious development at a certain stage corresponded to CRL. There were 187 specimens found to contain a morphologically normal embryo.

Embryos with isolated or combined external localized defects (Fig. 6) were seen in 7.8% of specimens. These defects were detected on external examination as internal dissection or serial histologic sectioning were not employed. Due to incomplete morphogenesis during the embryonic period, the diagnosis of a specific defect in an embryo depends heavily on the correct evaluation of the developmental stage. Table II shows 5 different types of specific localized defects described in embryos. Those listed as embryos with combined defects were more advanced in their development than typical GD4 embryos and had more than one developmental defect.

Degenerated and fragmented embryos (Fig. 7) represented 7.5% of total specimens; approximately 1/3 of specimens contained embryos without any evidence of growth disorganization.

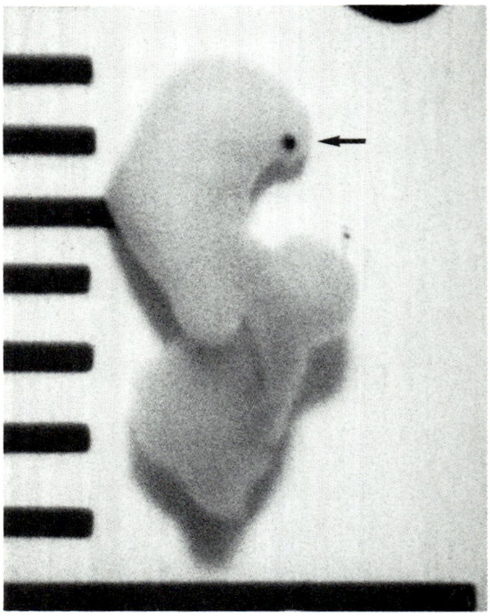

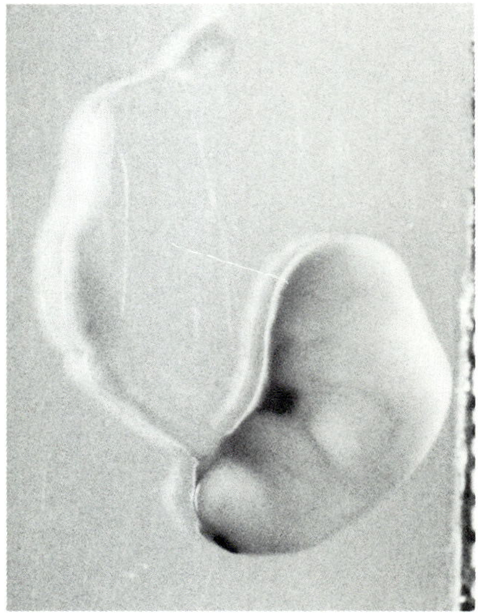

Fig. 3. GD3 specimen (left) presenting a typical polarization of nodular-shaped embryo with its cranial end marked by retinal pigment (arrow). The lack of any other differentiation in this 4-mm long embryo is obvious.

Fig. 4. GD4 embryo (right) showing the basic external structures such as head, rudimentary face, limb bud asynchrony. No specific localized defects are noted. Darkly pigmented areas represent subectodermal hemorrhages.

Specimen Morphology and Chromosome Anomalies

Of the 1794 specimens studied morphologically, 573 were set up in tissue culture and 460 (80.2%) were successfully grown and analyzed cytogenetically. The overall rate of chromosome anomalies was 59.1%. The highest rate of chromosome defects, 93.3%, was found in a category of embryos with one or more localized defects; the lowest rate, 20%, was found in the category of morphologically normal embryos. The data are detailed in Table III.

Table IV shows correlation of specimen morphology and cytogenetic findings. The different types of chromosome trisomies and their morphologic presentation are listed in Table V.

Table VI divides the chromosome defects into 3 major categories defined by their likelihood to be detected in liveborn infants and relates these 3 categories to specimen morphology. More embryos with localized defects and significantly less embryonic growth disorganization are seen in a group

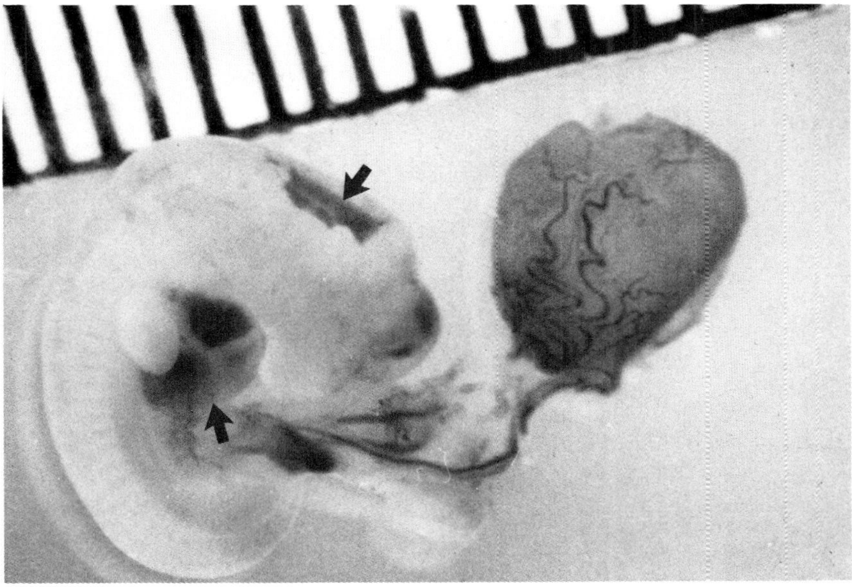

Fig. 5. C-shaped human embryo measuring 8 mm in length with cord and yolk sac. Lens vesicles are visible. Upper limb shows hand plate, lower limb is paddle shaped. Cervical sinus and heart bulge are marked with arrow. These morphologic features are consistent with stage 15, developmental age 33–36 days.

of chromosome defects compatible with intrauterine survival than among chromosome defects that generally do not allow survival to term. There is no significant difference in specimen morphology between the category of chromosome defects rarely compatible with intrauterine survival and surviving to term in significant percentage of gestations.

Specific chromosome rearrangements are listed in Table VII and are related to specimen morphology. The same is shown for double trisomies in Table VIII.

DISCUSSION

When a pregnancy fails and a spontaneous abortion results, the questions of "cause" and "risk of recurrence" are likely to arise. The detailed examination of early spontaneous abortion specimens by pathologists provides important information relating to the developmental age and morphology of the conceptus. It also allows for conclusions regarding the course of sponta-

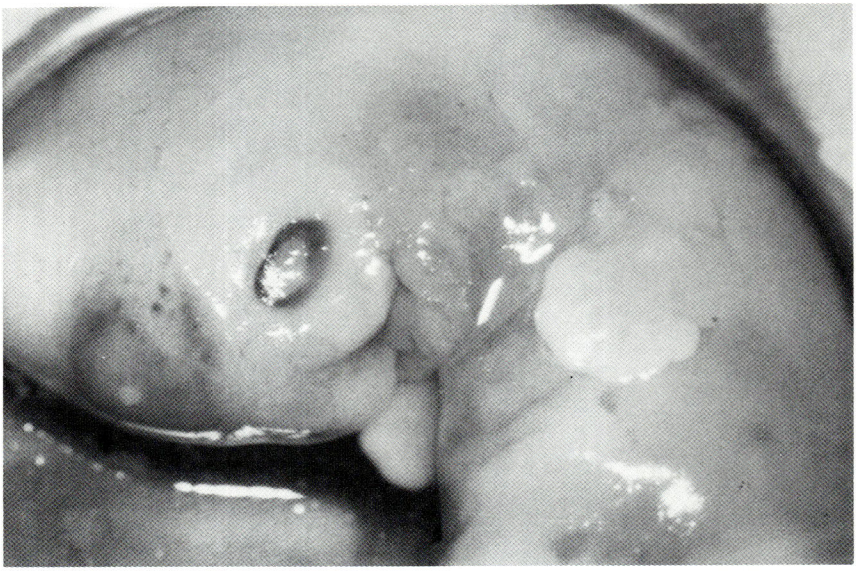

Fig. 6. Multiple defects consisting of digital polydactyly, facial midline cleft, and frontal encephalocoele are demonstrated. Embryo is stage 19, 45 developmental days, measures 17 mm CRL.

TABLE II. Spectrum of Localized Defects Observed in 140 Embryonic Specimens

Morphologic defect(s)	No.	%
Isolated CNS defects	40	28.6
Isolated facial cleft	6	4.3
Isolated limb defects	22	15.7
Combined defects*	64	45.7
Other unusual defects†	8	5.7

*Examples of combined defects are as follows: (1) spina bifida, absent cervical flexion, short cord; (2) microcephaly, absent cervical flexion, facial "dysplasia," delayed development of limb buds, bulge of neural tissue in lower lumbar area.

†Examples of other defects are as follows: (1) fused mouth; (2) amnion attached to anterior body wall starting at heart bulge and continuing to below body stalk.

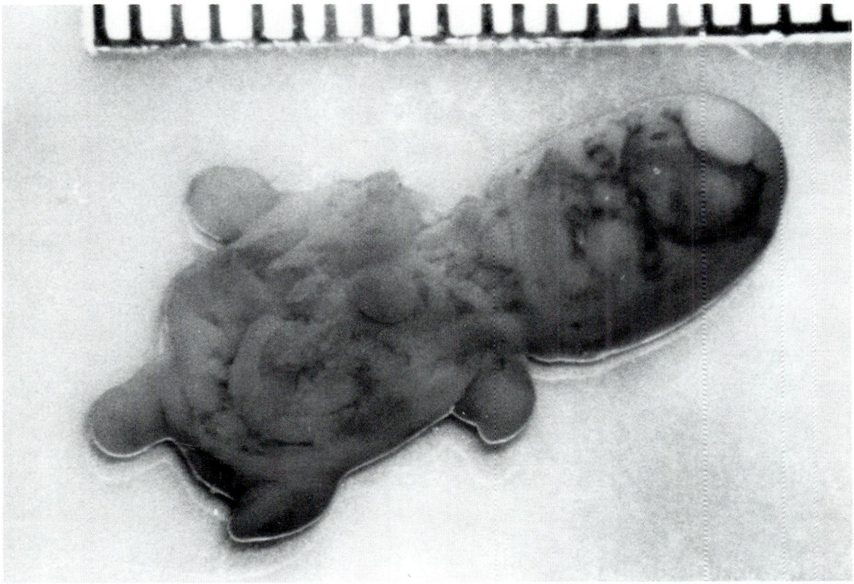

Fig. 7. Severe generalized damage due to maceration in embryo approximately stage 17, developmental age 39 days, CRL 12 mm.

neous pregnancy loss or failure of normal embryonic development and provides the basis for counseling the parents.

Examination of embryos is as important as performing perinatal postmortem examination. This can best be illustrated on example of specific localized defects such as neural tube defects, cleft lip, and limb defects. A much higher incidence of these defects has been described among embryos as compared to liveborn infants by several investigators [4,5,12]. The probability of recurrence of these defects in future pregnancies is generally around 2% to 5%, since they are most likely to be multifactorially determined. It may be much higher in case of autosomal dominant or recessive gene or lower if the defects represent an aneuploidy syndrome, such as a neural tube defect in triploidy. A complete investigation of these specimens is indicated to distinguish between nonchromosomal and chromosomal causes of malformation. Although the results in this study indicate a very high incidence of chromosome defects among embryos with specific localized defects, it must be remembered that specimens were selected for chromosome analysis on the basis of parental reproductive history rather than specimen morphology.

TABLE III. Summary of Specimen Morphology and Cytogenetic Findings

Morphology	Total specimens	Total specimens karyotyped		Specimen with abnormal karyotypes		Specimens with normal karyotypes	
		No.	%†	No.	%‡	No.	%*
GD1	190	37	19.5	22	59.4	15	40.6
GD2	128	22	17.2	16	72.7	6	27.3
GD3	97	21	21.6	11	52.4	10	47.6
GD4	15	8	53.3	3	37.5	5	62.5
Normal embryos	187	45	24.1	9	20.0	36	80.0
Embryos with localized defect(s)	140	90	64.3	84	93.3	6	6.7
Fragmented/degenerating embryos	134	32	23.9	24	75.0	8	25.0
Ruptured/fragmented sacs	690	205	29.7	103	50.2	102	49.8
Decidua	213	—	—	—	—	—	—
Total	1,794	460	25.5	272	59.1	188	40.9

†Percentage of each morphologic group successfully karyotyped.
‡Percentage of those karyotyped with an abnormal karyotype.
*Percentage of those karyotyped with a normal karyotype.

TABLE IV. Correlations of Morphology and Karyotype in 573 Specimens Submitted for Tissue Culture and Cytogenetics

Morphology	Normal karyotype	Trisomy	X Monosomy	Triploidy	Tetra-ploidy	Structural rearrangement	Double trisomy	Failure to grow in culture
GD1	15	12*	2	1	3	3	1	13
GD2	6	12		2	1			9
GD3	10	10				1	1	4
GD4	5	2	1					1
Normal embryos	32	4	5	3		1		12
Embryos with localized defect(s)	10	26	18	25		7	3	15
Fragmented/degenerating embryos	8	12	2	7		2	1	7
Ruptured/fragmented sacs	102	57	14	21	2	9	1	52
Total	188	135	42	59	6	23	7	113

*One with a marker chromosome

TABLE V. Correlations Between Specimen Morphology and Individual Chromosome Trisomies

Morphology	Trisomy* of chromosome																			
	2	3	4	6	7	8	9	10	11	13	14	15	16	18	19	20	21	22	X	Total
GD1	3		1			1		1				1	2			1		1		11[†]
GD2	1		2							1			4		1			3		12
GD3		2				1		1			1	1	3					1		10
GD4													1					1		2
Normal embryos													1	1			1	1		4
Embryos with localized defect(s)			1		1					7	3	1	3	1			2	7		26
Fragmented/ degenerating embryos										3	1	2					4	2		12
Ruptured/ fragmented sacs	1	1		1	2	1	3	1	2	4	2	4	18	2			2	12	1	57
Total	5	3	4	1	3	3	3	3	2	15	7	9	32	4	1	1	9	28	1	134

*Trisomies 1,5,12,17 not observed.
[†]Marker chromosome not included.

TABLE VI. Correlation of Three Categories of Chromosome Abnormalities Defined by Their Frequency of Survival to Term, with Degree of Embryonic Development as Indicated by Specimen Morphology

Frequency of survival to term		GD1-GD4	Normal embryos	Sacs with localized embryos	Fragmented/ degenerated embryos	Ruptured/ fragmented sacs	Total
Never survive to term*	N	30	1	9	3	34	77
	%	39.0	1.3	11.7	3.9	44.2	100
Rarely survive to term†	N	11	4	32	9	37	93
	%	18.0	4.3	34.4	9.7	39.8	100
Survive to term in significant percentage of gestations‡	N	4	7	28	9	23	71
	%	5.6	9.9	39.4	12.7	32.4	100

*Trisomies 2,3,4,6,7,10,11,14,15,16,19,20, tetraploidy.
†Trisomies 8,9,22, triploidy.
‡Trisomies 13,18,21,47,XXY, monosomy X.

TABLE VII. Correlation Between Specimen Morphology and Structural Rearrangements of Individual Chromosomes

Morphology	Structural rearrangement	
GD1	46,XY,4q+	
	46,XY,del(13q)	
	46,XY, −13, +der(13)t(3;13)(q24;q11)pat	
GD2	—	
GD3	47,XX, +4, −13, +t(13q;14q)	
GD4	—	
Normal embryos	46,XX,5p−	
Embryos with localized defect(s)	46,XY, −14, +t(13q;14q)mat	46,XX,del(6)(q13;q15)
	46,XX, −13, +t(13q;14)	46,XX,der(12),t(12p;?)
	46,XY,t(15;15)(cen;cen)	46,XX,iso(8q)
	67,XXY,t(13q;14q)mat,t(13q;14q)mat	
Fragmented/degenerating embryos	46,XY, −14, +der(14),t(6;14)(q15,p11)pat	
	46,XX,t(Yq;15p)	
Ruptured/fragmented sacs	46,XX,der(8),t(4;8)(q27*3)mat	46,XX, −14, +t(13q;14q)
	46,X,dic(Y)(p11)	46,XX, −14, +t(14q;21q)
	46,XX,t(3;5)(p13;p15)	46,XY, −21, +t(14q;21q)
	46,XX,del(10)(q24)/46,XX	46,XX,t(6;14)(q27;q32)
		46,XX,4p−

TABLE VIII. Correlation Between Specimen Morphology and Double Chromosomal Trisomies

Morphology	Double trisomy	
GD1	48,XX, +2, +7	
GD2	—	
GD3	47,XX, +4, −13, +t(13q;14q)	
GD4	—	
Normal embryos	—	
Embryos with localized defects(s)	48,XY, +21, +21	48,XXY, +4
	51,XYY, +8, +9, +18, +22	
Fragmented/degenerated embryos	48,XX, +18, +21	
Ruptured/fragmented sacs	48,XY, +18, +21	

The morphologic diagnosis of embryonic growth disorganization is less informative. It points to a very high possibility of several types of *de novo* chromosome abnormalities such as trisomy, monosomy, triploidy, and tetraploidy. These chromosome mutations either originating *de novo* in parental gametes (trisomy) or being the result of failure of normal fertilization (triploidy) and cleavage (tetraploidy) are not generally hereditary. However, the clear understanding of the pathologic condition of the conceptus in mothers with history of repeated abortions is important for the obstetrician and his/her counseling. Early pregnancy loss with chromosome trisomy places the couple at higher risk for repeated trisomy and pregnancy loss [13]. The detection of triploidy or tetraploidy indicates a more likely accidental and sporadic nature of that particular embryonic defect. The finding of normal chromosomes in a specimen with embryonic growth disorganization suggests the existence of submicroscopic lethal genetic defects preventing normal embryogenesis, or a possibility of a teratogenic effect interfering with a process of normal embryogenesis.

The identification of a well-developed, fresh, normal embryo in early spontaneous abortion specimen is highly suggestive of an abnormal hormonal function of corpus luteum or endometrial insufficiency [14].

The macerated and damaged embryos and incomplete specimens are difficult to evaluate meaningfully on morphologic examination. Unfortunately, these specimens generally represent more than one half of early spontaneous abortion specimens.

In spite of this obvious drawback, it is important to examine all early spontaneously aborted products of conception, as the information obtained from such an examination may identify the patients who can be offered counseling and procedures that may reduce their risk of a child with a birth defect in a subsequent pregnancy.

ACKNOWLEDGMENTS

The technical assistance of Mrs. Barbara Paradice and Mrs. Carol Thorp in the Embryopathology Laboratory is greatly appreciated. Special thanks to all members of the Cytogenetic Laboratory for their untiring cooperation.

REFERENCES

1. Warburton D, Fraser FC: Spontaneous abortion risks in man: Data from reproductive histories collected in a medical genetics unit. Am J Hum Genet 16:1–9, 1964.
2. Gilbert EF, Opitz JM: Developmental and other pathologic changes in syndromes caused by chromosome abnormalities. Perspect Pediatr Pathol 7:1–63, 1982.

3. Nelson T, Oakley GP, Shepard TH: Collection of human embryos and fetuses: A centralized laboratory for collection of human embryos and fetuses: Seven years experience. II. Classification and tabulation of conceptual wastage with observations on type of malformation, sex ratio and chromosome studies. In Hook EB, Janerich DT, Porter IH (eds): "Monitoring Birth Defects and Environment: The Problem of Surveillance." New York: Academic Press, pp 45–64, 1971.
4. Poland BJ, Miller JR, Harris M, Livingston J: Spontaneous abortion: A study of 1961 women and their conceptuses. Acta Obstet Gynecol Scand Suppl. 102:5–32, 1981.
5. Nishimura M, Takano K, Tanimura T, Yasuda M: Normal and abnormal development of human embryos. Teratology 1:281–290, 1968.
6. O'Rahilly R: "Developmental Stages of Human Embryos, Including a Survey of the Carnegie Collection." Part A: Embryos of the first three weeks (stages 1 to 9). Washington, Carnegie Institution of Washington, 1973.
7. Streeter GL: "Developmental Horizons in Human Embryos." Washington: Carnegie Institute of Embryology, 1951.
8. O'Rahilly R: Guide to the staging of human embryos. Anat Anz 130:556–558, 1972.
9. Moore KL: "The Developing Human - Clinically Oriented Embryology." Philadelphia: Saunders, 1980.
10. Poland BJ, Miller JR: Effect of karyotype in zygotic development. In Bouè A, Thibault C (eds): "Symposium on Chromosomal Errors in Relation to Reproductive Failure." Paris: INSERM, 1973, pp 111–118.
11. Kalousek DK, Poland JB: Embryonic and Fetal Pathology of Abortion. In Perrin EVDK (ed): "Pathology of the Placenta." New York: Churchill Livingstone, 1984, pp 37–56.
12. Nishimura H: Prenatal versus postnatal malformations based on the Japanese experience on induced abortions in the human being. In Blandon RJ (ed): "Aging Gametes, Their Biology and Pathology." Basel: Karger, 1975, pp 349–368.
13. Hassold JT: Cytogenetic study of repeated spontaneous abortion. Am J Hum Genet 32:723–730, 1980.
14. Poland B: Embryonic development in patients with a high risk of early pregnancy loss. In Persaud TVN (ed): "Genetic Disorders, Syndromology and Prenatal Diagnosis." Lancaster, England: MTP Press, 1982, pp 29–36.

The Value of Examining Spontaneously Aborted Human Embryos and Placentas

Harold J. Bruyere, Jr, PhD, Sunita Arya, MD, Joan S. Kozel, BS, Enid F. Gilbert, MD, Joan M. FitzGerald, MS, James F. Reynolds, Jr, MD, Susan O. Lewin, MB, BCh, and John M. Opitz, MD

Departments of Pathology and Laboratory Medicine, The University of Wisconsin Medical School, Madison, Wisconsin 53792 (HJB, SA, JSK, EFG) and Department of Medical Genetics, Shodair Children's Hospital, Helena, Montana 59604 (JMF, JFR, SOL, JMO)

INTRODUCTION

It is our impression that little time and attention are spent in many histopathology laboratories assessing the products of conception from early spontaneous abortions. This is unfortunate because much potentially valuable clinical, genetic, and epidemiologic information is not gathered. As a result, genetic counseling may not be conducted in cases where it is indicated and possible, clinical diagnoses may not be made to assist in the current and future management of the patient, and information that may prove helpful in detecting environmental teratogens is lost. The objectives of this paper are to inform the reader of a relatively simple method for staging and examining human embryos, to stress the importance of complete and accurate reporting of historic information related to each spontaneous abortion, and to demonstrate that it is possible to detect structural abnormalities in embryos that are at a 9-week stage of development, or younger.

EXAMINING THE SPONTANEOUSLY ABORTED HUMAN EMBRYO AND PLACENTA

The *embryonic* period of human development (as opposed to the *fetal* period) includes the first 8 weeks of development and is defined by a body

Birth Defects: Original Article Series, Volume 23, Number 1, pages 169–178

length less than 32 mm, eyes that have not begun to close, and a foot length less than 7 mm [1]. A number of good sources are available on staging of human embryos and describing abnormalities in both embryos and placentas [1–5]. However, there are inconsistencies in tables [1, 6, 7] used for determining the developmental age of embryos based on the greatest length of the embryo (Fig. 1A) or on crown-rump length (Fig. 1B). We have found that Moore's [1] measurements correspond well with the morphologic characteristics of normal embryos—especially those of handplate and footplate development—and, as a result, we have adopted and recommend his system for estimating embryonic age. Ages given by Streeter [6] were based on comparison with macaque embryos and are now known to be inaccurate. Furthermore, stages of normal embryonic development proposed by O'Rahilly [7] correlate well with those of Moore [1]. It is possible to assess accurately developmental age based solely on body length and morphogenesis of the hands and feet (Fig. 2). However, other traits [1] are helpful in determining more accurately developmental age of a normal embryo and should be noted:

1. The definite presence of retinal pigment indicates that the embryo is at least 37 days old.

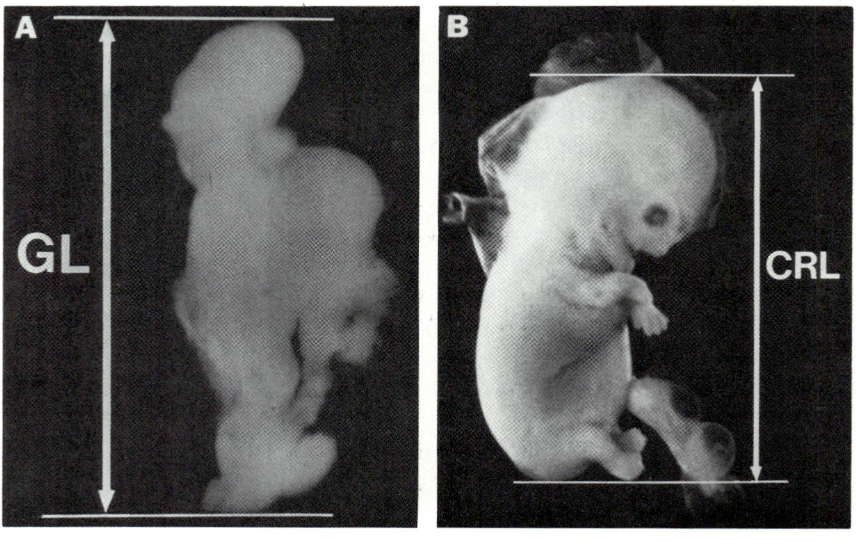

Fig. 1. (A) Measurement of greatest length (GL) in a 23–25 day embryo. (B) Measurement of crown-rump length (CRL) in a 7–8 week embryo.

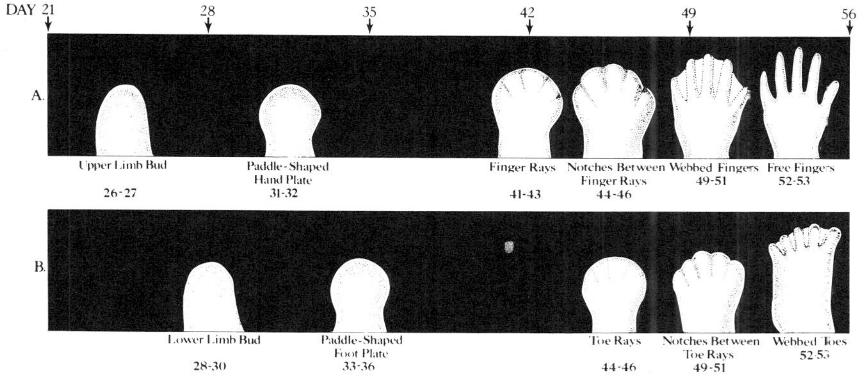

Fig. 2. Illustrations demonstrating development of the human hand (A) and foot (B).

2. Definite separation of a common aorticopulmonary trunk arising from the heart into an aorta and pulmonary artery indicates that the embryo is at least 6 weeks old.

3. Observation of a distinct elbow and/or developing eyelids suggests that the embryo is at least 44 days in development.

4. The presence of a scalp vascular plexus indicates that the embryo is at least 49 days old.

5. The presence of herniation of the intestines into the umbilical cord indicates that the conceptus is at 7–10 weeks of development.

6. Perforation of the anal membrane indicates that the embryo is at least 51 days old.

7. Lack of a short tail suggests that the embryo has reached at least 56 days of development.

8. The presence of fingernails and a well-defined neck indicate that the conceptus is at least 10–12 weeks old and ought to be referred to as a *fetus* rather than an *embryo*.

With the use of these criteria it is not difficult for even the novice embryopathologist to estimate the *developmental age* of the embryo within $\pm$ 1 day. If a complete historic record of the pregnancy accompanies the specimen, and it has not been done previously by the obstetrician, it is also possible to calculate both the gestational (menstrual) age and the fertilization age of the embryo. *Gestational age* is defined as the number of calendar days between the first day of the last menstrual period and the day of abortion [1]. *Fertilization age* is defined as 14 $\pm$ 2 days less than the gestational age [1]. These terms must be distinguished because the zygote does not form until approximately 2 weeks after the onset of the last normal menstrual period.

The difference between *fertilization age* and *developmental age* reflects the degree of growth retardation of the conceptus and/or the length of time that a nonviable embryo was retained before expulsion.

Early development of the external genitalia is similar in both sexes. Distinguishing sexual characteristics cannot be determined until early in the fetal period (9–12 weeks of developmental age) [1].

DESCRIBING DEVELOPMENTAL ABNORMALITIES OF THE EMBRYO

Only after one has established the developmental age of the embryo can structural malformations be described. It would be erroneous to note persistent truncus arteriosus in a 30-day embryo, since a common trunk at that stage of embryogenesis is simply a manifestation of normal development before aorticopulmonary septation has occurred. Several references [1,3] are excellent sources for determining the presence of external and internal malformations in the embryo.

Findings of *inconsistent morphologic development* in aborted embryos (ie, in which morphologic characteristics are not synchronous) are common. An example of this is a 17-mm crown-rump embryo with distinctly defined finger and toe rays, clearly an embryo with a developmental age of 44–46 days according to Moore [1]. However, absence of retinal pigment suggests that developing structures are not synchronous.

Growth disorganization (Fig. 3C) is also a common finding in spontaneous abortions, and degrees of growth disorganization have been established by Poland et al [5]. The authors defined GD1 as an intact chorionic or amniotic sac with no evidence of an embryo or a body stalk. They defined GD2 as a piece of embryonic tissue 1–4 mm long with no recognizable external structures and in which the caudal and cephalic poles could not be distinguished. GD3 was defined as a grossly disorganized embryo up to 10 mm long with some recognizable morphologic traits and in which the cephalic and caudal poles could be distinguished. GD4 was defined as an embryo with a major distortion of body shape, always involving the head. The head is often small, cervical flexion is absent or abnormal, and external morphologic characteristics are not consistent with any one stage of development. Crown-rump length ranges between 3–17 mm. The significance of growth disorganization lies in its high correlation (>50%) with abnormal chromosomes [5].

We wish to point out that not only can abnormalities be described in embryos, as shown in Figure 3, but that there is evidence that the developmental status of the aborted specimen is valuable in predicting the outcome of future pregnancies [8]. Furthermore, determinations of the developmental

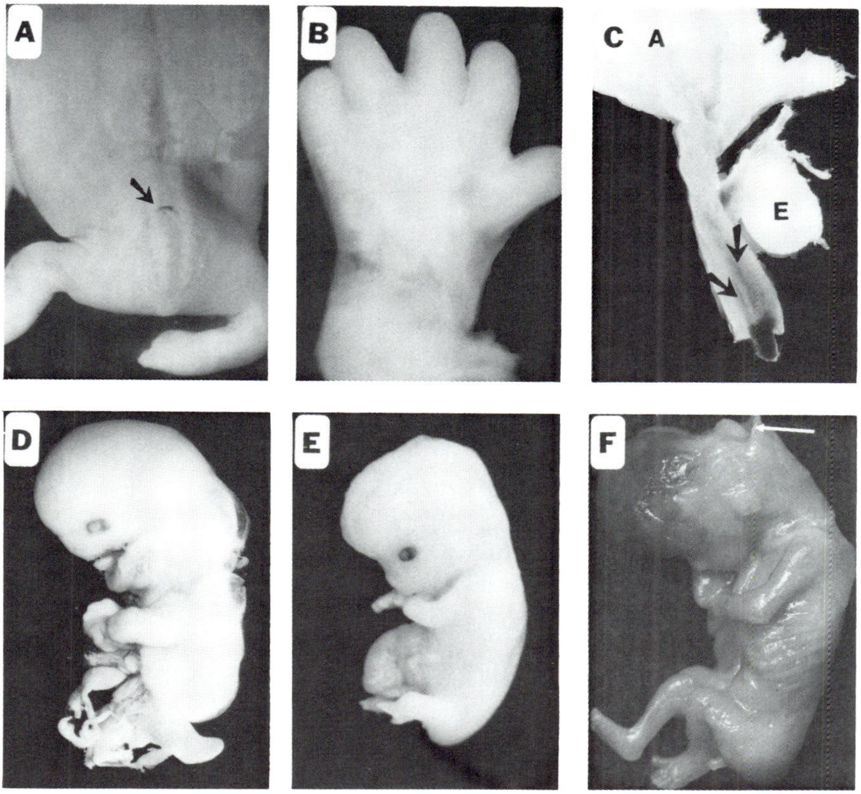

Fig. 3. Abnormalities in embryos observed among our 20 cases of spontaneous abortion. (A) Photograph showing the dorsal view of a 7-1/2-week human embryo with spina bifida (arrow). The caudal neuropore normally closes by the end of the fourth week of development. (B) Photograph showing the palmar view of the right hand from a 55-day human embryo. Note single syndactyly of the fourth and fifth digits. The digits of the developing hand are normally free by 53 days of development. (C) Photograph showing the amnion (A), 2 umbilical vessels (arrows), and disorganized embryonic tissue (E) observed following a gestational period of 9-1/2 weeks. The case was described as GD2 (Growth Disorganization type II) as there were no recognizable external features and the caudal and cephalic poles could not be distinguished. Growth disorganization is highly associated with chromosomal abnormalities. (D) Photograph showing the left lateral view of a 6-1/2-week human embryo with abnormal flexure of the left lower limb, micrognathia, and a defect in the coelomic wall. (E) Photograph showing a 7-1/2-week embryo with an omphalocele. (F) Photograph showing a 9-week fetus with cervical rachischisis (arrow) and cerebral hemorrhage.

status of embryos together with careful analyses of complete histories of pregnancy may be more helpful in detecting environmental teratogens and increasing our knowledge of the pathogenesis of developmental defects than epidemiologic and laboratory animal studies combined.

In our study of 20 spontaneously aborted human embryos from 1983–85 (Table I), we noted pathologic changes in 85% of the cases; in 75% we noted a structural defect, asynchronous development, or disorganized growth within embryonic tissue. Although the number of our cases was limited, the latter figure compares favorably with a frequency of abnormality in embryos of 84% cited by Poland et al [5].

X-irradiation of embryos is not an effective method of demonstrating the developing skeletal system. However, techniques are currently available [9,10] for preparing and examining embryos for cartilage development and early signs of ossification (Fig. 4). Furthermore, careful gross and/or microscopic examination of the placenta may offer an explanation for a spontaneous abortion as shown in Figure 5.

GATHERING INFORMATION RELATING TO EARLY PREGNANCY FAILURE

Clinically apparent spontaneous abortions (ie, after the first missed period) occur in a minimum of 15% of all recognized pregnancies [5, 11, 12]. The mechanisms of spontaneous abortion are not clear, nor is the relation between a malformation and a miscarriage except that over one-half of spontaneously lost embryos are malformed. The value of accurate and complete reporting of historic information concerning each pregnancy lies in the current and future management of patients and in increasing our knowledge of the pathogenesis of developmental defects and the major contributory factors to developmental morbidity and mortality. Since the theory of arrested devel-

TABLE I. Results Following Examination of 20 Spontaneously Aborted Human Embryos in Our Laboratory from 1983–85

	No. of cases (%)
Cases with at least one malformation	12 (60)
Cases with inconsistent morphologic development	2 (10)
Cases with disorganized growth of embryonic tissue	1 (5)
Cases with placental pathology	2 (10)
Total number of cases with pathology noted	17 (85)

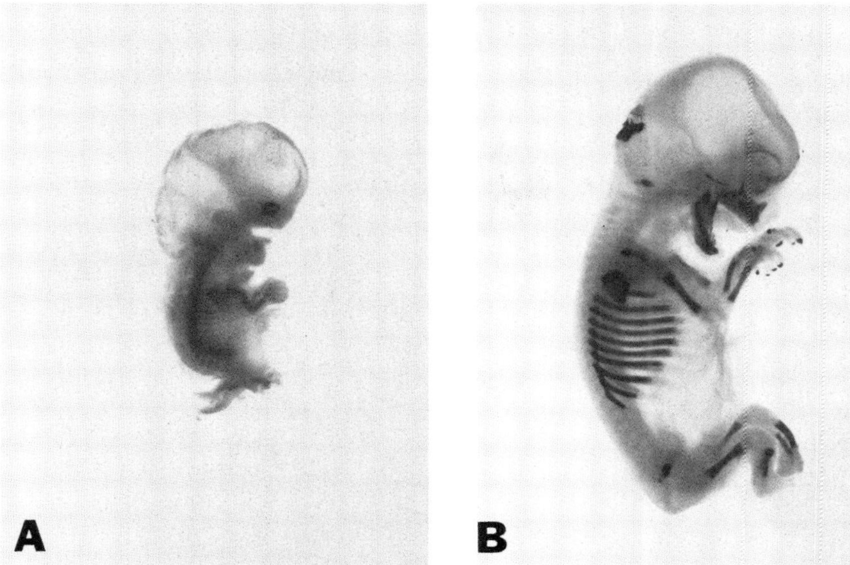

Fig. 4. Photographs showing application of a cartilage-bone stain (alcian blue-alizarin red S) to spontaneously aborted human embryos. (A) Left lateral view of a 6-1/2-week embryo (crown-rump length = 17 mm). Development of a cartilaginous skeleton lacking sites of ossification can be seen. (B) Right lateral view of a 9-week fetus (crown-rump length = 45 mm). Sites of ossification within the jaws, limbs, fingers, and rib cage are apparent.

opment still explains many types of congenital malformations, end stage pathology at the time of expulsion may closely reflect the timing of the insult to the developing conceptus.

Although the list below may be expanded, we recommend that the following information be made available to the embryopathologist at the time of his/her examination:

1. Dates of the first day of the last menstrual period and of the miscarriage
2. Maternal age at time of conception
3. A pregnancy history of drug ingestion (including smoking and the use of caffeine, alcohol, tranquilizers, and oral contraceptives)
4. Pregnancy illnesses
5. Occupational exposures
6. Previous reproductive history

Although there are probably few environmental teratogens today that have the widespread effects of rubella or thalidomide, there is increasing evidence that the interactive effects of certain agents may induce a synergism that

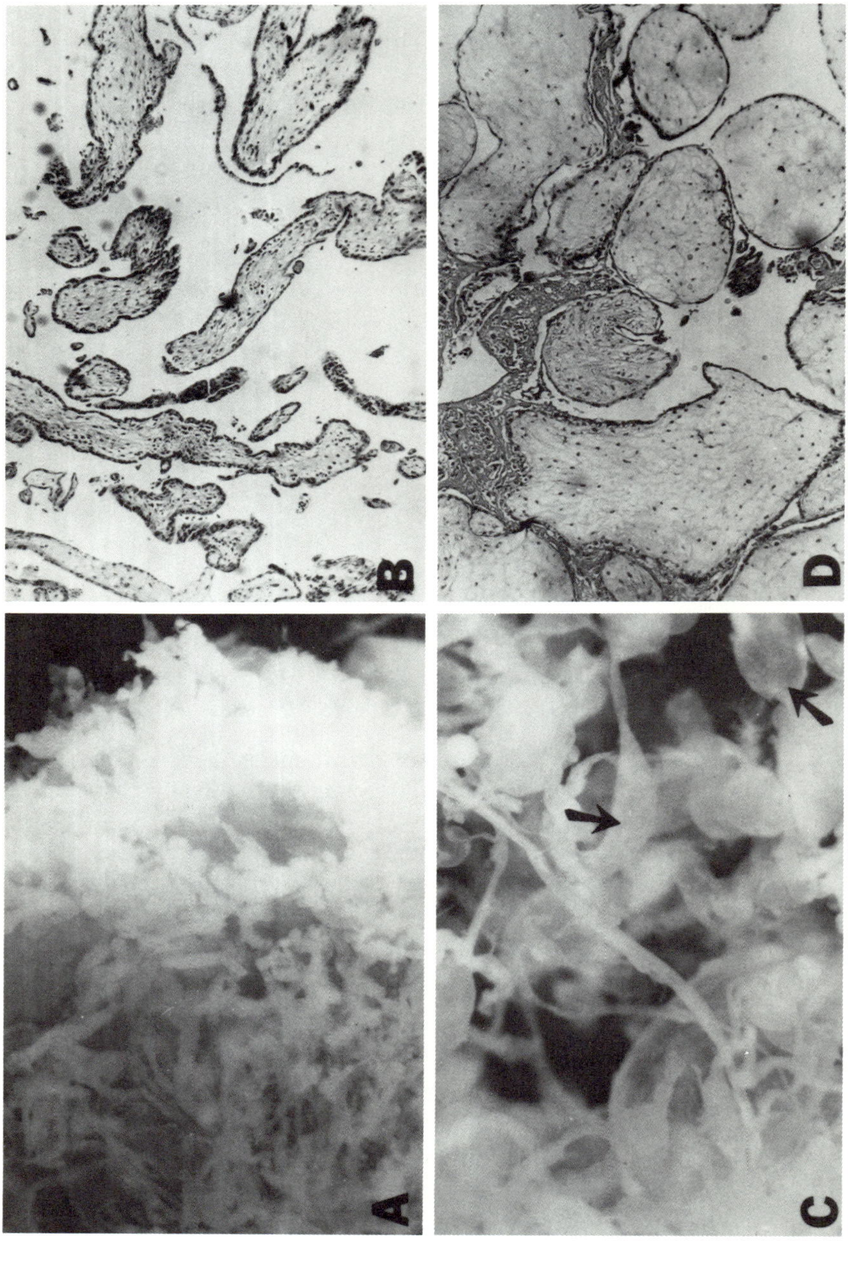
B
D
A
C

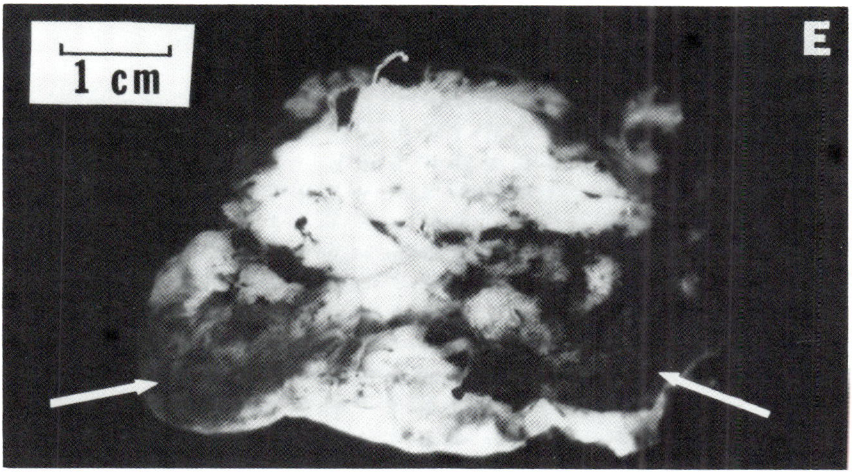

Fig. 5. Abnormalities in the placenta observed among our 20 cases of spontaneous abortion. (A) Photograph showing normally branching chorionic villi from pregnancy of 10 weeks gestation, magnification ×11. (B) Photograph showing light microscopic section of chorionic villi in Figure 5A, hematoxylin-eosin stain, magnification ×49. (C) Photograph showing marked hydropic swelling of chorionic villi (arrows) from a case in which no embryonic tissue was found after a gestational period of 13-1/2 weeks. A clinical diagnosis of partial molar pregnancy was made, magnification ×8. (D) Photograph showing light microscopic section of chorionic villi in Figure 5C. Note marked swelling of the villi when compared with Figure 5B, hematoxylin-eosin, magnification ×49. (E) Photograph showing placental products following a gestational period of 10-1/2 weeks. Extensive hemorrhage (arrows) was seen throughout the specimen extending from the decidua deep into the chorionic sac. Placental separation was suggested as an explanation for the death of the embryo.

mimics a potent teratogen [13, 14]. Thus, both complete and accurate documentation of pregnancy history, especially intake of drugs, is necessary.

CONCLUSION

We have attempted to demonstrate here the value of examining spontaneously aborted embryos and placentas and have presented a simple method for staging embryos. We contend that this practice should form part of the *normal* routine service commitment of hospital pathology laboratories, working in collaboration with obstetricians and clinical geneticists and, if possible and indicated, with anatomists, embryologists, and experimental teratologists.

REFERENCES

1. Moore KM: "The Developing Human—Clinically Oriented Embryology." 3rd ed. Philadelphia: W.B. Saunders, 1982.
2. Byrne JM: "Fetal Pathology Laboratory Manual." Vol. 19(2), BD:OAS, White Plains, New York: March of Dimes Birth Defects Foundation, 1983.
3. England MA: "Color Atlas of Life Before Birth—Normal Fetal Development." Chicago: Year Book Medical Publishers Inc., 1983.
4. Rushton DI: Examination of products of conception from previable human pregnancies. J Clin Pathol 34:819–835, 1981.
5. Poland BJ, Miller JR, Harris M, Livingston J: Spontaneous abortion. A study of 1,961 women and their conceptuses. Acta Obstet Gynecol Scand Suppl 102:1–32, 1981.
6. Streeter GL, Heuser CH, Corner GW: Developmental horizons in human embryos: Description of age groups XIX, XX, XXI, XXII and XXIII. Contrib Embryol Carnegie Inst 34:165-196, 1951.
7. O'Rahilly R: Developmental stages in human embryos. A. Embryos of the first three weeks (stages 1–9). Carnegie Institution of Washington Publication 631, Washington DC, 1973.
8. Poland BJ, Miller JR, Jones DC, Trimble BK: Reproductive counseling in patients who have had a spontaneous abortion. Am J Obstet Gynecol 127:685–691, 1977.
9. Peters PWJ: Double staining of fetal skeletons for cartilage and bone. In Neubert D, Merker HJ, Kwasigroch TE (eds): "Methods in Perinatal Toxicology." Stuttgart: Georg Thieme Publ., 1977, pp 153–154.
10. McLeod MJ: Differential staining of cartilage and bone in whole mouse fetuses by alcian blue and alizarin red S. Teratology 22:299–301, 1980.
11. Berry CL: The examination of embryonic and fetal material in diagnostic histopathology laboratories. J Clin Pathol 33:317–326, 1980.
12. Pettersson F: Epidemiology of Early Pregnancy Wastage. Stockholm: Norstedts-Bonniers, 1968.
13. Bracken MB, Holford TR: Exposure to prescribed drugs in pregnancy and association with congenital malformations. Obstet Gynecol 58:336–344, 1981.
14. Bracken MB, Holford TR, White C, Kelsey JL: Role of oral contraception in congenital malformations of offspring. Int J Epidemiol 7:309–317, 1978.
15. Ferencz C, Matanoski GM, Wilson PD, Rubin JD, Neill CA, Gutberlet R: Maternal hormone therapy and congenital heart disease. Teratology 21:225–239, 1980.

Acute Second Trimester EPH (Edema/Proteinuria/Hypertension) Gestosis as an Indicator of Fetal Anomaly

J.R. Colwill, MD, G.A. Machin, MD, PhD, J.S. Popkin, MD, and S.M. Styles, PhD

Departments of Obstetrics and Gynecology (JRC), Laboratory Medicine (GAM, SMS) and Pediatrics (JSP), Victoria General Hospital, Victoria, British Columbia, Canada V8Z 6R5

INTRODUCTION

Pregnancy-associated edema/proteinuria/hypertension (EPH gestosis) most commonly occurs in the mid to late third trimester. However, a few cases have an acute onset in the second trimester, and frequently are associated with a poor fetal prognosis. A number of abnormalities of the conceptus are known to be associated with, and presumably causative of, EPH. These include hydatidiform mole, partial mole (including triploidy), multiple gestation, and hydrops fetalis of whatever cause. In cases with placental molar changes there are frequent chromosome abnormalities, and the pathologic changes in the fetus are thought to be both primary (ie, associated with a chromosome abnormality) and also secondary to the abnormal feto-maternal endocrine environment induced by molar placental changes.

We present 3 cases of second trimester acute EPH gestosis with the following fetal anomalies: sacrococcygeal teratoma with hydrops fetalis, 13-trisomy, and triploidy. Comparison of the findings in the last two cases is instructive in distinguishing the traits that are intrinsic to the chromosome syndromes from those that are attributable to the abnormal endocrine status of the pregnancy.

Birth Defects: Original Article Series, Volume 23, Number 1, pages 179–190

Cases of acute second trimester EPH gestosis are reviewed in a literature survey.

CLINICAL HISTORIES

Case 1

Maternal age 25 years, G1, blood group A+, VSD repair at age 5 yrs. She was well at 4 prenatal visits up until 21 weeks' gestation when there was 2+ proteinuria, BP 150/70 mm Hg, fundal height 26 cm (normal 21 cm) with an 8-cm increase in 12 days, weight gain 6 kg in 12 days, and edema to mid-calf. When seen again 2 days later, there was further weight gain of 1 kg, edema to mid-thigh, hyperreflexia. On admission, BP was 170/95 mm Hg; there was hyperreflexia and the cervix was dilated 2–3 cm. She was treated with vasodilan and apresoline, but proceeded to spontaneous vaginal delivery of a 900 gm stillborn female hydropic fetus with a large sacrococcygeal teratoma (Fig. 1).The placenta weighed 645 g and was pale, fragmented and bulky.

There were no other congenital anomalies in the fetus. Histology showed an immature teratoma with a variety of tissues, predominantly immature

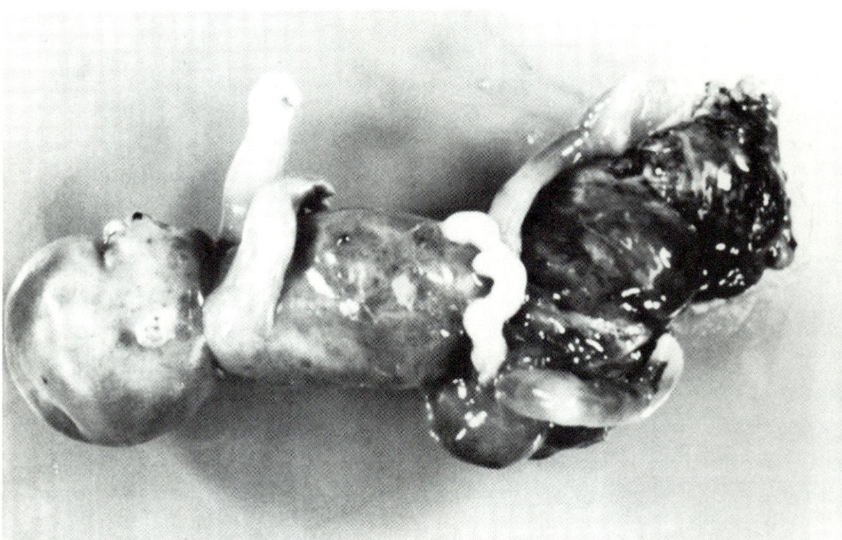

Fig. 1. Case 1. There is a large sacrococcygeal teratoma; ascites and generalized subcutaneous edema (hydrops) is also present.

neuroepithelium; the placenta showed marked hydropic changes (Fig. 2).

Case 2

Maternal age 31 years, G1, blood group O+. She was well at prenatal visits at 6 and 15 weeks' gestation. At 20 weeks, there was 1+ proteinuria, BP 140/100 mm Hg and 3 kg weight gain in 10 days with facial swelling. She was admitted the same day with uncontrolled hypertension, headaches, blurred vision, hyperreflexia, and edema to mid-thigh. Treatment with magnesium sulphate produced no response. Therefore an emergency hysterotomy was performed at 22 weeks of gestation. The placenta weighed 650 gm and was pale, friable, partially cystic, and fragmented. The fetus weighed 300 gm and had the following anomalies (Fig. 3): mild hydrops, extensive scalp defect (Fig. 4), large posterior fontanelle, hypertelorism and microphthalmia, posterior cleft palate, micrognathia, apparently low-set and malrotated ears, arrhinencephaly, cervical pterygia, flexion deformities at elbows, postaxial hexadactyly of both hands, cystic stroma of the umbilical cord, omphalocele, syndactyly 1-2 of the left foot, left diaphragmatic hernia, pulmonary hypoplasia, thymic hypoplasia, single umbilical artery, septum secundum ASD, VSD, pulmonary valve atresia, right aortic arch, intestinal malrotation,

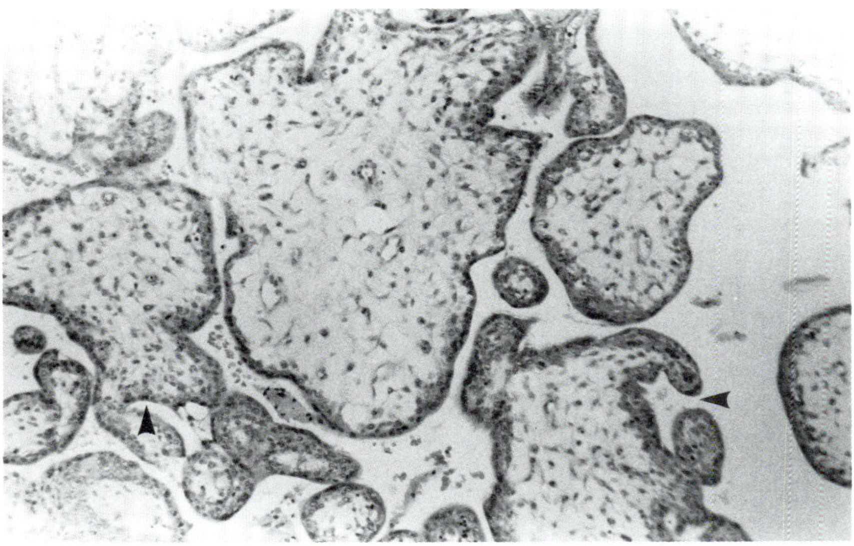

Fig. 2. Case 1. Placental villi are hydropic, and show trophoblastic clefts typical of hypergestosis (H&E ×250).

Meckel diverticulum, enlarged undescended testes (Fig. 5), large adenohypophysis, and hypoplastic adrenal glands with microcystic change. The placenta showed hydropic change (Fig. 6). Principal histologic changes were hepatic canalicular cholestasis with excessive extramedullary erythropoiesis (Fig. 7), Leydig cell hyperplasia of the testes (Fig. 8), and hydropic placental villi with trophoblastic clefting (Fig. 9). Cord blood peripheral lymphocyte chromosome analysis: 47,XY, +13.

Endocrine studies: Cord blood serum beta-hCG: 2060 IU/l.

Maternal serum values were as follows:

	Pre-hysterotomy	2 Days post-hysterotomy	3 Days post-hysterotomy	Normal 2nd trimester
Beta-hCG	>200,000 IU/l	160,000	40,000	6000–30,000
Estradiol	>1000 pg/ml	390	275	1240–1700
DHEA	360 ng/dl	235	425	416–1050
DHEA-S	50 ng/dl	30	25	12–75
Δ-4	610 ng/dl	180	170	96–552
Progesterone	207 ng/ml	19	9	80–200
Testosterone	100 ng/dl	—	—	60–220

Case 3

The mother was a 30-year-old gravida 2 woman who had had one previous spontaneous abortion; ultrasonic examination at 17 weeks' gestation showed a placenta that was large and multicystic but with no gross fetal anomalies. She was admitted at 24 weeks with vaginal bleeding, hypertension, proteinuria, and edema. She had an emergency cesarean section, and a 735 gm female infant was born with multiple anomalies suggestive of triploidy (Fig. 10). These included flexion contractures at elbows, knees, and fingers; mild syndactyly of 3-4 fingers; bulbous finger and toe pads, large tongue, and omphalocele. The infant survived 4 hours. Internal anomalies included agenesis of the corpus callosum, pulmonary valve stenosis, thymic hypoplasia, multiple renal cortical cysts, and a universal mesentery. Cord blood peripheral lymphocyte culture yielded a chromosome constitution of 69,XXX. The placenta weighed 880 gm and contained multiple cysts of hydatidiform type. Histologically, the villi showed hydropic change and typical trophoblastic clefting (Fig. 11).

DISCUSSION

The pathogenesis of edema/proteinuria/hypertension (EPH gestosis) remains largely unknown, but it clearly is caused by the presence of the implanted feto-placental unit, whether situated within or outside the uterus.

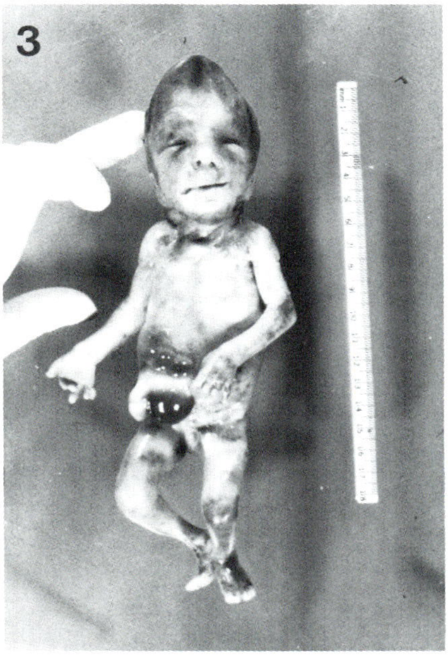

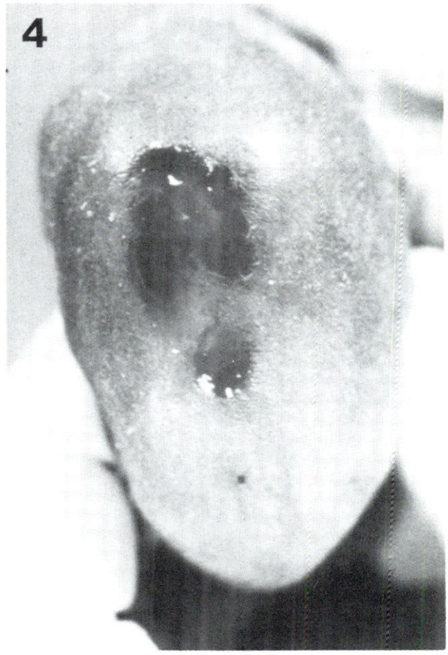

Fig. 3. Case 2. The trisomy 13 fetus shows hypertelorism, micrognathia, postaxial hexadactyly of right hand, omphalocele, and umbilical cord cysts.

Fig. 4. Case 2. Large scalp defect in this trisomy 13 fetus.

The concept of "hyperplacentosis" was introduced as a common factor in some cases of EPH-gestosis that appeared to be caused by the presence of relatively large amounts of placental tissue [1,2]. Examples include twinning and higher multiple gestations, maternal diabetes mellitus, hydrops fetalis, and complete and partial hydatidiform moles, with or without triploidy. The 3 cases presented here are examples of acute, severe 2nd trimester hyperplacentosis secondary to a variety of fetal anomalies; they suggest that early EPH-gestosis is a clinical syndrome that should arouse suspicion of fetal anomaly.

The mechanism whereby hyperplacentosis causes EPH is not understood, but raised maternal serum hCG appears to be a reliable marker as shown by the endocrinologic studies in case 2. It is interesting to note that maternal serum hCG is often raised in severe preeclampsia but normal in mild EPH-gestosis [3]. HCG may play a role as an immunosuppressor. It is well recognized that maternal serum hCG levels are high in pregnancies resulting

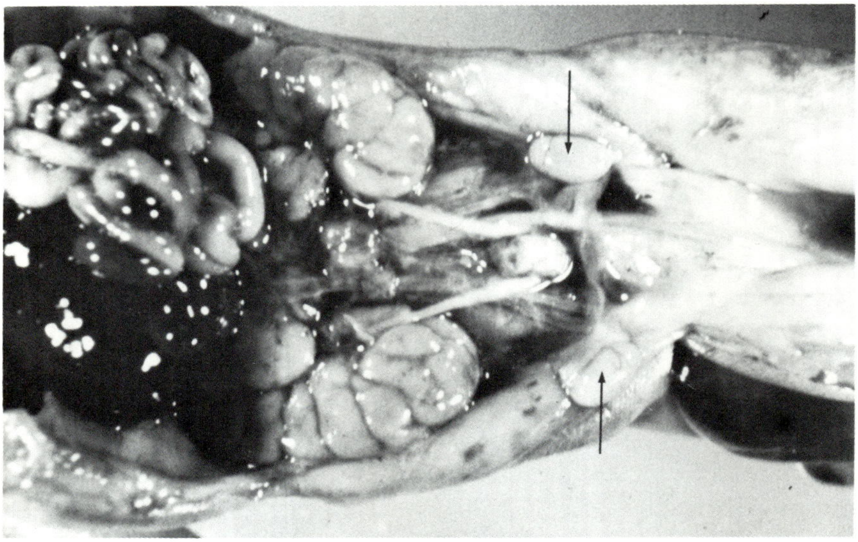

Fig. 5. Case 2. Dissection shows the enlarged testes (arrows).

in complete hydatidiform moles; partial molar pregnancies are usually associated with rather less markedly elevated maternal serum hCG levels, which also rise more slowly by gestational age [4,5]. A substantial proportion of partial molar conceptuses have a triploid constitution, with a characteristic clinical syndrome: hyperplacentosis with EPH-gestosis, enlarged placenta with hydatidiform change; hydropic fetus; cranial bone abnormalities, hydrocephalus, neural tube defect, microphthalmia, coloboma, hypertelorism; facial clefts, macroglossia; syndactyly and bulbous fingertips; congenital heart disease; obstructive renal disease; genital anomalies, depending on chromosome constitution; thymic hypoplasia; adrenal hypoplasia; and excessive extramedullary hepatic hemopoiesis [6,7]. Several authors have emphasized that hyperplacentosis is an important and frequent component of the triploidy syndrome [8–11]. Some of the anomalies in triploid fetuses are presumably true malformations, whereas others may be secondary to the abnormal endocrine environment of the hyperplacentotic pregnancy [12]. The latter authors have shown that the presence of placental molar changes correlates with testicular Leydig cell hyperplasia and increased extramedullary hemopoiesis, but not with adrenal or thymic hypoplasia.

Analysis of the 3 current cases suggests that the latter two manifestations are also correlated with hyperplacentosis, since they are not regular component anomalies of 13-trisomy.

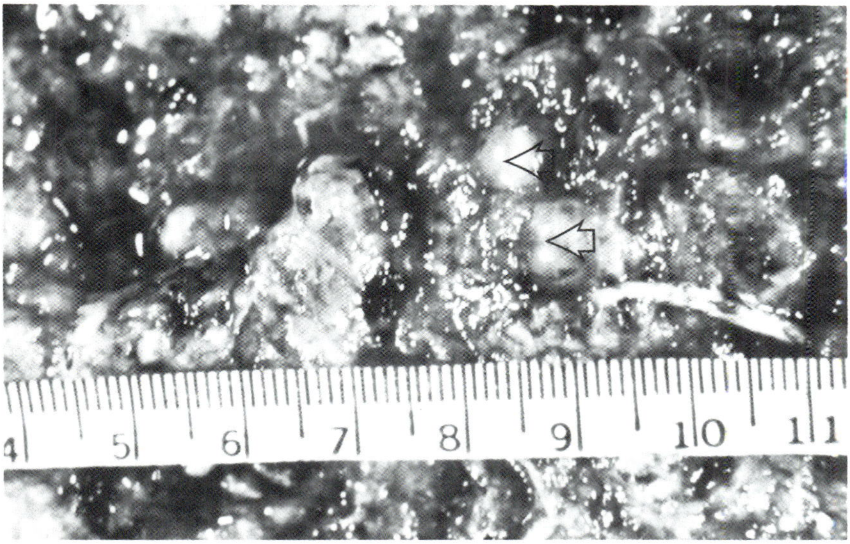

Fig. 6. Case 2. The placenta shows multiple hydatidiform cysts (arrows).

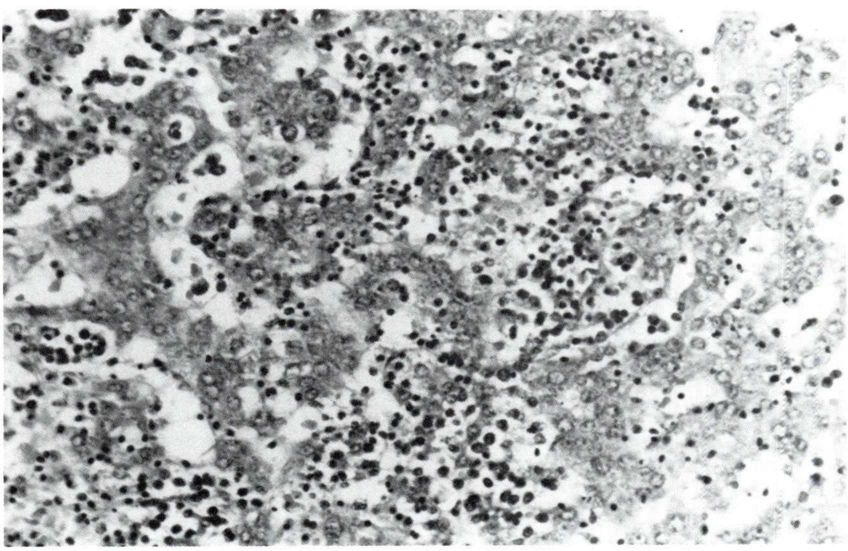

Fig. 7. Case 2. There is excessive extramedullary intrahepatic hemopoiesis (H&E ×400).

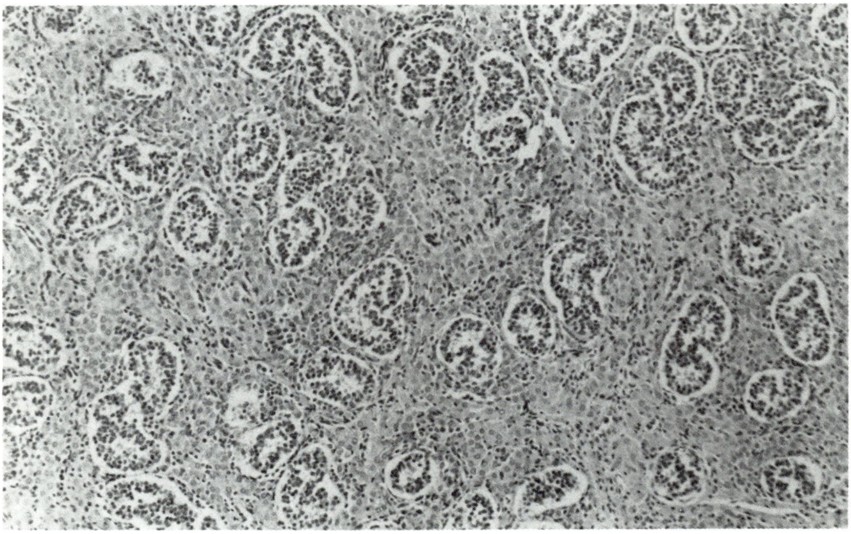

Fig. 8. Case 2. There is marked interstitial cell hyperplasia between seminiferous tubules (H&E ×400).

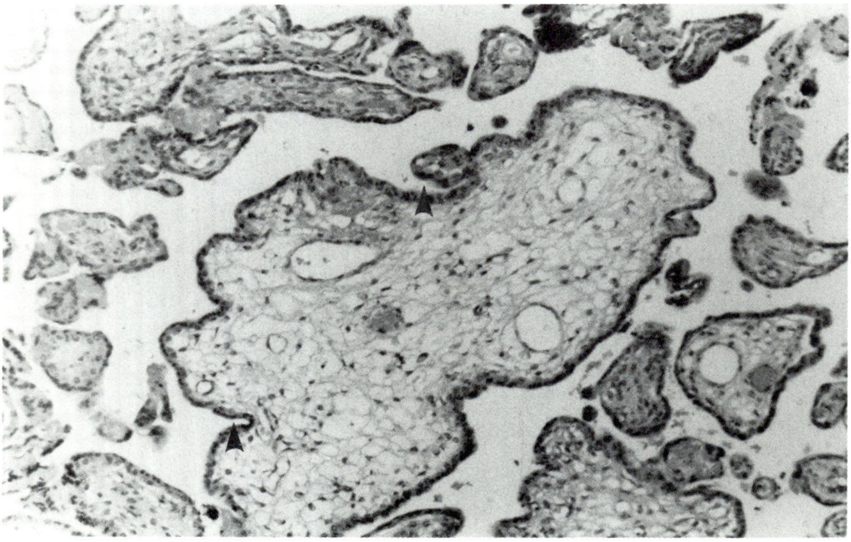

Fig. 9. Case 2. Placental villi are hydropic and show clefting (H&E ×250).

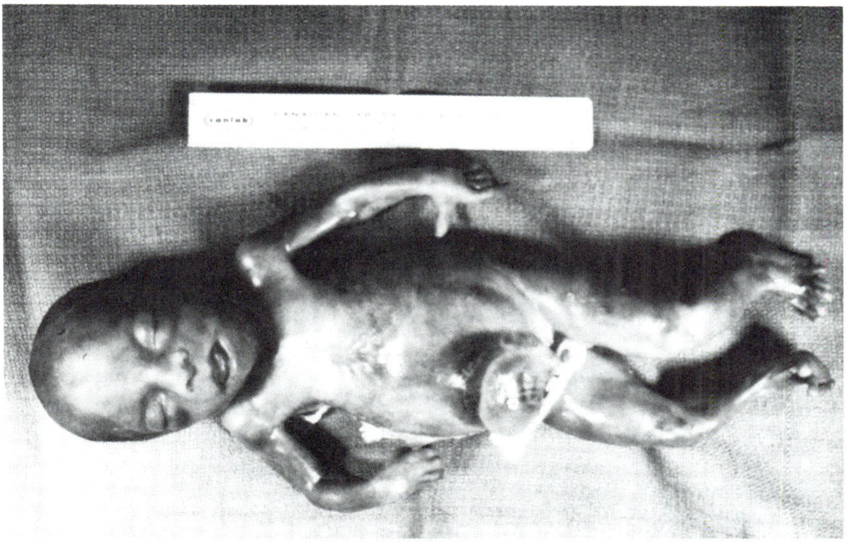

Fig. 10. Case 3. The fetus has several anomalies of triploidy—see text.

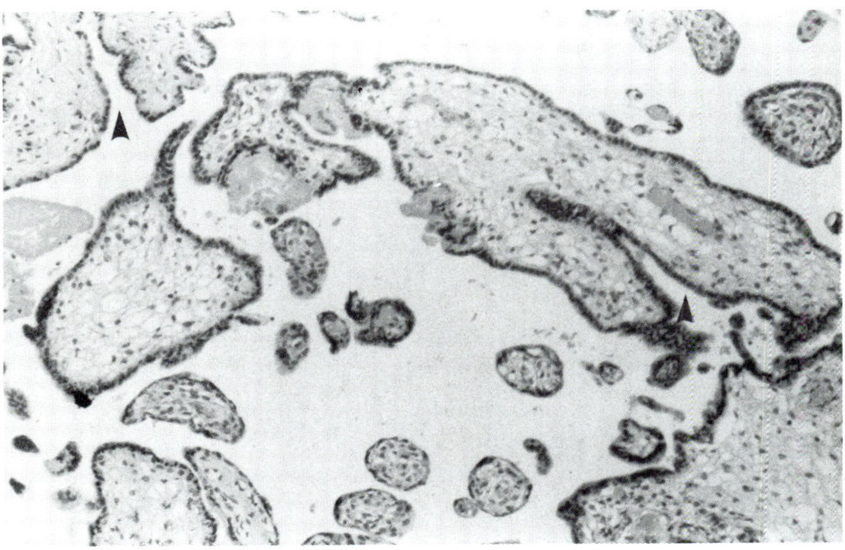

Fig. 11. Case 3. The placental villi are typical of triploidy, with hydropic change and deep trophoblastic clefts (H&E ×250).

TABLE I. Second Trimester EPH-Gestosis—Fetal Status*

Coexistent mole and fetus	24
Hydrops	20
Partial mole (nontriploid)	17
Complete mole	16
Normal fetus	9
Triploid fetus	9
Multiple pregnancy (feto-fetal transfusion, etc)	3
Other (2 sacrococcygeal teratomas, 1 exacerbation of pregestotic hypertension)	3
Total	101

*Data from Refs. 4, 8–11, 13–34, present series.

TABLE II. Cytogenetic Analysis of Partial Moles*

	n (%)
Triploid	199 (83)
Normal	16 (7)
Tetraploid	1
45,X	1
47,+2	1
47,+13	2
47,+16	14
47,+18	1
Double trisomy	1
Total	237

*Data from Refs. 8, 11, 16, 17, 25, 26, 34–37, present series.

Table I presents a literature survey of acute 2nd trimester EPH-gestosis with regard to fetal morphology [4,8–11,13–34]. Chromosome analysis of partial moles shows that most are triploid, but that a small proportion are aneuploid or chromosomally normal (Table II), [8,11,16,17,25,26,34–37].

SUMMARY

EPH gestosis in the second trimester suggests the likelihood of a number of fetal anomalies; the status of the fetus and risk to mother are such that spontaneous delivery or hysterotomy is usually the outcome, often without a full prenatal investigation. The types of fetal disorders encountered in this clinical setting are listed. Effects of abnormal endocrine environment as well as primary fetal malformations are distinguishable in these fetuses.

REFERENCES

1. Scott JS: Pregnancy toxemia associated with hydrops fetalis, hydatidiform mole and hydramnios. J Obstet Gynaecol Br Emp 55:689–701, 1958.
2. Jeffcoate TNA: Pre-eclampsia and eclampsia: The disease of theories. Proc R Soc Med 59:397–404, 1966.
3. Said ME, Campbell DM, Azzam ME, MacGillivray I: Beta-human chorionic gonadotropin levels before and after development of pre-eclampsia. Br J Obstet Gynaecol 91:772–775, 1984.
4. Czernobilsky B, Barash A, Lancet M: Partial moles: A clinicopathologic study of 25 cases. Obstet Gynecol 59:75–77, 1983.
5. Smith EB, Szulman AE, Hinshaw W, Tyrey L, Surti U, Hammond CB: Human chorionic gonadotropin levels in complete and partial hydatidiform moles and in non-molar abortuses. Am J Obstet Gynecol 149:129–132, 1984.
6. Wertelecki W, Graham JM, Sergovich FR: The clinical syndrome of triploidy. Obstet Gynecol 47:69–76, 1976.
7. Gilbert EF, Opitz JM: Developmental and other pathological changes in syndromes due to chromosome abnormalities. Perspect Pediatr Pathol 7:1–63, 1982.
8. Toaff R, Peyser MR: Midtrimester preeclamptic toxemia in triploid pregnancies. Israel J Med Sci 12: 234–239, 1976.
9. Lewis PE, Cefalo PC: Triploidy syndrome with theca lutein cysts and severe pre-eclampsia. Am J Obstet Gynecol 133: 110–111, 1979.
10. Broekhuizen FF, Elejalde R, Hamilton PR: Early-onset pre-eclampsia, triploidy and fetal hydrops. J Reprod Med 28: 223–226, 1983.
11. Hashimoto JS, Ling SH, Millerick JD, Kelley DJ: Mid-trimester pre-eclampsia associated with fetal triploidy: Report of a case. Am J Obstet Gynecol 116: 882–883, 1973.
12. Doshi N, Surti U, Szulman AE: Morphologic anomalies in triploid liveborn fetuses. Hum Pathol 14: 716–723, 1983.
13. Beischer NA: Hydatidiform mole with coexistent fetus. Aust NZ J Obstet Gynaecol 6: 127–141, 1966.
14. Benedetti TJ, Twiggs LB, Morrow CP: Pre- and post-evacuation hemodynamic and metabolic studies of hydatidiform mole and severe pregnancy-induced hypertension. A case report. J Reprod Med 25:133–135, 1980.
15. Santos-Ramos R, Forney JP, Schwarz BE: Sonographic findings and clinical correlations in molar pregnancy. Obstet Gynecol 56:186–192, 1980.
16. Lansing M, Mandel AK: Toxemic renal disease in incomplete molar pregnancy. Diagn Gynecol Obstet 4:45–51, 1982.
17. Szulman AE, Surti U: The clinicopathologic profile of the partial hydatidiform mole. Obstet Gynecol 59:597–602, 1982.
18. Goodlin RC, Cotton DB, Haesslein HC: Severe edema-proteinuria-hypertension gestosis. Am J Obstet Gynecol 132:595–598, 1978.
19. Macafee CAJ, Fortune DW, Beischer NA: Non-immunological hydrops fetalis. J Obstet Gynaecol Br Comm 77:226–237, 1970.
20. Lindheimer MD, Spargo BH, Katz AI: Eclampsia during the 16th gestational week. JAMA 230:1006–1008, 1974.
21. Jones WB, Lauerson NH: Hydatidiform mole with coexistent fetus. Am J Obstet Gynecol 122:267–272, 1975.
22. Sicuranza BJ, Tisdall LH: Hydatidiform mole and eclampsia with coexistent living fetus in the second trimester of pregnancy. Am J Obstet Gynecol 126:513–514, 1976.

23. Bree RL, Silver TM, Wicks JD, Evans E: Trophoblastic disease with coexistent fetus: A sonographic and clinical spectrum. J Clin Ultrasound 6:310–314, 1978.
24. Cohen AW, Burton HG: Nephrotic syndrome due to preeclamptic nephropathy in a hydatidiform mole and coexistent fetus. Obstet Gynecol 53:130–134, 1979.
25. Sauerbrei EE, Salem S, Fayle B: Coexistent hydatidiform mole and live fetus in the second trimester. Radiology 135:415–417, 1980.
26. Block MF, Merrill JA: Hydatidiform mole with coexistent fetus. Obstet Gynecol 60:129–134, 1982.
27. Yee Tu B, Platt LD: Coexisting hydatidiform mole with a live fetus presenting as placenta previa on ultrasound. Am J Obstet Gynecol 144:726–728, 1982.
28. Graves GR, Baskett TF: Nonimmune hydrops fetalis: Antenatal diagnosis and management. Am J Obstet Gynecol 148:563–565, 1984.
29. Van Praagh I, Jones JSP: Benign fetal sacrococcygeal teratoma associated with hydramnios and premature labor. Obstet Gynecol 23:912–914, 1964.
30. Hallgrimsson JT: Case report. Sacro-coccygeal teratoma with acute hydramnios. Acta Obstet Gynecol Scand 60:517–518, 1981.
31. Cousins L, Benirschke K, Porreco R, Resnik R: Placentomegaly due to fetal congestive failure in a pregnancy with a sacrococcygeal teratoma. J Reprod Med 25:142–144, 1980.
32. Hutchison AA, Drew JH, Yu VYH, Williams ML, Fortune DW, Beischer NA: Nonimmunologic hydrops fetalis: A review of 61 cases. Obstet Gynecol 59:347–352, 1982.
33. Sibai BM, Abdella TH, Taylor HA: Eclampsia in the first half of pregnancy. A report of three cases and review of the literature. J Reprod Med 27:706–708, 1982.
34. Ballas S, Peyser MR, Toaff R: Diagnosis of hydatidiform mole with and without coexistent fetus by nonstored image echography. Obstet Gynecol 50:182–185, 1977.
35. Jacobs PA, Hunt PA, Matsuura JS, Wilson CI, Szulman AE: Complete and partial hydatidiform mole in Hawaii: Cytogenetics, morphology and epidemiology. Br J Obstet Gynaecol 89:256–266, 1982.
36. Vassilakos P, Riotton G, Kajii T: Hydatidiform mole: Two entities. Am J Obstet Gynecol 127:167–170, 1977.
37. Szulman AE, Phillipe E, Boué JG, Boué A: Human triploidy: Association with partial hydatidiform moles and non-molar conceptuses. Hum Pathol 12:1016–1021, 1981.

The Short Umbilical Cord

Dorothy K. Grange, MD, Sunita Arya, MBBS, John M. Opitz, MD, Renata Laxova, MD, Jürgen Herrmann, MD, and Enid F. Gilbert, MD

Departments of Pathology (DKG, SA, EFG), Medical Genetics (JMO, RL), and Pediatrics (JMO, RL, EFG), University of Wisconsin Medical School, Madison, Wisconsin 53792, Department of Medical Genetics, Shodair Children's Hospital Helena, Montana 59604 (JMO), and Great Lakes Genetics (JH), S.C. Wauwatosa, Wisconsin 53226

INTRODUCTION

The length of the normal umbilical cord is extremely variable, although a cord less than 35 cm has been defined as abnormally short [1,2]. Both short and long cords are known to be associated with an increased risk of complications during labor and delivery [3–7]. A short umbilical cord is highly correlated with other major developmental anomalies. Attempts have been made to determine factors influencing cord length and the etiology of a short cord, both in experimental animal models and by retrospective analysis of human infants.

We think that a short umbilical cord can arise from several different pathogenetic mechanisms, in some cases, in association with several previously well-described malformation syndromes. We have studied 15 fetuses with a short umbilical cord and multiple associated anomalies, and have divided the cases into 6 groups, based on similarities in the constellation of anomalies and the proposed pathogenesis.

Birth Defects: Original Article Series, Volume 23, Number 1, pages 191–214

The 6 groups include (1) ADAM sequence, (2) cyllosomus/pleurosomus, (3) acephalus-acardia, (4) presumed primary defect of umbilical cord and abdominal wall formation, (5) schisis association, and (6) reduced fetal movement.

We found 15 cases in the University of Wisconsin Pathology Department and Great Lakes Genetics Center with an umbilical cord length less than 30 cm. All of the infants were stillborn or died shortly after birth due to multiple severe anomalies. Autopsies were performed on all of the patients. Multiple severe malformations and/or disruptions were present in association with a short umbilical cord.

CLINICAL CASE REPORTS

ADAM Sequence

Case 1 was a stillborn 930 g, 40.5 cm male fetus, born at 31 weeks' gestation with multiple amniotic band abnormalities, including anencephaly, facial cleft and cleft palate, and limb deficiencies. The cord was 30 cm long and the abdominal wall was intact. There was right thoracic scoliosis. The left lower leg and the right index finger were amputated with evidence of adherent amniotic bands. The left index finger was attached to the posterior neck by an aberrant tissue band. The internal organs were normally formed and had their proper relationships. The right testis was undescended (Fig. 1).

Case 2 was a stillborn white female infant who weighed 2490 g and was 38 cm long. At autopsy, the infant was found to have a large left-sided thoracoabdominal defect through which the liver, spleen, left lung, and small and large bowel protruded. The umbilical cord was short (estimated 15 cm), and was stretched over and adherent to the exposed abdominal contents. Other defects included cleft palate, skull defect (8 × 10 cm), and severe left scoliosis. The left arm was short with absent thumb and radius and syndactyly of the fingers. Pseudosyndactyly of the right toes due to amniotic band was also present. There was bilateral clubfoot (Fig. 2).

Case 3 was a term infant with encephalocele and an overlying scalp defect. There was a left cleft lip and cleft face with visible amniotic bands. The left eye was also involved. There was a huge right abdominal mid-thoracic defect with extrusion of the internal organs and absence of the right arm. The short umbilical cord came off the left side of the defect and was wrapped tightly around the body causing a narrow compressed thorax and upper abdomen (Fig. 3) (Table I).

Cyllosomus/Pleurosomus

Case 4 was a stillborn 490 g, 28 cm male fetus, born at 24 weeks of gestation to a 20-year-old primigravida. Ultrasonography documented poly-

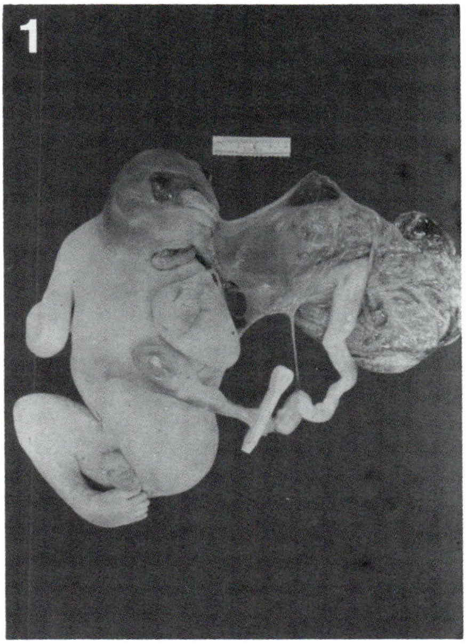

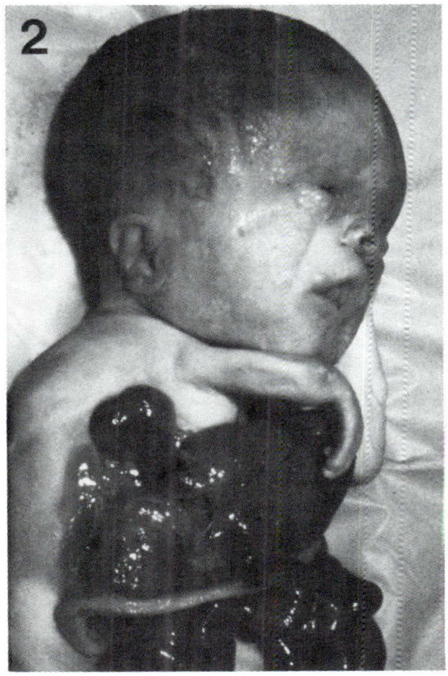

Fig. 1. Case 1. An example of ADAM sequence, with anencephaly and limb reduction defects. The placenta was adherent to the head and the cord was 30 cm long.

Fig. 2. Case 2. A female infant with ADAM sequence who had limb anomalies, body wall defect, and a short cord stretched over the extruded abdominal contents.

hydramnios, intrauterine growth retardation, and multiple malformations. At autopsy, a huge anterior abdominal wall defect was present through which the bowel, liver, spleen, and bladder protruded. The umbilical cord was only 3 cm long and adhered to the placenta. The right hemidiaphragm was absent. The right leg was entirely absent and there were severe reduction defects of the left leg. The external genitalia were rudimentary and there was an imperforate anus (Fig. 4).

Case 5 was a 1550 g, 32 cm female infant born at 31 weeks by C-section because of abruptio placenta. The mother was a 42-year-old G_2P_1 woman with no known complications of pregnancy. The infant died shortly after birth with multiple anomalies. At autopsy, there was a large abdominal wall defect with extrusion of liver, spleen, and small and large intestine. The three-vessel umbilical cord was only 10 cm long. In addition, the right arm was almost entirely absent, with a hypoplastic right subclavian artery, and containing only a tiny remnant of humerus on x-ray examination. The right

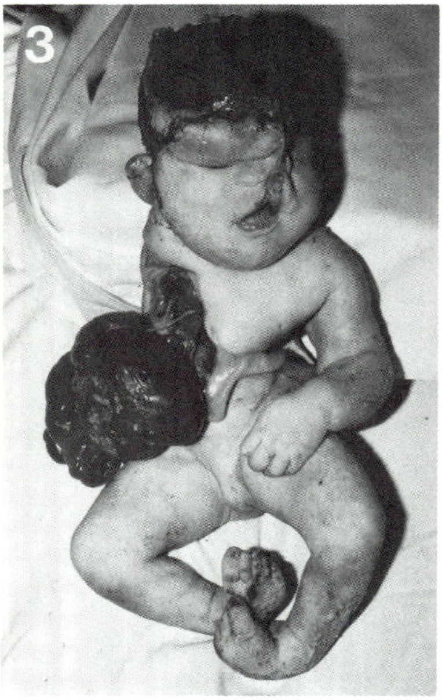

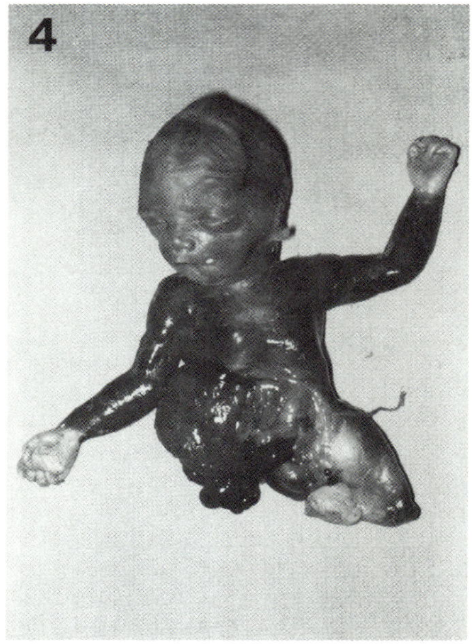

Fig. 3. Case 3. ADAM sequence with encephalocele, cleft face and lip, body wall defect, and a short cord constricting the mid-torso.

Fig. 4. Case 4. Cyllosomus with lateral body wall defect, absent lower limb, and a 3-cm cord.

radius, ulna, and hand were missing except for a single digit. Severe right scoliosis was present. The brain, organs of the chest, genitalia, and lower limbs were normal (Fig. 5).

Case 6 was a 1070 g fetus, estimated at 32.5 weeks gestational age, of undetermined sex. There was a very extensive abdominal wall defect with exteriorization of abdominal organs. The left lower limb was entirely absent and the right lower limb was abnormal. Severe scoliosis was present. The umbilical cord was extremely short. Head, arms, chest, heart were normal. However, there was absence of the internal and external genitalia, imperforate anus, and agenesis of one kidney, the pancreas, and the gallbladder. (Table II)

Acephalus-Acardia (Twinning Defect)

Case 7 was a 400 g stillborn female fetus born at 29 weeks of gestation with a normal twin. The mother was a 35-year-old G_2 white woman who underwent ultrasonography for investigation of polyhydramnios; a twin preg-

TABLE I. ADAM Sequence

Case	Cord length (cm)	Abdominal wall	Limbs	Back	Cranium	Other
1	30	Normal	Amputation left leg at knee; Absent right index finger; amniotic bands	Right scoliosis, C1-T4	"Anencephaly"	Cleft palate; undescended right testis; dextroversion of heart
2	15, adherent to abdomen	Large gastroschisis with extruded liver, spleen, bowel, left lung	Absent left thumb and radius; syndactyly right toes with amniotic bands	Left scoliosis with absent left rib cage	Large skull defect	Cleft palate; absent left ovary and tube
3	Very short, adherent to abdomen	Large gastroschisis with extruded liver, bowel	Absent right arm; bilateral clubfoot	Scoliosis	Encephalocele with scalp defect	Cleft lip and cleft side of face

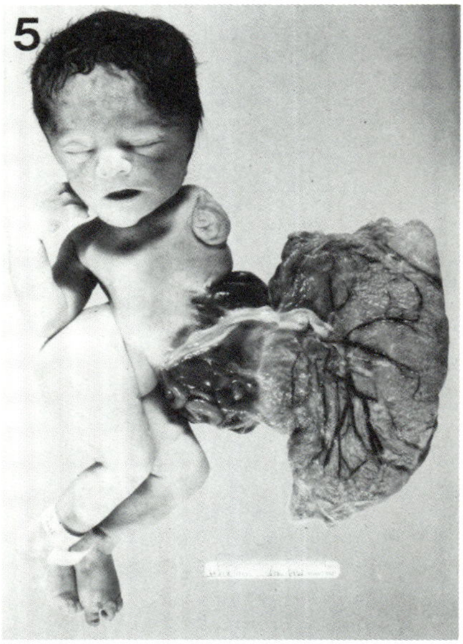

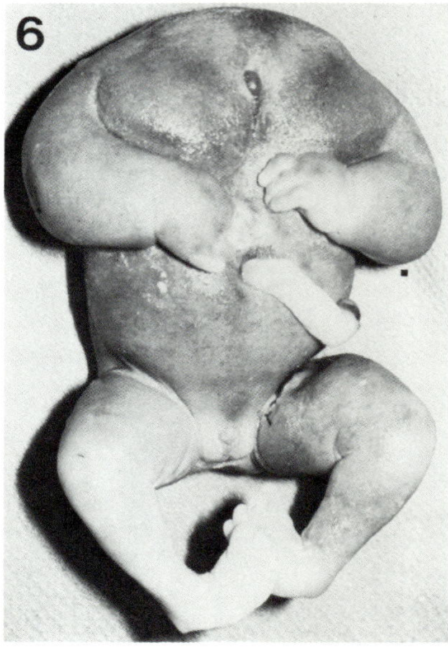

Fig. 5. Case 5. Pleurosomus, with severe reduction deformity of the upper limb, lateral body wall defect, and 10-cm cord.

Fig. 6. Case 7. Acephalus-acardia with a short umbilical cord.

nancy was diagnosed, and one twin was noted to have multiple anomalies. At autopsy, the fetus was found to have acephalus-acardia, with only a "thoracic cleft" containing a rudimentary mouth and atretic esophagus. Head, neck, heart, lungs, and liver were absent. All 4 limbs were present, with several missing digits. The stomach, intestine, pancreas, spleen, and female reproductive organs were normal. The twin placenta was diamniotic, monochorionic, and the acardiac twin's umbilical cord was short (less than 15 cm) and much smaller than the normal twin's cord. Double vascular anastomoses (artery-to-artery and vein-to-vein) were found (Figs. 6, 7) (Table III).

Presumed Primary Defect of Umbilical Cord Formation

Case 8 was an 1860 g, 29 cm male infant, born at 37 weeks of gestation to a 16-year-old primigravida. The umbilical cord was abnormal with only a single artery and was markedly reduced in length (11 cm). There was a large omphalocele, bilateral simian crease, severe scoliosis, bilateral clubfoot de-

TABLE II. Cyllosomus/ Pleurosomus

Case	Cord length (cm)	Abdominal wall	Limbs	Back	Cranium	Other
4	3	Anterior abdominal wall defect with evisceration of liver, spleen, bowel, bladder	Absent right leg; reduction defect left leg	Normal	Normal	Imperforate anus; rudimentary external genitalia
5	10	Omphalocele with evisceration of liver, spleen, bowel	Absent right arm except for nubbin of humerus	Scoliosis	Normal	
6	"Very short"	Large abdominal wall defect with evisceration of organs	Absent left leg; reduction defect of right leg	Scoliosis	Normal	Imperforate anus; absent genitalia; unilateral renal agenesis; absent pancreas and gallbladder

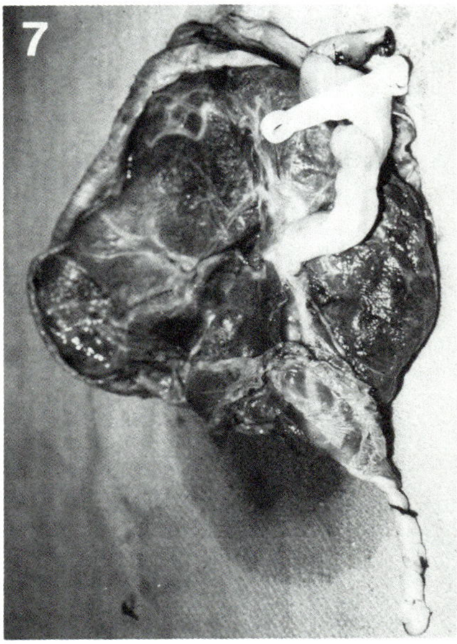

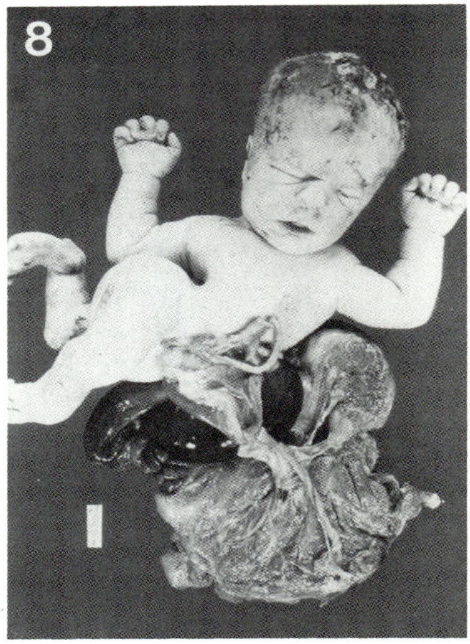

Fig. 7. The twin placenta from case 7 with the cord of the normal twin on the right and the smaller, shorter cord of the acardiac twin on the left.

Fig. 8. Case 8. A primary defect of umbilical cord formation, with body wall defect and an 11-cm cord with single umbilical artery.

TABLE III. Acephalus-Acardia

Case	Cord length (cm)	Abdominal Wall	Limbs	Other
7	15, thin	Normal	Absent left finger and left toe; syndactyly of right toes	Absent heart, lungs, head, neck; rudimentary mouth in thoracic cleft

formity, pterygium of the right leg, absent right fibula, and malformed right foot. The thorax, head, neck and upper limbs were normal, although there was a suggestion of a Potter oligohydramnios sequence facial appearance. Chromosomes were 46,XY (Fig. 8)

Case 9 was a 20.5 week male fetus born by spontaneous vaginal delivery to a 38-year-old G_3P_0 woman. The mother had previously had a spontaneous abortion at 15 weeks and a stillbirth at 32 weeks. Elevated alpha-fetoprotein and pseudocholinesterase levels were found on amniocentesis, and an open spinal defect was suspected. At autopsy, the fetus was found to have a large omphalocele with extrusion of bowel and liver. There was no discrete umbilical cord and the 3 umbilical vessels passed through the covering of the abdominal defect. The placenta was adherent to the abdomen. A left diaphragmatic defect was present with left lung and heart pulled down into the abdomen. The cranium, face, and limbs were normal (Fig. 9).

Case 10 was a 375 g, 22.5 cm male fetus, born at 22–23 weeks of gestation. An elevated alpha-fetoprotein level was found on amniocentesis

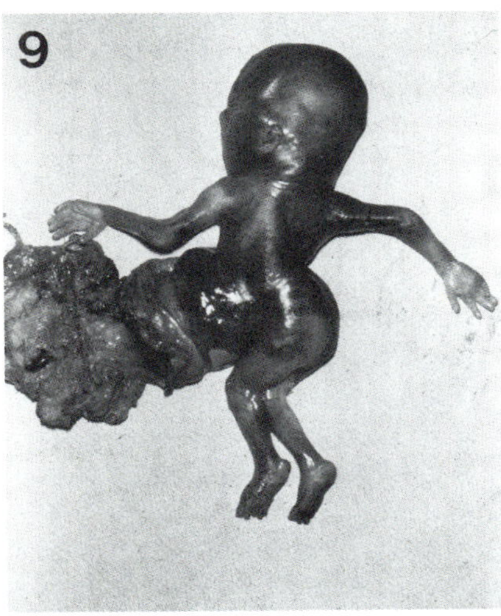

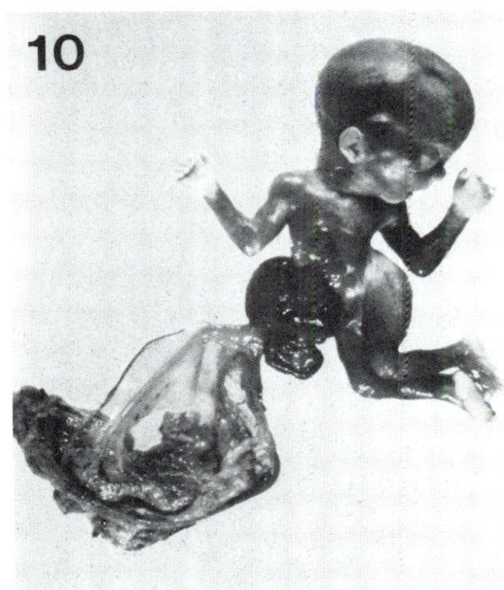

Fig. 9. Case 9. This represents a primary umbilical cord defect with no discrete cord. The omphalocele was directly adherent to the placenta.

Fig. 10. Case 10. A primary umbilical cord defect with a 15-cm cord invested in the amniotic membranes and an abdominal wall defect.

and an abdominal wall defect was seen on ultrasound. At autopsy, there was a large omphalocele containing liver, small intestine, and most of the large intestine. A 15 cm umbilical cord with a single umbilical artery ran through the amniotic membranes. The heart protruded through a diaphragmatic defect into the abdomen due to traction from the short cord. There was severe thoraco-lumbar scoliosis with near obliteration of the left thoracic cavity. The cranium and limbs were normal (Fig. 10).

Case 11 was a 2100 g white female infant born by C-section at 39 weeks of gestation to a 25-year-old primigravid woman. The baby was noted to have multiple anomalies and died shortly after birth. At autopsy, a 10 cm right abdominal wall defect was seen, with extrusion of liver and bowel. The umbilical cord was only 10 cm long. Severe right thoraco-lumbar scoliosis was present. No other anomalies of head, chest, or limbs were found (Table IV).

Schisis Association

Case 12 was a 520 g, 25 cm stillborn female fetus born spontaneously to a 23-year-old G_2P_1 woman. An elevated alpha-fetoprotein level was present in the maternal blood and amniotic fluid. At autopsy, the fetus had a large abdominal wall defect, through which the liver and small bowel protruded. The 3-vessel umbilical cord was 22 cm long. Partial agenesis of both hemi-diaphragms, scoliosis, coarctation of the aorta, and abnormal lobation of the lungs were also present.

Case 13 was a 36-week-female infant with omphalocele and exstrophy of the cloaca. The abdominal contents protruded through the body wall defect. The umbilical cord was extremely short (less than 10 cm) and had a cleft dividing umbilical vein and left umbilical artery. There was duplication of the colon and apendix with a common cloacal-colonic opening, bicornuate uterus with duplication of the vagina, meningocele with aqueductal stenosis, and mild hydrocephalus. The left hemidiaphragm was absent with herniation of heart and left lung into the abdominal cavity. There were severe deformities of both lower limbs. The head, neck, and upper limbs were normal (Figs. 11, 12).

Case 14 was a 1250 g, 32 cm stillborn female fetus, born at 32 weeks of gestation to a 29-year-old G_2P_1 white woman. At autopsy, the fetus was found to have a short cleft umbilical cord with a single artery. There was also a large abdominal wall defect, imperforate anus, absence of the left hemidiaphragm and partial agenesis of the right hemidiaphragm, agenesis of the bladder with a common cloacal-colonic opening, bicornuate uterus, and scoliosis (Table V).

TABLE IV. Presumed Primary Defect of Umbilical Cord Formation

Case	Cord length (cm)	Abdominal wall	Limbs	Back	Other
8	11, SUA*	Omphalocele with liver, bowel extruded	Absent right fibula; absent right foot; bilateral clubfoot; pterygium right leg	Scoliosis	Flattening and torsion of right chest
9	*No* discrete cord	Omphalocele with liver, bowel extruded	Abnormal right toe	Scoliosis	Left diaphragmatic defect
10	15, SUA	Omphalocele with liver, bowel extruded	Normal	Scoliosis	Diaphragmatic defect
11	10	Abdominal wall defect with liver, bowel extruded	Normal	Scoliosis	

*SUA: Single umbilical artery.

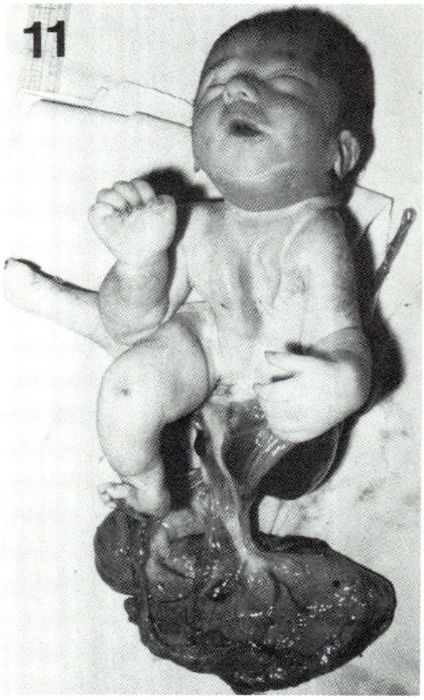

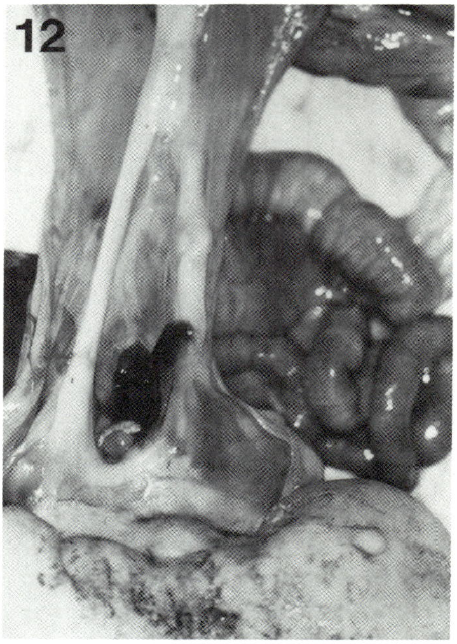

Fig. 11. Case 12. Female infant with schisis association. There was omphalocele, exstrophy of the cloaca, diaphragmatic hernia, hydrocephalus, and meningocele. The cord was extremely short.

Fig. 12. Case 12. A closer view of the short, cleft umbilical cord.

Reduced Fetal Activity

Case 15 was a 270 g, 22 cm male fetus, born at 19 weeks of gestation to a 26-year-old G_2P_0 woman. At autopsy, the fetus was found to have a 12-cm umbilical cord. The cord contained 3 vessels and microscopically was normal. There was a large retroplacental hemorrhage, which was probably responsible for the death of the fetus.

DISCUSSION

Review of Embryology and Development of Cord

To understand the pathogenesis of defects of the umbilical cord, it is important to review the embryology of the abdominal wall.

At the beginning of the 2nd week of development, the embryo is a bilaminar disc, composed of ectoderm and entoderm between the yolk sac

TABLE V. Schisis Association

Case	Cord length (cm)	Abdominal wall	Limbs	Back	Cranium	Other
12	22	Abdominal wall defect with extrusion of liver, bowel	Normal	Scoliosis	Normal	Coarctation of aorta; bilateral partial absence of diaphragm
13	"Short" with cleft	Omphalocele	Ankylosis of knees; rotated left hip; "deformed feet"	Meningocele	Arnold-Chiari with hydro-cephalus and aqueductal stenosis	Exstrophy of cloaca; agenesis of bladder; right cystic dysplastic kidney; agenesis left diaphragm; bicornuate uterus with duplication of vagina
14	"Short" with cleft	Abdominal wall defect with liver, bowel	Left leg "deformed"	Scoliosis	Normal	Exstrophy of cloaca; agenesis of bladder; agenesis left diaphragm and partial agenesis of right diaphragm; bicornuate uterus; imperforate anus

and amniotic cavity [8,9]. Mesoderm eventually separates the layers of ectoderm and entoderm. At day 16, the mesoderm splits into an outer somatic layer and an inner splanchnic layer, forming a cavity known as the primitive coelom.

These two mesodermal layers extend beyond the limits of the embryo, reinforcing the amnion and the yolk sac. Where the body wall opens ventrally, the amnion attaches to the body of the embryo. This ventral opening gradually closes as development progresses, forming the umbilical ring. As the yolk sac disappears, the yolk stalk becomes part of the extraembryonic mesoderm, eventually elongating to form the umbilical cord. The amnion provides an epithelial covering for the cord extending to the placenta and then beyond as a free membrane to form the amniotic cavity.

Closure of the ventral body wall opening is also occurring at this time. The intraembryonic mesoderm forms 4 folds that close over the ventral surface of the embryo; these include the cephalic fold, which forms the thoracic and epigastric walls and closes the foregut; two lateral folds, which form the lateral abdominal walls and close the midgut; and the central fold, which forms the hypogastric wall and closes the hindgut. The apex of these 4 folds forms the umbilical ring.

The midgut loop protrudes through the umbilical ring temporarily between the 5th and 10th weeks of gestation producing the physiologic hernia. By the end of the 10th week the embryonic abdomen has enlarged considerably and the intestine withdraws through the umbilical ring into the abdominal cavity.

At this point of development, there are no further changes in the umbilical opening until after birth. Following birth and ligation of the cord, the umbilical ring is closed by fibrous tissue and forms a scar.

Therefore, most primary abdominal wall defects must occur before the tenth week of gestation, either from a failure of closure of the ventral wall of the embryo by the mesodermal folds, or due to failure of the intestines to return to the abdominal cavity at the end of the 10th week [10–12]. In association with defects in the formation of the anterior abdominal wall, abnormal development of the umbilical cord may occur, resulting in a short or malformed cord.

Cord Length

What is the normal length of the umbilical cord? Gardiner concluded that the normal umbilical cord has an average length of 55 cm [2]. He also stated that the cord must be at least 32 cm long in order to allow for normal progression of labor and delivery. Any cord shorter than 35 cm may result in abnormal progression of labor and delivery. Other more recent studies have confirmed that the normal cord ranges from 50–60 cm for infants delivered at term. Walker and Pye suggested that cords from 20 to 120 cm could all be associated with normal labor and delivery, but that the mean length was 54 cm [13]. A study in 1972 by the US Department of Health, Education and Welfare reviewed over 19,000 deliveries and concluded that the median cord length was 54.5 cm in white and black infants [14]. Most recently, a standard curve for umbilical cord length was developed by Mills et al [15]. They showed that on the average males have longer cords than females, ranging from 38–90 cm with a mean of 60 cm. Females had cords from 36–86 cm with a mean of 57 cm. These male/female differences may be related only to average body weight and length.

From all of these studies, one may safely conclude that an umbilical cord less than 35 cm is abnormal and that the average normal cord of the term infant is 50–60 in length [16, 17].

It has also been shown that there is little change in the length of the cord during the third trimester; viable premature infants and infants born at term have essentially the same length umbilical cord [1]. This fact supports the theory proposed by Miller et al, that the length of the umbilical cord is determined by fetal activity and the tension placed on the cord during growth [18]. During the third trimester the fetus is so large that movement is more limited. Factors that retard fetal movement for whatever reason, either intrauterine compression or fetal malformation resulting in decreased limb movement could result in a short umbilical cord. Miller et al reviewed 37 patients with umbilical cords 1–43 cm long [1]. One group had early amnion rupture with limitation of fetal motion presumably due to temporary oligohydramnios and tethering of the fetus by amniotic bands. A second group of patients had limitation of motion during the second trimester due to oligohydramnios, maternal uterine malformation, or late amnion rupture. The third group had a short cord due to presumed decreased fetal movement from structural or functional limb defects, including amelia, acardia, arthrogryposis, Pena-Shokeir syndrome, and Werdnig-Hoffman disease.

Animal studies performed by Moessinger et al support the hypothesis that cord length is primarily a function of cord tension [19]. In these studies, oligohydramnios was produced experimentally in pregnant rats on day 15 of gestation (approximately corresponding to the 6th week of gestation in humans) by puncture of the fetal membranes. Another group of animals was paralyzed during the last few days of gestation by daily injections of tubocurarine. A third group of rat fetuses was removed from the uterus for the last few days of gestation and the fetuses were allowed to float free in the abdominal cavity. All rats were delivered abdominally at term and the umbilical cords were measured. Rats subjected to oligohydramnios had cords 65% of control cord length. Those that were paralyzed had cords 85% of control length. But those who had increased tensile forces on the umbilical cord due to extrauterine pregnancy, had cords 144% of the control length. These results were thought to confirm the concept that umbilical cord length is directly related to the degree of fetal activity and tension on the cord.

In a similar animal study by Moessinger, newborn rats were examined for both umbilical cord length and other associated anomalies following experimental induction of paralysis during the last 3 days of gestation [20]. The rats had polyhydramnios, presumably due to decreased fetal swallowing, and short umbilical cords, as well as low body weight, pulmonary hypoplasia, and multiple joint contractures. These findings bear a striking resemblance to those seen in the Pena-Shokeir syndrome. Moessinger proposed that the Pena-Shokeir syndrome results from prolonged fetal immobilization and that a more appropriate choice of title would be the "fetal akinesia deformation sequence." Again, these experiments support the idea that a short umbilical cord may be seen in situations where there is decreased fetal movement.

ADAM Sequence

Early amniotic rupture during pregnancy has been well described as a cause for multiple congenital abnormalities [21]. The spectrum of defects has been enlarged to include not only limb reduction defects and pseudosyndactyly, but also craniofacial defects, body wall defects, cleft lip and palate, and scoliosis [22–26]. Short umbilical cord has also been an associated finding [1]. The particular defects found in each case are highly variable and depend on the time during gestation at which amnion rupture occurs and on the extent of fetal entrapment in the strands of amnion. It has been postulated that amnion rupture must occur sometime before the 12th week of gestation, since until then a space exists between the amnion and chorion, allowing rupture of amnion while sparing the chorion [23]. The umbilical cord and anterior abdominal wall should be completely formed by the end of the 10th week. If amnion rupture occurs before completion of cord formation, defects in the cord and body wall may result by several possible mechanisms. There may be temporary oligohydramnios following amnion rupture, leading to decreased fetal movement and therefore shortened cord. A better explanation is that the fetus becomes entangled in the amniotic bands and various adhesions form, decreasing fetal movement and also preventing return of the bowel to the abdominal cavity.

In case 1, the cord was much shorter than normal. However, the anterior abdominal wall was intact and the cord was structurally normal. One could postulate that in this case, the short cord was primarily due to decreased fetal movement, secondary to anencephaly, scoliosis, and limb reduction defects. However, in cases 2 and 3, in which an abdominal wall defect was present, the cord was extremely short and adhered to the abdominal contents. Therefore, it is reasonable to suggest that the cord was short due to severe tethering and entanglement in the extruded abdominal organs, preventing tensile forces from lengthening the cord.

Cyllosomus/Pleurosomus

The terms cyllosomus and pleurosomus have been used to describe infants with body wall defects and limb reductions, first by Geoffroy St. Hilaire in 1837 [27]. Cyllosomus refers to a lateral body wall defect with ipsilateral lower limb deficiency. Pleurosomus refers to lateral body wall defect associated with upper limb deficiency [28]. Pagon et al described 15 infants with body wall defects and limb reduction anomalies [29]. Five cases had thoracogastroschisis with anomalies of the left arm and major CNS malformations. Ten cases had lateral or midline abdominal defects with absent or rudimentary lower limb and abnormal ipsilateral kidney. No mention of umbilical cord development or length is made. Aberrant tissue bands were observed in 4 of the 15 cases, but were not considered causative of the multiple anomalies, since they involved only well-differentiated structures; they concluded that these bands must have occurred some time later than the major malformations. Results of chromosome studies were all normal and no history of teratogens or other exposures could be elucidated.

Miller et al report 3 cases of cyllosomus and 4 cases of pleurosomus in which they observed body wall and limb defects associated with a short umbilical cord [1]. Although no aberrant tissue bands were found, they concluded that these fetuses probably suffered early intrauterine constraint from amnion rupture before 6 weeks' gestation. Decreased fetal movement was thought to contribute to the short umbilical cord.

Other studies have also suggested that limb deficiency, body wall deficiency, scoliosis, neural tube defects, and short umbilical cord could all result from very early amnion rupture and the subsequent combination of fetal compression due to loss of amniotic fluid and tethering by amniotic bands [30–32]. Miller et al reported 10 cases of limb/body wall deficiency; the mean length of the umbilical cord was 7 ± 3 cm (range 5–15 cm) and 2-vessel cords were common [32]. Evidence for amniotic bands was found in 41% of the cases, supporting the theory of early amnion rupture.

A number of animal experiments have been performed to demonstrate the effects of amniotic sac puncture and subsequent fetal abnormalities induced by oligohydramnios and intrauterine pressure. DeMyer and Baird showed that rats subjected to amniocentesis on days 14.5, 15.5, and 16.5 of gestation had various malformations including cleft palate, clubfeet, adactyly, microstoma, short trunks and necks, and short umbilical cords [33].

Love and Vickers did similar rat experiments and coined the term "amniocentesis dysmelia" to describe their findings [34]. They showed that amniocentesis performed on pregnant rats on day 15.5 (6th week of gestation in humans) produced reduction defects of the limbs, more often involving the hind limbs than the forelimbs and more common on the left side. The rats also had cleft palate, anomalies of the abdominal wall, genitourinary tract defects, and short umbilical cord.

A third study by Kennedy and Persaud using the rat showed that after amniotic sac puncture, severe venous stasis in the compressed body parts resulted in dilation and disruption of the local blood vessels with surrounding hemorrhage into the tissues [35]. Tissue hypoxia, necrosis, and repair then occurred, causing the observed limb defects and other associated anomalies.

Our cases 4 and 6 had changes of cyllosomus, with large abdominal wall defects associated with absence of a lower limb. Case 5 had pleurosomus, with a severe reduction defect of the right upper limb and abdominal wall defect. All patients had very short cords (3–10 cm). No evidence of amniotic bands was found in any of the cases. The right subclavian artery was considered hypoplastic in case 5, perhaps the cause of the reduction defect of the right arm. Reduction defects and abdominal wall disruption may occur as a result of vascular accidents early in gestation or secondary to early compression of developing fetal parts [36, 37]. Whatever the cause may be, the short umbilical cord is probably due to decreased fetal movement and to disruption of the developing umbilical stalk by the abdominal wall defect.

Acephalus-Acardia

Acephalus-acardia results from a defect in twinning caused by umbilical artery-to-artery and vein-to-vein anastomoses. Van Allen et al proposed the term TRAP (Twin Reversed Arterial Perfusion) sequence to better describe the pathophysiology of this defect [38]. The "pump twin" is usually normal except for evidence of heart failure. However, the "perfused twin" will show a variety of malformations, depending on which organs and tissues have the most normal vascular supply. The abdominal aorta and iliac arteries are usually the best developed, explaining the better formation of the lower half of the body in most acardiac fetuses. Most acardiac fetuses will have a primitive vascular plexus of some kind in lieu of a heart. Of the 14 cases described by Van Allen, 6 had a 2-vessel cord, but no mention of cord length was made. Limb reduction defects were extremely common.

Miller et al collected 13 cases of acardiac fetuses, in which all cords were less than 30 cm long [1]. They postulated that the umbilical cord is primarily short due to the inactivity of the acardiac twin. These fetuses do not move as vigorously *in utero* as do normal fetuses due to severe limb reductions.

In case 7, the umbilical cord was not only short, but also was smaller and narrower than usual. Abnormal vascular connections were easily demonstrated in the placenta. Cord abnormalities in the acephalus-acardiac fetus may be related both to decreased fetal movement and to an intrinsic defect in cord formation associated with the abnormal vascular communications.

Primary Defect of Umbilical Cord Formation

Ullrich and Böhm have described a malformation complex with maldevelopment of the umbilical cord, defect of the abdominal wall, and other severe malformations, which they termed "dysplasia umbilico-fetalis" [39]. They postulate that this defect must occur in early embryonic life (7 mm stage, or the end of the 3rd week of gestation). In this disorder, the abdominal wall, umbilicus, and umbilical cord do not develop. The umbilical vessels are only a few centimeters long and are contained in the mesodermal layer of the amnion-mesoderm tube. There may be limb anomalies and secondary scoliosis.

Böhm reported an additional 7 cases with similar abnormalities, which he referred to as "the missing cord syndrome" [40]. Again, the defect was thought to occur at 3 weeks of gestation, but the cause is unknown. A more recent article by Barr and Heidelberger reports 2 cases that had virtually no umbilical cord, with a large omphalocele adherent to the placenta [41]. No evidence of amniotic disruption was seen. They proposed that the extremely short cord may be a primary malformation that produces extensive deformation and disruption.

We have included 4 cases that may represent "the missing cord syndrome," or proposed primary defect of umbilical cord development. In all cases, the cord was very short (0–15 cm), and 2 of the 4 cases had a single artery. One case had no discrete cord, and the vessels passed through the abdominal wall defect directly to the adherent placenta. In contrast to those cases included under ADAM sequence, cyllosomus/pleurosomus, or schisis association, these fetuses in general had normal CNS development, normal head and neck, and the limb abnormalities could be related to secondary effects of the massive anterior body wall defect. Cases 9, 10, and 11 had normal upper and lower limbs, while case 8 had bilateral clubfoot deformity, bowing of the legs, and pterygium formation of the right knee. All cases had scoliosis.

Schisis Association

Czeizel described a group of infants with nonrandom combinations of "schisis-type" abnormalities [42,43]. These abnormalities include neural tube defects (anencephaly, encephalocele, spina bifida), cleft lip and palate, abdominal wall defects, and diaphragmatic hernia. He studied a total of 210 infants with combinations of 2 or more schisis-type abnormalities and showed that there was greater-than-chance concurrence for these malformations. In his review of the literature, he found mention of a number of other cases that demonstrated multiple schisis abnormalities [44–47]. Another case described by Pratt and Sutton may represent schisis association occurring in only 1 fetus of a set of twins [48]. The "OEIS Complex" of defects proposed by Carey et al overlaps with several of the abnormalities of the schisis association. The OEIS complex includes the midline abdominal and pelvic defects of omphalocele, exstrophy of the bladder, imperforate anus, and spine abnormalities [45]. OEIS is considered a distinct entity, different from isolated exstrophy of the bladder, resulting from an arrest in embryonic development of the cloaca and adjacent structures, which normally become the anterior abdominal wall and lower gastrointestinal genitourinary tracts. Some authors have suggested cloacal exstrophy results from failure of closure of the caudal fold, overgrowth of the cloacal membrane, and caudal placement of the genital tubercles [49].

No mention is made in the studies of schisis association or OEIS complex regarding abnormalities of the umbilical cord, but with the extensive nature of the midline defects, it is reasonable to suggest that the cord may be affected. We have included 3 cases with 2 or more schisis-type abnormalities. Case 12 had abdominal wall defect and diaphragmatic hernia with a 22-cm cord. Cases 13 and 14 had more extensive defects, including abdominal wall deficiency, exstrophy of the cloaca, agenesis of the diaphragm, and other major malformations; in both cases the cord was very short and cleft.

Reduced Fetal Activity

It has been shown that infants with neuromuscular disorders may have a variety of deformational defects, including multiple joint contractures, clubfoot, congenital hip dislocation, and scoliosis, presumably all explained by decreased intrauterine fetal movement [50]. It has been documented in the literature that infants with neuromuscular disorders, arthrogryposis, and severe limb deficiencies may also have short umbilical cords [51]. Miller et al collected a number of patients with short umbilical cords with a variety of disorders/malformations leading to decreased fetal activity [1]. They included cases of arthrogryposis, Pena-Shokeir syndrome, amelia secondary to thalidomide, maternal uterine malformation, prenatal onset of Werdnig-Hoffmann disease, and acardia. Pena and Shokeir have described a syndrome that is generally a lethal condition and includes camptodactyly, multiple ankyloses, facial anomalies, and pulmonary hypoplasia, but umbilical cord length was not specified [52]. Additional cases described by Punnett et al did have short umbilical cords [53]. However, in cases of reduced fetal activity the cords may not be as short as those found in instances where the abdominal wall and umbilical stalk are disrupted (ie, schisis association or primary cord defect).

We have included one case who had no anomalies at birth aside from the fact that the umbilical cord was only 12 cm long. One could postulate that this fetus had a neuromuscular disorder, leading to decreased fetal movement and, thus, a short cord.

CONCLUSION

We have described 15 fetuses with short umbilical cords and have divided them with varying degrees of certainty into 6 groups based on the proposed pathogenetic mechanisms. Short cord in ADAM sequence probably occurs as a consequence of both decreased fetal movement and entanglement in aberrant tissue bands, resulting in decreased tensile forces on the cord. Short cord is seen in fetuses with cyllosomus and pleurosomus, the etiology of which is not clear, but may result from very early amnion rupture with subsequent compression-related defects. Fetuses with acephalus-acardia may have short cords due to both decreased fetal movement and intrinsic cord defect due to abnormal twinning. Short cord is described in fetuses with schisis association, perhaps as a part of the extensive midline field defect. Fetuses with decreased *in utero* movement from a variety of causes, including neuromuscular disorders, Pena-Shokeir syndrome, arthyrogryposis, and other limb defects, are known to have short cords. Finally, we have described several fetuses that may have short cords due to a primary defect of umbilical cord and abdominal wall formation.

REFERENCES

1. Miller ME, Higginbottom M, Smith DW: Short umbilical cord: Its origin and relevance. Pediatrics 67: 618–621, 1981.
2. Gardiner JP: The umbilical cord: Normal length; Length in cord complications; Etiology and frequency of coiling. Surg Gynecol Obstet 34: 252–256, 1922.
3. Benirschke K, Driscoll SG: "The Pathology of the Human Placenta." Berlin-Heidelberg-New York: Springer-Verlag, 1967, pp 63–64.

4. Pal SK, Bhattacharya B: Absolute short umbilical cord (A case report): J Obstet Gynecol India 27: 442–444, 1977.
5. Pal SK: Absolute short cord dystocia. J Indian MA 74: 134–136, 1980.
6. Rayburn WF, Beynen A, Brinkman DL: Umbilical cord length and intrapartum complications. Obstet Gynecol 57: 450–452, 1981.
7. Rosen RH, Hills KG: The short umbilical cord. Am J Obstet Gynecol 66: 1253–1259, 1953.
8. Janosko EO, Jona JZ, Belin RP: Congenital anomalies of the umbilicus. Am Surg 43: 177–185, 1977.
9. Hutchins P: Somatic anomalies of the umbilicus and anterior abdominal wall. Surg Gynecol Obstet 120: 1075–1090, 1965.
10. Klein MS, Hertzler JH: Congenital defects of the abdominal wall. Surg Gynecol Obstet 152: 805–808, 1981.
11. Baird PA, MacDonald EC: An epidemiologic study of congenital malformations of the anterior abdominal wall in more than half a million consecutive live births. Am J Hum Genet 33: 470–478, 1981.
12. Duhamel B: Embryology of exomphalos and allied malformation. Arch Dis Child 38: 142–147, 1963.
13. Walker CW, Pye BG: The length of human umbilical cord: A statistical report. Br Med J 1: 546–548, 1960.
14. Blanc WA: Pathology of the placenta and of perinatal deaths. In Niswander KR, Gordon M (eds): "The Women and Their Pregnancies." Philadelphia: WB Saunders, 1972, pp 440–445.
15. Mills JL, Harley EE, Moessinger AC: Standards for measuring umbilical cord length. Placenta 4: 423–426, 1983.
16. Malpas P: Length of the human umbilical cord at term. Br Med J 1: 673–674, 1964.
17. Agboola A: Correlates of human umbilical cord length. Int J Gynecol Obstet 16: 238–239, 1978.
18. Miller ME, Jones MC, Smith DW: Tension: The basis of umbilical cord length. J Pediatr 101: 844, 1982.
19. Moessinger AC, Blanc WA, Marone PA, Polsen DC: Umbilical cord length as an index of fetal activity: Experimental study and clinical implications. Pediatr Res 16: 109–112, 1982.
20. Moessinger AC. Fetal akinesia deformation sequence: An animal model. Pediatrics 72: 857–863, 1983.
21. Torpin R: "Fetal Malformations Caused by Amnion Rupture During Pregnancy." Springfield (Illinois): Charles C Thomas, 1968.
22. Keller H, Neuhauser G, Durkin-Stamm MV, Kaveggia EG, Schaaff A, Sitzmann F: "ADAM Complex" (Amniotic Deformity, Adhesions, Mutations)—A pattern of craniofacial and limb defects. Am J Med Genet 2: 81–98, 1978.
23. Jones MC: The spectrum of structural defects produced as a result of amnion rupture. Semin Perinatol 7: 281–284, 1983.
24. Graham JM, Higginbottom MC, Smith DW: Preaxial polydactyly of the foot associated with early amnion rupture: Evidence for mechanical teratogenesis. J Pediatr 98: 943–945, 1981.
25. Chappard D, Lauras B: Unusual morphodysplasia as a result of early amnion rupture: Umbilico-cephalic adherence. J Genet Hum 31: 329–339, 1983.
26. Khudr G, Benirschke K: Discordant monozygous twins associated with amnion rupture. Obstet Gynecol 39: 713–716, 1972.

27. Geoffroy Saint-Hilaire I: Histoire Générale et Particulière Des Anomalies De L'Organisation Chez L'Homme et Les Animaux, Vol 2. Bruxelles: Société Belge de Librairie, 1837, pp 193–212.
28. Ballantyne JW: Manual of Antenatal Pathology and Hygiene, Vol 2. Edinburgh: Wm Green and Sons, 1904, pp 514–520.
29. Pagon RA, Stephens TD, McGillivray BC, Siebert JR, Wright VJ, Hsu LL, Poland BJ, Emanuel I, Hall JG: Body wall defects with reduction limb anomalies: A report of fifteen cases. March of Dimes Birth Defects Foundations BD:OAS 15(5A): 171–185, 1979.
30. Miller ME: Structural defects as a consequence of early intrauterine constraint: Limb deficiency, polydactyly, and body wall defects. Semin Perinatol 7: 274–277, 1983.
31. Graham JM, Miller ME, Stephan MJ, Smith DW: Limb reduction anomalies and early in utero limb compression. J Pediatr 96: 1052–1056, 1980.
32. Miller ME, Graham JM, Higginbottom MC, Smith DW: Compression-related defects from early amnion rupture: Evidence for mechanical teratogenesis. J Pediatr 98: 292–297, 1981.
33. DeMyer W, Baird I: Mortality and skeletal malformations from amniocentesis and oligohydramnios in rats: Cleft palate, clubfoot, microstomia, and adactyly. Teratology 2: 33–38, 1969.
34. Love AM, Vickers TH: Amniocentesis dysmelia in rats. Br J Exp Pathol 53: 435–444, 1972.
35. Kennedy LA, Persaud TVN: Pathogenesis of developmental defects induced in the rat by amniotic sac puncture. Acta Anat 97: 23–35, 1977.
36. Hoyme HE, Van Allen MI, Jones KL: The vascular pathogenesis of some sporadically occurring limb defects. Semin Perinatal 7: 299–306, 1983.
37. Hoyme HE, Jones MC, Jones KL: Gastroschisis: Abdominal wall disruption secondary to early gestational interruption of the omphalomesenteric artery. Semin Perinatol 7: 294–298, 1983.
38. Van Allen MI, Smith DW, Shepard TH: Twin reversed arterial perfusion (TRAP) sequence: A study of 14 twin pregnancies with acardius. Semin Perinatol 7: 285–293, 1983.
39. Ullrich K, Böhm N: Early embryonal maldevelopment of the umbilical cord with defect of the abdominal wall and severe body malformations (Dysplasia umbilico-fetalis). Beitr Pathol 160: 286–297, 1977.
40. Böhm N: The missing cord syndrome: A typical malformation sequence. Verhandlungen Der Deutschen Gesellschaft Für Pathologie 88: 436–439, 1982.
41. Barr M, Heidelberger KP: Short umbilical cord: Cause or effect of fetal anomalies? Proc Greenwood Genetic Center 2: 100–101, 1983.
42. Czeizel A: Schisis-Association. Am J Med Genet 10: 25–35, 1981.
43. Czeizel A, Pazsy A, Telegdi L, Tusnady G: Classification and registration of multiple congenital abnormalities. Acta Morph Acad Sci Hung 29: 377–390, 1981.
44. Kajii T, Oikawa K, Itakura K, Ohsawa T: A probable 17–18 trisomy syndrome with phocomelia, exomphalos, and agenesis of hemidiaphragm. Arch Dis Child 39: 519–522, 1964.
45. Carey JC, Greenbaum B, Hall BD: The OEIS Complex (Omphalocele, exstrophy, imperforate anus, spinal defects). March of Dimes Birth Defects Foundation BD:OAS 14(6B): 253–263, 1978.
46. Hayden PW, Chapman WH, Stevenson JK: Exstrophy of the cloaca. Am J Dis Child 125: 879–883, 1973.

47. Rukstinat GJ, Balfour JD: Hypogastro-etroschisis, spina bifida, diaphragmatic hernia and left renal agenesis in a viable full term child. Arch Pathol 6: 48–53, 1928.
48. McKenzie-Pratt R, McLean JH, Sutton PD: Foetal abnormality in twins with an unusual presentation causing dystocia. J Obstet Gynecol Br Emp 66: 452–456, 1959.
49. Wyburn GM: The development of the infra-umbilical portion of the abdominal wall, with remarks on the aetiology of ectopia vesicae. J Anat 71: 201–230, 1937.
50. Trauner DA: Neuromuscular abnormalities as a cause of deformational defects. Semin Perinatol 7: 250–252, 1983.
51. Jones MC: Intrinsic versus extrinsically derived deformation defects: A clinical approach. Semin Perinatol 7: 247–249, 1983.
52. Pena SDJ, Shokeir MHK: Syndrome of camptodactyly, multiple ankyloses, facial anomalies, and pulmonary hypoplasia: A lethal condition. J Pediatr 85: 373–375, 1974.
53. Punnett HH, Kistenmacher ML, Valdes-Dapena M, Ellison RT: Syndrome of ankylosis, facial anomalies, and pulmonary hypoplasia. J Pediatr 85: 375–377, 1974.

Abnormalities of Brain Differentiation

Lucy Balian Rorke, MD

Department of Pathology, The Children's Hospital of Philadelphia, Philadelphia, Pennsylvania 19104

INTRODUCTION

Evaluation of central nervous system malformations is a task primarily for the pediatric pathologist, as many individuals with major malformations are stillborn, or aborted, or die early in life.

As the range of possibilities for disordered neural development is wide indeed, the pathologic anatomist is often presented with an infant whose malformations do not appear to resemble any of the many types that have already been described. At the same time, some who have a clearly delineated defect, such as the Arnold-Chiari malformation, frequently have other gross or microscopic neural lesions that have no apparent relationship to the primary abnormality [1]. For example, 25 infants and children who came to necropsy with a clinical diagnosis of Arnold-Chiari malformation were found to have numerous anomalies in other parts of the brain that have little obvious relationship to the cerebellar-brain stem-lumbosacral defects [2] (Table I).

PATHOGENESIS

There is a widespread misconception that all malformations are consequent to some noxious factor operating at sensitive periods of embryologic development; in fact, an enormous body of experimental data support this notion [3]. Thus, it is often assumed that knowledge of the time of formation of the malformed part, eg, cerebellum, provides a clue to the operation of a noxious factor during that period in gestation. For example, Hicks subjected pregnant rats to a single dose of ionizing radiation and found "stage specific"

Birth Defects: Original Article Series, Volume 23, Number 1, pages 215–224

TABLE I. CNS Abnormalities Associated With Arnold-Chiari Malformation, Meningomyelocele and Hydrocephalus, 25 Postmortem Studies [2]

Defect	No.	%
1. Cerebral dysplasias		
a. White matter and subependymal heterotopias	11	44
b. Subependymal heterotopias only	2	8
2. Disordered cortical lamination		
a. Polymicrogyria	10	40
b. Microgyria	3	12
3. Polygyria	1	4
4. ''Primitive'' cortical development	6	24
5. Cerebellar dysplasia		
a. Heterotaxias	12	48
b. Heterotopias	10	40
c. Immature germinal cell collections	5	20
d. Mature neuronal groups	4	16
6. Ventricular-aqueductal abnormalities		
a. Atresia of third ventricle	2	8
b. Aqueductal atresia	2	8
c. Aqueductal forking	11	44
d. Aqueductal stenosis	13	52
7. Brain stem abnormalities		
a. Hypoplasia of cranial nerve nuclei	5	20
b. Hypoplasia of basal pontine nuclei	4	16
c. Aplasia/hypoplasia of olivary nuclei	5	20
d. Tegmental aplasia	1	4
e. Delayed or absent myelination	11	44

TABLE II. CNS Malformations in Rat Pups Following Maternal Irradiation [4–7]

Day of exposure	Anomaly
9	Severe head defects and anencephaly
11	Aqueductal stenosis
13–18	Cortical striatal malformation; agenesis of corpus callosum
19–20	Cerebellar malformations

malformations in the pups [4–7]. He established a timetable of these malformations, as noted in Table II.

These data must of course be accepted as valid scientific observations; however, the pathologist knows that any given human infant may have aqueductal stenosis, cerebral and cerebellar malformations, *and* agenesis of the corpus callosum. Moreover, it is also known that a single teratogen may produce different malformations in any given litter and in human twins as well [8].

There is no doubt that sensitive periods of embryologic development exist but we rarely know what went awry at that time — indeed, whether some extrinsic noxious agent was involved at one point in time or continuously, or whether the disordered development was under genetic control.

CNS malformations uncommonly occur in isolation; in fact, when present they are usually multiple, and under these circumstances it appears that the cause or causes must have operated at or throughout *several* critical periods of development.

EVALUATION OF ANOMALOUS NEURAL DEVELOPMENT

The range of possibilities of abnormal brain development is almost limitless, and, indeed, the textbooks and current medical journals bulge with case reports of individuals with malformations that appear to be unique or, at best, share only a few characteristics with other more well-established entities. Thus, it is best to approach each case as an individual "experiment of nature," and examine the specimen in a methodic manner unhampered by preconceived ideas as to what might be present. At the same time, knowledge of the range of possibilities is helpful in dealing with infants or children with established entities such as the chromosome disorders of the trisomy type or the Arnold-Chiari malformation.

Preparation of a detailed gross description following careful dissection, and photography at critical stages of the dissection should be routine in evaluation of infants or children who come to necropsy with a diagnosis of CNS malformation. If radiologic studies have been done, they should be reviewed before proceeding with the postmortem examination. Scalp, skull, and vertebral abnormalities are largely destroyed in the process of gaining access to the brain and spinal cord; thus, photographs of the intact defects taken at various stages of the dissection allow reconstruction of the entire case after the brain and cord have been studied. Figures 1–6 illustrate a series of photographs taken in process of one such dissection. The complex combination of skull and brain anomalies in this infant have not previously been described.

In those cases in which the malformations are complex or which do not clearly fall into a recognized "syndrome," it is helpful to list the anomaly along with the embryonic origin of the malformed structure. This brings into focus groups of malformations that may have resulted from a defect in a

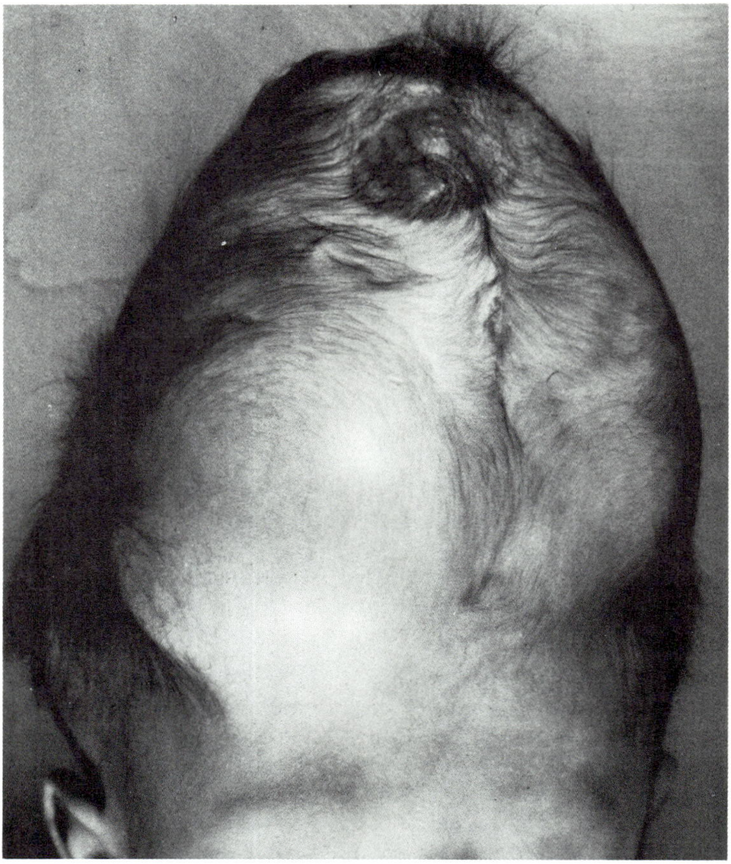

Fig. 1. Front view of head of 13-day-old infant showing "tower skull" deformity, right frontal bulge, abnormal hair pattern, and right paramedian galeal bulge.

given anlage, ie, defective development of alar plate leading to olivo-ponto-cerebellar hypoplasia.

PRENATAL DIAGNOSIS OF VENTRICULOMEGALY AND AQUEDUCTAL STENOSIS

Increasing use of ultrasound examination of women during high-risk pregnancies has led to the diagnosis of many types of fetal abnormalities for which therapeutic abortion has often been performed. A wide variety of CNS

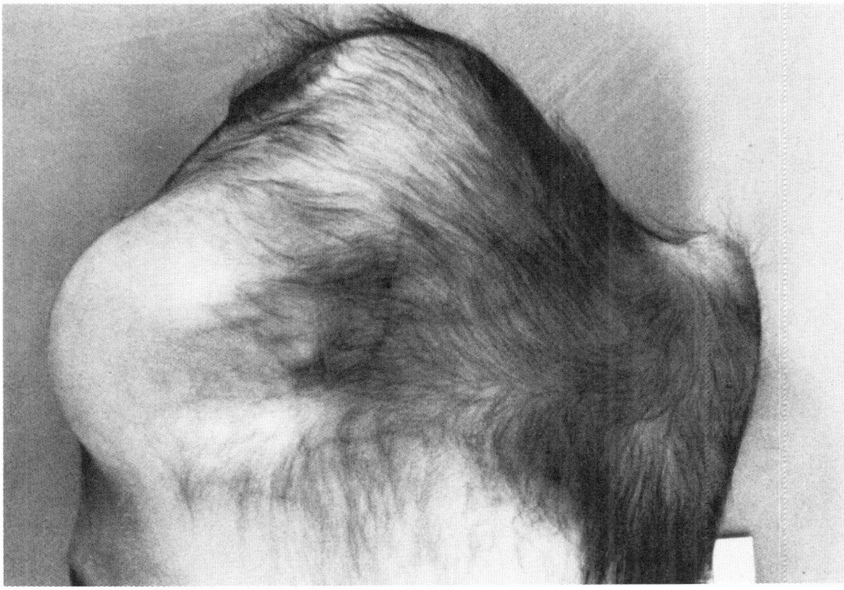

Fig. 2. Lateral view of head showing abnormal configuration produced by frontal and vertex bulges and by posterior, clifflike protuberance.

lesions has been found, of these, one of the most important is ventriculomegaly and hydrocephalus. Under the circumstances, some have advocated placement of a ventricular shunt *in utero* to minimize craniofacial disfigurement, to maximize the developmental potential of the brain and to allow safer delivery [9].

The usefulness of this procedure is a subject of lively debate among pediatric neurosurgeons, as well it might be. Cochrane et al [9] reviewed 156 fetuses and newborn infants (41 of their own and 115 from the literature) in whom fetal diagnostic techniques indicated ventriculomegaly. They found that approximately 75% had other CNS anomalies and other system malformations, some of which proved fatal. Approximately 1/3 of the fetuses survived to be treated postnatally, and only 7.5% were considered to have attained normal psychomotor development.

Diagnosis of ventriculomegaly must be made with caution as the ventricles are normally relatively large in early fetal life and diminish progressively in size as cerebral tissue grows.

When a diagnosis of hydrocephalus is made on the basis of ultrasonography, examination of the brain may show no obvious malformations and ventricular size may be borderline normal. Under the circumstances, a diagnosis of isolated aqueductal stenosis is entertained and the pathologist must determine whether it is justified.

The aqueduct and central canal of the spinal cord are remnants of the primitive neural tube; both are narrowed during development by thickening of surrounding structures [10]. The decrease in size is most marked in the ampulla and medial segment during fetal life. The ampulla is the portion at the level of the oculomotor nuclei and middle part of the superior colliculi, whereas the medial portion is between the oculomotor and trochlear nuclei anteriorly and intercollicular region posteriorly. As the fetus grows, the aqueduct increases in length, and in postnatal life enlarges in all directions to reach its maximum size in late adolescence [1].

The diameter and configuration of the aqueduct vary from level to level as it traverses the midbrain. Absolute measurements of aqueductal diameter during life have not been done, but use of the MRI scan technique now

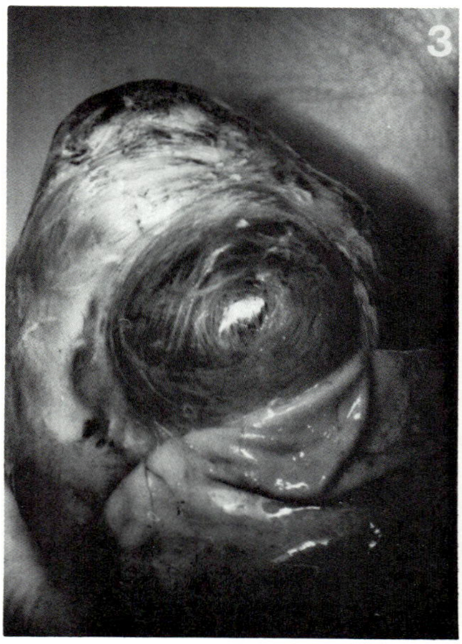

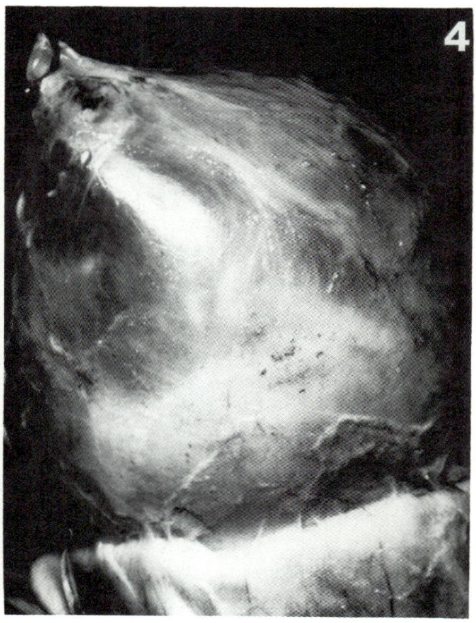

Fig. 3. The scalp has been carefully dissected away from the skull to demonstrate absence of bone to account for the soft right anterior bulge consisting of a meningocele. Note more posterior bone abnormality.

Fig. 4. Posterior aspect of head following reflection of the scalp to show formation of only the posterior parietal and occipital bones.

makes it possible to do so. It has been suggested [12] that a cross-sectional area of 0.0001 cm or less is necessary to reduce flow of the CSF, and that the normal cross-sectional area ranges from 0.009 to 0.0015 cm^2[10].

It has long been taught that abnormalities of aqueductal configuration are developmental malformations in the same sense as spina bifida or lissencephaly. In her classic monograph on the pathology of hydrocephalus, Russell [13] separated aqueductal malformations into 3 types: stenosis, forking ("atresia"), and membrane formation. However, Williams [10] argues that nontumorous obstruction of the aqueduct is almost always the *result,* not the cause, of hydrocephalus, but admits that the causes of hydrocephalus leading to these aqueductal abnormalities are generally unknown. He suggests that mechanical compression and distortion of the midbrain consequent to the dilated ventricles and excessive CSF produce the forking, stenosis, and atresia seen in most individuals with severe hydrocephalus [10].

Although his arguments have merit, they do not satisfactorily explain the pathogenetic mechanisms involved in well-documented cases of hydrocephalus associated with sporadic, familial, and X-linked aqueductal stenosis [14–17]. In these cases, the hydrocephalus is much more likely the conse-

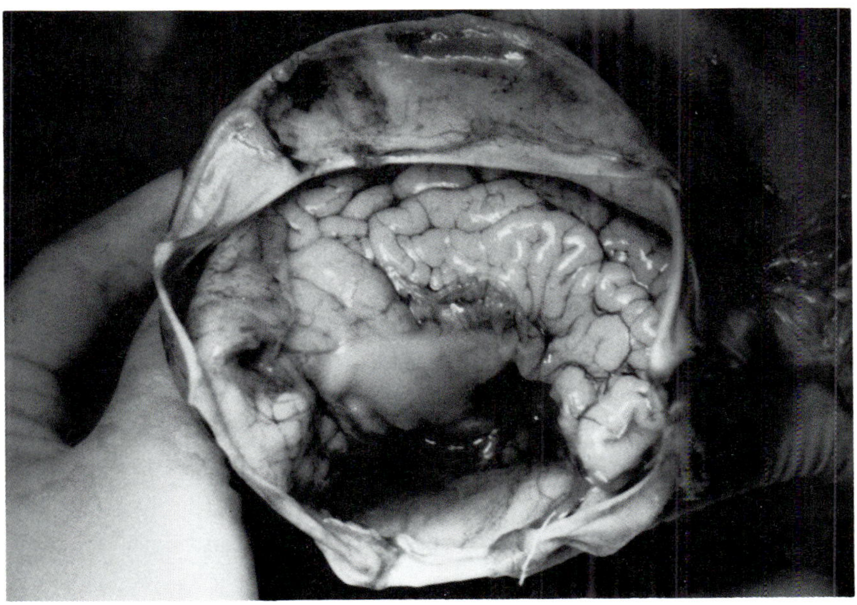

Fig. 5. Removal of dura forming the "cranial vault" shows partially fused abnormally formed brain and abnormal bone shelf of the frontal bone.

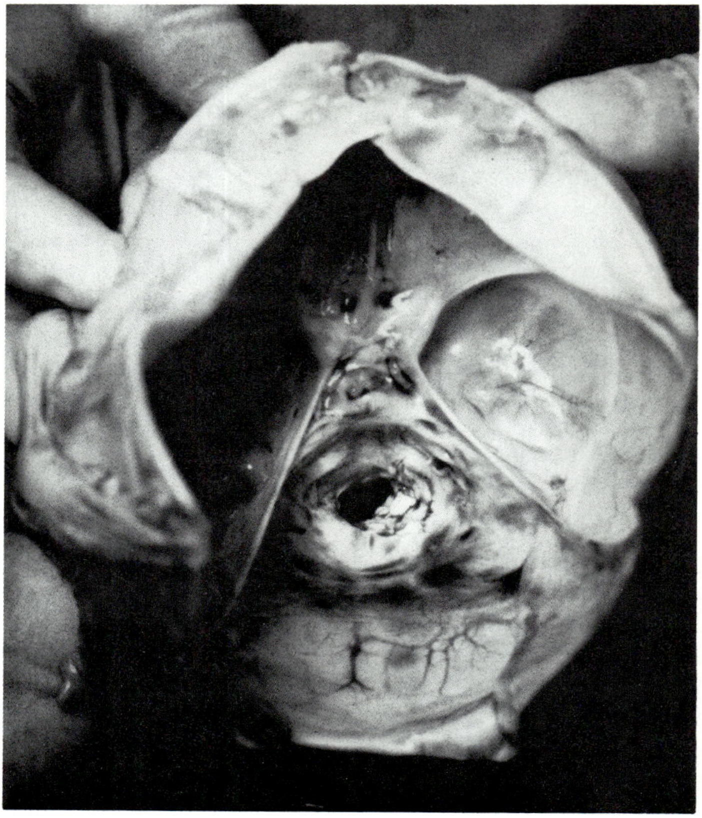

Fig. 6. Cranium following removal of brain discloses abnormal bone shelf arising from frontal bone, large anterior and posterior fossa, and formation of only the anterior portion of the middle fossae.

quence than the cause of an aqueductal lesion. In this connection it has been established that a number of viruses may produce aqueductal stenosis then followed by hydrocephalus, and there seems to be no difficulty in accepting this sequence of events [18]. Moreover, aqueductal gliosis following bacterial infections or intraventricular hemorrhages are known causes of hydrocephalus [13].

Williams's compression theory is also unsatisfactory in what appears to be forking, atresia, or stenosis of the third ventricle. This abnormality was found in 2 of 25 infants with Arnold-Chiari malformation noted above (Table

I), and it may be suspected when gross examination discloses apparent fusion of the thalamus, deep grey masses, and no identifiable foramina of Monro. The choroid plexus usually rests on the floor of the dilated body of the lateral ventricles.

In these cases, microscopic study discloses a few tiny canals lined with beautifully preserved ependymal cells without adjacent evidence of tissue destruction or gliosis. The architecture of the fiber tracts and deep nuclear structures is abnormal, suggesting that some complex disturbance of organogenesis occurred early in development.

It is conceivable that "overgrowth" of deep cerebral structures is responsible for forking or atresia of the foramina of Monro and the third ventricle, ie, these channels are originally present but later are squeezed out of existence. The possibility that dilatation of the lateral ventricles produces mechanical compression and distortion similar to that presumed to be responsible for aqueductal abnormalities is much less attractive.

It is clear at this point that the number of unanswered questions relating to even common CNS malformations far exceeds the puny amount of information that has been accumulated to date. Moreover, the possibility is great that the flimsy collection of facts we treasure today may become next year's scientific flotsam and jetsam.

Perhaps we would do well to share Phyllis McGinley's [19] lament:

> Ah, snug lie those that slumber
> Beneath conviction's roof.
> Their floors are sturdy lumber,
> Their windows weatherproof.
> But I sleep cold forever
> And cold sleep all my kind,
> For I was born to shiver
> In the draft from an open mind.

REFERENCES

1. Alvord EC Jr: The pathology of hydrocephalus. In Fields WS, Desmond MM (eds): "Disorders of the Developing Nervous System," Springfield: CC Thomas, 1961.
2. Gilbert JN, Jones KL, Rorke LB, Chernoff GF, James HE: Associated CNS anomalies with meningomyelocele, hydrocephalus and the Arnold-Chiari malformation: Reappraisal of theories regarding pathogenesis of posterior neural tube closure defects. J Neurosurg, in Press.
3. Kalter H: "Teratology of the Central Nervous System: Induced and Spontaneous Malformations of Laboratory, Agricultural and Domestic Mammals." Chicago: University of Chicago Press, 1968.

4. Hicks SP: Symposium on cerebral palsy: Some effects of ionizing radiation and metabolic inhibition on developing mammalian nervous system. J Pediatr 40:489–513, 1952.
5. Hicks SP: Developmental brain metabolism: Effects of cortisone, anoxia, fluoroacetate, radiation, insulin and other inhibitors on the embryo, newborn and adult. Arch Pathol 55:302–327, 1953.
6. Hicks SP: Developmental malformations produced by radiation. Am J Roentgen 69:272–293, 1953.
7. Hicks SP: Mechanism of radiation anencephaly, anophthalmia and pituitary anomalies in the mammalian embryo. Arch Pathol 57:363–378, 1954.
8. Warkany J: "Congenital Malformations." Chicago: Year Book Medical Publishers, 1971, p 50.
9. Cochrane DD, Myles ST, Nimrod C, Still DK, Sugarman RG, Wittman BK: Intrauterine hydrocephalus and ventriculomegaly: Associated abnormalities and fetal outcome. Can J Neurol Sci 12:51–59, 1985.
10. Williams B: Aqueduct stenosis. In Smith WT, Cavanaugh JB (eds): "Recent Advances in Neuropathology," Vol. 2. London: Churchill Livingstone, 1982.
11. Salam MZ: Stenosis of the aqueduct of Sylvius. In "Handbook of Clinical Neurology. Congenital Malformations of the Brain and Skull," Part I, Vol. 30. Amsterdam: Elsevier, 1977.
12. Masters CL: The pathogenesis of human post-infective hydrocephalus: The significance of aqueductal changes. Zeit Kinderchir Grenzgeb 22:395–412, 1977.
13. Russell DS: "Observations on the Pathology of Hydrocephalus." London: Her Majesty's Stationery Office, 1949, pp 11–19.
14. Edwards JH, Norman RM, Roberts JM: Sex-linked hydrocephalus. Report of a family with 15 affected members. Arch Dis Child 36:481–485, 1961.
15. Edwards JH: The syndrome of sex-linked hydrocephalus. Arch Dis Child 36:486–493, 1961.
16. Holmes LB, Nash A, ZuRhein GM, Levin M, Opitz JM: X-linked aqueductal stenosis: Clinical and neuropathological findings in two families. Pediatrics 51:697–704, 1973.
17. Adams C, Johnston WP, Nevin NL: Familial study of congenital hydrocephalus. Dev Med Child Neurol 24:493–498, 1982.
18. Johnston RT: Hydrocephalus and viral infections. Dev Med Child Neurol 17:807–816, 1975.
19. McGinley P: "A Pocketful of Wry: Lament for a Wavering Viewpoint," In Tripp RT (ed): "The International Thesaurus of Quotations." New York: Thomas Y Crowell, 1970, p 445.

Developmental Aspects of Lissencephaly and the Lissencephaly Syndromes

William B. Dobyns, MD

Department of Neurology, Medical College of Wisconsin, Milwaukee, Wisconsin 53201

INTRODUCTION

Lissencephaly, or "smooth-brain," is a developmental defect of the brain caused by failure of normal neuronal migration. Most pathologists use the term synonymously with "agyria." I prefer to define lissencephaly as complete (grade 1) or nearly complete (grade 2) agyria, or mixed agyria/pachygyria (grade 3) for two reasons: (1) very few cases of truly complete agyria have been reported; and (2) I think that the clinical implications are different than for less severe gyral/migrational defects such as pachygyria alone, polymicrogyria, or other unclassified cortical dysplasias.

Lissencephaly has been observed in a variety of different clinical settings: (1) alone except for a group of secondary brain and craniofacial malformations; (2) as part of complex malformation syndromes including the above and several apparently unrelated malformations of the face and other organ systems; and (3) associated with other structural brain and craniofacial abnormalities *not* explicable by a migration defect. In all types, prior stages of brain development (ie, neural tube closure, prosencephalic cleavage) are normal and the degree of the gyral/migrational defect may vary. Taking all groups together, significant causal heterogeneity has been proven including (1) several autosomal recessive disorders, (2) chromosomal "aneuploidy," (3) a recognized teratogen, and (4) many sporadic cases suggesting extrinsic causes, new mutation, and/or multifactorial determination.

Birth Defects: Original Article Series, Volume 23, Number 1, pages 225–241

Thus, the process of neuronal migration meets developmental field criteria for a specific morphogenetic series of events, and defects of this process may be "primary malformations" [1]. In discussing the "lissencephaly syndromes" we are restricted to the more severe gyral/migrational defects and, accordingly, might expect a greater proportion of familial and complex cases than if all types of migrational defects were included. Further discussion regarding the various types and syndromes requires a brief review.

TYPES OF LISSENCEPHALY

In type I lissencephaly, the gyral abnormality varies from grade 1 to grade 3, and the opercula are hypoplastic, creating a "figure-8" appearance to the brain. Coronal sections show a thick cortex, thin white matter with many heterotopic cells and rests, colpocephaly (fetal ventricular configuration with posterior regions disproportionately enlarged), and, frequently, hypoplasia of the corpus callosum. The brainstem is small, primarily due to hypoplasia of corticospinal tract (peduncles, basis pontis, pyramids) and of lateral rhombic lip (pontine nuclei, inferior olives; also external granular layer of the cerebellum) derivatives. In most patients, olivary heterotopias extend dorsally toward the embryonic site of origin. Cerebellar size is normal or only slightly small. Microscopically, the cerebral cortex is often described as "4-layered" including (1) marginal, (2) superficial cellular, (3) cell-sparse, and (4) deep cellular layers. However, the cell-sparse layer varies greatly in thickness and may be absent, and early lamination within the superficial cellular layer (the "true" cortex) is sometimes present.

In cerebro-cerebellar lissencephaly (CCL), the cerebellum is much smaller and more dysplastic than in type I, consisting of two apparently separate masses on either side of the brainstem; the vermis is not grossly visible. In the 3 patients on whom detailed pathologic descriptions are available, the cerebral surface was agyric (grade 1), and all rhombic lip and corticospinal structures were absent. Microscopically, the widened cortex appeared more primitive than in type I lissencephaly with no evidence of layering.

In type II lissencephaly, the surface is agyric (grade 1 to 3) but also pebbled or verrucous with occasional regions of atypical pachygyria or polymicrogyria. The opercula are hypoplastic. Coronal sections show a thick cortex and thin, edematous white matter with numerous scattered heterotopic cells (not in rests). The cerebellum, especially the vermis, is small and there may be a Dandy-Walker malformation. The associated cyst sometimes protrudes through the posterior skull as a cephalocele. Microscopically, there is complete disorganization of the cerebral cortex with no observable lamination and disturbed (irregular, oblique) orientation of neurons and neuronal columns. In addition to the migratory defects, there is widespread and severe glial, vascular, and mesodermal proliferation, which frequently obstructs the subarachnoid space and aqueduct (secondarily causing obstructive hydrocephalus in most patients), fuses the cerebral hemispheres especially frontally, and distorts and divides the cortex by formation of gliovascular bundles or septa that extend deep into the cortex. The latter pathologic changes have not been observed in other types of lissencephaly.

Further details regarding the pathologic and radiologic changes in the above types are available elsewhere [2–6].

DEVELOPMENTAL ASPECTS

The array of different types of lissencephaly described above may seem confusing at first. Do they represent separate pathologic processes or different points along the spectrum of a single process? If the latter, why separate them? My explanation rests on the clinical utility of the separation in determining cause and diagnosis, prognosis, and recurrence risk. A detailed explanation follows (embryologic data from Sidman and Rakic [7]).

In a developing embryo, the stage is set for the beginning of neuronal migration by a series of critical steps. Late in the 5th gestational (postconceptual) week, the cerebral hemispheres form as lateral evaginations of the prosencephalic cavity and quickly differentiate into a thick basal and thin upper or pallial region. The cerebellar tubercle forms as a V-shaped mass of tissue (apex pointing rostrally) in the roof of the rostral 4th ventricle. The lateral rhombic lips form as tissue masses at the junction of the roof and the floor of the 4th ventricle; rostrally, they lie immediately ventral to the cerebellar tubercle.

The process of neuronal migration begins in earnest in the 6th gestational week. The upper part of the cerebral vesicle or "pallium" consists of a thin cellular zone adjacent to the ventricle and covered by a marginal layer. During the ensuing week, a substantial, cellular subventricular zone is formed and the first young neurons begin climbing the recently formed radial glia fibers to reach the site of the future cortex. The cortical plate, homogeneous in appearance, slowly thickens with later-migrating neurons climbing past earlier cells to reach a more superficial position. Thus, some early cortical layering may be observed by 11–13 weeks. By 15 weeks, the ventricular and subventricular zones are mostly depleted of cells.

The basal part of the cerebral vesicles thickens substantially to form the ganglionic eminences in the floor of the lateral ventricles and walls of the

3rd ventricle. By 6 weeks, distinct lateral and medial ridges are present, which will give rise to the striatum, amygdala, and claustrum, and to the globus pallidus, nucleus accumbens, and hemispheric stalk, respectively. Little migration is required relative to the pallium. However, a distinct tongue of cells, the corpus gangliothalamicum, emanates from the ganglionic region at about 16 weeks and migrates to the posterior pole of the thalamus to form the pulvinar and related structures.

The cerebellar tubercle begins as a *single* distinct mass at the rostral end of the 4th ventricle. During the 6th week, the two caudal limbs thicken rapidly but little growth occurs in the rostral midline region. During the 7th and 8th weeks, the lateral/caudal limbs bulge dorsally above the roof of the 4th ventricle and come to resemble paired masses on either side of the brainstem. The rostral midline region or future vermis is present but small and inapparent. At 9–10 weeks, the relatively dormant midline component begins a phase of rapid growth and quickly fills the space between the lateral masses, converting the cerebellum into a prominent band of tissue overlying the 4th ventricle. Surface fissures begin to appear at about the same time.

During the 6th and 7th weeks, the lateral rhombic lips thicken rapidly. At 8 weeks, cells begin to migrate along several specialized pathways. One is directed dorsally and spreads out over the surface of the cerebellum to form the external granular layer. The others turn ventrally to follow a superficial or deep route through the pons and upper medulla. The superficial pathway or corpus pontobulbare courses visibly over the surface to form the inferior olives and pontine nuclei (by 15–22 weeks). The deep pathway forms the accessory olives and related structures.

Thus, migrational events in different brain regions share many similarities but also possess specific unique attributes, and different pathologic processes (or similar processes at different times) should cause a spectrum of related but not identical structural defects. By definition, all patients with lissencephaly have significant involvement of the cerebral (pallial, especially neopallial) pathway. Involvement of the other major pathways is virtually always present but very variable in extent.

In type I (classic) lissencephaly, the pallial and rhombic lip pathways are most prominently affected with less severe or no involvement of the cerebellar and ganglionic pathways. The presence of early lamination in the cortex is most comparable to the developing brain at 11–13 weeks. The cerebellum is usually normal or only slightly small with intact midline structure, also most consistent with 11–13 weeks development.

In CCL, cerebellar migration is also severely affected and cortical lamination is more primitive with no evidence of lamination and a lower brain weight. These changes are most comparable to those of a developing brain at 8–9 weeks gestation. Also, pathologic changes in structures derived from the lateral rhombic lips are more severe (present data based on only 3 patients). Thus, it seems possible that type I and CCL may be caused by similar pathologic processes affecting migration at slightly different times in addition to their occurrence in distinct disorders.

The basis for separation is entirely empiric. All patients with Miller-Dieker syndrome and del(17)(p13.3) (Table I) have had typical type I lissencephaly. The affected sibs with CCL reported by Barth et al [8] had identical neuropathologic changes, suggesting that at the moment CCL is specific for this syndrome. The clinical manifestations of isolated lissencephaly sequence (Table I) have been observed in patients with type I lissencephaly; patients with CCL have usually had additional malformations [5].

In type II lissencephaly, migration defects involve all major pathways beginning no later than 6 weeks, and are associated with a spectrum of defects not clearly attributable to a defect in migration (persistent embryonic vascular structures in the eye, gliovascular/mesodermal proliferation in the subarachnoid space and brain). To date, all observed cases may be explained on the basis of one or a few specific autosomal recessive disorders. It probably does not occur as an isolated developmental defect. Thus, it is probable that type I and CCL are *not* caused by the same pathologic process as type II, and making this distinction seems critical for correct evaluation and genetic counseling.

SYNDROMES WITH LISSENCEPHALY

Because of clinical, pathologic, and causal heterogeneity in the lissencephaly syndromes, a detailed evaluation is essential to provide diagnoses, prognoses, and recurrence risk estimates. Routine evaluation of all patients suspected or proven to have lissencephaly should include a good CT scan with low and thin cuts, a complete eye examination, and high-resolution chromosome analysis with attention to 17p13. If type II is suspected, a serum creatine kinase, electromyogram, and muscle biopsy are also indicated. Pathologic confirmation should be obtained when possible.

A brief review of clinical syndromes associated with lissencephaly follows (Table I). Two syndromes with unusual clinical presentation and inadequately described pathologic changes (Neu-Laxova and XK-aprosencephaly syndromes) are excluded but have been discussed elsewhere [5].

Isolated Lissencephaly Sequence

Isolated lissencephaly sequence (ILS) comprises a heterogeneous group of patients with type I lissencephaly and its direct sequelae, including secondary

TABLE I. Classification of Lissencephaly Syndromes

Syndrome	Type	Grade	Cause*
Isolated lissencephaly sequence (ILS)	I	1–3	Unknown or AR
Miller-Dieker syndrome (MDS)	I	2	del(17)(p13.3) or unknown
Norman-Roberts syndrome (NRS)	I	1	AR
Isotretinoin embryopathy (IE)	I	3	In utero exposure
Cerebro-cerebellar lissencephaly (CCL)	CCL	1–?	Unknown or AR
Walker-Warburg syndrome (WWS)	II	1–3	AR
Neu-Laxova syndrome (NLS)	?	1?	AR
XK aprosencephaly syndrome	a/a†	1	Unknown

*AR, autosomal recessive.
†a/a, aprosencephaly/atelencephaly.

brain malformations, abnormal brain function, and craniofacial changes (Table II, Figs. 1, 2) but without other malformations. Some patients with CCL may have similar clinical manifestations but are classified separately. The causes of ILS are not known but are probably heterogeneous. Results of chromosome analysis, when done, have been normal. The mothers of several patients had well-documented abnormalities at about 3 months gestation. Recently I evaluated a patient with typical manifestations born to first cousins. The empiric recurrence risk figure is probably between 5 and 12%, though admittedly based on inadequate data [5].

Miller-Dieker Syndrome

Miller-Dieker syndrome (MDS) is a complex malformation syndrome which includes lissencephaly (usually grade 2), the lissencephaly sequence, and additional craniofacial and somatic abnormalities (Table III, Figs. 3, 4) [2]. More than 20 patients have been reported. Recently, chromosome abnormalities resulting in deficiency of the subterminal part of band 17p13.3 have been detected in most patients [9,10]. The few patients with apparently normal chromosomes have had nearly identical brain and craniofacial changes but fewer somatic malformations. The cause of MDS in patients with normal chromosome studies is not known but a submicroscopic deletion in band 17p13.3 is possible. Familial recurrence of MDS has been observed only in

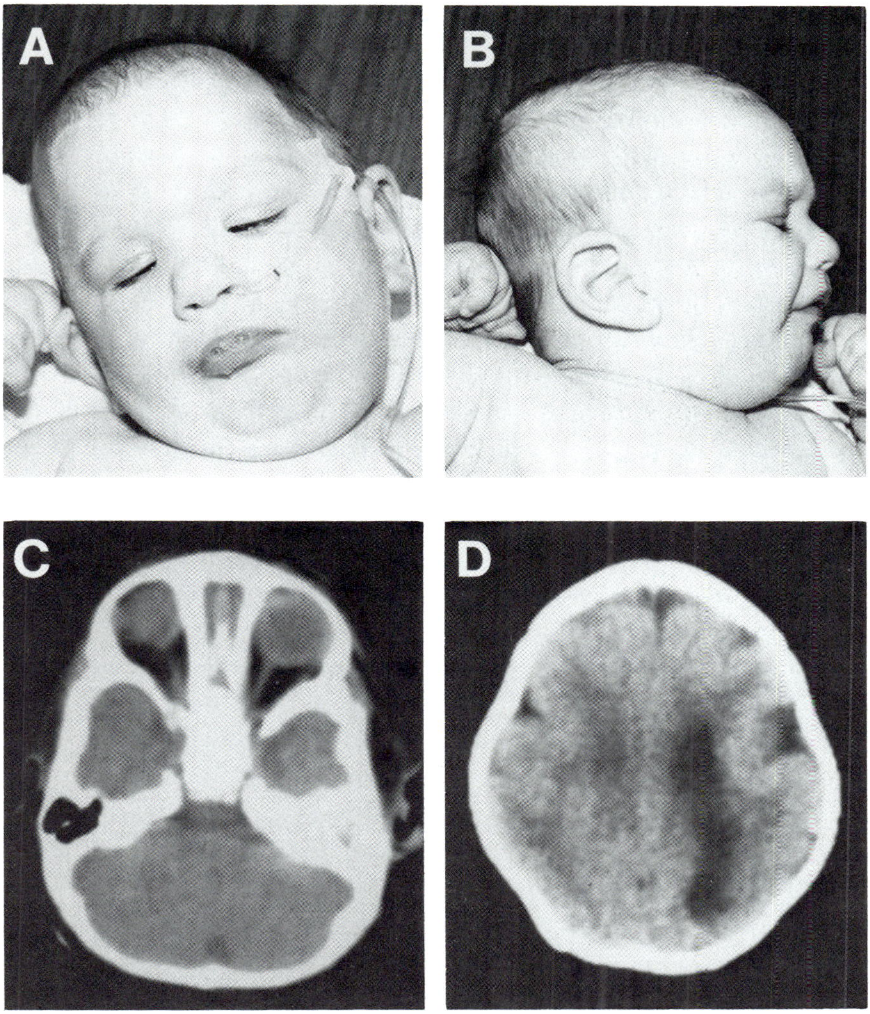

Fig. 1. Patient ILS-2 (patient 8 in [2]). Frontal (A) and lateral (B) views at 5 months show craniofacial changes of the lissencephaly sequence (LS) plus small epicanthal folds. CT scans show type I (grade 3) lissencephaly with an apparently normal cerebellum (C); and hypoplastic opercula, regions of agyria (frontal area) and pachygyria (temporo-parietal area), and asymmetric ventricular enlargement (D). Additional cuts published previously [2,3].

families in which one parent carries a balanced rearrangement involving 17p13.

Norman-Roberts Syndrome

Norman-Roberts syndrome (NRS) is based on detailed observations of a single patient from a highly inbred French Canadian family; several older sibs and first cousins were probably affected [2,11]. Clinical and pathologic manifestations differed from MDS and ILS (Table IV).

Isotretinoin Embryopathy

Isotretinoin embryopathy (IE) has been observed in at least 20 infants exposed to the drug Accutane® in utero, usually the result of an unexpected pregnancy in a woman being treated for cystic acne. In a few patients,

TABLE II. The Lissencephaly Sequence

Abnormality	Manifestations
Frequent	
Brain	Type I or cerebro-cerebellar lissencephaly, hypoplastic opercula, subcortical heterotopias, colpocephaly, hypoplasia of the corticospinal tracts, pontine nuclei, inferior olives, olivary heterotopias
Brain function	Severe or profound mental retardation, decreased spontaneous activity, early hypotonia, subsequent hypertonia, seizures, poor feeding
Craniofacial	Microcephaly, bitemporal hollowing, prominent occiput, micrognathia
Occasional	
Brain	Small cerebellum with cortical dysplasia, hypoplasia of corpus callosum
Brain function	Infantile spasms
Prenatal	Polyhydramnios, decreased fetal movement
Perinatal	May require resuscitation, contractures
Cause	
Chromosomes	Normal except in MDS
Other	Heterogeneous including some autosomal recessive

Fig. 2. Patient ILS-3 (unreported). Frontal (A) and lateral (B) views at 7 and 11 months, respectively, show changes of LS. CT scans show type I (grade 3) lissencephaly with normal midline structures (C); and figure-8 shape due to hypoplastic opercula, regions of agyria (frontal area) and probable pachygyria (parietal area), and colpocephaly (D). MRI scan shows a normal cerebellum and confirms frontal agyria and parietal pachygyria (E).

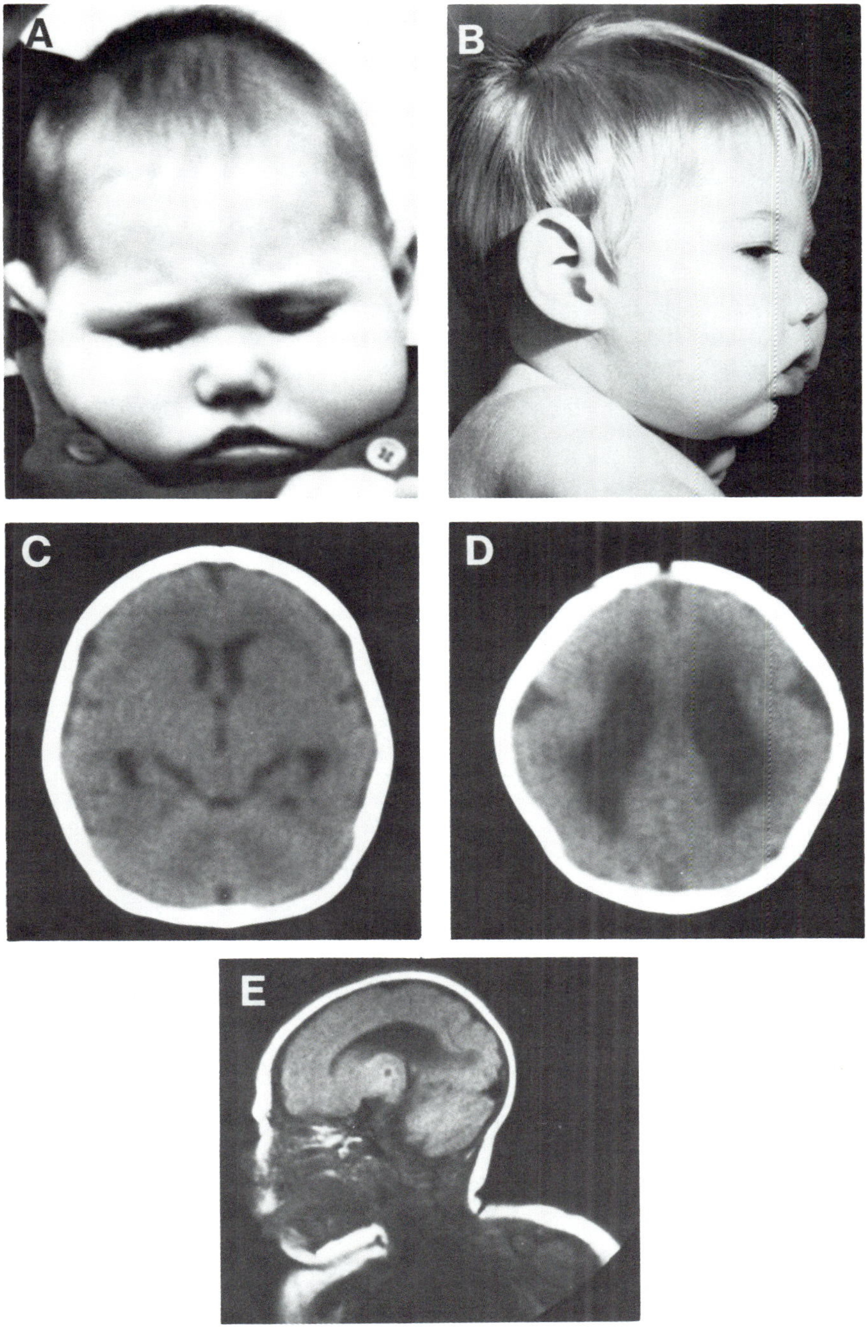
A
B
C
D
E

regions of pachygyria and sometimes agyria have been observed [12]. Histologic changes have been most similar to type I lissencephaly in patients with gyral defects (D. Armstrong, personal communication, 1985), although most patients do not have gyral defects [13]. The craniofacial and cardiac abnormalities (Table V) are hypothesized to result from defective migration of cephalic neural crest [12].

Cerebro-Cerebellar Lissencephaly

CCL (Fig. 5) has been reported in only 5 patients. Associated clinical abnormalities have included polydactyly, the lissencephaly sequence, and other somatic and craniofacial abnormalities including malformed ears, and minor genital abnormalities [5]. The reports suggest causal heterogeneity. However, based on the concurrence of CCL in sibs [8], a recurrence risk of up to 25% should be given pending further experience.

Walker-Warburg Syndrome

Walker-Warburg syndrome (WWS) is an autosomal recessive malformation syndrome characterized by type II lissencephaly and associated brain

TABLE III. Manifestations in Miller-Dieker Syndrome

Abnormality	Manifestations
Frequent	
Brain	Type I (grade 1–2) lissencephaly, lissencephaly sequence, midline calcification
Brain function	Lissencephaly sequence
Craniofacial	Lissencephaly sequence, relatively high forehead. Abnormal irides, tortuous fundal vessels. Low nasal bridge, telecanthus, epicanthal folds, upturned nares. Long, thin upper lip, late eruption of primary teeth, prominent alveolar ridges
Body	Abnormal palmar creases, clinodactyly, camptodactyly. Cryptorchidism, sacral dimples
Growth	Small at birth, severe postnatal growth deficiency
Occasional	
Brain and brain function	Lissencephaly sequence
Prenatal, perinatal	Lissencephaly sequence, prolonged neonatal jaundice
Craniofacial	Vertical wrinkling of forehead
Body	Congenital heart defect, polydactyly, visceral anomalies, sacral tail
Cause	
Chromosomes	del(17)(p13.3) in > 50%
Other	Unknown

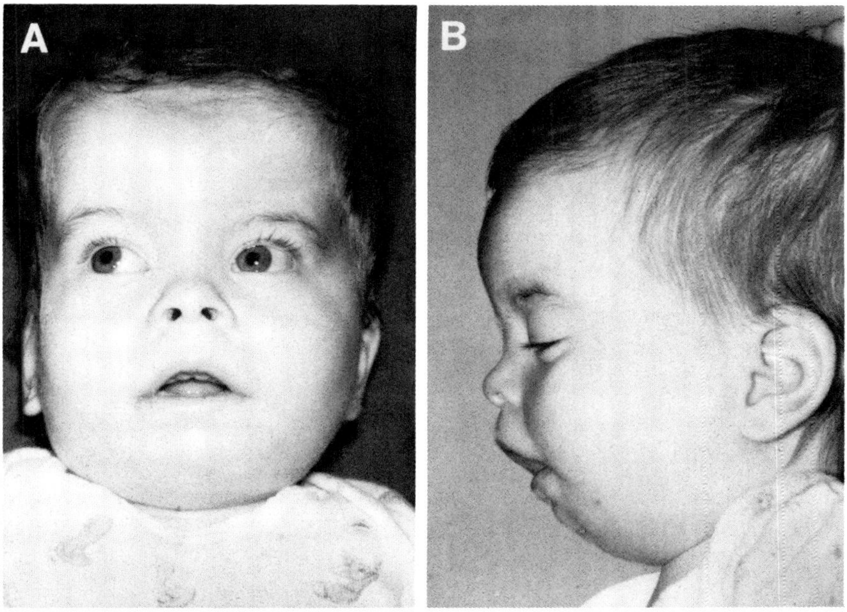

Fig. 3. Patient MDS-3 (patient 3 in [9]). Frontal (A) and lateral (B) views at 9 months show typical craniofacial changes of MDS. CT scans published previously [2] show type I (grade 1 or 2) lissencephaly, hypoplasia of the corpus callosum, and a small midline calcification. Chromosome analysis was abnormal [46,XX,−17,+der(17),t(7;17)(p22.3;p13.2)pat].

TABLE IV. Manifestations in Norman-Roberts Syndrome

Abnormality	Manifestations
Brain	Type I lissencephaly, lissencephaly sequence, no olivary heterotopias
Brain function	Lissencephaly sequence
Craniofacial	Lissencephaly sequence, low, sloping forehead. Telecanthus, prominent nasal root. Nares not upturned, eyes normal
Body	Low birthweight, clinodactyly, chordee
Cause	
Chromosomes	Normal
Other	Autosomal recessive

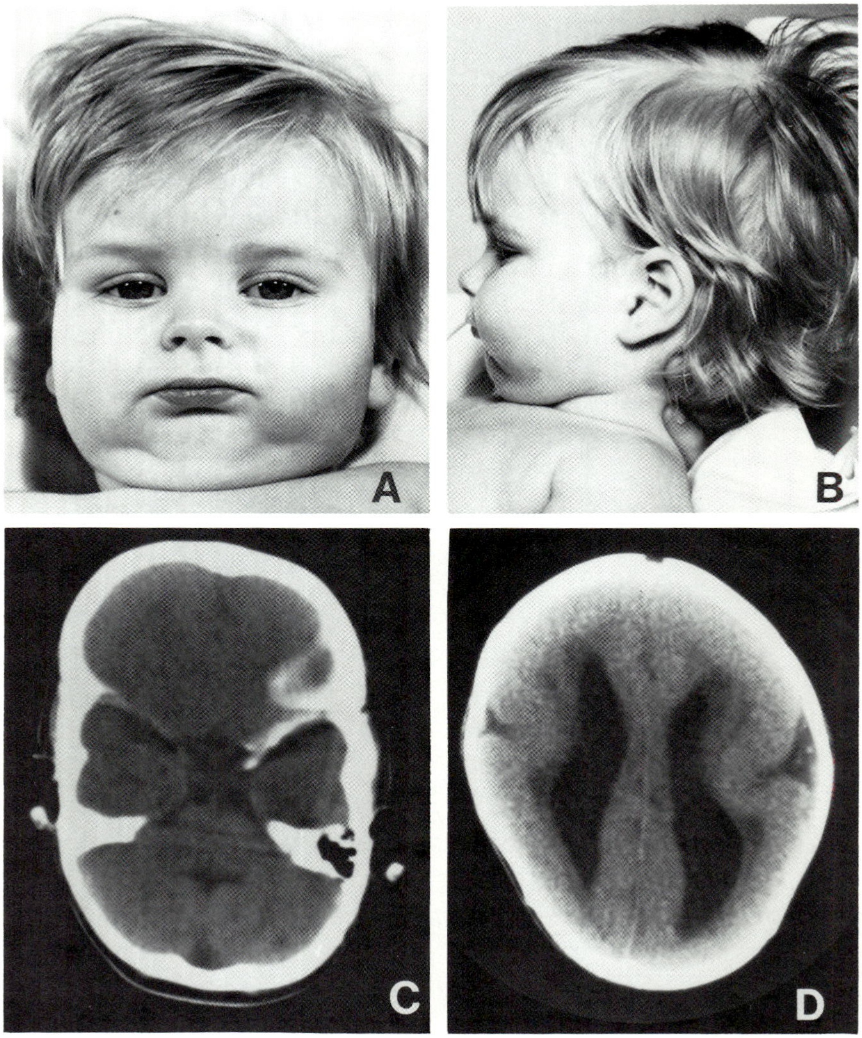

Fig. 4. Patient MDS-9 (unreported). Frontal (A) and lateral (B) views at 25 months show typical but more subtle changes of MDS. CT scans show type I (grade 1 or 2) lissencephaly with a normal cerebellum (C); and figure-8 shape due to opercular hypoplasia, smooth subsurface lines indicating widespread agyria, and colpocephaly (D). Other cuts showed hypoplasia of the corpus callosum. No midline calcification was seen. Chromosome analysis was normal. The parents are double third cousins.

TABLE V. Manifestations in Isotretinoin Embryopathy

Abnormality	Manifestations
Brain	Hydrocephalus, leptomeningeal heterotopias, vermis hypoplasia, Dandy-Walker malformation, corticospinal tract malformations
Brain (occasional)	Gyral defects including grade 3 lissencephaly, regional pachygyria, subcortical heterotopias
Brain function	Severe or profound mental retardation, hypotonia, diminished deep tendon reflexes, absent or abnormal primitive reflexes, hypoactive
Craniofacial	Low-set, small or atretic, malformed ears, small or atretic external auditory meatus, microphthalmia, telecanthus, epicanthal folds, low nasal bridge, small jaw sometimes with U-shaped cleft palate (Robin sequence)
Heart	Ventricular septal defect, truncus arteriosus, double-outlet right ventricle, interrupted aortic arch, patent ductus arteriosus
Cause	
Chromosomes	Normal
Other	Exposure at 2–8 weeks gestation

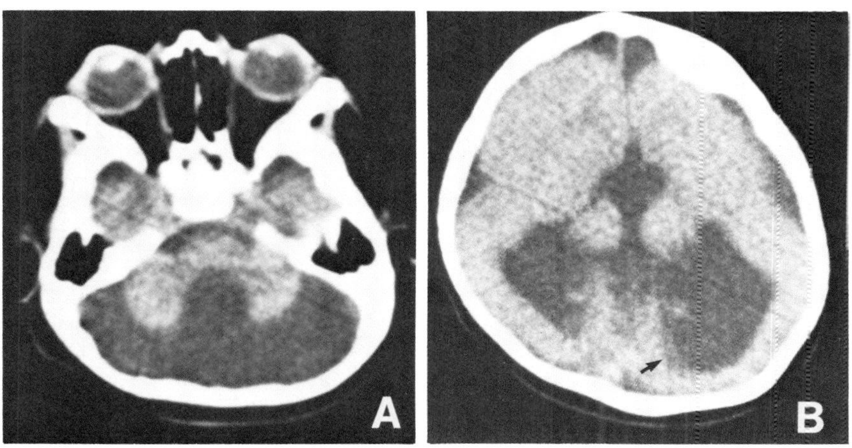

Fig. 5. Patient CCL-2 (patient 2 in [5]). CT scans show striking hypoplasia of cerebellar hemispheres with apparently absent vermis (A); and typical figure-8 appearance of cerebrum with smooth subsurface lines consistent with agyria. A and B reprinted from [3] and [5] with permission.

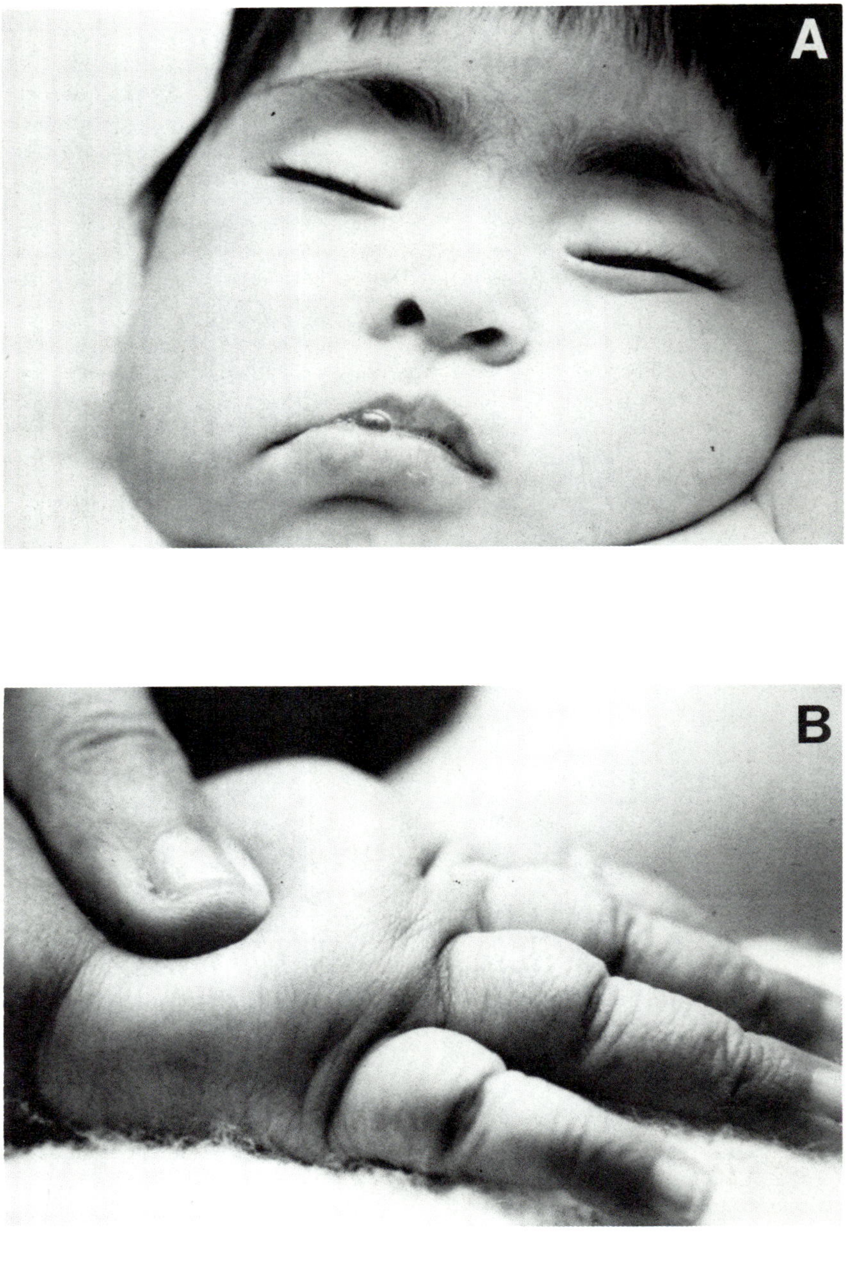
A
B

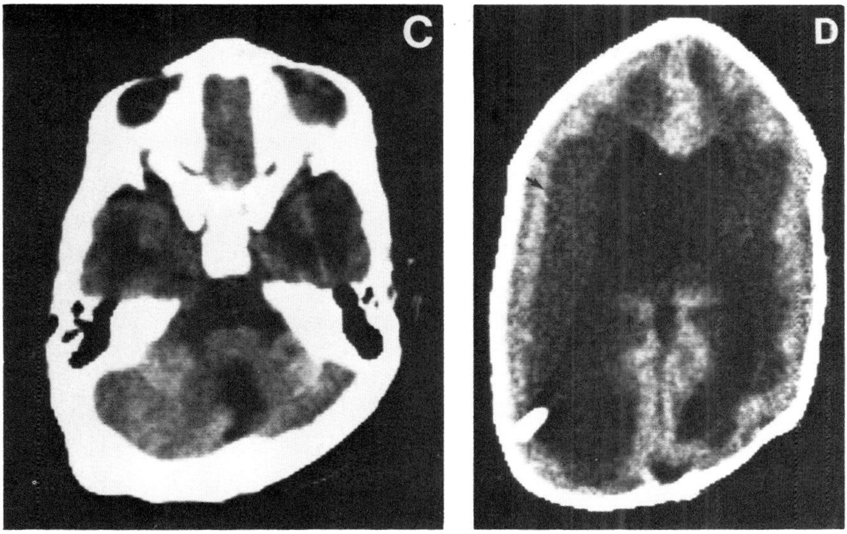

Fig. 6. Patient WWS-3 (patient 1 in [4]). Frontal (A) and hand (B) views at 6 months show a low anterior hairline, wide and low nasal bridge with epicanthal folds, upslanting palpebral fissures, upturnal nares, small jaw, and "puffiness" of both face and hand. CT scans show type II lissencephaly with Dandy-Walker malformation (C); and hydrocephalus, lucent white matter, smooth white-gray interface, and radiodense tissue obscuring the anterior interhemispheric fissure (D). C reprinted from [4]; D reprinted from [3] and [4] with permission.

defects, anterior chamber and retinal changes, and other abnormalities (Table VI, Fig. 6) [4,6]. Many patients (all?) also have a type of congenital muscular dystrophy and a few cleft lip/palate [6,14]. Similar but not identical clinical and pathologic changes have been described in one other syndrome—Fukuyama congenital muscular dystrophy [4].

CLINICAL COURSE

All patients with lissencephaly are severely or profoundly mentally retarded and at risk for frequent infections, especially recurrent aspiration pneumonia (caused by reduced and/or abnormal neuromuscular control of coughing and swallowing) and urinary tract infections. Most patients with grade 1 or 2 lissencephaly and some with grade 3 are very hypoactive and make little or no developmental progress; a few have been able to visually fix and follow, and smile briefly. Some patients with grade 3 lissencephaly have learned to sit and crawl (late), and a few have learned to walk (at 3–7 years) [15]; none have developed useful speech.

TABLE VI. Manifestations in Walker-Warburg Syndrome

Abnormality	Manifestations
Frequent	
Prenatal	Polyhydramnios, decreased fetal movements
Perinatal	Frequent cesarean section, low Apgar scores, often require resuscitation
Brain	Type II lissencephaly, hydrocephalus, small or absent corpus callosum, septum pellucidum. Vermis hypoplasia with or without Dandy-Walker malformation, posterior cephalocele
Muscle	Congenital muscular dystrophy in many, perhaps all
Brain function	Profound mental retardation, decreased spontaneous activity, severe and unremitting hypotonia, seizures
Eye	Microphthalmia, corneal opacity, Peter anomaly, other anterior chamber mesenchymal dysgenesis, cataracts, persistent hyperplastic primary vitreous, retinal dysplasia, optic nerve hypoplasia
Craniofacial	Frequent macrocephaly, apparently low-set malformed ears, low nasal bridge, small jaw, prominent alveolar ridges, puffy appearance
Body	Puffy appearance (?)
Growth	Normal at birth, subsequent growth deficiency in some
Occasional	
Brain function	Abnormal temperature regulation
Eye	Buphthalmos, iris and retinal colobomas
Craniofacial	Cleft lip, palate
Body	Congenital contractures, abnormal palmar creases, cryptorchidism, small genitalia. Several other abnormalities in one patient each
Cause	
Chromosomes	Normal
Other	Autosomal recessive

Almost all patients are hypotonic at birth. Most with type I lissencephaly become hypertonic (or mixed hypertonia/central hypotonia) with opisthotonus. Most with type II are profoundly hypotonic and remain so. At least 1 developed some signs of hypertonia (patient 4 in [4]).

Seizures usually begin before age 6 months and may progress to (or begin with) infantile spasms in at least 20 to 30% of patients (probably an underestimate). ACTH therapy for infantile spasms results in improvement in about half the patients with this type of seizure, and may lead to a relatively prolonged seizure-free period. However, most patients continue to have seizures that may be refractory to treatment. Status epilepticus seems to be uncommon.

The lifespan of patients with lissencephaly is shortened. Most patients with type II (WWS) die during the first year. Patients with MDS often die before age 2 years, especially if congenital heart defects are present, but some live longer. The oldest child known to me is now 4 years old. Patients with ILS (especially those with grade 3 lissencephaly) have lived much longer; the oldest reported patient died at 11 years [15]. Others have died within the first few years. The most common cause of death is aspiration pneumonia.

ACKNOWLEDGMENTS

I wish to thank Dr. William Rhead for providing information on patient ILS-3 (Fig. 2) and Janet Jacobs for manuscript preparation.

REFERENCES

1. Opitz JM: The developmental field concept. Am J Med Genet 21:1–11, 1985.
2. Dobyns WB, Stratton RF, Greenberg F: Syndromes with lissencephaly. I: Miller-Dieker and Norman-Roberts syndromes and isolated lissencephaly. Am J Med Genet 18:509–526, 1984.
3. Dobyns WB, McCluggage CW: Computed tomographic appearance of lissencephaly syndromes. Am J Neurorad 6:545–550, 1985.
4. Dobyns WB, Kirkpatrick JB, Hittner HM, Roberts RM, Kretzer FL: Syndromes with lissencephaly. II: Walker-Warburg and cerebro-oculo-muscular syndromes and a new syndrome with type II lissencephaly. Am J Med Genet 22:157–195, 1985.
5. Dobyns WB, Gilbert EF, Opitz JM: Further comments on the lissencephaly syndromes. Am J Med Genet 22:197–211, 1985.
6. Towfighi J, Sassani JW, Suzuki K, Ladda RL: Cerebro-ocular dysplasia—muscular dystrophy (COD-MD) syndrome. Acta Neuropathol (Berl) 65:110–123, 1984.
7. Sidman RL, Rakic P: Development of the human central nervous system. In Haymaker W, Adams RD (eds): "Histology and Histopathology of the Nervous System." Springfield, IL: Thomas, 1982, pp 3–145.
8. Barth PG, Mullaart R, Stam FC, Sloof JL: Familial lissencephaly with extreme neopallial hypoplasia. Brain Dev 4:145–151, 1982.
9. Dobyns WB, Stratton RF, Parke JT, Greenberg F, Nussbaum RL, Ledbetter DH: Miller-Dieker syndrome and monosomy 17p. J Pediatr 102:552–558, 1983.
10. Stratton RF, Dobyns WB, Airhart SD, Ledbetter DH: New chromosomal syndrome: Miller-Dieker syndrome and monosomy 17p13. Hum Genet 67:193–200, 1984.
11. Norman MG, Roberts M, Sirois J, Tremblay LJM: Lissencephaly. Can J Neurol Sci 3:39–46, 1976.
12. Lammer EJ: Retinoic acid embryopathy: A neural crest migrational abnormality. Am J Hum Genet 36:61S (Abstract), 1984.
13. Hansen LA, Pearl GS: Isotretinoin teratogenicity: Case report with neuropathologic findings. Acta Neuropathol (Berl) 65:335–337, 1985.
14. Zimmerman RL, Hanson RD, Blomberg DJ, Nollet DJ: The lissencephaly syndrome. Minnesota Medicine 65:223–224, 1982.
15. Paskind HA, Stone TT: Familial spastic paralysis: Report of 3 cases in one family and observation at necropsy. Arch Neurol Psych 30:481–500, 1933.

Microscopic Study of Midline Determinants in Janiceps Twins

G.H. Sperber, PhD, and G.A. Machin, MD, PhD

Department of Oral Biology, Faculty of Dentistry, University of Alberta, Edmonton, Alberta, Canada (GHS) and Department of Laboratory Medicine, Victoria General Hospital, Victoria, British Columbia, Canada (GAM)

"Monstrosities contribute to rectify our opinions . . . . From wrong construction of parts arises unnatural action, which by studying we may discover the natural action" [1].

INTRODUCTION

Cephalothoracopagus conjoined twins (so-called janiceps, after the two-faced Greek god, Janus) are an uncommon type of conjoined twins, and there are few detailed descriptions in the literature [2–4]. This type of conjoined twinning is of interest for several reasons, primarily with regard to pathogenesis and anatomic pathology, particularly concerning midline organization of organs and tissues. We have had the opportunity to study spontaneously aborted janiceps fetuses that were sufficiently small to permit serial horizontal sections to be cut through the entire specimen for microscopic study. We report the findings of this study and the conclusions we have drawn concerning the pathogenesis of janiceps twinning, the key anatomic regions involved in and affected by the conjoined head regions, and compare these with previously reported cases. The present specimen is at the earliest developmental stage of janiceps twinning reported to date.

CLINICAL HISTORY

The fetus was spontaneously aborted by a 28-year-old gravida 2, para 1 woman, whose first child was born normally at term, but died suddenly in

Birth Defects: Original Article Series, Volume 23, Number 1, pages 243–275

the postneonatal period. The current pregnancy was clinically normal until nearly 14 weeks of gestation by menstrual age, when there was an episode of vaginal bleeding. Ultrasound examination at exactly 14 weeks' gestation showed an apparently single fetus that measured 33 mm crown-rump length (corresponding with a menstrual age of 10 weeks). The biparietal diameter was 13 mm and it was noted that the head region appeared bilobed, with suspicion of an occipital encephalocele. The amniotic fluid volume appeared normal. The fetus was thought to be dead because there was no visible heart beat, and spontaneous abortion took place at 14 weeks and 4 days of gestation. There was no known exposure to teratogenic agents early in the pregnancy.

MATERIALS AND METHODS

The fetus was received intact without the placenta, in formalin, precluding chromosome study. It was 33 mm long, corresponding exactly with the ultrasonic measurement. Roentgenograms (CT scans and Grenz rays) showed no detectable ossification centers. After photography, "faces" and "bodies" were designated (Figs. 1, 2), and the fetus was then processed routinely for histologic sections at 7 μ intervals in the horizontal (transverse) plane so as to maximize the correlation of facial structures with each other and with the bodies. Interval sections were stained with hematoxylin and eosin, while intervening sections were kept for special stains, and for the elucidation of areas of rapid or critically important change in orientation of midline structures. The histologic sections were cut and mounted so as to correlate with the macroscopic "faces" and "bodies." All the illustrations in this paper are oriented according to the designations shown in Figures 3 and 4.

RESULTS

The fetuses were conjoined cephalothoracopagus males, with a nearly perfect symmetrical janiceps configuration. As far as could be judged from external appearance, the longitudinal (vertebral) axes of the fetuses were almost exactly at 180 degrees ventroventrally, since both faces were apparently fully represented.

Ossification of clavicles and frontal bones was compatible with a conception age of at least 8 weeks. The brains and spinal cords were autolysed, but other organs were moderately well preserved, suggesting that intrauterine death had occurred only a few days before spontaneous abortion.

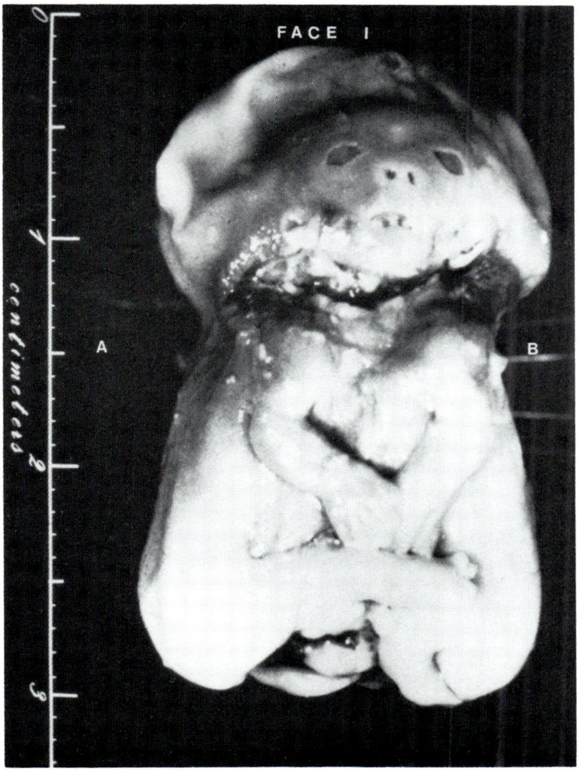

Fig. 1. View of face 1, which is identified by the hemorrhagic laceration in the cervical region. This is also seen in the histologic sections. Bodies A and B are designated as shown.

Central Nervous System

The orientation of the brains was complex; the septum separating the 2 halves of the cerebrum of face 1 (brain 1A/1B in Fig. 5) was regarded as a true falx cerebri orientated at a right angle to face 1. The cerebrum of face 2 appeared undivided into hemispheres because of virtual absence of the falx cerebri. It is therefore presumed to be holoprosencephalic. Remnants of a hypoplastic falx were seen as indicated in Figure 5.

The midbrains and hindbrains were oriented to the vertebral axes of bodies A and B (Fig. 5), and there was a definite impression that face 1 was subtended by a reflex angle and face 2 by an obtuse angle between the vertebral axes. The autolytic condition of the brain prevented assessment of the presence of a corpus callosum in the brain of face 1.

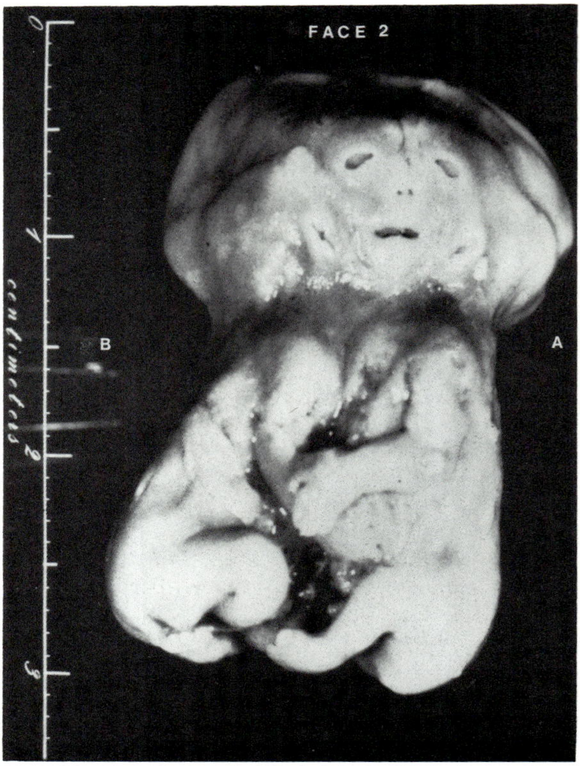

Fig. 2. Face 2 and the orientations of the bodies. The nostrils appear slightly closer than in face 1, and there is also mild relative hypotelorism. Ears of both faces are low-set.

Orientation of the eyes and other cranial nerves was studied in some detail. Olfactory nerves were not identified, but this does not preclude their presence. The eyes of both faces appeared normal, and the courses taken by the optic nerves were not fully determined because of autolysis. The optic nerves of both faces ran toward the common central diencephalon/mesencephalon. The optic nerves of face 1 are shown in Figure 6 A and B. The orientation of the optic nerves and the presence of a rudimentary dividing septum (Fig. 6, item 4) suggests that there probably was no optic chiasm of face 1. The trigeminal nerve ganglia seen in Figures 3 and 6 received their tracts from the midbrain in the corresponding quadrants, as did the acoustic nerves (Fig. 7). In this specimen, no cranial nerves were observed to cross the facial midlines. Thus, each cerebrum was a compound structure in which

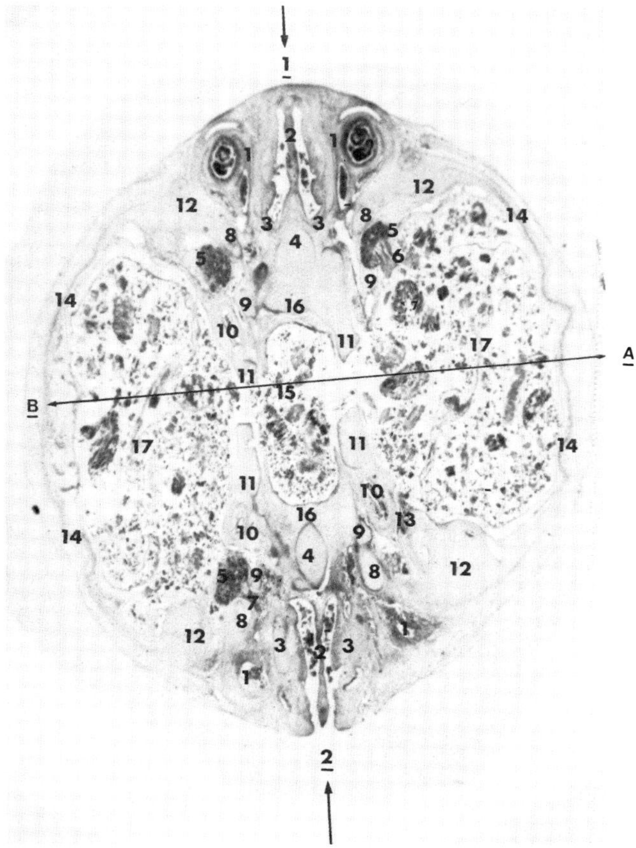

Fig. 3. A typical horizontal section at the level of the eyes of face 1 (× 10.5). This orientation of faces and bodies applies to all the subsequent histologic illustrations. 1: eyes, 2: nasal septa, 3: nasal capsules, 4: mesethmoid cartilages, 5: trigeminal ganglia, 6: trigeminal tract, 7: ophthalmic nerve, 8: orbitosphenoid cartilages, 9: alisphenoid cartilages, 10: cochleae, 11: postsphenoid cartilages, 12: otic capsules, 13: internal acoustic meatus, 14: occipital sclerotomal cartilages, 15: diencephalon, 16: presphenoid cartilages, 17: posterior cranial fossae.

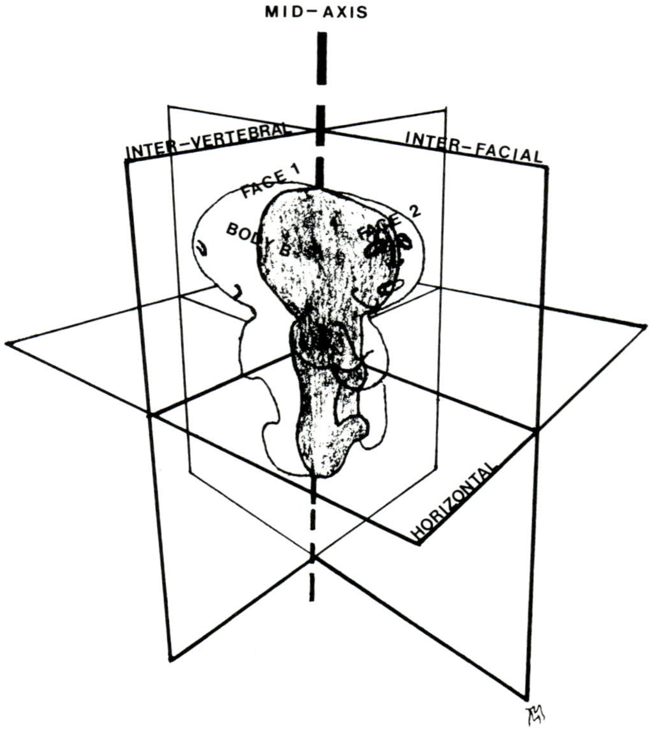

Fig. 4. Line drawing depicts axes and planes of the twins.

each half was derived from the central nervous systems of different conjoined fetuses as defined by their vertebral axes. The presence of a cerebral holosphere corresponding with face 2 indicates that close fusion or failure of complete fission of the central nervous systems occurred at the lines of meeting of the hemifaces.

Faces

Microscopic examination confirmed the macroscopic observation that there were minimal differences between the faces, and that these were less marked than might have been expected from the presence of holoprosencephaly of the brain of face 2. The nasal septum of face 2 contained no cartilage, while that of face 1 contained normal cartilage (Fig. 6). In other respects, the nasal capsules appeared very similar. In particular, both faces 1 and 2 appeared to

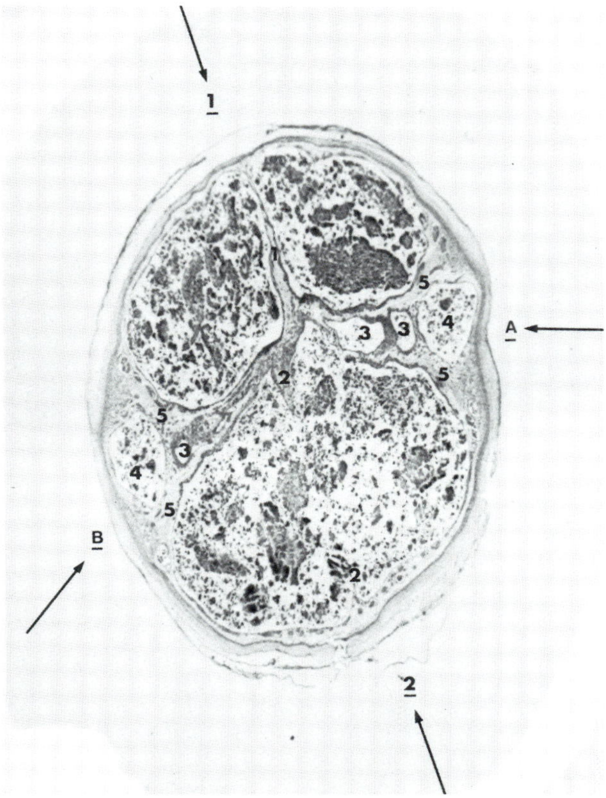

Fig. 5. Horizontal section to show orientation of cerebra (× 10.5). 1: falx cerebri of brain 1, 2: remnants of falx cerebri of brain 2, 3: midbrains, 4: hindbrains, 5: tentoria cerebelli.

have mesethmoid cartilages (Figs. 3, 6). Thus, absence of a nasal septal cartilage was the only perceptible "reduction" abnormality of face 2.

The 2 stomatodea gave rise to oral cavities that led to an undivided midaxial pharyngeal cavity, which was bounded on its vertebral aspects by artefactually ruptured postsphenoid cartilages (Fig. 8). The common pharynx was continuous superiorly with a dilated single Rathke pouch, the roof of which could not be identified. There was a large central defect of the chondrocranial floor in this region, with presumed close apposition of the roof of the Rathke pouch and the hypothalamic regions of the brains (Figs.

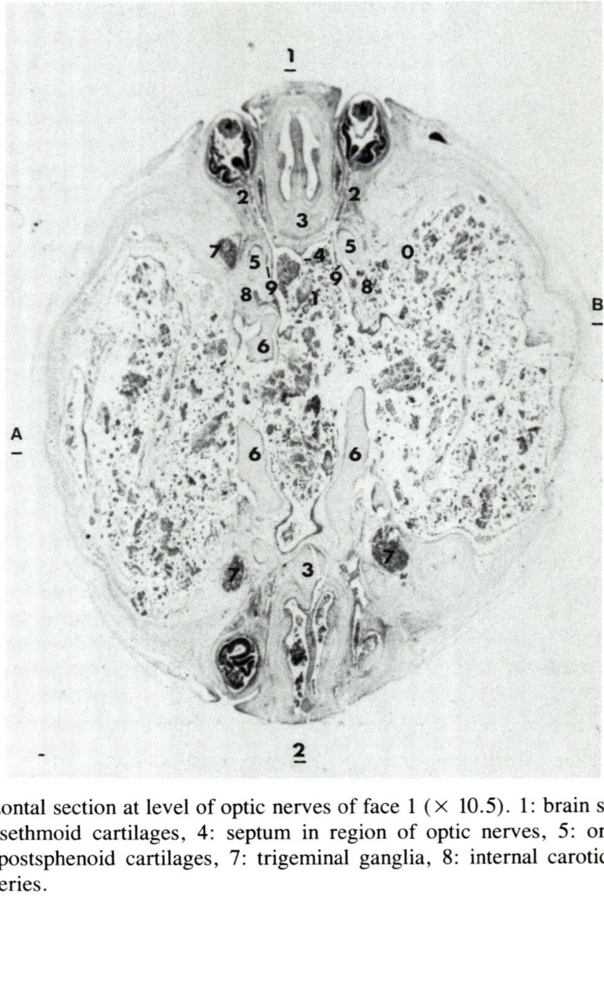

Fig. 6. Horizontal section at level of optic nerves of face 1 (× 10.5). 1: brain stem, 2: optic nerves, 3: mesethmoid cartilages, 4: septum in region of optic nerves, 5: orbitosphenoid cartilages, 6: postsphenoid cartilages, 7: trigeminal ganglia, 8: internal carotid arteries, 9: ophthalmic arteries.

7–9). Pre- and postsphenoid cartilages were arranged at right angles around the rim of the defect (Fig. 3). It appeared that the roof of the Rathke pouch had ruptured, allowing autolytic brain tissue to escape from the cranial cavity into the pharynx (Figs. 7, 8). No adenohypophysis was identified. The palatal shelves were incompletely fused; since they normally fuse by day 56, a cleft palate was present in each mouth. A normal complement of first and second branchial arch, groove and pharyngeal pouch derivatives (ear ossicles, Meckel cartilage, external acoustic meatus, Eustachian tube, and tonsillar fossa) was

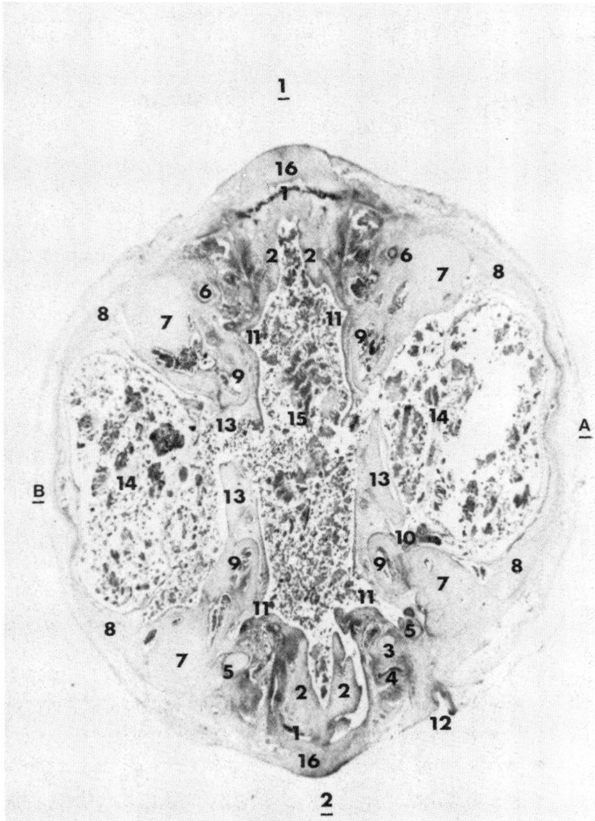

Fig. 7. Horizontal section at the level of the palatal shelves and inner ears (× 10.5). 1: maxillae, 2: palatal shelves, 3: Meckel cartilage, 4: mandible, 5: ear ossicles, 6: second arch cartilages, 7: otic capsules, 8: occipital sclerotomes, 9: cochleae, 10: acoustic nerve, 11: auditory tubes, 12: external acoustic meatus with hillocks, 13: postsphenoid cartilages, 14: posterior cranial fossae, 15: common pharyngeal cavity, 16: upper lips.

present in each hemiface (Figs. 7–9). However, no maxillary or mandibular tooth buds were present.

Foregut

Between the posterior aspects of the two tongues there was a single foregut cavity that more resembled respiratory than gastrointestinal tract (Fig. 10). The lumen was bounded at its 4 corners by the second and third branchial

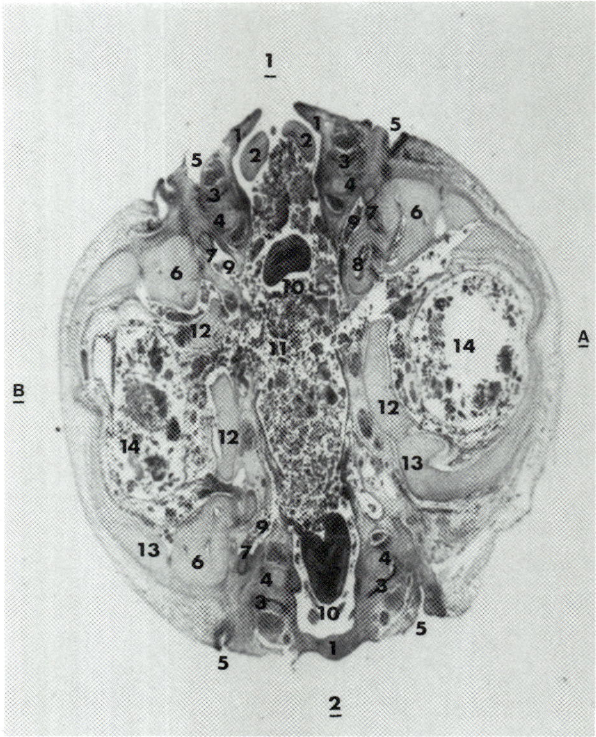

Fig. 8. Horizontal section through upper mouth region (× 10.5). 1: upper lips, 2: palatal shelves, 3: mandibles, 4: Meckel cartilages, 5: external acoustic meatus, 6: otic capsules, 7: ear ossicles, 8: cochlea, 9: auditory tubes, 10: tongues, 11: common pharynx, 12: parachordal cartilages, 13: occipital sclerotomal cartilages, 14: brain stems.

arch cartilages. Further caudad, septation led to 2 larynges oriented to the vertebral axes (Fig. 11). The hyoid cartilages adopted a highly abnormal orientation with fusion according to facial orientation but with inclination to the vertebral axes (Fig. 11). Immediately below the larynges, the lumen was reduced again to a single canal, not totally surrounded by cartilage (Fig. 12). From this level, the two tracheae budded obliquely between strict vertebral and facial axes (Fig. 13), but soon became oriented to the faces, running inferiorly close to and parallel to the single midaxial esophagus. The latter

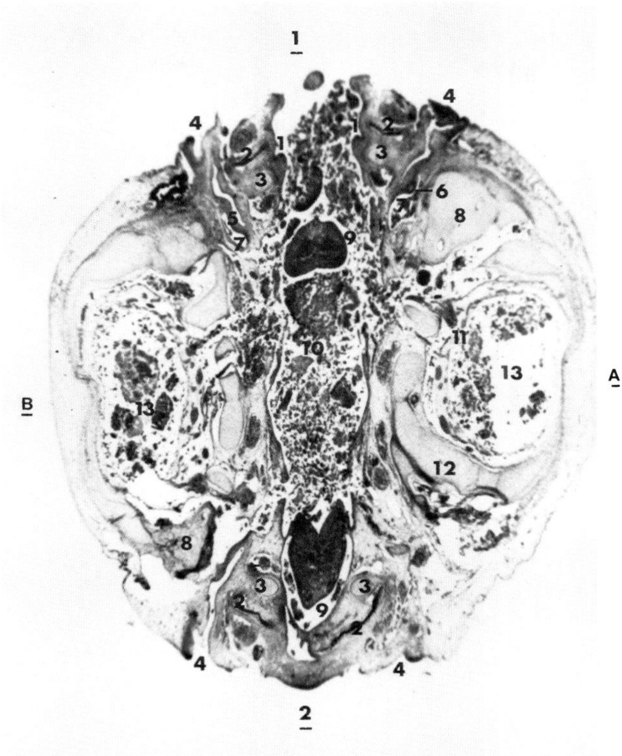

Fig. 9. Horizontal section through lower mouth region showing derivatives of first and second branchial arches and grooves, and pharyngeal pouches (× 10.5). 1: tonsillar fossae (second pharyngeal pouches), 2: mandibles, 3: Meckel cartilages, 4: external acoustic meatus, 5: tympanic membrane, 6: ear ossicle, 7: auditory tubes, 8: otic capsules, 9: tongues, 10: common pharynx, 11: hypoglossal nerve, 12: occipital sclerotomal cartilages, 13: medulla oblongata.

was continuous with the sublaryngeal foregut, and was "left" in the midline after the tracheae had budded off (Fig. 14). The lungs were normally oriented with respect to the faces, and each trachea bifurcated into main bronchi at the appropriate level, with recognizable right and left bronchi, as demonstrated by eparterial bronchi (Figs. 14 and 15). The esophagus led to a single

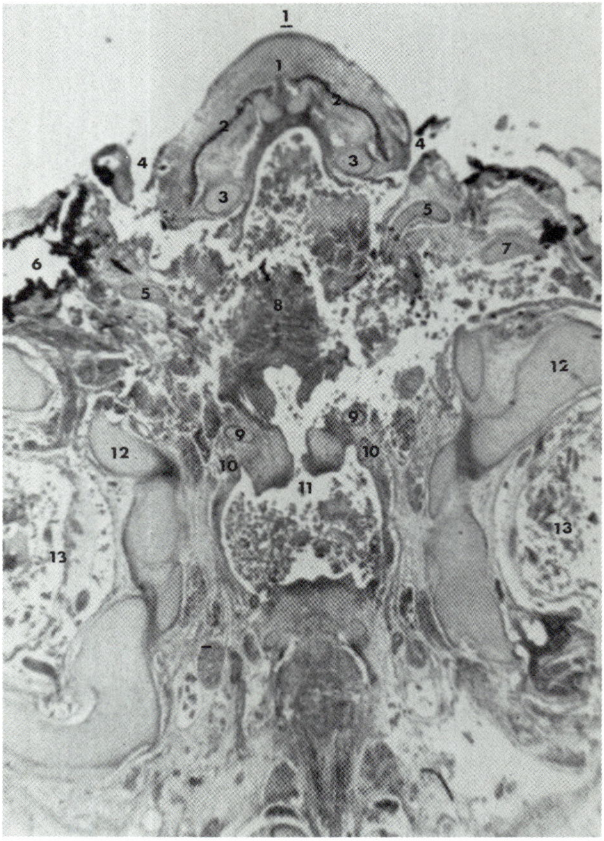

Fig. 10. Horizontal section through face 1 at upper cervical level (× 14). At this level, the orientation of the 1st, 2nd and 3rd branchial arch cartilages around the foregut is depicted. The cervical hemorrhage in face 1 is conspicuous. 1: lower lip, 2: mandibles, 3: Meckel cartilages, 4: external acoustic meatus, 5: styloid process (branchial arch 2), 6: hemorrhage, 7: branchial arch cartilage (?3rd), 8: infrahyoid muscles, 9: hyoid cartilages, 10: thyroid cartilages, 11: common pharynx, 12: cervical vertebral arch cartilages, 13: spinal cords.

midaxial stomach, and the small bowel remained single until the level of the vitellointestinal duct, at which point it duplicated. The arrangement of the remainder of the gastrointestinal canal was typical of conjoined thoracoomphalopagus twins.

Cardiovascular System

The hearts were oriented normally to the faces, and communicated appropriately with the pulmonary circulations. There was an interaortic anasto-

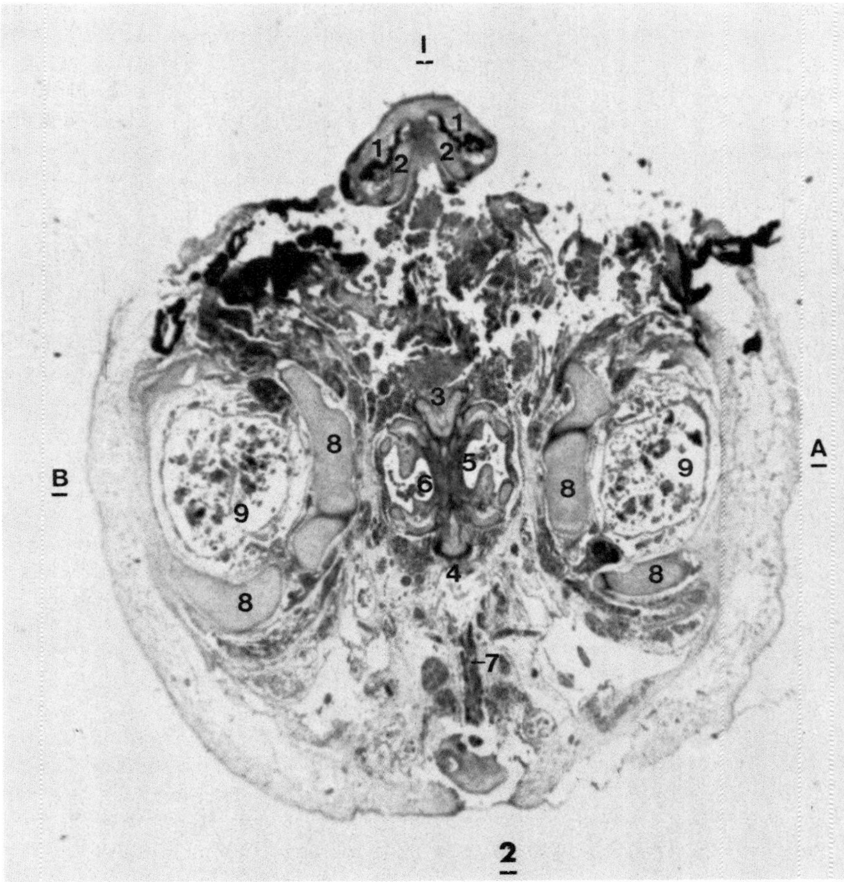

Fig. 11. Horizontal section at the level of the hyoid cartilages to show their abnormal location and shape (× 10.5); they fuse bilaterally appropriately in the midfacial planes, but also show the influence of vertebral orientation by their "inverted" orientation to the faces. The cervical hemorrhage in face 1 is conspicuous. Note the absence of midaxial esophagus. 1: mandibles, 2: Meckel cartilages, 3: hyoid cartilage of face 1, 4: hyoid cartilage of face 2, 5: larynx A, 6: larynx B, 7: infrahyoid muscles, 8: vertebral cartilages, 9: cervical spinal cords.

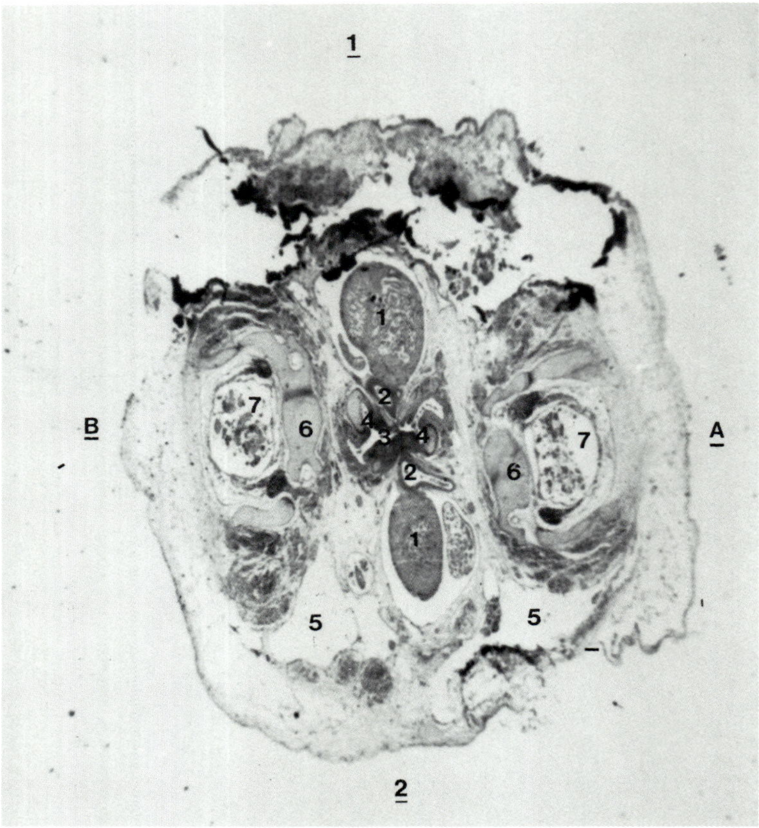

Fig. 12. Horizontal section at a level below the larynges to show the common foregut lumen reestablished, and the obliquely budding tracheae (× 10.5). Note the obliquity of the vertebro-vertebral plane to the facio-facial plane (cf Fig. 3). 1: hearts, 2: aortae, 3: common foregut canal, 4: obliquely budding tracheae, 5: pleural cavities, 6: vertebral cartilages, 7: spinal cords.

mosing vessel connecting the two aortic arches (Fig. 16). The hearts of faces 1 and 2 gave rise to the descending aortae of vertebral axes B and A, respectively. The descending aorta of vertebral axis B was hypoplastic in comparison with that of A (Fig. 14). The pericardial sacs were deficient anteriorly, but the pleuroperitoneal canals were closed. There were two livers oriented to the faces.

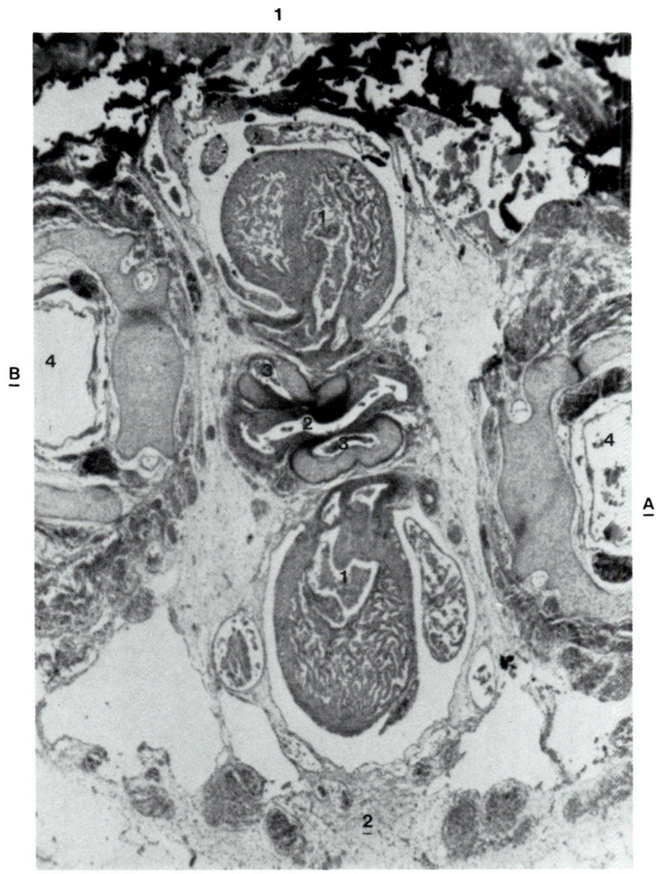

Fig. 13. Horizontal section shows separation of tracheal lumina from the esophagus (× 14). 1: hearts, 2: esophagus, 3: tracheae, 4: spinal cords.

Abdominal Viscera

The findings in the abdominal cavity were typical of those previously described in thoracoomphalopagus twins. The lower gastrointestinal tracts and the entire genitourinary systems were oriented to the vertebrae. Normal male external genitalia were present. There was fusion of the superior poles of the adrenal glands of vertebral fetus A. An omphalocele was present below the insertion of the single umbilical cord.

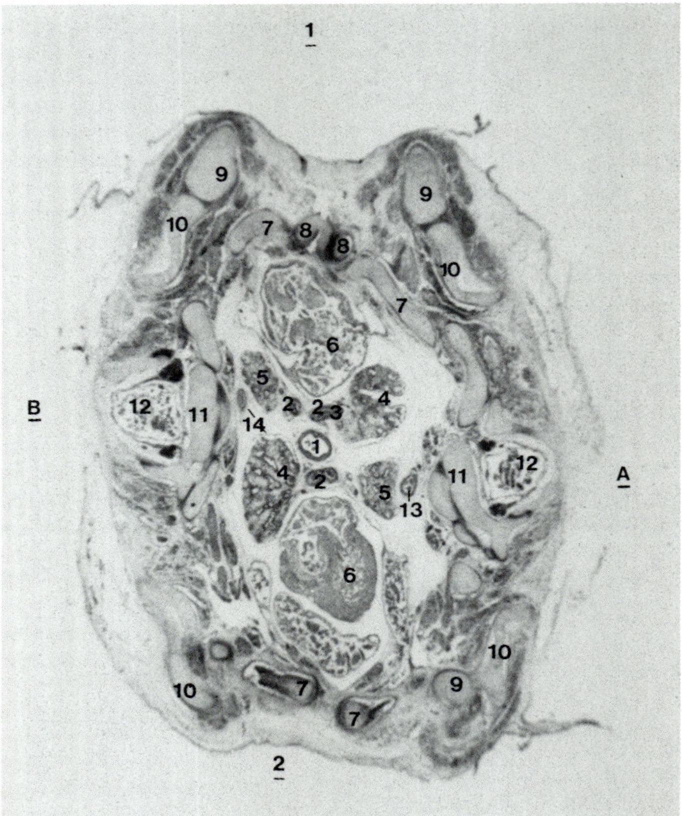

Fig. 14. Horizontal section to show tracheae bifurcating into bronchi (× 10.5); the aorta of body B is hypoplastic. 1: midaxial esophagus, 2: bronchi, 3: eparterial bronchus, 4: right lungs, 5: left lungs, 6: hearts, 7: clavicles (ossified in face 2 only), 8: sternal cartilages, 9: heads of humeri, 10: scapulae, 11: vertebral cartilages, 12: spinal cords, 13: aorta A/2, 14: aorta B/1.

DISCUSSION

It is generally agreed that conjoined twins represent incomplete fission of an originally single zygote, thereby forming an apparent coalescence of more or less closely apposed embryonic areas in the embryonic plate [5]. Indeed, it is difficult to envision how partial fusion of previously completely separated embryos could account for the phenomenon of conjoined twinning. The

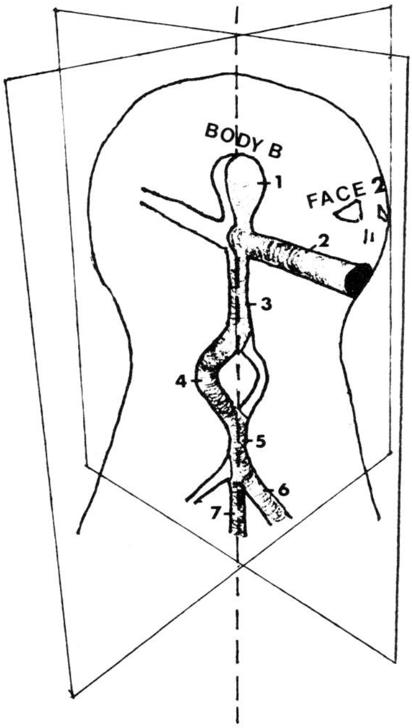

Fig. 15. Diagrammatic representation of the abnormal configuration of the foregut. 1: dilated Rathke pouch, 2: oropharynx oriented to face 2, 3: midaxial canal above larynges, 4: larynx oriented to body B, 5: midaxial canal below larynges, 6: trachea oriented to face 2, 7: midaxial esophagus.

incomplete fission that occurs in the janiceps configuration offers a number of interesting problems because of the conflicting influences of two sets of midline planes defined by the vertebrae and faces. It seems clear that such an anatomic arrangement could give valuable clues to the inductive relationships between various organs in the head and neck regions. The present case is unusual in two respects, since it is very nearly disymmetric and was spontaneously aborted at an earlier age than any previously described specimen; this allowed detailed microscopic study of an earlier stage of morphogenesis of organ systems than previously observed in janiceps twins.

In contrast with the standard orientation of the singleton conceptus in the embryonic plate, conjoined cephalothoracopagus twins are rotated on their longitudinal axes such that their ventral surfaces are apposed, and their dorsoventral axes are set at varying angles to one another, up to and including 180 degrees. At the same time, their longitudinal axes diverge caudally, thus

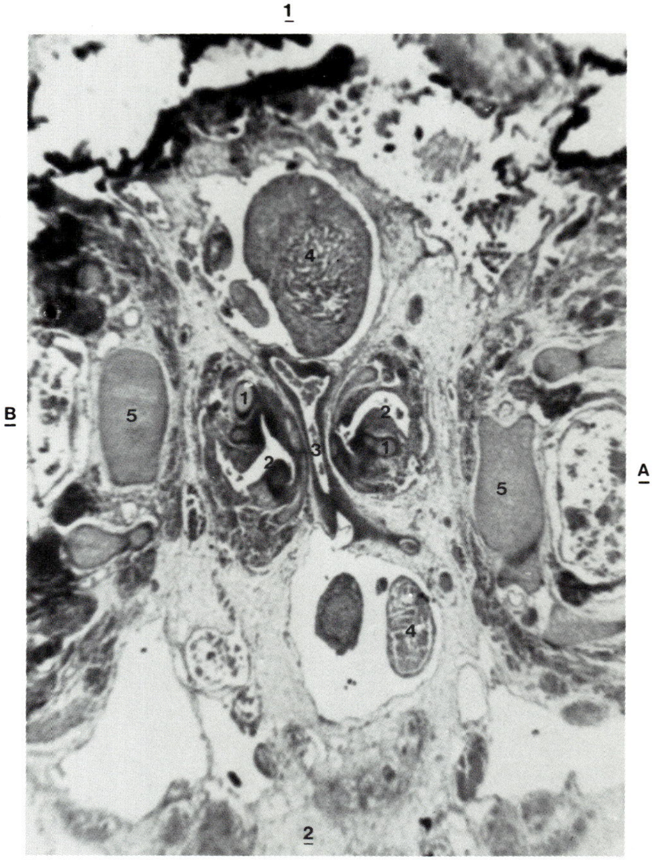

Fig. 16. Horizontal section to show the interaortic anastomosing vessel passing between the 2 larynges (× 14). 1: laryngeal cartilages, 2: vocal folds, 3: interaortic anastomosing vessel, 4: hearts, 5: vertebral cartilages.

accounting for the greater degree of fission caudad than craniad. Steadily increasing degrees of fission are seen as the caudal end is approached, with critical zones where organs and organ systems revert from a facial to a vertebral orientation. The discontinuity of facial and vertebral orientations occurs because the notochord can be regarded as a true midline, unpaired, dorsal-determining inducing influence. There is no comparably dominant ventral inducer, and normal formation of the ventral midline of the face, neck, and trunk results from the fusion of bilaterally paired structures, eg, the frontonasal, maxillary, and mandibular neural crest-derived prominences in the face. It seems reasonable to regard the midline dorsoventral planes set by the notochordal axes as the true axes of the conjoined fetuses, whereas the facial structures merely reflect the bilateral origins of all faces, singleton, twin, or conjoined twin. In janiceps twins, the faces cannot be constructed in the normal location because the apposed heads have remained interposed ventroventrally to the depth of the common Rathke pouch, so that the facial prominences meet each other laterally. Each face of the cephalothoracopagus twin is compounded of two "hemifaces," each derived from a different fetus. The two hemifaces combine to form a "bridge" or "synthesis" of bilateral structures forming a "compound" or "bifetogenic" face on each lateral aspect of the head region of the conjoined fetuses. The ability of these hemifaces to form perfect or variably reduced faces oriented at right angles to the true, vertebral axes of the fetuses is not as unlikely an event as might at first appear, since they are merely recapitulating the "midline" adjustment normally undergone by structures approaching the ventral region. However, there are various degrees of disorientation of internal organ systems, since the "synthetic" facial axes weaken in their inductive effects caudally as the vertebral axes diverge from one another. The ability to form a corpus callosum, optic chiasm, and holospheric brain attests to the degree to which this fusion of structures from two fetuses can occur. In the present case, the anatomy of the disorientations has been described in detail in order to gain insight into the relative inductive influences of the conflicting vertebral and facial axes. The findings are in broad agreement with those previously reported, but the microscopic study allowed the orientation of most of the organs to be appreciated in a cross-sectional *in situ* manner without disturbance by dissection.

There are 3 situations in which conjoined twins have 2 faces: (1) Craniopagus, in which cranial union at any site; the union is often quite asymmetric with minimal penetration, and the bodies are otherwise quite separate. (2) Fission beginning at the cranial end whereby the head is split to a variable degree, but there is only 1 body from the neck region caudally. There are two broad categories, (a) monocephalus diprosopus, with a single head bearing two faces, and (b) dicephalus, with two heads, each with its own face. (3) Cephalothoracopagus twinning, in which fission begins at the caudal end so that there are discrete bodies caudal to the umbilicus, but varying degrees of lack of ventroventral fission of upper abdomens, thoraces, and heads. Ventroventral orientation is usually only approximately at 180 degrees on the longitudinal axes so that one of the faces is hypoplastic. There are three types: (a) deradelphus, with a single face and cerebrum, but with fission from brainstems caudally; (b) syncephalus, in which the lesser face is represented by ears only, but with a variable cerebral component to the lesser face; (c) janiceps configuration, with faces on opposite sides of the head, and a greater degree of representation of the cerebrum of the lesser face.

The cephalothoracopagus configuration is among the rarer types of conjoined twinning. In 4 series of conjoined twins, totaling 132 sets, there were only 6 cases of syncephalus and cephalothoracopagus twinning [6–9]. Conjoined twins as a whole have a M:F ratio of 0.48:1; for cephalothoracopagus twins, the sex ratio is 0.11:1. There are now several reports of the prenatal diagnosis of conjoined twins [10–33]; only 3 of these concerned thoracopagus twinning [15,27,28]. Conjoined twins are seldom described among spontaneously aborted fetuses; none were found in one series of 55 pairs [34], while 2 were reported in another series of 15 pairs [35], 1 being a thoracopagus and the other dicephalic; it is noteworthy that both these pairs of aborted conjoined twins were male.

Few cases of janiceps twins have been reported in detail, and truly symmetrical (disymmetros) configuration is extremely rare, although it probably exists [4,36]. It is interesting to note that, while the case illustrated by Potter and Craig [36] appears to have 2 normal faces, close inspection of the other disymmetric case [4] strongly suggests that both the faces are cebocephalic, and the brains were reported to be holoprosencephalic. Most cases of craniothoracopagus show varying degrees of differences in the completeness of 1 of the faces, and are termed monosymmetros. They fall into a continuous spectrum of degrees of dissimilarity of the 2 faces, in which 1 face is practically normal, while the opposite face shows degrees of "reduction" through typical holoprosencephalic configurations to cases with no external representation of the second face; this appears to be caused by differing degrees of longitudinal axial rotation away from a precise 180 degrees ventroventral orientation. The definition of what does or does not constitute a facial component leads to somewhat arbitrary exclusions of some cases from the janiceps group. It seems logical to define cephalothoracopagus twins as having separate central nervous systems, at least from the brain stems caudally, with degrees of external expression of the second face from zero to expression equal to that of the first face. Internal pharyngeal components of the second face are always present. Whereas the first face is usually virtually normal, there are cases at the extreme end of the spectrum of monosymmetry in which the first face fails to fuse in the midline because of "overstretching"; it also appears that the second face may "break through" to be partially expressed in the midline of the split first face.

In the present case, critical points of "conversion" from facial to vertebral orientation were identified at varying levels of the body in the serial horizontal sections. There were levels at which the facial orientations "unraveled" to assume vertebral orientations. There were several of these critical points:

Critical point 1. In the area of the Rathke pouch (future hypophyseal fossa), there was a large central defect in the chondrocranium, where the postsphenoid and presphenoid cartilages were oriented (at right angles to one another) to the vertebral and facial axes, respectively. The absence of the adenohypophysis could indicate confused or absent inductive capacity of the roof of the stomatodeum, and the same could apply to the absent central base of the chondrocranium of the skull in this position.

Critical point 2. This specimen allowed little delineation of brain anatomy, but some clues were available from dural supporting structures. Face 1 had an apparently normal cerebrum, but we were unable to assess the status of the corpus callosum; it seems unlikely that there was an optic chiasm. Absence of full falx cerebri development in face 2 was strongly suggestive of holoprosencephaly, and this is supported by the very mild midfacial hypoplasia, viz, the absence of cartilage in the nasal septum. The components of a cerebral holosphere and a midfacial hypoplasia have 2 consequences in this case; first, they are supportive evidence of the orientation of the cerebra to the faces rather than the vertebrae; second, the cause of the hypoplasia of face 2 is presumed to be the obtuse (slightly less than 180 degrees) angulation of the vertebral axes on this side of the conjoined twins, with overlapping (or overfusion) of the midface of face 2. Although the mechanism of production of midfacial hypoplasia is thus probably different from that found in singletons, the implication for the brain is the same, viz, a cerebral holosphere. It should be noted that it seems probable that no truly symmetric janiceps could have a normal brain on either side; if the vertebral axes are oriented at exactly 180 degrees, convergence cranially of the 2 apposed notochordal axes will result in overfusion of the cerebra, even if the faces were perfectly fused, with no evidence of midfacial hypoplasia. Indeed, by this argument, a criterion for disymmetric janiceps would be holoprosencephaly of both brains; this criterion is met by the case of Wedburg et al [4]. It is harder to explain why 1 face of monosymmetric cephalothoracopagus twins is usually normal, while the other face shows varying degrees of midfacial hypoplasia. Study of reported cases, such as that of Hioki et al [48] suggests that the hemifaces may "cut the corner" to reach the midline, since the whole facial contour appears flattened, with the impression that the hemifaces may meet end-on rather than by side-to-side fusion. While lack of fission of the fetuses at vertebral angles of less than 180 degrees leads to progressive hypoplasia of the reduced face, the other face remains substantially normal in most cases. However, the stage is ultimately reached where fusion of face 1 does not occur, and face 2 may even be expressed in the midline of face 1. No cases have been described in which faces on opposite sides of the common head are both severely reduced, for example to the level of ears only. In other words, fission of the 2 head zones is somehow limited. The internal correlation of this observation is that all reported cases, including ours, show fission as far as the Rathke pouch, which is frequently noted to be dilated, often associated with absent or abnormal adenohypophysis, and anatomically related to a central basal chondrocranial defect. Various hypotheses can be advanced as to why this is so, and these are discussed below. With regard to conversion of the orientation of the central nervous system from facially oriented cerebra to vertebrally oriented hindbrains, our material was too autolytic to allow a definitive opinion; however, it seems likely that reorientation occurred at or near the mesencephalon.

Critical point 3. Orientation of the branchial and pharyngeal derivatives was particularly informative. The first and second branchial arch and pharyngeal pouch derivatives were unequivocally oriented to the faces. However, the greater horn of the hyoid bone (branchial arch 3) showed evidence of conflicting facial and vertebral influences. Whereas ventral (ie, facially induced) fusion of the bilateral arches took place across the midlines of the faces in normal manner, the bodies of the hyoid cartilages were deformed, with the proximal ends deviated toward the vertebrally determined midlines by the virtue of the "inverted" orientation of the hyoid cartilages (Fig. 11). The thyroid cartilages (branchial arch 4) were unequivocally oriented to the vertebrae. Branchial pouch derivatives were variously oriented; auditory tubes and tonsillar fossae (pouches 1 and 2) were oriented to the faces but thymus glands (third pouch) were not found. This is interpreted to imply severely conflicting inducing influences, with resultant organ aplasia. It was not expected that fourth and fifth pouch derivatives would be identified. The orientation of the thyroid glands was to the larynges. However, the thyroid gland is primarily derived from the thyroglossal duct bud in the base of the tongue. No thyroglossal duct remnants were seen, so that it is not possible to discern the way in which the facially derived thyroid glands came to be vertebrally oriented.

In view of the fact that all other neural crest tissue derivatives were present in the faces, the absence of dental anlagen is difficult to explain; however, the aplasia of the complete dentition suggests an orientation conflict early in the organogenesis of the fields of dental development. The dental aplasia may be attributed to the confusion of a specific (dental) area of neural crest histogenesis at the level of the Rathke pouch where conflicting facial and vertebral influences led to nonproduction or lack of migration of "dental" neural crest tissue.

Critical point 4. The anatomy of the postpharyngeal foregut was complex, and sets some problems in interpretation. There was fission into 2 larynges which were oriented to the vertebrae (Fig. 11); the tracheae were likewise divided but supplied facially oriented lungs, having arisen rather obliquely from an undivided sublaryngeal foregut tube. The fixation of the larynges might appear anomalous, although it is clear that reorientation of the branchial arch cartilages was occurring at the level of the greater horn of the hyoid cartilage. There is nevertheless disorientation and discontinuity between the larynges and tracheae, with the latter only budding from the foregut tube below a further segment of midaxial, common foregut tube (Figs. 12, 13). Since the hearts and livers were facially oriented (septum transversum derivatives), and had originated high in the neck of the embryo prior to caudal migration, it seems reasonable to infer that lung orientation is largely induced by the pulmonary circulatory connections rather than the foregut orientation, should those two inductive influences be opposed. The gastrointestinal tract was not fully differentiated until the point where the 2 tracheal diverticula emerged from the common esophagotracheal canal caudal to the larynges. The most cranial component of the foregut was identifiable as respiratory tract, without a gastrointestinal contribution. This is quite contrary to normal embryogenesis. Complex anatomy somewhat resembling the present case was described by Gunter [37]. Much of the cranial foregut was represented by an undivided midaxial canal. The respiratory tract underwent fission at 2 separate levels, laryngeal and tracheal. The trachea and lungs, together with the hearts and livers, were oriented to the faces, and the larynges were the only respiratory components oriented to the vertebral axes. The facial orientation, so caudal in the body, of the hepato-cardio-respiratory complex is explicable by the migration of the septum transversum from its facially oriented origin in the upper cervical region. The conversion of facially oriented ascending and arch aortae to vertebrally oriented descending aortae occurs at the same level as the conversion of the branchial arch derivatives. The interaortic anastomotic vessel probably represented abnormal orientation at the level of branchial arch 3.

LITERATURE REVIEW

Published cases of cephalothoracopagus were studied in detail as far as the illustrations and descriptions permitted [2–4,36–53]. The cases were placed on points of the spectrum of loss of disymmetry, reduction in the expression of the second face, and eventual cleavage of the first face. These cases are shown diagrammatically in Figure 17. From these studies, the following observations and hypotheses were made:

Control of facial structures in janiceps twins depends on two principal mechanisms: (1) The degree of fission and separation of the head regions. The central defect in the basal chondrocranium is reported in several cases of cephalothoracopagus twins, and is well seen in the present specimen. It may give valuable clues to the mechanisms whereby the range of anomalies arises in janiceps twins. No cases have been described in which there is apposition of the heads to such an extent that both faces are severely reduced, eg, so as to consist of two sets of ears only. This supports the concept of incomplete fission rather than partial fusion of structures. It appears that the region of the Rathke pouch marks a point of relative equilibrium, and has the following characteristics: (a) it is the point that marks the minimal degree of fission of the apposed vertebral axes, (b) it is the point around which there is a 90 degree conversion of the 2 sets of pre- and postsphenoid cartilages, (c) it is the point at which the 2 dorsoventral axes of the apposed fetuses intersect when set at angles of less than 180 degrees, (d) cranial to this point, there is continued convergence of the longitudinal (vertebral) fetal axes, which diverge caudal to this point. It is not clear whether these properties are intrinsic to the region of the Rathke pouch or merely mark the most craniad extent of the mutually repulsive notochordal inductive influences. It is possible that both alternatives apply, since the Rathke pouch is close to the oropharyngeal membrane, a point where ectoderm and endoderm are apposed without intervening mesoderm. In a simple mechanical way it is possible to regard this a "sticking point" in the structure of the fetuses, and parallels may be drawn with sticking points in and around the cloacal membrane in xiphopagus and ischiopagus conjoined twins.

(2) The second principal mechanism of face formation depends on the varying degree to which there is deviation of the longitudinal (vertebral) axes from a true 180 degrees ventroventral fusion. On the assumption that the area of the Rathke pouch is a hiatus, equilibrium point or pivot, it is possible to

---

Fig. 17. Diagrammatic representations of the vertebro-vertebral orientations of published cases of janiceps monosymmetros twins. The figures are oriented so that the normal face (N) is above the horizontal section of the brain. The reduced face is shown below the brain. Where there is no information about the brain structure, the brain area is left blank.

Fig. 17A. Holmes F [36]. 2 probably normal faces. No other details.

Fig. 17B. Jackson and Twomey [38]. Cebocephaly of face 2.

Fig. 17C. Wedberg et al [4]. 2 cebocephalic faces, 2 cerebral holospheres, large sella turcica.

Fig. 17D. Present case. Minimal external asymmetry, nearly identical faces; cerebral holosphere, face 2.

Fig. 17E. Sturrock and McKenzie [39]. Holoprosencephaly, cebocephaly; large sella turcica.

Fig. 17F. Nishimura and Okamoto [40]. Cyclops, no proboscis; no other details.

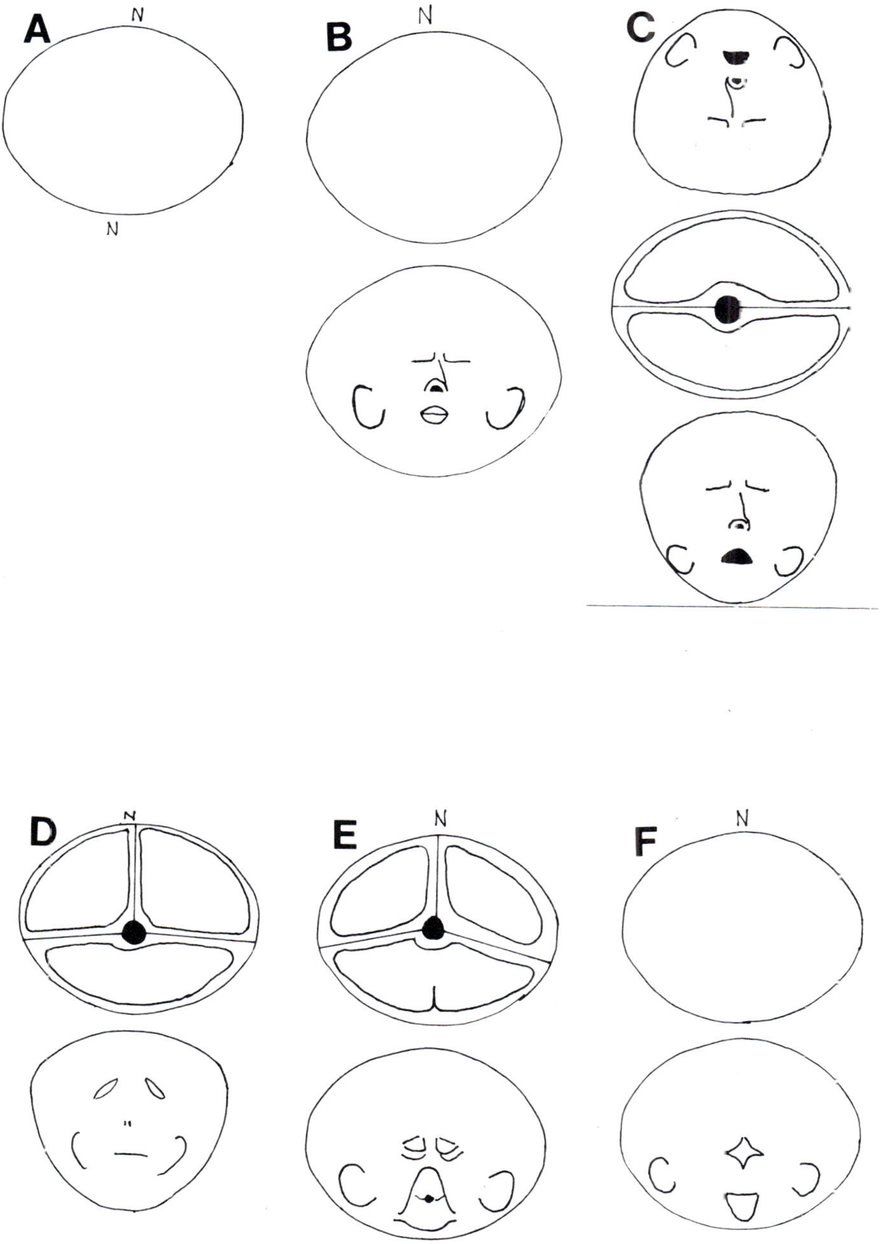
A
N
N
B
N
C
D
N
E
N
F
N

construct a continuous spectrum of the types of syncephaly, and to freeze the degree of orientation of the dorsoventral (vertebral) axes to produce models for the published cases of cephalothoracopagus twins. A true ventroventral orientation gives rise to disymmetric janiceps, with reduction anomalies craniad to the Rathke pouch expressed in the double holoprosencephalic case of Wedburg et al [4]. At the other extreme are cases where the hypoplastic face is not externally expressed or consists, at most, of a single ear. It is not clear whether the so-called lateral cephalothoracopagus twins arise by other mechanisms that do not involve ventroventral apposition of notochordal influences, since central chondrocranial defects are not described in these cases. Lateral cases usually have anencephaly, which is only described in janiceps twins at the extreme end of the monosymmetric spectrum. However, the criterion for janiceps is the presence of pharyngeal derivatives of the second face even if there is complete suppression of external expression of that face.

The topology is complex, but semidiagrammatic representations can be drawn up, as in Figure 17. It has to be reiterated that, except in the case of disymmetric janiceps, most other cases show one "perfect" face, and a spectrum of increasing degrees of hypoplasia of the opposite face. It is not clear why face 1 does not usually show evidence of "stretching," but 2 possible mechanisms could be invoked: (a) there is continuing convergence of whatever is the notochord-equivalent cause of dorsoventral orientation in the cranial region, thus ensuring that face 1 does close in the midline, (b) the point of midline hemifacial fusion may be a fairly strong "equilibrating point" in its own right; some published cases with severe hypoplasia of face 2 showed marked flattening of face 1, as if the hemifaces had "cut the corner" of the increased distance required to achieve fusion, and had met end-on instead of by the normal side-to-side fusion. Definite facial splitting does occur [37,50–53]; it is interesting to speculate whether some cases of marked facial splitting, with extra midline facial structures such as mandible,

---

Fig. 17G. Bedawy and Shahata [41]. Cyclops, one cerebrum. L - larynx of face 2.
Fig. 17H. Slager et al [2]. Holoprosencephaly, large sella turcica.
Fig. 17I. Abbott and Kaufmann [42]. Holoprosencephaly.
Fig. 17J. Hartung et al [15]. Cyclops, no other details.
Fig. 17K. Pack and Berrey [43]. Holoprosencephaly, large sella turcica.
Fig. 17L. Weingast et al [28]. Holoprosencephaly.
Fig. 17M. Edwin [44]. Cyclops, no other details.
Fig. 17N. Bartlett [45]. Single cerebrum, 2 sellae turcicae.
Fig. 17O. Priddle and Stevenson [46]. 2 ears only, no other details.

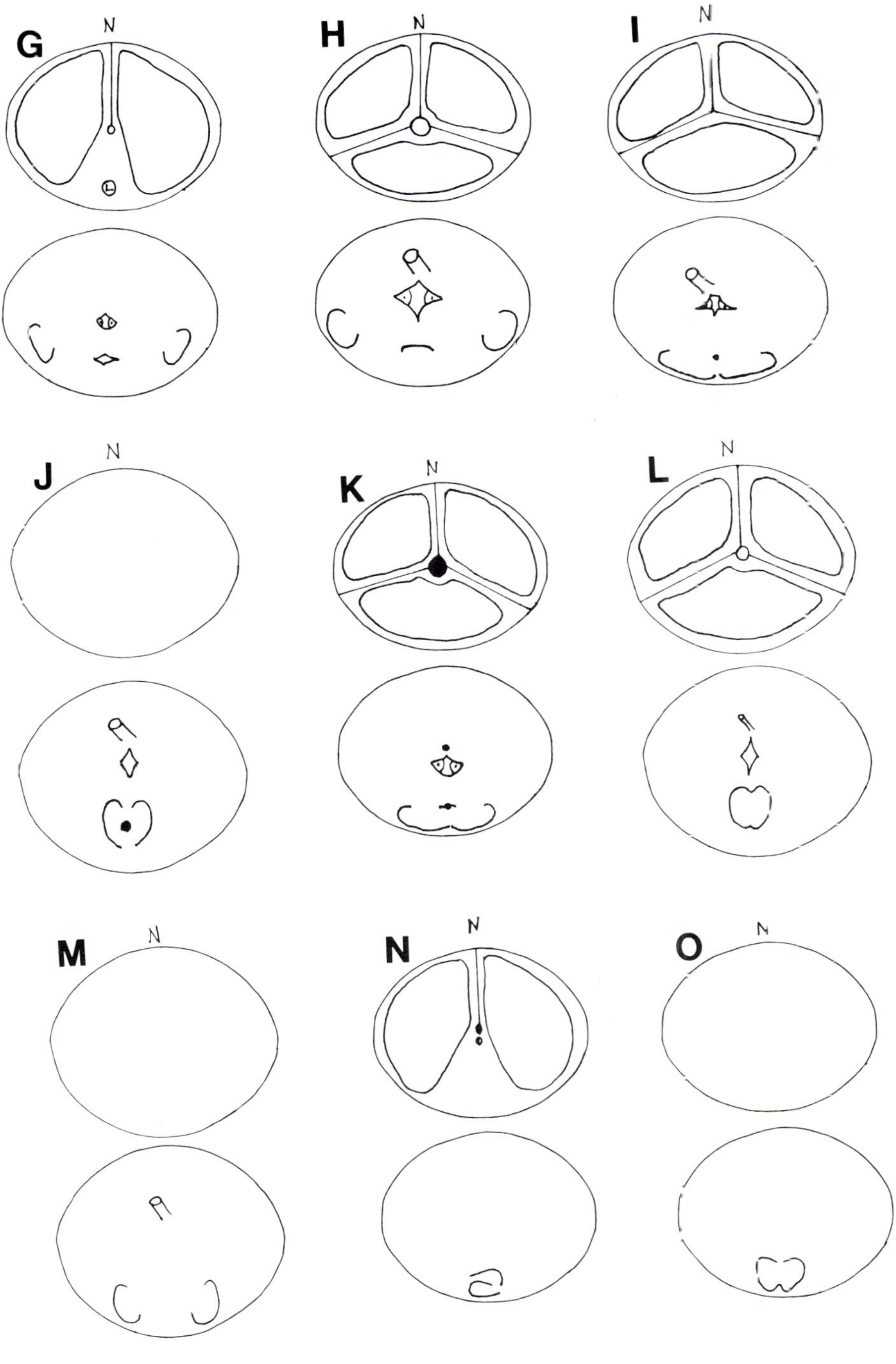
G
N
H
N
I
N
J
N
K
N
L
N
M
N
N
N
O
N

eye, tongue, etc, actually represent a side-by-side arrangement in which there is fusion of the right side of the left face with the left side of the right face. This is presumably not so if there are vestigial pharyngeal structures of face 2, and the presence of parts of a second face on the same side of the fetus as face 1 must imply that face 2 is now represented in the midline of face 1. In this event, there will be severe disorientation, since there will be attempted fusion of the right side of fetus A (originally right side of face 2) with the left side of fetus B (originally left side of face 2), with the former to the left of the latter.

The hypothesis of rotation of dorsoventral axes illustrates the concept of "vector" forces that delineate the dorsoventral axes and the midline. The asymmetry of most cases of janiceps has been attributed by others to vascular "steal" across the interaortic anastomotic vessel [2], or [47] to the general principle of discordance for midline malformations in monozygotic twins [54]. However, this latter argument seems fallacious, since each face is synthesized from 2 hemifaces, 1 from each hemizygote. Hence, if there were discordance between the fetuses, the halves of a synthetic face would be discordant, reflecting the origin of the hemifaces from discordant monozygotic conceptuses. If 1 fetus had a predisposition for holoprosencephaly but the other did not, then holoprosencephaly would be expressed in 1 side of each face by the contribution of holoprosencephalic hemifaces to each face by the holoprosencephalic twin. While the "holoprosencephaly-equivalent" defects seen in cephalothoracopagus twins may represent inadequacy of neural crest-derived frontonasal prominences, resulting in hypotelorism, other reduction malformations may be due to "bifetal midline interaction hypopla-

---

Fig. 17P. Delprado and Baird [47]. Holoprosencephaly; 2 ears only.

Fig. 17Q. Hioki et al [48]. Single cerebrum, 1 ear only.

Fig. 17R. Carlson et al [3]. Single cerebrum, 1 ear only.

Fig. 17S. Mudaliar [49]. No second face, no other details.

Fig. 17T. Plumer and Scheffer [50]. Single cerebrum, 1st face stretched, unfused mandibles, lower cleft lip, no 2nd face. Arrows show stretching: L - larynx, T - trachea.

Fig. 17U. O'Toole [51]. Anencephalic, 2 mouths, no 2nd face, no other details. Arrows to show split face and central expression of face 2 in face 1.

Fig. 17V. Herring and Rowlatt [52]. Anencephalic, 3rd midfacial mandible cleft palate, sellar abnormality, no 2nd face. Arrows suggest mode of migration of face 2 into midline of face 1.

Fig. 17W. Buchta [53]. Anencephalic, cleft lip and palate, no 2nd face. Arrows show facial splitting and mode of migration of face 2 into face 1.

Fig. 17X. Gunter [37]. Anencephalic, 1st face has cyclopic 3rd eye, 2 noses and mouths; no 2nd face. Arrows show path of migration of face 2 into face 1.

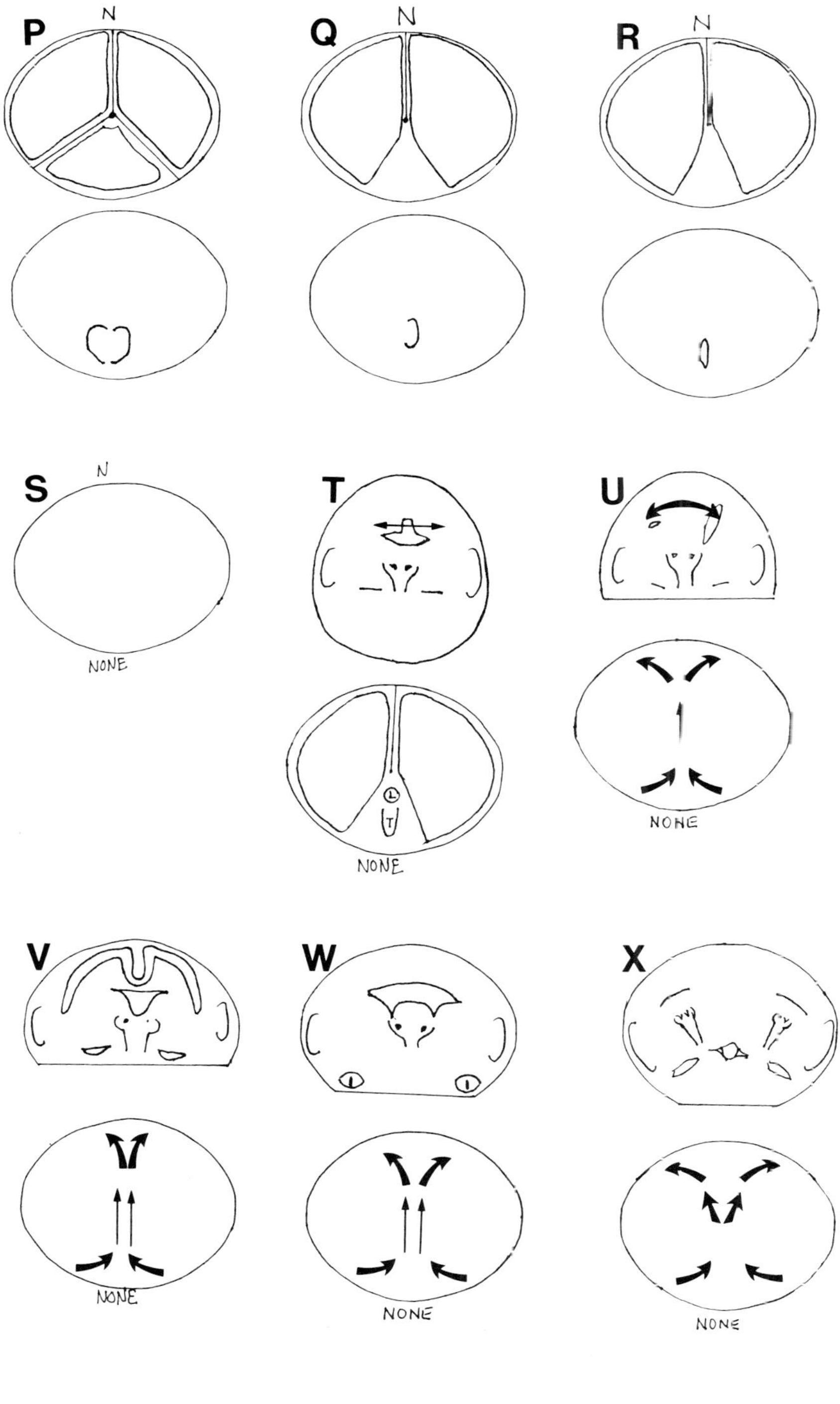
P
N
Q
N
R
N
S
N
NONE
T
L
T
NONE
U
NONE
V
NONE
W
NONE
X
NONE

sia or aplasia." This arises because of conflict in the development of regions of the fetus in the presence of conflicting messages from 2 sets of axes concerning the location of the midline and the vertebrofacial axis. When the vectorial forces are not critically opposed, severe disorganizations are found, eg, the hyoid bone, which is developed, albeit abnormally; but too severe a conflict between axes results in aplasia, eg, the central chondrocranium, adenohypophysis, thymus gland, and, possibly, the dental anlagen. Anencephaly in extreme cases of monosymmetry could be explained by appositional aplasia of the dorsal neuropores of the 2 fetuses.

It is not clear whether these proposed mechanisms could also be implicated in the genesis of similar midline malformations in singletons and in nonconjoined monozygotic twins, or whether the circumstances are unique to conjoined twinning. It has been proposed that holoprosencephaly results from a lack of the most cranial influence of the notochord [55], although this model assumes that the notochord does have influence in a craniocaudal dimension rather than purely in the dorsoventral plane. Parallels with frontonasal dysplasia [56–60] are even less close, since the clefting of overstretched faces in janiceps twins clearly involves many facial midline structures, not only those derived from the frontonasal prominences. A minor point of interest is that the report of 4 pituitary glands around a single cranial base defect [2] raises the possibility that the adenohypophysis is a paired midline organ. By implication, the stomatodeum would also be a paired organ, as would the cloaca. If this observation is true, it would be important in the delineation of malformations in and around the stomatodeum and cloaca.

SUMMARY

The earliest hitherto recorded developmental stage of human cephalothoracopagus (janiceps) twins, at 8 weeks of conceptional age, is described macroscopically and microscopically. The nearly perfect disymmetrical configuration of the 2 faces was compared with previously reported cases, and horizontal sectioning of the entire conceptus allowed detailed histologic description of the internal orientation of most organs and systems. The concept of conflicting facial and vertebral axes was explored to account for shared cerebral, facial, pharyngeal, and esophageal structures, and for aplasia of the pituitary and thymus glands and of the teeth. Critical points of changing axial orientation were identified at the mesencephalon, the Rathke pouch and third branchial arch, and with the hepato-cardio-respiratory complex split between the 2 axes. The caudal components conformed with previously reported cases.

ACKNOWLEDGMENTS

The technical expertise of Colleen Murdoch and the graphic draftsmanship of Tim Machin are gratefully acknowledged. Appreciation is expressed for grant support of this project by the Canadian Fund for Dental Education.

REFERENCES

1. Hunter J: In Palmer JF (ed) "Lectures on the Principles of Surgery, the Collected Works of J Hunter." London: Longman, 1835.
2. Slager UT, Anderson VM, Handmaker SD: Cephalothoracopagus janiceps malformation. Contribution to the pathogenesis of cerebral malformation. Arch Neurol 38:103–108, 1981.
3. Carlson DH, Hamburger R, Yeransian J: Cephalothoracopagus syncephalus: Pre-natal roentgenographic diagnosis. Pediatr Radiol 3:50–52, 1975.
4. Wedberg R, Kaplan C, Leopold G, Porreco R, Resnick R, Benirschke K: Cephalothoracopagus (Janiceps) twinning. Obstet Gynecol 54:392–396, 1979.
5. Willis RA: "The Borderland of Embryology and Pathology," 2nd edition. London: Butterworths, 1962, p 144.
6. Milham S: Symmetrical conjoined twins. An analysis of the birth records of twenty-two sets. J Pediatr 69:643–647, 1966.
7. Viljoen DI, Nelson MM, Beighton P: The epidemiology of conjoined twinning in Southern Africa. Clin Genet 24:15–21, 1983.
8. Edmonds LD, Layde PM: Conjoined twins in the United States, 1970–1977. Teratology 25:301–308, 1982.
9. Zake EZN: Case reports of 16 sets of conjoined twins from a Uganda hospital. Acta Genet Gemellol 33:75–80, 1984.
10. Appuzio JJ, Ganesh V, Landau I, Pelosi M: Prenatal diagnosis of conjoined twins. Am J Obstet Gynecol 148:343–344, 1984.
11. Chatterjee MS, Weiss RR, Verma UL, Tejani MA, Macri J: Prenatal diagnosis of conjoined twins. Prenatal Diagn 3:357–361, 1983.
12. Fagan CJ: Antepartum diagnosis of conjoined twins by ultrasonagraphy. Am J Roentgenol 129:921–922, 1977.
13. Garten KJ, Rawlinson KF, Pulliam RP: Sonographic antepartum diagnosis of dicephalus dipus dibrachius: Two case reports. W Va Med J 79:218–220, 1983.
14. Gore RM, Filley RA, Parer JT: Sonographic antepartum diagnosis of conjoined twins. JAMA 247:3351–3353, 1982.
15. Hartung RW, Yiu-Chiu V, Aschenbrenner CA: Sonographic diagnosis of cephalothoracopagus in a triplet pregnancy. J Ultrasound Med 3:139–141, 1984.
16. Hubinont C, Pratola D, Rothschild E, Rodesch F, Schwers J: Dicephalus: Unusual case of conjoined twins and its prepartum diagnosis. Am J Obstet Gynecol 149:693–694, 1984.
17. Koontz WL, Herbert WNP, Seeds JH, Cefalo RC: Ultrasonography in the antepartum diagnosis of conjoined twins. J Reprod Med 28:627–630, 1983.
18. Morgan CL, Trought WS, Sheldon G, Barton TK: B-scan and real-time ultrasound in the antepartum diagnosis of conjoined twins and pericardial effusion. Am J Roentgenol 130:578–580, 1978.
19. Schmidt W, Heberling D, Kubli F: Antepartum sonographic diagnosis of conjoined twins in early pregnancy. Am J Obstet Gynecol 139:961–963, 1981.

20. Siegfried MS, Koptik GF: Prenatal sonographic diagnosis of conjoined twins. Postgrad Med 73:317–319, 1983.
21. Wilson RL, Shaub MS, Cetrulo CJ: The antepartum findings of conjoined twins. J Clin Ultrasound 5:35–39, 1977.
22. Wood MJ, Thompson HE, Robertson FM: Real-time ultrasound diagnosis of conjoined twins. J Clin Ultrasound 9:195–197, 1981.
23. Wiegenstein L, Iozzo RV: Unusual findings in a conjoined ("Siamese") twin placenta. Am J Obstet Gynecol 137:744–745, 1980.
24. Socol ML, Tamura RK, Sabbagha RE: Multiple gestation. Clin Obstet Gynecol 27:352–358, 1984.
25. Chervenak FA, Pinto MM, Heller CI, Norooz H: Obstetric significance of fetal craniofacial duplication. A case report. J Reprod Med 30:74–76, 1985.
26. Chew SC: Prenatal diagnosis of cephalo-thoraco-pagus (conjoined twin) by ultrasound. Singapore Med J 25:248–250, 1984.
27. Preziosi P, Medici D, Maiorana A: Sonographic findings in cephalothoracopagus-conjoined twins. Pediatr Radiol 14:453–454, 1984.
28. Weingast GR, Johnson ML, Pretorius DH, Porreco RP, Waldstein G, Foley C, Appareti K: Difficulty in sonographic diagnosis of cephalothoracopagus. J Ultrasound Med 3:421–423, 1984.
29. Wilson DA, Young GZ, Crumley CS: Antepartum ultrasonographic diagnosis of ischiopagus: A rare variety of conjoined twins. J Ultrasound Med 2:281–282, 1983.
30. Chen HY, Hsieh FJ, Huang LH: Prenatal diagnosis of conjoined twins by real-time sonography: A case report. J Clin Ultrasound 11:94–96, 1983.
31. Wilson RL, Cetrulo C, Shaub MS: The prepartum diagnosis of conjoined twins by the use of diagnostic ultrasound. Am J Obstet Gynecol 126:737, 1976.
32. Austin E, Schifrin BS, Pomerance JJ, Gans SL, Komaiko MS: The antepartum diagnosis of conjoined twins. J Pediatr Surg 15:332–334, 1980.
33. Hahmann K, Issel EP, Steinbach C: Prenatal diagnosis of anterior duplication anomaly (dicephalus diauchenos) by ultrasonography. J Perinat Med 10:93–98, 1982.
34. Livingstone JE, Poland BJ: A study of spontaneously aborted twins. Teratology 21:139–148, 1980.
35. Uchida IA, Freeman VC, Gedeon M, Goldmaker J: Twinning rate in spontaneous abortions. Am J Hum Genet 35:987–993, 1983.
36. Case of Holmes F. In Potter EL, Craig JM: "Pathology of the Fetus and the Infant," 3rd Ed. London: Lloyd Luke Ltd, 1976, p 233.
37. Gunter JU: Cephalothoracopagus monosymmetros. Report of a case. Am J Pathol 22:855–861, 1946.
38. Jackson MCH, Twomey JC: Janiceps. A case of conjoined twins. Roy Nav Med Serv J 61:33–40, 1975.
39. Sturrock MM, McKenzie J: The abnormalities and genesis of cephalo-thoracopagus (Janiceps) twins - report of a case. Anat Anz 133, S:350–362, 1973.
40. Case in: Nishimura H, Okamoto N: "Sequential Atlas of Human Congenital Malformations." Baltimore: University Park Press, 1976, p 19.
41. Badawy AH, Shehata R: Cephalothoracopagus: Clinical and anatomic study of a case. Obstet Gynecol 18:106–112, 1961.
42. Abbott ME, Kaufman J: Double monster of janus type: Cephalothoracopagus monosymmetros cyclops synotus. Bull Int Assoc Med Museums 6:95–107, 1916.
43. Pack GT, Berrey IC: Janiceps asymmetros with the report of a case. Am J Obstet Gynecol 11:779–788, 1926.

44. Edwin N: Craniopagus and thoracopagus (Janiceps). Indian J Pediatr 44:20–21, 1977.
45. Bartlett RC: Cephalothoracopagus. Arch Pathol 68:292–298, 1959.
46. Priddle HC, Stevenson CS: Case in: Potter EL, Craig JM: "Pathology of the Fetus and the Infant," 3rd Ed. London: Lloyd Luke Ltd, 1976, p 231.
47. Delprado WJ, Baird PJ: Cephalothoracopagus syncephalus: A case report with previously unreported anatomical abnormalities and chromosomal analysis. Teratology 29:1–9, 1984.
48. Hioki T, Tominaga Y, Maeda K, Matsui K: A craniothoracopagus associated with a normally developed newborn infant in uniovular triplets: a case report with autopsy findings. Asia-Oceania J Obstet Gynaecol 8:29–35, 1982.
49. Mudaliar AL: Double monsters - a study of their circulatory system and some other anatomical abnormalities - and the complications of labour. J Obstet Gynaecol Br Emp 37:753–768, 1930.
50. Plumer JS, Scheffer CJ: Report on a case of cephalothoracopagus monosymmetros. Bull Int Assoc Med Museums 6:101–107, 1916.
51. O'Toole VEJ: Anencephalic conjoined twins. Br J Obstet Gynaecol 83:908–909, 1976.
52. Herring SW, Rowlatt UF: Anatomy and embryology in cephalothoracopagus twins. Teratology 23:159–173, 1981.
53. Buchta RM: Anencephaly in female thoracopagus conjoined twins. Clin Pediatr 12:598–599, 1973.
54. Schinzel AAGL, Smith DW, Miller JL: Monozygotic twinning and structural defects. J Pediatr 95:921–930, 1979.
55. Cohen MM, Jirasek JE, Guzman RT, Gorlin RJ, Peterson MQ: Holoprosencephaly and facial dysmorphia: Nosology, etiology and pathogenesis. March of Dimes-Birth Defects Foundation:BD:OAS VII(7):125–135, 1971.
56. Barr M: Facial duplication: Case, review, and embryogenesis. Teratology 25:153–159, 1982.
57. Cohen MM, Sedano HO, Gorlin RJ, Jirasek JE: Frontonasal dysplasia (median cleft face syndrome): Comments on etiology and pathogenesis. March of Dimes-Birth Defects Foundation:BD:OAS VII(7):117–119, 1971.
58. Sedano HO, Cohen MM, Jirasek J, Gorlin RJ: Frontonasal dysplasia. J Pediatr 76:906–913, 1970.
59. Mazzola RF: Congenital malformations in the frontonasal area: Their pathogenesis and classification. Clin Plast Surg 3:573–609, 1976.
60. DeMeyer W: The median cleft face syndrome. Neurology 17:961–971, 1967.

The Developmental Field Concept in Pediatric Pathology—Especially With Respect to Fibular A/Hypoplasia and the DiGeorge Anomaly*

John M. Opitz, MD, and Susan O. Lewin, MB, BCH, FRCP(C)

Shodair Children's Hospital, Helena, Montana (JMO, SOL), the Universities of Washington/Seattle and Wisconsin/Madison, and Montana State University, Bozeman, Montana (JMO)

INTRODUCTION

Those in "our field" not led to exclaim in wonder at the daily new discoveries in molecular genetics, or who doubt that these are surely the most exciting times in the history of biology and medicine, can perhaps be said not to have really lived. Nor those who think that these developments have no pertinence to pathology, for they shall be taught better on the front pages of the *Wall Street Journal*, their children in ninth grade biology texts, and their patients on nightly television programs. For example, they may soon experience with astonishment, and some chagrin, the rather easy confirmation of a pathogenetic hypothesis about cystic fibrosis made by molecular biologists who have already succeeded in producing a probe to the mutant gene and in localizing it on the long arm of chromosome 7. This is a feat that has become commonplace in the field and will soon allow isolation of the gene, accurate analysis of its complete DNA message, and comparison of

*Dedicated to Enid F. Gilbert, gracious lady and eminent investigator, with highest admiration, respect, and gratitude for her friendship, collaboration, and leadership in bridging developmental and pediatric pathology and genetics.

Birth Defects: Original Article Series, Volume 23, Number 1, pages 277–292

DNA of mutant and nonmutant alleles in a manner that was first pioneered for the hemoglobinopathies and that opened our understanding of the many mechanisms whereby alterations of the substance of heredity influences human structure and function in health and in "disease." We said above "with chagrin"—for when the answer about cystic fibrosis is in hand at last, it may turn out that it had been staring us in the face for decades, on the basis of available, known facts, had we only seen more clearly and thought rightly about them.

Is it therefore time to cease work on morphology and to turn the field of developmental pathology over to molecular biologists? At the moment, the answer is clearly no—for several reasons. First, we should not be swept away with unwarranted reductionist enthusiasm, for it will be a long time before molecular biologists are going to come up with a testable model of multifactorial determination (or of a polygene*), which is postulated as the cause of most single malformations in vertebrates, or of the developmental effects of aneuploidy. Second, we must avoid at all costs repeating the mistake made a half-century ago when morphology began to be abandoned and denigrated as a second-class intellectual endeavor in the wake of the many wonderful discoveries in physiology and finally in biochemistry as applied to normal and abnormal development. Otto Warburg, Jean Brachet, Joseph Needham, Gavin de Beer, Julian Huxley, and the biochemists and molecular biologists who entered the field later are not to blame for that abandonment and denigration; the morphologists themselves thought that starting with the chemical substances of life would provide the answers and more quickly than with the anatomic, embryologic, teratologic, and developmental genetic methods they had learned in graduate school.

By isolating and "working around" morphology (as a necessary evil confined to autopsy rooms and the dissection tanks of medical students), the theory of vertebrate development never progressed beyond its essentially tautologic beginnings as defined by the experimental embryologists of a half-century ago, namely, that the developmental field is what they observed it to be on the basis of grafting and transplantation experiments. These experiments suggested that "organizers" produced in one tissue were responsible for inducing in another development not necessarily related to its "innate," ie, genetic, potential. Also, that the outcome of the experiments depended to a greater or lesser extent on the nature of the tissues used, timing (ie, stage

*A necessary intellectual construct, which may not have a basis in reality and which may turn out to be nothing more than a pleiotropic attribute of small effect of "oligogenes."

of differentiation), location (ie, certain spatial considerations), and possible distance from a "center of organization" (Spemann)—ie, a morphogenetic gradient. These are all conclusions that foreshadowed later, more concrete formulations of field theory.

Now is the time in morphology to pick up where we left off a half-century ago and to face freshly the challenges of developmental mechanisms and theory posed by our daily exposure to malformed humans before and after birth. In doing so, we must apply *all* of the methods that seem appropriate to yield answers, including histochemistry, electron and scanning electron microscopy, molecular approaches, and the genetic and teratologic study of animal models.

THE DEVELOPMENTAL FIELD

The insight that breathed a new life into the developmental field concept came from clinical genetics and is so startlingly simple as to be intuitively obvious—namely, that documentation of causal heterogeneity of a given malformation defines a *dys*morphogenetically reactive embryonic unit, ie, a set of embryonic primordia that reacted together in identical manner to different causes. It then follows that these primordia must also constitute a morphogenetically reactive unit under *normal* circumstances. Fields then are the morphogenetically reactive structural units of the embryo.

This view of development seems so obvious that it would surprise if it had not been formulated in a like or similar manner by earlier workers. Meckel may have done so as early as 1802 (in his inaugural thesis on congenital heart defects), in work that was first published in 1805 in which he stated: "The constant involvement of certain organs together in congenital malformations allows the conclusion that their development is coordinated under normal conditions" (translated from a quotation in Schierhorn [1]).

And incorporating the concepts of classic and experimental embryology, we can define a field as "that part of an embryo that reacts as a temporally and spatially coordinated and epimorphically hierarchical unit to normal localized forces of organization and differentiation . . . ." These forces may ultimately all turn out to be mediated by cell adhesion molecules (CAMs) as studied in most elegant work by Edelman [2, 3] and Rutishauser [4].

The occurrence of the "same" malformations (eg, cleft palate, cyclopia, polydactyly) and the extensive similarity of structure and function of these units during ontogeny of vertebrate species of diverse lineages must also indicate (1) descent from a common ancestor with a prototypic developmental plan, and (2) participation in normal and abnormal morphogenesis of the genetic changes responsible for the phylogenetic changes over the millennia.

PRIMARY AND SECONDARY MALFORMATIONS

Primary malformations are all of those errors of organogenesis due to an *intrinsic* defect of the developing primordia. They include all dysmorphogenetic abnormalities due to mendelian mutations, chromosome abnormalities, and multifactorial determination whose action is inferred from the presence of the anomaly and additional genetic evidence but whose presence in a zygote does not make the occurrence of the malformation inevitable. This probabilistic statement refers to two observations: (1) the nonobligatory nature of the component malformations of syndromes, and (2) the phenomenon of nonpenetrance of nonsyndromal malformations caused by mendelian oligogenes. A primary malformation can be viewed as an intrinsic defect OF the developmental field.

On the other hand, secondary malformations, now called *disruptions*, are due to an exogenous dysmorphogenetic disturbance acting IN a field that was initially (intrinsically) destined to develop normally, or, in any event, to do so with much greater likelihood than in the case of primary malformation. The reason for the qualification in the last sentence is the fact that all events of organogenesis are probabilistic threshold phenomena that result in only 2 classes of outcome—the morphogenetic process either did or did not occur. That is to say, events of organogenesis are all-or-none phenomena.

Three other facts about organogenesis must be remembered in this context: (1) most gross morphogenetic events during embryogenesis involve the midline; (2) most dysmorphogenetic anomalies of vertebrates are defects of incomplete, not of abnormal differentiation (cleft palate vs polydactyly); and (3) while organogenesis precedes histogenesis, the latter, ie, events of cellular differentiation, do play an important role in the morphogenesis of the brain, kidneys, and gonads, which continues after the organogenetic period of embryogenesis into fetal and, to some extent, postnatal life. Thus, (dysplastic) tumors are more likely to occur in these organs—especially if they are malformed (eg, Wilms tumor in horseshoe kidneys), an exception to the rule that histologic normality in postnatal life allows the cautious inference of histologic normality during organogenesis as the explanation for the observation that, on the whole, malformed organs are *not* more likely to develop cancers than their nonmalformed counterparts.

DEVELOPMENTAL TERMINOLOGY

Early in the nineteenth century, the distinctions between ontogeny, phylogeny, and growth were not carefully drawn, since all of them could be called *evolutio*. It was not until 1866 and 1886, respectively, that Haeckel coined the terms "phylogeny" and "ontogeny," which Herbert Spencer then insisted on using in English scientific writing to make the distinction crystal clear between the development of species on one hand and the development of individual organisms on the other. It took almost 70 years after Goethe's introduction of the term "morphology" before the term "morphogenesis," or "morphogeny," as Haeckel used to call it, became established in English biologic writing. No one seems to have difficulties with the term "organogenesis" (ie, the gross morphogenetic events during embryogenesis); however, the term "phenogenesis," coined by Eugen Fischer in 1939 and derived from Haeckel's "phenogenetics," is unfamiliar to most pathologists and clinical geneticists. We propose that it be restricted to all morphogenetic events occurring *after* organogenesis. This results in the following terminologic outline (adapted from Opitz [5, 6]):

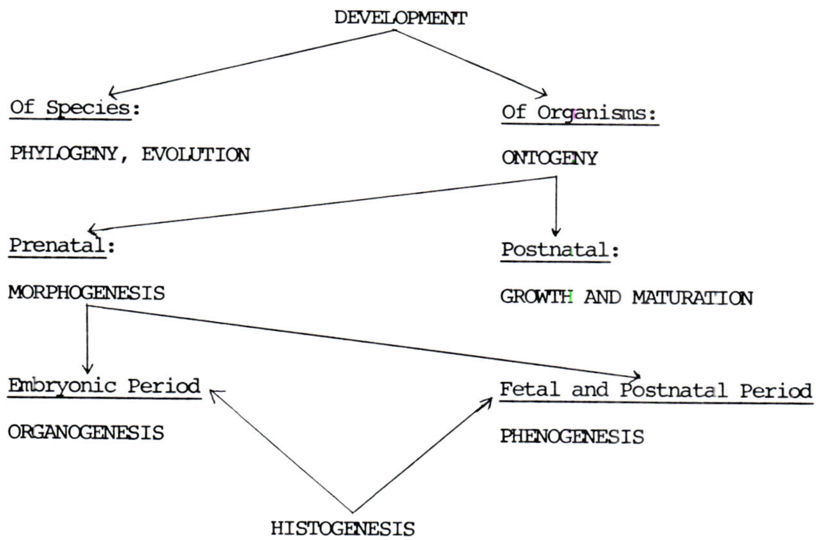

Heuristically, then, organogenesis can be contrasted with phenogenesis as follows:

1. Organogenesis leads to qualitatively different developmental end products *within* an individual, whereas phenogenesis leads to quantitatively documentable differences *between* individuals.

2. Organogenesis is controlled by oligogenes and "polygenes," the latter mostly to "buffer" development; phenogenesis, in the language of Waddington, represents the process of developmental "fine-tuning" and is controlled by polygenes.

3. Whereas organogenesis involves thresholds, ie, all-or-none traits, phenogenesis does *not* involve developmental threshold decisions, but only "shades" of difference.

4. Defects of organogenesis are malformations, either primary or secondary (disruptions), whereas defects of phenogenesis mostly result in *minor anomalies** and growth disturbances.

5. Since mild malformations always involve defects of organogenesis, they are always abnormal, even though common in the "normal population," and frequently clinically benign. Minor anomalies, ie, defects of phenogenesis, are phenotypically indistinguishable, hence, developmentally identical to so-called *normal variants*, which are the basis of ethnic variability of the population and intrafamilial variability.

6. Severe and mild malformations are studied clinically, pathologically, and anatomically, whereas minor anomalies are also studied anthropometrically and by radiometry and cephalometry, photography, and subjective description.

7. With respect to multiple congenital anomalies (MCA) syndromes, defects of organogenesis are responsible for true malformation syndromes, a type of discontinuous, abnormal variability. On the other hand, the so-called funny-looking kid (FLK) either has (1) a multiple minor anomalies syndrome (a form of abnormal variability) or (2) a variant familial developmental pattern (VFDP), ie, unusual but normal variability, the difference between these two being established by examination of first-degree relatives for family resemblance before a chromosome study is done.

8. Examples contrasting severe and mild abnormalities of *organogenesis* are cleft palate/cleft uvula; asternia/cleft xiphisternum; radius aplasia/triphalangeal thumb, or notched distal thumb phalanx; micr(an)ophthalmia/coloboma of the iris; omphalocele/umbilical hernia; alobar holoprosencephaly/single upper central incisor; and hemifacial microsomia/contralateral preauricular tag.

Examples of abnormalities of *phenogenesis* are a reduced total ridge count (10 low arches in trisomy 18 syndrome), increased total ridge count (10 whorls) in the Ullrich-Turner syndrome, a head circumference or height 3 or more standard deviations above or below the mean; a head length 3 or more standard deviations below the mean (as in Down syndrome, hyperbrachycephaly), increased *atd* angle (in Down syndrome), increased *ab* and *cd* ridge counts (in the Ullrich-Turner syndrome), etc.

*Also called "dysmetric" traits by Newton Freire-Maia [7, 8].

Another class of anomalies that may be regarded as defects of phenogenesis can be called *dysmaturational*. They may involve muscle (eg, persistence of myoblasts in muscle of newborn infants with the Wiedemann-Beckwith syndrome), endocrine glands (ie, the common occurrence of apparent neuroblastoma *in situ* in the adrenals of newborn infants), heart valves (as in the persistence of "embryonic" vascular/mesenchymal tissue on valve leaflets in the 18-trisomy syndrome), and lymph and venous channels (as in the persistence of more or less severe degrees of fetal lymphedema in many aneuploidy states, the prominence of venous channels in cutis marmorata telangiectatica congenita, and forehead capillary hemangiomatosis in many normal and abnormally formed newborn infants). Thus, many dysmaturational abnormalities are also properly spoken of as dysplasias.

In a word, mild malformations are defects of organogenesis; minor anomalies are defects of phenogenesis, and dysplasias are defects of histogenesis. Mild malformations and minor anomalies are *not* synonymous. Developmentally and anatomically, individual minor anomalies and normal morphologic variants are identical but causally have totally different implications, the former being the most common effects of aneuploidy but with each minor anomaly individually also occurring in the normal population. Thus, 10 low arches on the fingertips may represent normal variability, but on the fingertips of a child with intrauterine growth retardation and many other minor anomalies are an indication of trisomy 18 until proven otherwise.

WHAT IS GAINED BY VIEWING MALFORMATIONS AS DEVELOPMENTAL FIELD DEFECTS?

For one, we gain an appreciation of the fact that, though the causes are many, final dysmorphogenetic paths in vertebrates are few. From this it follows that there probably is no such thing as a causally specific malformation.

Second, the classic method of clinical genetics—searching for causal heterogeneity and actually finding it—automatically makes a given set of abnormalities, regardless of how complex, a single malformation rather than a syndrome or an association. As can be imagined, this conclusion has rather important consequences for genetic counseling.

Third, the insight so gained implies automatically that *all* malformations are developmentally complex, whether we are speaking of a single upper central incisor or the anophthalmic form of alobar holoprosencephaly.

Fourth, it teaches one respect for and reemphasizes a point made by Wright and Waddington, among others, that a tremendous amount of gene interaction must occur in the development of a given trait. This idea is of the most important consequence in thinking about the developmental effects of aneuploidy. It follows that oligogenes participating in development must exert complex pleiotropic effects.

WHAT INSIGHT IS GAINED INTO NORMAL DEVELOPMENT FROM THE DEVELOPMENTAL FIELD CONCEPT?

Most important, we gain the insight that an individual anatomic part is not developmentally autonomous, but is intimately interrelated with that of contiguous and frequently more distantly located structures.

In this connection the terms "monotopic" and "polytopic" (developmental field defects) refer to clinical outcome and *not* to initial morphogenetic relationships. In monotopic anomalies the defects are all in closely contiguous anatomic structures - eg, the extra bones, muscles, nerves, blood and lymph vessels, and nail of a duplication of the thumb, or the related nasal, maxillary, and palatal defects of a bilateral cleft lip and palate. In polytopic field defects, the correlated anomalies are more distantly located, depending on the nature of the inductive or developmental relationship between the primordia. Thus, in acrorenal field defects the limb anomalies are thought to be due to deficiency or production of an abnormal limb inductor by the mesonephros; in the Bartsocas-Pappas, Hanhart, and focal dermal hypoplasia syndromes due to defective interrelationship between the ectoderm and underlying mesoderm of the ectoderm ring; and in correlated renal and cerebellar anomalies due to defective production of a common CAM or inability of cell surface receptors to bind it.

Polytopic field defects must be distinguished from *sequences* (a cascade of consequences of a single developmental defect) and *pleiotropy* (multiple effects of a single gene acting at various times on different tissues of organs during pre- and postnatal development).

It is an axiom of developmental genetics that the attributes of incomplete penetrance and reduced expressivity are *not* intrinsic characteristics of the mutant gene. A striking example of this is the family reported by Freire-Maia et al [7] and Freire-Maia [8] in whom the effect of a mutant gene affecting limb development ranged from amelia with severe underdevelopment of the zonoskeleton to monodactylous phocomelia to radius aplasia to mild abnormality of the thumb. Since the mutant gene is identical in all affected individuals in the family, these differences in expressivity obviously are not an attribute of the mutant gene but rather of "epistatic" factors. This family also shows that progressive differentiation, as in the proximodistal development of the limb, gradually reduces the size of the epimorphic field in which a dysmorphogenetic cause can act: thus, early action of the gene segregating in the aforementioned family reported by Freire-Maia [7] leads to amelia and severe developmental defects of the pectoral girdle, latest action of that same gene may possibly produce a triphalangeal thumb. This is responsible for the observation of "nested" anomalies, eg, pituitary hypoplasia, arrhinencephaly with hypotelorism, coloboma of iris, and central upper incisor as anomalies "contained" in the alobar holoprosencephaly field defect, or triphalangeal thumb "contained" in the radius a/hypoplasia field defect.

WHAT IS GAINED BY A PHYLOGENETIC VIEW OF THE DEVELOPMENTAL FIELD CONCEPT?

First, it allows us to postulate that developmental integration into fields may be the consequence of the reduction of metamerism that occurred during the evolution of vertebrates.

Second, we realize that atavisms (a term coined by Charles Darwin) are real biologic entities that have allowed a unique and important insight into the developmental effects of aneuploidy [Barash et al, [9]; Aziz, [10]].

Third, we understand that the vertebrate midline is not just an imaginary sagittal plane dividing right from left half of body but is a biologically real entity of profound morphogenetic importance in early development, related, among other ways, to the dynein arms of ciliated epithelia as demonstrated in the Kartagener syndrome [11]. Since most malformations are midline defects, the midline must partake of some of the characteristics of developmental fields, namely, at least temporal synchronization and an epimorphically hierarchical progression of development. The third cardinal attribute of developmental fields, spatial organization, seems to be the attribute that most clearly sets the midline apart from paramedian structure; it is a subject of investigation by our former Madison co-worker, Dr. Mark Lubinsky of Omaha.

Fourth, we know that at least 2 different kinds of temporal developmental instructions must be coded in mammalian development: the timing of species-specific ontogenetic events and the phylogenetically more general genetic history leading to the increasing diversity of form during advanced stages of development in related but different species.

The participation in normal morphogenesis of genetic changes responsible for phylogenetic changes is illustrated by the fact that persistence of webs between digits and presence of a tail are malformations in humans when they are perfectly normal attributes of most lower mammals. An even more striking example of this is the gene *Px*, which in heterozygous form can restore the pentadactyl foot of the ancestors of hystricomorph mammals (ie, release the genetic restriction placed on first and fifth digit development that occurred during the descent of guinea pigs from their pentadactylous rodent ancestors). The effect of the gene *Px* and the dramatic results of making it homozygous were described in a classic of modern developmental genetics by Sewall Wright in 1935 [12]. It was also Sewall Wright who, a half-century ago, produced a sophisticated but simple mathematic model of morphogenetic events as threshold phenomena and of primary malformations as failure to cross the threshold toward completion [13].

Last, a phylogenetic perspective of the developmental field gives respect for and confidence in developmental defects ("animal models") seen or produced in other mammals.

Two examples have been chosen to illustrate the process of identifying developmental fields on the basis of causal heterogeneity of malformations. The first, fibular a/hypoplasia and the "fibular" developmental field, has been inferred principally on the basis of clinical and anatomic evidence; the delineation of the second, namely, the DiGeorge anomaly, is a brilliant example of the synergistic effects of investigations by many workers in different fields, including in this case a.o. pathologists (Rössle and Lobdell), clinicians, endocrinologists (Angelo DiGeorge), immunologists (Robert Good), cytogeneticists (Albert de la Chapelle), experimental embryologists (Nicole Le Douarin and Margaret Kirby), and teratologists (eg, Malcolm Johnston, Kathleen Sulik, Bill Webster, and Ed Lammer).

FIBULAR A/HYPOPLASIA (q.v. Lewin and Opitz [14])

Fibular a/hypoplasia is the commonest of the mesomelic paraxial hemimelias. It is usually nonsyndromal and in most instances is an apparently isolated, sporadic event. About 1/3 of cases have bilateral, 2/3 have unilateral involvement. In unilateral cases the right side is more frequently involved than the left. Complete absence is more common than partial absence. Overall, the sex ratio is equal, though it differs in individual reports, and some investigators are impressed with a (slight) male preponderance. The virtual lack of recurrence suggests that most cases of fibular a/hypoplasia are of nongenetic origin; however, this does not exclude multifactorial determination in some cases. There exist virtually no twin data to aid genetic analysis of the nonsyndromal cases. Reviews of fibular hypoplasia have confirmed it to be part of the same spectrum of leg-foot malformations as fibular aplasia, supported by the observation of hypoplasia and aplasia occurring in the same individual.

Individuals ascertained on the basis of fibular aplasia have absence of the talus (36%), cuboid (23%), and metatarsals 2–5 in, respectively 19%, 22%, 61%, and 67% of cases; frequent absence of ipsilateral patella and of anterior cruciate ligament; together with (secondary) shortness and bowing of tibia and involvement of proximal femur, acetabulum, and capital femoral epiphysis, which some orthopedists note in most cases of congenital absence of the fibula. In some syndromes, fibular a/hypoplasia is associated with defects of the ulna, in others with ectrodactyly of the foot (rather than just oligodactyly of fibular rays). Very little is said in the literature regarding the renal status in most cases of fibular a/hypoplasia, and at the moment we are not excluding the possibility that fibular a/hypoplasia may also turn out to be a polytopic acrorenal developmental field defect as is the case with radial a/hypoplasia in all its forms.

CAUSAL HETEROGENEITY

Aneuploid Form

Curiously, only 1 example of fibular a/hypoplasia is known to be due to aneuploidy—in this case as part of a complex MCA/MR syndrome due to del (21q) with bilateral fibular a/hypoplasia and ulnar involvement [15].

Nonaneuploid Forms

Autosomal dominant mutations. Of all mutations causing fibular a/hypoplasia, the best known is the condition known as Volkmann dysostosis, which was inherited in the family of the master-tailor Georg Bernhard over 5 generations. The eponym "Volkmann," as well as being attached to the ischemic contracture of the thumb, also refers to any causally nonspecific ankle deformity involving lateral and upward dislocation of the foot due to upward-outward slant of the distal articular surface of the tibia with or without fibular defect. In the case of Volkmann dysostosis, both fibular and ankle defects were present to variable degrees in all affected individuals. This is probably a nonsyndromal form of fibular a/hypoplasia.

Several syndromal autosomal dominant forms of fibular a/hypoplasia are known, including Reinhard-Pfeiffer mesomelic dysostosis, the ectrodactyly-fibular a/hypoplasia (EFA) dysostosis of Deragna-Zucco-Ferrante, the fibular-ulnar dimelia syndrome of Sandrow-Sullivan-Steel, and Nievergelt dysplasia/dysostosis.

Autosomal (or ?X-linked) recessive mutations include the Lowry craniosynostosis-fibular a/hypoplasia syndrome, Herrmann-Pallister craniosynostosis-fibular agenesis syndrome, Al-Awadi syndrome, Fuhrmann syndrome, Pfeiffer oto-onycho-peroneal syndrome, 1 known case of familial femoral-fibular-ulnar (FFU) dysostosis, the SC-Roberts syndrome, Langer mesomelic dysostosis, postaxial acrofacial dysostosis syndrome of Genée and Wiedemann, DuPan-Grebe-Hunter syndrome, Grebe-Quelce-Salgado acromesomelic dysostosis or syndrome, and the fibula aplasia and complex brachydactyly syndrome of Grebe.

Fibular a/hypoplasia also occurs in a number of sporadic dysostoses and syndromes including atelosteogenesis, the Walbaum-Titran syndrome, Ulbright-Hodes syndrome, "boomerang" syndrome, amelia/phocomelia, Hanhart dysostosis, FFU dysostosis and proximal focal femoral deficiency (PFFD).

Teratologic considerations involve a possible recent FFU epidemic observed in southern France, occurrence of unilateral proximal fibular deficiency in a case of presumed congenital vaccinia, fibular a/hypoplasia in a child born to a diabetic mother, and the production of this defect in experimental animals with busulfan, retinoic acid, and N-fluoro-uracil.

The most severely affected cases, the virtually constant hypoplasia of the proximal femur and occasional involvement of the ulna, lead to the conclusions that (1) the "fibular" developmental field includes the pubic portion of the pelvis and acetabulum, the proximal femur, patella, anterior cruciate ligament, fibula (and secondarily all the nerves, muscles, and vessels intimately associated with fibular development), and axial and/or lateral foot rays (but never the first); and (2) fibula and ulna are developmentally homologous structures.

THE DIGEORGE ANOMALY (q.v. Lammer and Opitz [16])

This condition is paradigmatic of how certain complex developmental disorders, formerly considered syndromes and their component manifestations as evidence of pleiotropy, come to be viewed instead as developmental field defects.

Observations of lethal tetany in infants with absence of the thymus antedate the work of DiGeorge and were documented as early as 1829. It was the great merit of DiGeorge to have recognized the pertinence of the revolutionary 2-compartment view of the development of immunocompetence in vertebrates to human patients with combined functional and structural defects of thymus and of parathyroid glands—both derivatives of the third and fourth pharyngeal pouches. The "full" DiGeorge syndrome was an even more complex condition with high incidence of congenital heart defects of a specific type involving developmental defects of the paired branchial arch arteries and of conotruncal septation, hypoplasia, aplasia or ectopic position of thymus, partial or complete absence or dystopia of parathyroids, a characteristic constellation of minor facial anomalies, and frequent mild mental retardation. In contradistinction to children with fibular a/hypoplasia who are the picture of health, infants and toddlers with the DiGeorge anomaly commonly tend to be wretchedly unhappy and chronically, miserably ill with a high death rate.

What is the evidence for causal heterogeneity of this complex constellation of developmental defects? Most cases of DiGeorge anomaly represent sporadic occurrence with apparently low empiric recurrence risk, hence presumed multifactorial determination. However, many genetically and teratologically different forms of the anomaly are known.

Aneuploid Forms

The most common chromosome anomaly observed in the DiGeorge anomaly is deletion of the proximal long arm of chromosome 22, rarely monosomy 22. It has also been seen in dup (9) (q22→qter), del (5) (p13), and dup (1q?).

Nonaneuploid Forms

Autosomal dominant mutations. Besides a few observations of affected children born to less severely involved parents, the most common autosomal dominant disorder with DiGeorge anomaly is the velo-cardio-facial syndrome, which may be identical to the "conotruncal anomaly face syndrome" described in Japan. Several other familial observations are compatible either with X-linked or autosomal recessive determination, or autosomal dominant inheritance with incomplete penetrance.

However, some of the most important contributions to the analysis of causal heterogeneity of the DiGeorge anomaly have come from teratologic studies in humans and animals. The most important of these contributions are the fetal alcohol syndrome, induction of craniofacial, cardiac, and thymic malformations completely analogous to the DiGeorge anomaly with vitamin A in mice by Kalter and Warkany over a quarter of a century ago, followed by the subsequent unhappy discovery of the teratogenicity in humans of 13-cis-retinoic acid (Accutane ®) and the production of isotretinoin embryopathy in mice. The DiGeorge complex has also been produced in rats and hamsters with bisdiamine ("Fertilysin" or bis-dichloroacetyl-diamine).

Several workers, most prominently Margaret Kirby and her coworkers, have now demonstrated that the unifying pathogenetic explanation of all developmental defects in the DiGeorge anomaly (with the possible exception of the commonly observed MR) is an injury to migrating neural crest, which is not only postulated to "induce" but to participate actively in the morphogenesis of the craniofacial, branchial arch, and conotruncal cardiac structures that are involved in the DiGeorge complex. Thus, the DiGeorge anomaly emerges as another neurocristopathy—perhaps not so much in the sense best understood by pathologists, of dysplasias and tumors of tissues derived from neural crest cells, but of defects of organogenesis involving cells of neural crest origin.

SUMMARY

Identical anomalies produced by different causes such as aneuploidy, gene mutation, teratogenic chemicals, and certain surgical procedures are a clear indication that embryonic primordia respond as units in the production of developmental anomalies of anatomic structure. Hence, they must also act as units during normal ontogeny. The presence of identical malformations in different mammalian species identifies developmental and anatomic homology by virtue of descent from a common ancestor. These dys- and orthomorphogenetically reactive units are the equivalents of the classic experimental embryologist's epimorphic fields, which are those units of the embryo in which the development of complex structures appropriate to the species is determined and controlled in a spatially coordinated, temporarily synchronous, and epimorphically hierarchical manner that expresses both species-nonspecific (that is, phylogenetic) and species-specific genetically coded developmental information.

Thus, it is as important for pathologists as it is for clinical geneticists to steep themselves in the art and science of phenotype analysis and to be able to do all of those studies, including anthropometry, dermatoglyphics, and growth analysis, that are required to arrive at inferences of cause and pathogenesis from the phenotype. There is probably one other incentive besides the ethical and intellectual ones to do this and to do it as well as possible, namely, the medico-legal consequences. If pathologists fail to illuminate the causal genesis of a given case to aid in preventing recurrence, then, in short order, they might be held equally as liable as clinicians for missing high recurrence risk genetic diagnoses.

These depressing considerations aside, it is important to close on a positive note. As at the outset, we want to emphasize once more that, without question, this is the most exciting time to be working in the field of developmental pathology. In this specialty a marriage is occurring of several types of investigational methods, ranging from humble morphologic studies to metabolic analysis to the most sophisticated designs of molecular biology, to produce new interdisciplinary approaches to the solution of the oldest intellectual problem confronting medicine—how does the "fabric of the human body" (in the immortal words of Vesalius) come about? Proceeding, as we are, from study of the abnormal, we should be able—in the same way as biochemists elucidated normal intermediary metabolism from "the inborn errors"—to construct a developmental field map of the human body; and ultimately to discover the forces that guarantee its integrity, in most cases in faithful obedience to the ontogenic orders and phylogenetic legacy "written" into its genes.

ACKNOWLEDGMENTS

This research was supported, in part, by a grant from the State of Montana Department of Health and Environmental Sciences. Susan O. Lewin is supported by a grant from the Alberta Heritage Foundation. I am grateful to Melanie Matson for expert secretarial collaboration.

REFERENCES

1. Schierhorn H: Johann Friedrich Meckel d. J. ahs Begrunder der wissenschaftlichen Teratologie. Gegenbaur's Morph Jahrb 130:399–439, 1984.
2. Edelman GM: Cell-adhesion molecules. Science 219:450–457, 1983.
3. Edelman GM: Cell-adhesion molecules: A molecular basis for animal form. Sci Am 250:118–129, 1984.
4. Rutishauser U: Developmental biology of a neural adhesion molecule. Nature 310:549–554, 1984.
5. Opitz JM: Invited Editorial Comment: Study of minor anomalies in childhood malignancy. Eur J Pediatr 144:252–254, 1985.
6. Opitz JM: Editorial Comment: The developmental field concept. Am J Med Genet 21:1–11, 1985.
7. Freire-Maia N, Quelce-Salgado A, Amundsen-Kohler R: Hereditary bone aplasias and hypoplasias of the upper extremities. Acta Genet Statist Med 9:33–40, 1959.
8. Freire-Maia N: A heterozygote expression of a "recessive" gene. Hum Hered 25:302–304, 1975.
9. Barash BA, Freedman L, Opitz JM: Anatomic studies in the 18-trisomy syndrome. White Plains, NY: The National Foundation-March of Dimes, BD:OAS VI(4):3–15, 1970.
10. Aziz MS: Possible "atavistic structures" in human aneuploids. Am J Physiol 54:347–353, 1981.
11. Opitz JM, Gilbert EF: Editorial Comment: CNS anomalies and the midline as a development field. Am J Med Genet 12:443–455, 1982.
12. Wright S: A mutation in the guinea pig, tending to restore the pentadactyl foot when heterozygous, producing a monstrosity when homozygous. Genetics 20:84–107, 1935.
13. Wright S: Are results of crosses between inbred strains of guinea pigs different in numbers of digits? Genetics 19:537–551, 1934.

14. Lewin SO, Opitz JM: Fibular a/hypoplasia: Review and preliminary documentation of a fibular developmental field. Am J Med Genet (in press).
15. Reynolds JF, Wyandt HE, Kelly TE: De novo 21q interstitial deletion in a retarded boy with ulno-fibular dysostosis. Am J Med Genet 20:173–180, 1985.
16. Lammar EJ, Opitz JM: The DiGeorge anomaly as a developmental field defect. Am J Med Genet (in press).

Pathology of Chromosome Abnormalities in the Fetus—Pathologic Markers

Enid F. Gilbert, MD, Sunita Arya, MD, Renata Laxova, MD, and John M. Opitz, MD

Departments of Pathology and Genetics (EFG, SA, RL), University of Wisconsin Medical School, Madison, Wisconsin 53792 and Department of Genetics, Shodair Children's Hospital (JMD), Helena, Montana 59604

Chromosome abnormalities represent the largest category of causes of death in humans. Abortuses that have reached a 2-week stage of development are estimated to have a 78.3% rate of chromosome abnormalities [1,2]. However, this rate declines to 62.1% for abortions occurring after the first missed period, but before the 20th week [1,2]. The proportion of fetuses with chromosome defects drops continuously, with only 5.8% of stillborn infants having a chromosome defect [3–5]. In liveborn infants the rate of chromosome defects is 5.9 per 1000 [6].

The phenotypic expression of chromosome abnormalities can be readily observed in the fetus [7]. Dermatoglyphics are also discernible by 13 weeks of gestation. The pathologic changes can be recognized and some pathologic markers for specific chromosome abnormalities may be apparent in early fetal life such as cystic and calcified Hassal corpuscles in trisomy 21 [8], gelatinous multivalvular disease in trisomy 18 [9,10], partial hydatidiform mole of the placenta in triploidy [11–14], and cystic hygromas in Ullrich-Turner (45,X) syndrome [15,16]. Although chromosome studies confirm the diagnosis, if the specimen has been placed in fixative or is autolyzed (precluding chromosome analysis) pathologic studies are helpful in the recognition of chromosome abnormalities.

The fate of fertilized human ova is shown in Table I. It has been estimated that the total reproductive loss due to aneuploidy or polyploidy approaches 50%. The incidence and types of chromosome abnormalities in spontaneous

Birth Defects: Original Article Series, Volume 23, Number 1, pages 293–306

TABLE I. Fate of Fertilized Ova

About 16% of ova exposed to sperm fail to divide.
Another 15% fail to implant.
Some 27% are aborted spontaneously at previllous stages, presumably because they are grossly abnormal.
Of the 42% of fertilized human ova that survive the first missed menstrual period, about one-fourth are aborted spontaneously.
68.5% total reproductive loss. 31.5% of ova exposed to sperm in women of proven fertility survive to be born alive.

TABLE II. Incidence of the Types of Chromosome Abnormalities in 1500 Spontaneous Abortions*

	Percent
Autosomal trisomies	52.00
Triploidy	19.86
45,X	15.30
Tetraploidy	6.18
Double trisomy	1.73
Translocations	3.80
Mosaicism	1.08

*Boué J, Boué A, Lazar P: Retrospective and prospective epidemiological studies of 1500 karyotyped spontaneous human abortions. Teratology 12:11, 1975.

TABLE III. Chromosome Defects

At birth 1:200 have chromosome defects.
38% of all 2-week embryos have chromosome defects.
50% of all embryos from the time of conception are estimated to have chromosome defects.
High percentage of chromosome defects represent trisomies.
The commonest trisomy is trisomy 16, which is lethal.
Most aneuploid embryos are aborted at 7–8 weeks, although they usually stop their development at approximately 4 weeks.

abortions are listed in Table II. The incidence and fate of chromosome defects at various gestational ages is seen in Table III and the developmental effects of aneuploidy are shown in Table IV. These include multiple minor and major malformations with the most severe effects being on the central nervous system with frequent gross malformation prenatally and mental retardation postnatally. Disturbance of growth results in intrauterine growth retardation or a small-for-gestational-age (SGA) infant. Aneuploidy has more or less severely deleterious developmental effects on gonads [10]. The Ullrich-Turner syndrome is associated with gonadal dysgenesis or late fetal ovarian

TABLE IV. Aneuploidy

Developmental effects of aneuploidy include:
- Multiple congenital anomalies—minor and major
- Multiple mild malformations
- Most effect CNS function with mental retardation
- Frequent severe effect on gonads
- Increased number of dysplasias → increased risk of cancer
- Disturbance of growth → intrauterine growth retardation

TABLE V. Mild Malformations in Chromosome Defects

Bipartite uvula	Megaureters and megapelvis
Abnormal lobation of lungs	Renal microcysts
Intrahepatic gallbladder	Single umbilical artery
Stenosis and abnormal branching of bile ducts	Mingling of different organ tissues
Annular pancreas	Abnormal lobulation of spleen
Malrotation of gut	Accessory spleens
Meckel diverticulum	Abnormal lobation of liver
Kinky ureters	Costal and sternal defects

degeneration, and the Klinefelter syndrome with congenital microorchidism. The increased incidence of dysplasias in aneuploidy results in a greater risk for the development of neoplasia; for example, there is an association of del (13q) with retinoblastoma; del (11p) with Wilms tumor; trisomy 21 with leukemia, retinoblastoma and CNS and testicular tumors; the Klinefelter syndrome with breast cancer; trisomy 13 with retinal dysplasia, retinoblastoma, and leukemia; and trisomy 18 with Wilms tumor.

Mild malformations are also common in aneuploidy syndromes. A mild malformation is an anomaly of morphogenesis and should be viewed as a reduced expression of a major anomaly. They are all-or-none traits. A list of the more common mild malformations seen in chromosomal defects is shown in Table V.

Some pathologic markers can be identified in some of the aneuploidy syndromes. The characteristic appearance of trisomy 21 is evident in the fetus (Fig.1) and can be identified by 14 weeks' gestation. Cystic and calcified Hassal corpuscles in the thymus (Fig. 2) in trisomy 21 appear to be a constant anomaly. In trisomy 13, in addition to the typical phenotype in the fetus (Fig. 3) retinal dysplasia has been a constant anomaly (Fig. 4). In trisomy 18, by 13 weeks' gestation, the phenotype is easily recognized (Fig. 5). Matsuoka [9] has found gelatinous valvular tissue in the heart. This involves all valves (multivalvular) (Fig. 6) and represents persistence of early fetal valvular tissue. In triploidy (Fig. 7) (Table VI) partial hydatidiform mole is constantly present (Fig. 8) [17–19]; the microscopic appearance of

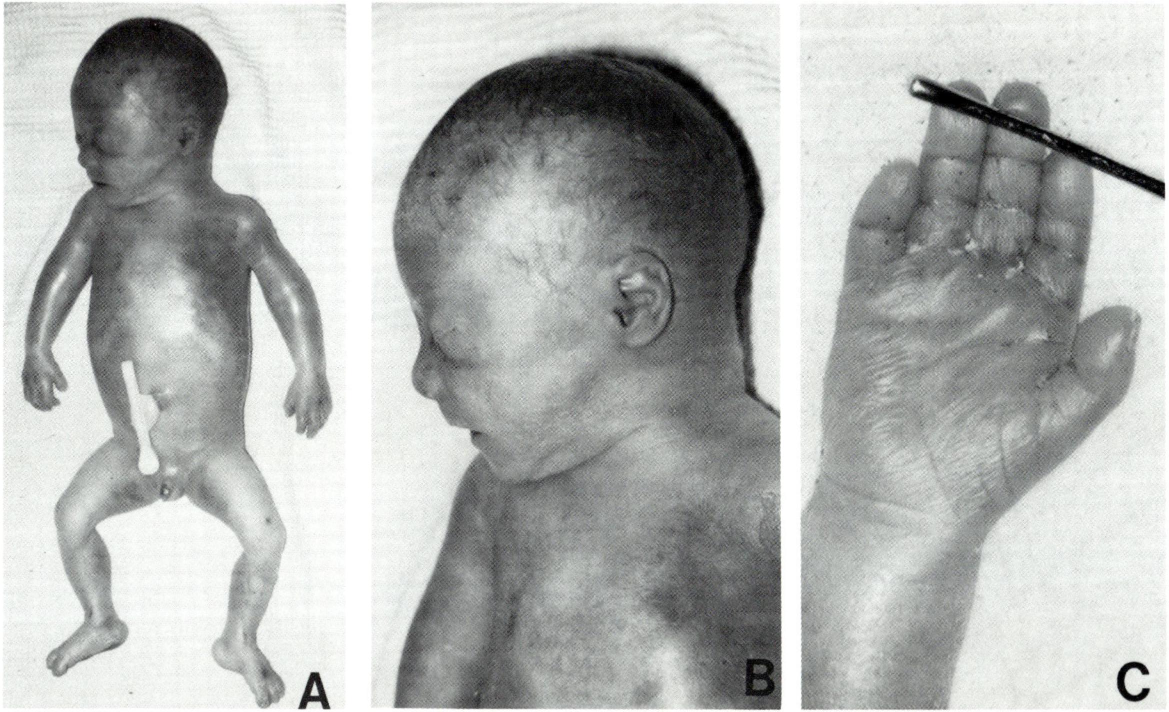

Fig. 1. Trisomy 21. (A) Typical manifestations of trisomy 21 in a 26-week fetus, brachycephaly and slanting palpebral fissures. (B) Lateral view of head: flat face with hypoplastic maxilla. (C) Simian crease on palm.

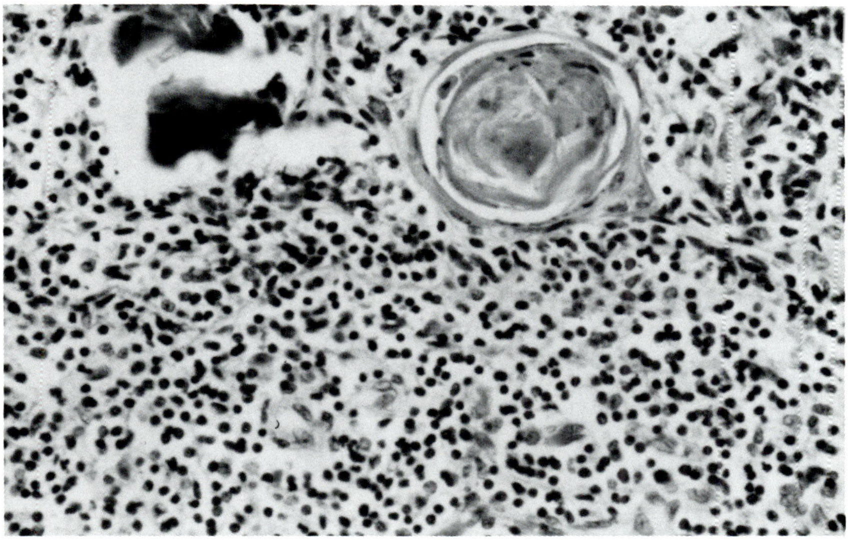

Fig. 2. Cystic and calcified Hassall corpuscles (from E.F. Gilbert and J.M. Opitz: Perspectives in Pediatric Pathology 7:1–63, 1982. Reprinted with permission of Masson Publishing Co., New York), H&E magnification ×100.

the placenta is also characteristic with large edematous chorionic villi with peripheral scalloping of their margins (Fig. 9) [20–23]. Another pathologic change in triploidy is the presence of large bizarre hyperchromatic cells in the pancreatic islets that stain positively for somatostatin by immunoperoxidase (Fig. 10). In the fetus with the Ullrich-Turner (45,X) syndrome, cystic hygromas (Fig. 11) are characteristic [15, 24], usually associated with generalized lymphedema that results from generalized hypoplasia and partial agenesis of the lymphatic system that ceases to extend peripherally at an early embryonic stage [25]. Other conditions in which cystic hygromas are seen are listed in Table VII.

Pathologic studies are helpful in the study of chromosome abnormalities and in some cases there appear to be markers that may be particularly helpful in their recognition.

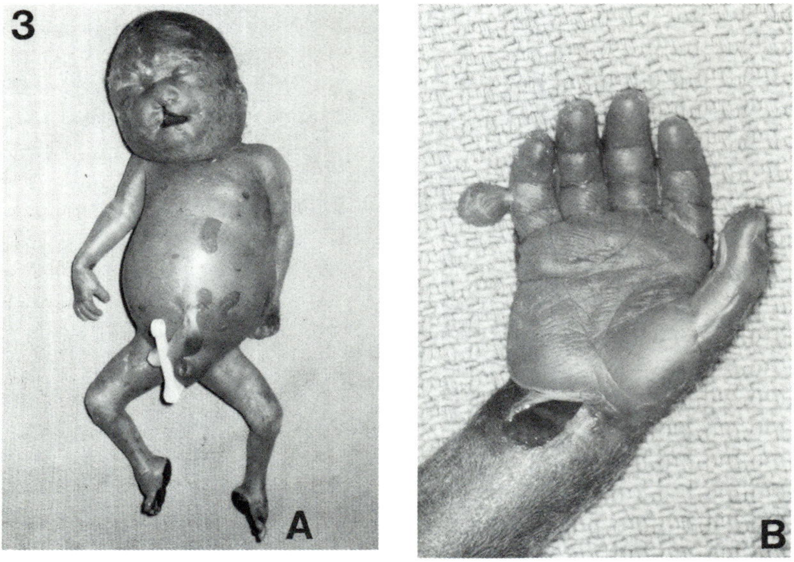

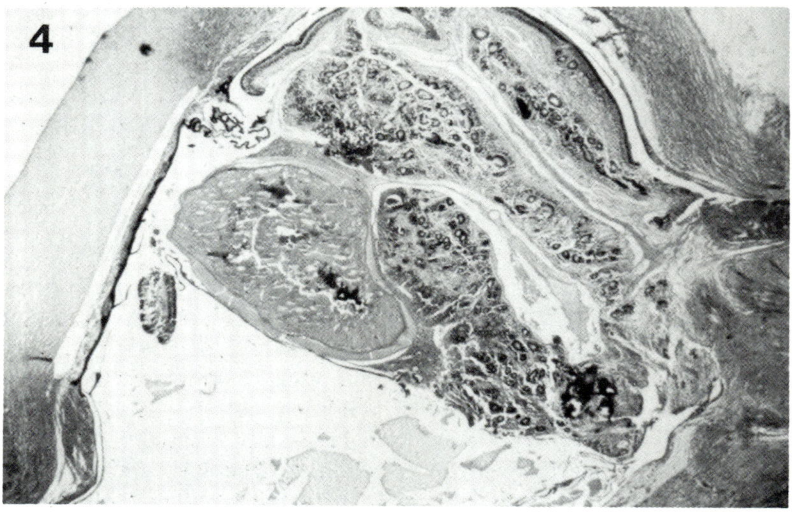

Fig. 3. Trisomy 13. (A) Typical appearance of trisomy 13 in 26-week fetus. Microcephaly, hypotelorism, and midline facial defect. (B) Postaxial hexadactyly.

Fig. 4. Retinal dysplasia: a marker for trisomy 13. (From E.F. Gilbert and J.M. Opitz: Perspectives in Pediatric Pathology 7:1–63, 1982.)

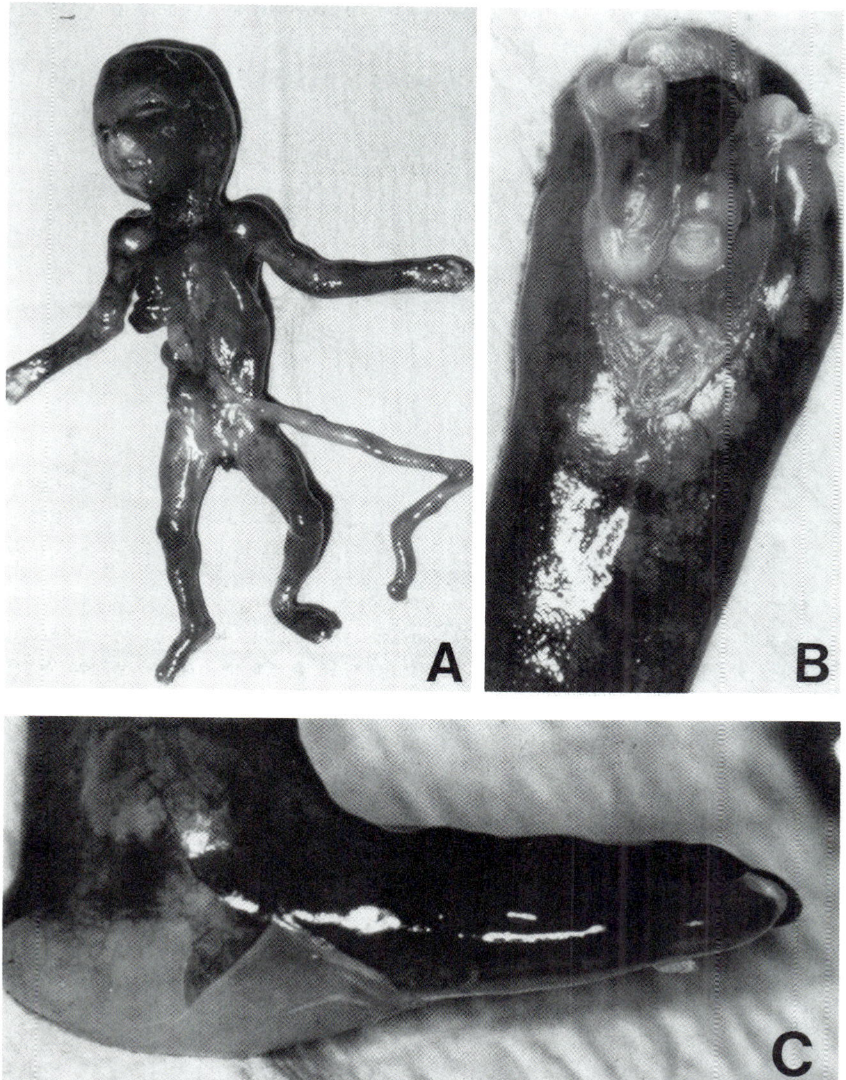

Fig. 5. Trisomy 18. (A) Typical appearance of trisomy 18-dolicocephalic head and clenched hands. (B) Clenched hand with overlapping of index finger over middle finger. (C) Rocker-bottom foot.

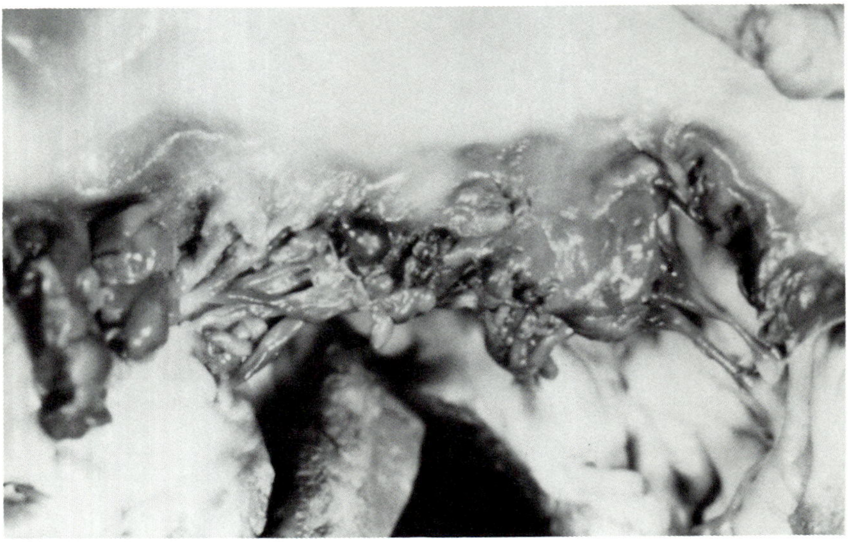

Fig. 6. Thick gelatinous mitral valve: a marker for trisomy 18. (From E.F. Gilbert and J. M. Opitz: Perspectives in Pediatric Pathology 7:1-63, 1982. Reprinted with permission of Masson Publishing Co., New York.)

TABLE VI. Triploidy
Usually spontaneous abortion
Some stillborn—rarely liveborn
Meningomyelocele
Congential heart defects
Cleft lip/palate
Syndactyly of fingers and/or toes
Growth retardation
Hydatidiform degeneration of placenta

Fig. 7 Triploidy. (A) Karyotype 69,XXY. (B) Typical appearance of triploidy: large bulbous nose, large head, and limb abnormalities. (C) Feet with abnormal length and displacement of toes. (From E.F. Gilbert and J.M. Opitz: Chromosomal abnormalities. Chapter 14. In Wigglesworth J, Singer D (eds): "Perinatal Pathology." Courtesy of Blackwell Scientific Publications, Inc.)

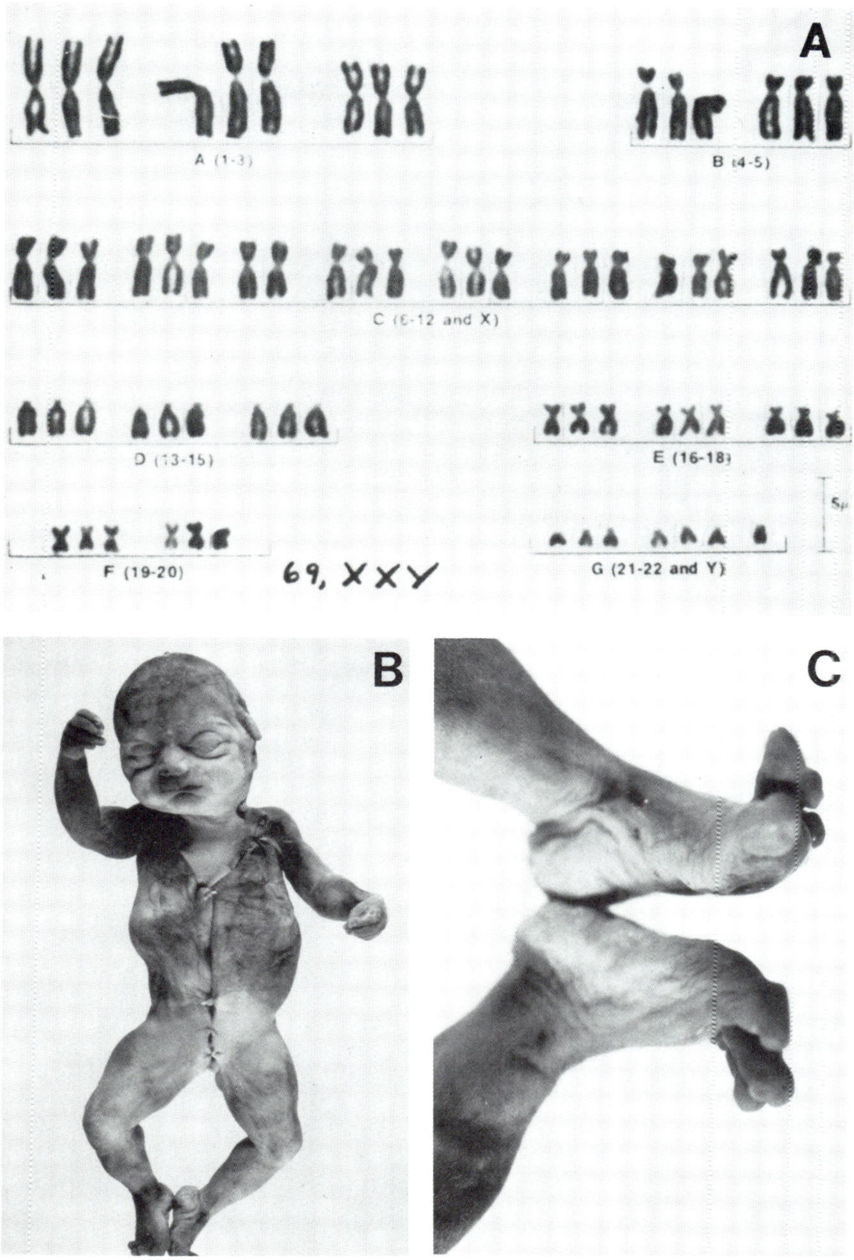
A
A (1-3)
B (4-5)
C (6-12 and X)
D (13-15)
E (16-18)
F (19-20)
G (21-22 and Y)
69, XXY
B
C

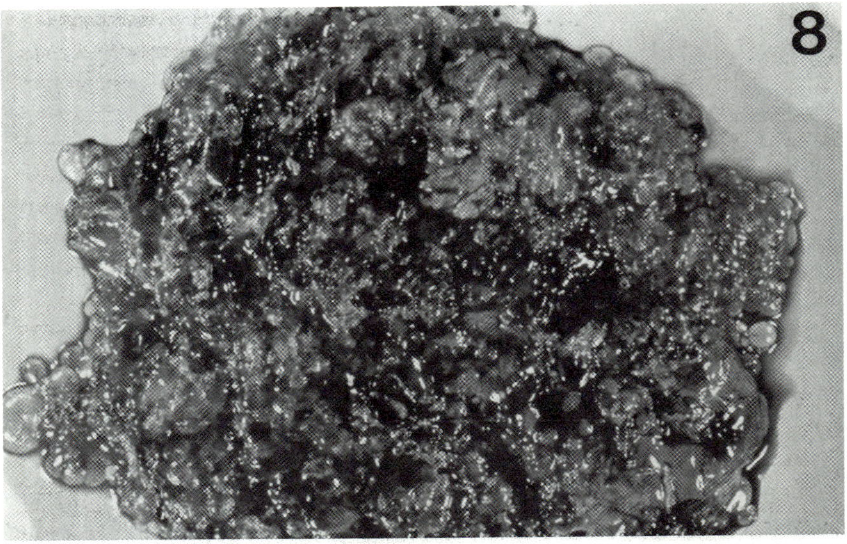

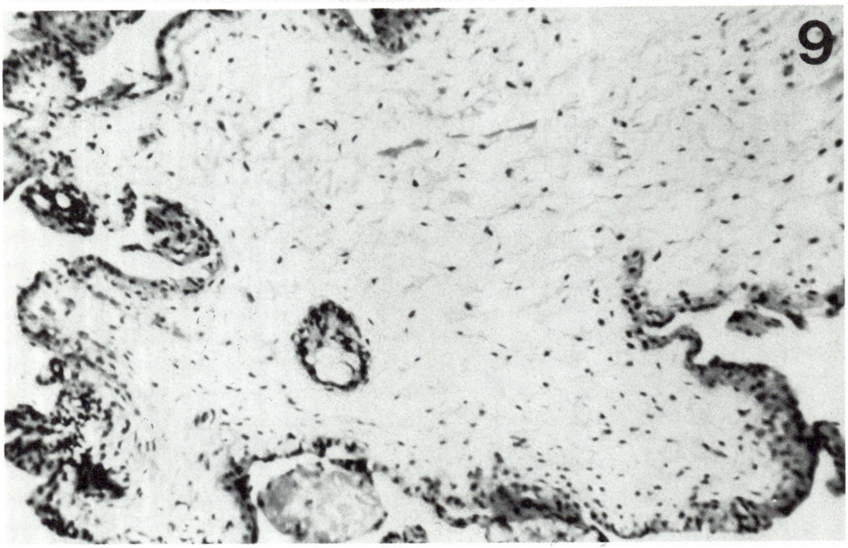

Fig. 8. Placenta with partial hydatidiform mole.

Fig. 9. Large hydropic chorionic villus with scalloping of margin and mild trophoblastic hyperplasia.

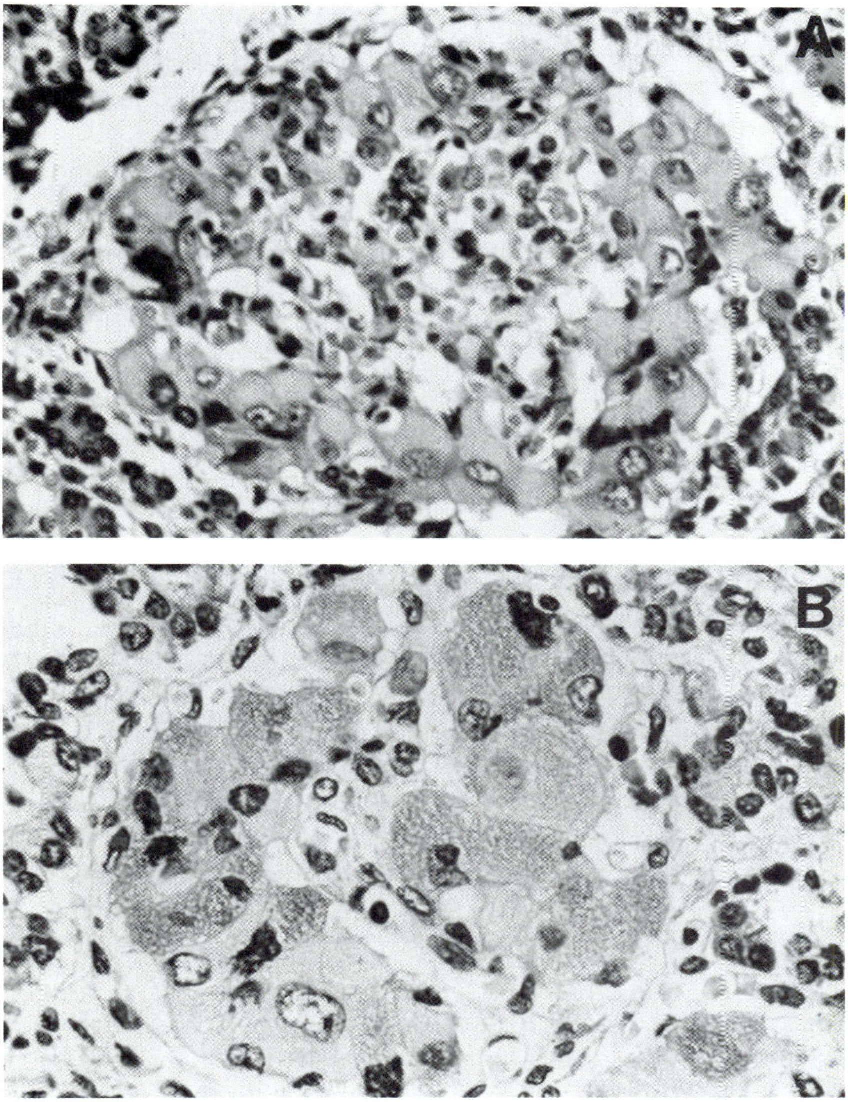

Fig. 10. (A) Islet of Langerhans showing large atypical cells with giant hyperchromatic nuclei in triploidy. (B) Immunoperoxidase stain for somatostatin showing positive reaction of giant cells in triploidy. (A & B courtesy of Dr. Donald Singer.)

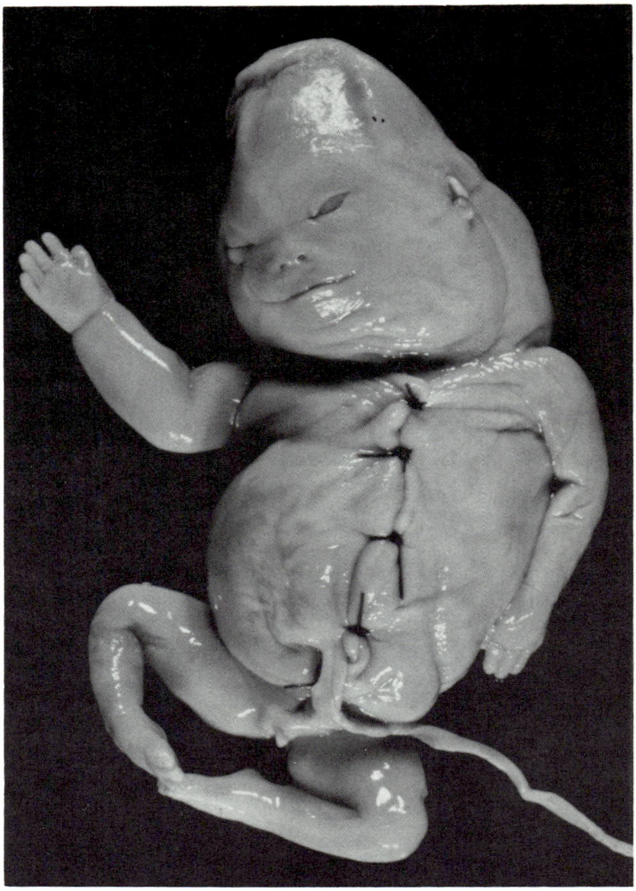

Fig. 11. 45,X, Ullrich-Turner syndrome: Lymphedema and cystic hygromas in a 14-week fetus.

TABLE VII. Conditions Associated With Cystic Nuchal Hygromas

Single gene disorders	Chromosome disorders (continued)
Familial neck webbing (autosomal dominant)	dup(11p) syndrome
Lymphedema distichiasis syndrome (autosomal dominant)	Trisomy 18 syndrome
Roberts syndrome (autosomal recessive)	Trisomy 21 syndrome
Cowchock syndrome (? autosomal recessive)	Trisomy 22 mosaicism syndrome
Chromosome disorders	Teratogenic disorders
45,X Ullrich-Turner syndrome	Fetal alcohol syndrome
X-chromosome polysomy	Fetal aminopterin syndrome
del(13q) syndrome	Fetal trimethadione syndrome
del(18p) syndrome	Disorders of unknown cause
	Noonan syndrome

REFERENCES

1. Boué J, Boué A: Anomalies chromosomiques dans les avortements spontanés. In Boué A, Thibault CD (eds): "Les Accidents Chromosomiques de la Reproduction." Paris: INSERM, 1973, p 29.
2. Boué J, Philippe E, Giroud A et al: Phenotypic expression of lethal chromosomal anomalies in human abortuses. Teratology 14:3, 1976.
3. Bauld R, Sutherland GR, Bain AD: Chromosome constitution of 500 infants dying during the perinatal period. Humangenetik 23:183, 1974.
4. Machin GA, Crolla JA: Chromosome constitution of 500 infants dying during the perinatal period. Humangenetik 23:183–198, 1974.
5. Kuleshov NP, Alekhin VI, Egoliana NA, et al: Frequency of chromosomal anomalies in children dying in the perinatal period (Plenum translation). Genetika 11:107, 1975.
6. Jacobs PA: Epidemiology of chromosome abnormalities in man. Am J Epidemiol 105:180, 1977.
7. Baldwin VJ, Kalousek DK, Dimmick JE, Applegarth DA, Hardwick DF: Diagnostic pathologic investigation of malformed conceptus. Perspect Pediatr Pathol 7 65–108, 1982.
8. Hubbard JD: Down's syndrome—Dilated Hassall's corpuscles as a histopathologic marker. Pediatric Pathology Club Interim Meeting, Providence, Rhode Island, October 11-13, 1979.
9. Matsuoka R, Matsuyama S, Yamamoto Y et al: Trisomy 18q: A case report and review on karyotype-phenotype correlations. Hum Genet 57:78, 1981.
10. Gilbert EF, Opitz JM: Developmental and other pathologic changes in syndromes caused by chromosome abnormalities. Persp Pediatr Pathol 7:1–63, 1982.
11. Le Marec B, Senecal J: Sex ratio et age maternel dans la trisomie 18. J Genet Hum 23:119, 1975 (suppl).
12. Moerman P, Fryns JP, Goddeeris P, Lauweryns JM: Spectrum of clinical and autopsy findings in trisomy 18 syndrome. J Genet Hum 30:17, 1982.
13. Rodrigues MM, Punnet HH, Valdes-Dapena M et al: Retinal pigment epithelium in a case of trisomy 18. Am J Ophthalmol 76:265, 1973.
14. Karayalcin G, Shanske A, Honigman R: Wilms' tumor in a 13-year-old girl with trisomy 18. Am J Dis Child 135:665, 1981.
15. Rushton DI, Faed M, Richards S, et al: The fetal manifestations of the 45,XO karyotype. J Obstet Gynaec Br Cwith 76:266, 1969.
16. Vander Putte SCJ: Lymphatic malformations in human fetuses. A study of fetuses with Turner's syndrome or status Bonnevie-Ullrich. Virch Arch Path Anat 376:233, 1977.
17. Jacobs PA, Hunt PA, Matsuura JS, Wilson CC: Complete and partial hydatidiform moles in Hawaii: Cytogenetics, morphology and epidemiology. Br J Obstet Gynaecol 89:258, 1982.
18. Szulman AE, Philippe E, Boué JG, Boué A: Human triploidy: Association with partial hydatidiform moles and nonmolar conceptuses. Human Pathol 12:1016, 1981.
19. Jacobs PA, Szulman AE, Funkhouser J, Matsuura JS, Wilson CC: Human triploidy: Relationship between parental origin of the additional haploid complement and development of partial hydatidiform mole. Ann Hum Genet 46:223, 1982.
20. Szulman AE, Surti U: The syndromes of hydatidiform mole. II. Morphologic evolution of the complete and partial mole. Am J Obstet Gynecol 132:20, 1978.
21. Philippe E, Boué JG: Le placenta des aberrations chromosomiques létales. Ann Anat Pathol (Paris) 14:249, 1969.

22. Philippe E: "Histopathologie Placentaire." Paris: Masson et Cie, 1974.
23. Honore LH, Dill FJ, Poland BJ: Placental morphology in spontaneous human abortuses with normal and abnormal karyotypes. Teratology 14:151, 1976.
24. Singh RP, Carr DH: The anatomy and histology of XO human embryos and fetuses. Anat Rec 155:369, 1966.
25. Cowchock FS, Wapner RJ, Kurtz A, Chatzkel S, Barnhart SB Jr, Lesnick DC: Brief clinical report: Not all cystic hygromas occur in the Ullrich-Turner syndrome. Am J Med Gen 12:327–331, 1982.

Diagnostic Trends in Childhood Chromosome Abnormalities and Their Implications—A Total Population Eight-Year Survey From Queensland, Australia

J.A. Bell, DIP MED TECH, **J.R. Bell,** MD, **and J.H. Pearn,** MD

State Health Department, Mater Misericordiae Hospital and University Department of Child Health, Brisbane, Queensland, Australia

INTRODUCTION

This study is part of an ongoing total population survey in which all chromosome abnormalities diagnosed in the state of Queensland, Australia are recorded in a central register [1,2]. Absolute numbers of each type of chromosome anomaly, along with age at diagnosis, are readily derived from the database, permitting construction of relative frequency histograms. It also becomes possible to compare the "observed" rate for each chromosome abnormality with the "expected" rate by utilizing data from the neonatal period. Such comparisons may well provide an index of the diagnostic efficiency of clinicians serving the target population. Extension of the analysis to all anomalies diagnosed up to the age of 14 years provides estimates of the size and nature of the pool of unrecognized chromosome disorders in childhood.

This long-term study permits annual monitoring and provides information on secular trends. Thus, changes in observed versus known rates of abnormality may be detected, along with any alterations of mean age at diagnosis. It is possible to monitor clinical awareness of cytogenetic conditions and to detect any changes in true incidence. The data permit comparisons between different time periods and also other populations. The information allows

Birth Defects: Original Article Series, Volume 23, Number 1, pages 307–314

guidelines to be provided for formulation of policies concerning prenatal population screening programs.

MATERIALS AND METHODS

Queensland is a subtropical state situated in the northeast of Australia. The area is 1.7 million square kilometers and the population, at mid-survey point, was 2.4 million. Ninety percent are Caucasion and 85% are of Anglo-Saxon origin. Total live births numbered 296,548 during the 8 years of the study (1976–83) [3]. Six cytogenetic laboratories operate in the state, with each contributing yearly listings of all diagnosed chromosome abnormalities to a central register [2]. Information is recorded on source of report, date of referral, age and sex of patient, karyotype, and maternal age when the abnormality was diagnosed in infancy.

RESULTS

Table I illustrates that of 760 cases, 431 (60%) were autosomal trisomies and 126 (16%) were sex chromosome anomalies. Table II provides an analysis of age at diagnosis and shows that nearly half (49%) of all chromosome disorders diagnosed up to age 14 years are detected in the first week. If one considers only the diagnoses made in the neonatal period (0–4 weeks), comparisons can be made between rates of cytogenetically confirmed cases and the expected incidence (Table III). Over the 8 years of the study, 351 cases of autosomal trisomy were diagnosed in the neonatal period, giving an incidence of 0.118 per 100 live births. This figure is not significantly different from the estimated true incidence of 0.144, the value obtained from unselected newborn data [4]. Table III shows that with the exception of unbalanced translocations, detection rates for other abnormalities in the neonatal

TABLE I. Chromosome Abnormalities in Children (0–14 Yrs) Queensland 1976–1983 (760 Cases)

Type of Abnormality	Absolute Numbers
Autosomal trisomies (AT)	431
Sex chromosome abnormalities (SC)	126
Balanced translocations (BT)	37
Unbalanced translocations (UT)	41
Duplications/deletions (D/D)	58
Miscellaneous (M)	67
Total	760

TABLE II. Age of Children at Diagnosis of Chromosome Abnormalities Queensland 1976–1983 (760 Cases)

	Type of Abnormality						
Age at Diagnosis	AT	SC	BT	UT	D/D	M	Total
0–6 days	295	23	6	19	14	17	374
1–4 weeks	56	9	3	8	8	3	87
1–5 months	31	8	7	5	2	6	59
6–11 months	11	3	3	2	2	1	22
1–4 years	11	12	4	3	14	11	55
5–9 years	12	34	6	3	11	19	85
10–14 years	15	37	8	1	7	10	78
	431	126	37	41	58	67	760

TABLE III. Comparative Study of Observed and Expected Chromosome Abnormalities: Eight Year Total Population Study, Queensland, Australia 1976–1983

Type of Abnormality	Elevated True Incidence (4)	Expected Total Number (296,000 births)	Number Diagnosed by 4 Weeks
Autosomal trisomies	0.144	426	351 (0.118)
Sex chromosome abnormalities	0.223	661	32
Balanced translocations	0.193	571	9
Unbalanced translocations	0.021	62	27
Miscellaneous	0.039	115	42
All types	0.620	1,835	461(0.156)

period are very low. Figure 1 charts the relative frequency histograms for age at diagnosis and shows that almost all the chromosome anomalies detected in newborn infants are autosomal trisomies.

DISCUSSION

The relative frequency of sex chromosome abnormalities in a population is known to be higher than that of autosomal trisomies by a factor of 1.5 [4]. Data derived from this study show the relative frequency of diagnosed versus expected cases of sex chromosome disorder to be low. If it is accepted that the 431 diagnosed cases of autosomal trisomy in this study approximate the expected number, one would anticipate the existence of approximately 646 cases (× 1.5) of sex chromosome abnormality. Diagnosed cases number only 126, indicating the large number of undetected patients with this condition in the target population (Table IV). It also becomes apparent from Table III that most patients with balanced translocation, minor deletions and duplications,

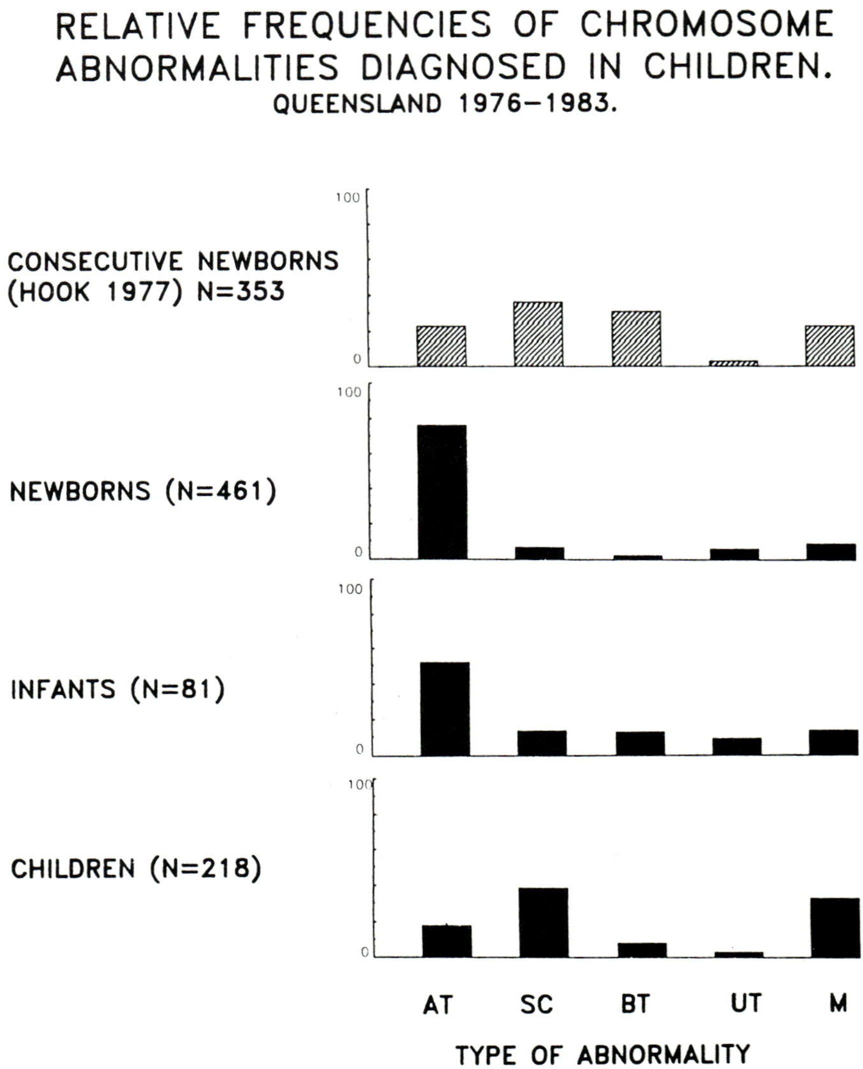

Fig. 1. AT = autosomal trisomy; SC = sex chromosome abnormality; BT = balanced translocation; UT = unbalanced translocation; M = miscellaneous.

TABLE IV. Frequency of Abnormalities

	Known Relative Frequency (4)	Relative Frequency in Study Cases
Autosomal trisomies	23.2	56.7
Sex chromosome abnormalities	36.0	16.6

rings, fragments, and other chromosome rearrangements remain undiagnosed during the childhood years.

Documentation of the size and nature of the pool of unrecognized chromosome abnormalities in childhood allows for a consideration of the clinical implications. It can be argued that balanced translocations [5–7] and fragments or microchromosomes [8,9] are infrequently associated with significant sequelae. However, the presence of sex chromosome disorders, small deletions or duplications, and ring chromosomes may be associated with major clinical effects [10–14]. The data from this study suggest a need for the careful scrutiny of indications for cytogenetic investigation. Target groups should include small-for-dates babies [15], infants with minor anomalies, and children with developmental delay [10].

The largest component of the unrecognized chromosome abnormality pool in childhood is the sex chromosome group, and it is pertinent to consider the implications for these patients in greater detail. In the absence of ambiguous sex, hypospadias or lymph stasis in the newborn infant, diagnosis is rarely made before puberty. Shortness of stature, neck webbing, and abnormal nails may arouse suspicion of the Ullrich-Turner syndrome (UTS). There has been recent interest in hormone supplementation, attempting to increase final height [16–19]. The efficacy of anabolic steroids remains indeterminate, with one study showing negative results [16] and another claiming considerable benefit [17]. There is further controversy regarding effects on final height of estrogens prescribed for the development of secondary sex characteristics [18]. Finally, recent studies indicate that many UTS patients have a relative deficiency of growth hormone before puberty, and this may contribute to their short adult stature [19]. There are clearly cogent reasons for making the diagnosis of the UTS as early in life as possible.

Testosterone treatment of boys with Klinefelter syndrome is indicated at 12–13 years in order to secure normal pubertal development. Such treatment, which is generally without undesirable side effects, may also have a stabilizing effect on emotional development. There is no indication for hormone treatment of any kind in girls with the 47, XXX or boys with the 47, XYY constitution [10].

Early diagnosis is indicated in all conditions involving abnormalities of the sex chromosomes—whether amenable to hormone treatment or not. Deviations from normal in growth patterns, educational difficulties, and behavior disorders may be explained by the diagnosis of sex chromosome aneuploidy [10].

Many patients with sex chromosome anomalies are at increased risk for the development of neoplasia [20,21]. This particularly applies to patients with dysgenetic gonads and a Y chromosome, where tumors may occur as early as the first decade. Gonadoblastomas are the commonest lesions, frequently with transformation to a malignant germ cell tumor. Early diagnosis of underlying sex chromosome anomaly permits gonadal ablation and also prevents virilization of a phenotypically female patient at puberty. Reports of gonadal tumors in patients with a 45,X karyotype are very rare, but there is a propensity to develop extragonadal neoplasms, often of neurogenic origin, both in children and adults [20,21]. Klinefelter syndrome patients are at increased risk for the development of extragonadal germ cell neoplasms [20,21], and an association with mixed gonadal dysgenesis and Wilms tumor has been described.

While the major responsibility for improving rates of diagnosis of chromosomal abnormalities in childhood falls on pediatricians, pathologists too have responsibilities. Recent surveys have demonstrated the value of cytogenetic studies in perinatal autopsies, with detection rates near 5% [22,23]. Cytogenetic studies can easily be overlooked when infants present more pressing problems of immaturity, sepsis, and respiratory distress syndrome. The autopsy clearly represents the last change for a specific chromosome diagnosis and subsequent informed genetic counseling.

SUMMARY

The data from an ongoing total population survey of all diagnosed chromosome anomalies in Queensland, Australia have been presented for an 8-year period (1976–83). A total of 760 patients was diagnosed, principally autosomal trisomies (431) and sex chromosome abnormalities (126). Nearly half of total childhood diagnoses (up to 14 years) were made in the first week. Virtually all expected cases of autosomal trisomies were detected in the first month. The largest component of the pool of unrecognized childhood disorders in this study was the sex chromosome group. This failure of detection has implications in terms of potentially beneficial hormone treatment and predisposition to neoplasia.

ACKNOWLEDGMENTS

Members of the Queensland Cytogenetics Group, who contributed data from their laboratories to the Chromosome Abnormality Register.

REFERENCES

1. Bell J, Pearn J, McCarthy C, Jones L, Trouten C, Hunt F, Berry L: A total population study of undiagnosed chromosome abnormalities in Queensland, Australia. Clin Genet 22:49–56, 1982.
2. Bell JA, Bowling FG, Pearn JH et al.: Register of chromosome abnormalities in Queensland. Med J Aust 2:186–189, 1983.
3. Australian Bureau of Statistics. 1976–1983. Queensland Demography. Cat. No. 3101 3. Brisbane, Aust Bureau Stat (Qld).
4. Hook EB, Hamerton JL: The frequency of chromosome abnormalities detected in consecutive newborn studies—differences between studies—results by sex and by severity of phenotypic involvement. In Hook EB, Porter IH (Eds): "Population Cytogenetics: Studies in Humans," New York: Academic Press, 1977, pp 63–79.
5. Hecht F, Kaiser-McCaw B, Patil S, Wyandt HE: Are balanced translocations really balanced? Preliminary evidence for position effect in man. March of Dimes: Birth Defects Foundation BD: OAS 14:(6C):281–286, 1978.
6. Aymé S, Mattei MG, Mattei JF, Giraud F: Abnormal childhood phenotypes associated with the same balanced chromosome rearrangements as in the parents. Hum Genet 48:7–12, 1979.
7. Warburton D: Outcome of cases of de novo structural rearrangements diagnosed at amniocentesis. Prenat Diag 4:69–70, 1984.
8. Fryns JP, Kleczkowska A, Van Den Berghe H: Small accessory chromosomes (SAC) and their genotype-phenotype correlation. J Genet Hum 30:215–232, 1982.
9. Benn PA, Hsu LYF: Incidence and significance of supernumerary marker chromosomes in prenatal diagnosis. Am J Hum Genet 36:1092–1102, 1984.
10. Nielsen J, Sorensen AM, Sorensen K: Follow-up until age 7 to 11 of 25 unselected children with sex chromosome abnormalities. In Stewart DA (Ed) "Children With Sex Chromosome Aneuploidy: Follow-Up Studies. New York: Alan R. Liss, Inc. for the March of Dimes Birth Defects Foundation, BD:OAS 18(4):61–97, 1982.
11. deGrouchy J, Turleau C: Turner's syndrome. "Clinical Atlas of Human Chromosomes." 2nd Ed. New York: John Wiley and Sons, 1984, pp 375–383.
12. Cowchock FS, Wapner RJ, Kurtz A, Chatzkel S, Barnhart JS, Lesnick DC: Not all cystic hygromas occur in the Ullrich-Turner syndrome. Am J Med Genet 12:327–331, 1982.
13. Fryns JP, Kleczkowska A, Van den Berghe K, Moerman F, Van Den Berghe H: Cystic hygroma and hydrops fetalis in dup(11p) syndrome. Am J Med Genet 22:287–289, 1985.
14. Martin NJ, Harvey PJ, Pearn JH: The ring chromosome 13 syndrome. Hum Genet 61(1):18–23, 1982.
15. Anderson NG: A five year survey of small for dates infants for chromosomal abnormalities. Aust Paediatr J 12:19–23, 1976.
16. Sybert VP: Adult height in Turner syndrome with and without androgen therapy. J Pediatr 104:365–369, 1984.
17. Joss E, Zuppinger K: Oxandrolone in girls with Turner's syndrome. A pair-matched controlled study up to final height. Acta Paediatr Scand 73:674–679, 1984.

18. Demetriou E, Emans SJ, Crigler JS: Final height in estrogen-treated patients with Turner syndrome. Obstet Gynecol 64:459–464, 1984.
19. Ross JL, Long LM, Loriaux DL, Cutler GB: Growth hormone secretory dynamics in Turner's syndrome. J Pediatr 106:202–206, 1985.
20. Scully RE: Neoplasia associated with anomalous sexual development and abnormal sex chromosomes. In Josso N (Ed): "The Intersex Child." Basel: Karger, 1981, pp 203–217.
21. Welch WR, Robboy SJ: Abnormal sexual development: A classification with emphasis on pathology and neoplastic conditions. In Kogan SJ, Hafez ESE (eds): "Pediatric Andrology," The Hague: Martinus Nijhoff, 1981, pp 71–85.
22. Sutherland GR, Carter RF: Cytogenetic studies; An essential part of the pediatric necropsy. J Clin Pathol 36:140–142, 1983.
23. Angell RR, Sandison A, Bain AD: Chromosome variation in perinatal mortality: A survey of 500 cases. J Med Genet 21:39–44, 1984.

Anatomical Defects and Variations Due to Aneuploidy

James C. Pettersen, PhD, and Edward T. Bersu, PhD

Department of Anatomy, University of Wisconsin, Madison, Wisconsin 53706

INTRODUCTION

For a number of years our laboratory has been studying the gross anatomic variations and defects associated with human multiple congenital anomaly syndromes. This effort was stimulated by Dr. John M. Opitz, who encouraged the parents of children with multiple congenital anomaly syndromes to donate the bodies of these children at the time of death to the Department of Anatomy, University of Wisconsin, for detailed anatomic study. These bodies were embalmed arterially and stored until such time dissection could be performed. Efforts were made to dissect several subjects for each syndrome so that the anatomic phenotypes would reflect the range of variation within each syndrome. Such anatomic phenotypes have been described for trisomy 13 [1,2] based on 8 cases, trisomy 18 [3,4] based on 9 cases, and trisomy 21 [5] based on 5 cases. Additional subjects with trisomy 18 and with trisomy 13 have been studied by Aziz [6,7] who consulted with the authors. His findings are in essential agreement with our own, although each additional subject contributes something new to the total range of variations.

Historic recognition should be given to Barash [8] who was the first person in our program to dissect a cytogenetically confirmed aneuploid infant in detail. The subject, a girl with trisomy 18, showed a wide spectrum of muscle defects and variations. Her study suggested that an "anatomic phenotype" might be definable for a trisomy syndrome if one could study enough subjects so that the "background noise" could be eliminated.

Birth Defects: Original Article Series, Volume 23, Number 1, pages 315–331

It is apparent to us now that each of the 3 most common human trisomies that can survive to the neonatal period may be characterized by a unique combination of anatomic defects and variations in addition to the constellations based on physical examination and autopsy data. Thus, physical examination, autopsy, and anatomic data each contribute to the delineation of trisomies 13, 18, and 21. In the following subsections we present anatomic phenotypes, with emphasis on the musculature, for these 3 human trisomy syndromes in a greatly condensed fashion made possible by eliminating much of the "background noise." The reader is advised that there is much more variation present in each individual subject than is indicated by the composite summary data. Following these subsections we present more recent anatomic findings for a subject with dup (6p), a fetus with del (18p), several subjects with triploidy, and some summary information on our work with murine trisomies 1, 16, and 19. The latter were studied on serial sections at various stages of embryonic development.

TRISOMY 13

Trisomy 13 is characterized by variations of the muscles of all body regions. Six variations occur with such remarkable consistency that they appear from our present body of information to form a diagnostically conclusive cluster: 1) absence of palmaris longus (16 of 16 limbs); 2) absence of peroneus tertius (16 of 16 limbs); 3) absence of palmaris brevis (13 of 14 limbs); 4) absence of plantaris (13 of 16 limbs); 5) presence of pectorodorsalis (14 of 16 limbs, Fig. 1); 6) variations in extensor indicis (14 of 16 limbs, Fig. 2).

None of the above variations is remarkable in itself, although the palmaris brevis has been reported as absent in only 2% of the normal population [9]. Its presence was not sought in 1 of the 2 fetuses dissected, so that only 14 limbs are reported. In the 1 limb where it was present, it was aberrant. Its fibers passed obliquely distalward from the fascia over the pisiform bone to the palmar fascia and the ulnar artery and nerve passed superficial rather than deep to its belly. The plantaris muscle, which is absent in about 7% of persons in the normal population, was present in 3 limbs but in 2 of these it was hypoplastic. One subject lacked pectorodorsalis muscles and 1 subject possessed normal extensor indicis muscles.

The muscle phenotype can be expanded to include variations in the biceps brachii and coracobrachialis; fusion of the bellies of the radial extensors of the wrist; variations in stylohyoideus, posterior belly of digastricus, and the anterior belly of digastricus in conjunction with mylohyoideus; missing

1

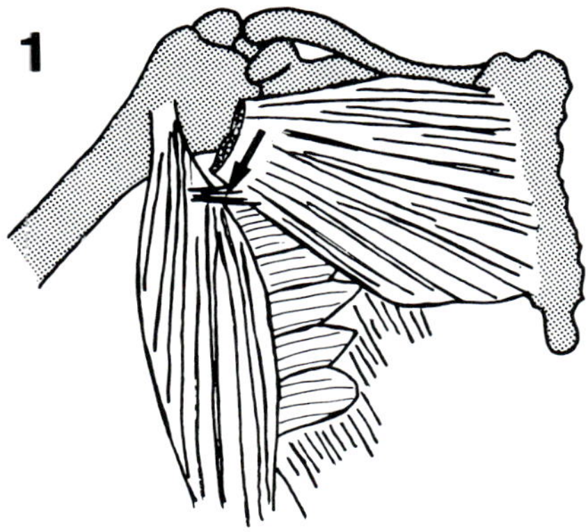

2

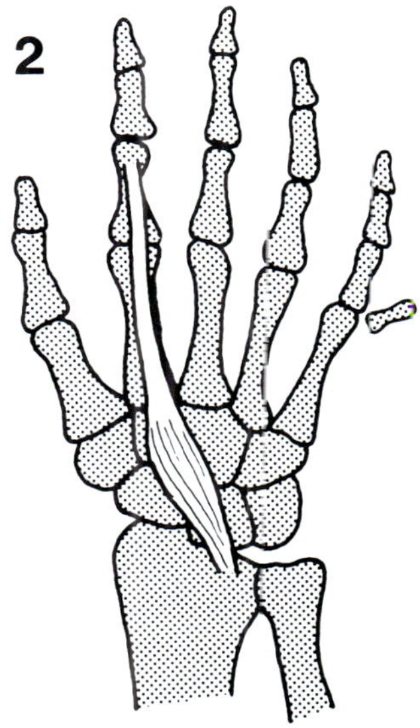

Fig. 1. Arrow indicates a small pectorodorsalis muscle extending from pectoralis major to latissimus dorsi.

Fig. 2. Extensor indicis muscle arising distal to its usual origin. This was the most common variation of this muscle seen in trisomy 13. This muscle normally arises from the ulna about 10 cm proximal to the wrist.

tendons of flexor digitorum brevis in the foot; and presence of an occipital platysma muscle [10]. The above variations occur about 50% of the time. Other less diagnostic variations occur less frequently.

A 6-year-old male trisomic for 13q12→qter was similarly studied, and it was obvious that he did not fit well the muscle phenotype defined above [11]. Overall he had *more* muscle variations than did any of the 8 complete 13-trisomy subjects, but palmaris longus, palmaris brevis, plantaris, and peroneus tertius were all present bilaterally. However, he possessed 1 pectorodorsalis muscle and his extensor indicis muscles showed variations. He possessed 9 muscle variations not found in any of the complete trisomy 13 subjects. Other than the presence of 4 muscles usually absent in complete trisomy 13, his muscle phenotype corresponded quite well in other respects to that seen in complete trisomy 13.

TRISOMY 18

Muscle variations in trisomy 18 cluster around the otomandibular and preaxial forearm and hand regions. These regions also present the most diagnostically important findings on physical examination such as apparently low-set, malformed ears and small jaw and a tendency toward radius and thumb aplasia. The muscle variations tend to be more bizarre than in trisomy 13 and a bit less uniform. However, one can expect small occipital platysma muscles (Fig. 3) to be uniformly present, some variation in the supra- and infrahyoid muscles and in the muscles on the preaxial side of the forearm and hand, and absence of the palmaris longus in all subjects with this

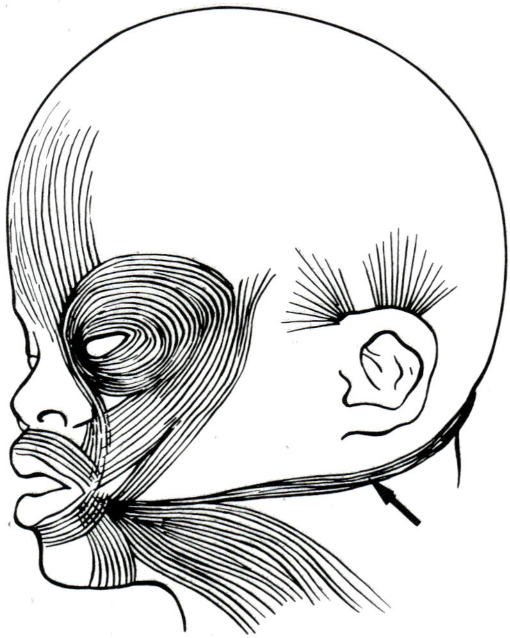

Fig. 3. Arrow indicates an occipital platysma muscle, which is an embryonic muscle retained characteristically in trisomy 21 and also found routinely in trisomy 18 and frequently in trisomy 13. The muscles to the upper lip, as shown in the drawing, illustrate the condition of the midfacial muscles in trisomy 21, ie, they represent a relatively unsegregated sheet of muscle.

syndrome. In 9 carefully dissected subjects, there were no significant exceptions. Other less clustered muscle variations occur in all body regions so that, in this respect, it is similar to trisomy 13.

It is more difficult to define a muscle phenotype for trisomy 18 due, perhaps, to the underlying skeletal defects in the 2 predominantly affected regions. One must assume that some of these deviations from the normal represent defects caused by developmental field disturbances that are likely to be of vascular origin. We suggest that hemorrhaging of the regional arteries to the otomandibular and preaxial upper limb areas may have occurred early in development with subsequent healing. The result is sometimes a severe disturbance of the musculoskeletal system, which can be compared to the normal situation only on the basis of painstaking analysis and with some speculation. Characteristically, the radial artery is absent and is replaced by a neighboring artery. The musculocutaneous nerve is uniformly absent and its territory is supplied by direct branches from the median nerve. Other common findings in the otomandibular region, such as absence of salivary glands, middle ear defects, and mandibular hypoplasia, are consistent with a developmental field defect hypothesis.

TRISOMY 21

Three muscle variations found almost uniformly in 5 dissected subjects with the Down syndrome were: presence of a well-developed occipital platysma muscle; failure of the muscles of facial expression to separate into individual discrete muscles in the midface (Fig. 3), absence of palmaris longus. In somewhat less than 50% of the instances, the superficial flexor tendon to the fifth finger and the flexor digitorum brevis tendon to the fifth toe were absent. Other than these, we encountered only a slightly increased tendency toward muscle variation in this syndrome.

Based on complete gross anatomic data from the 5 subjects, a characteristic anatomic phenotype for the Down syndrome includes the following: 1) presence of a well-developed occipital platysma muscle (10 of 10 sides), 2) a continuous undifferentiated sheet of muscles of facial expression in the midfacial region (10 of 10 sides), 3) presence of dorsal root ganglia associated with the first cervical dorsal roots and the spinal accessory nerve (4 of 5 bodies), 4) multiple roots of the vertebral artery (3 of 5 bodies), 5) origin of the definitive middle colic artery from the inferior mesenteric artery (5 of 5 bodies), 6) absence of palmaris longus muscle (8 of 10 sides, but bilaterally aberrant in the one body where it was present).

The first 4 of these variations represent failure in the progression of normal differentiation. An occipital platysma muscle is uniformly present in human fetuses from 7–12 weeks [10] but regresses thereafter and is never seen in a euploid neonate or adult. The muscles of facial expression arise from a common embryonic sheet of mesenchyme but in the normal situation they separate into discrete entities. Dorsal root ganglia are present on the dorsal roots of the first cervical nerve through the first trimester, but they normally degenerate and are not observed grossly beyond that time [12–14]. Vertebral arteries form from several roots initially, and all but 1 of these normally regress [15,16].

No explanation is offered for the aberrant middle colic artery. Its incidence in normal persons is not known and we could find no evidence that its presence in this form has ever been reported. Thus, it is a consistent curiosity. The absence of palmaris longus is of interest because, aside from muscles such as psoas minor and pyramidalis, which are so frequently absent as normal variations, it is the most frequently absent muscle in the body. Its absence in the "mildest" of the 3 trisomy syndromes considered here seems consistent with a mild degree of developmental instability.

DUP(6p)

A subject trisomic for the distal segment of 6p from 6p21→6pter was donated for anatomic study at the time of her death at 17 11/12 years. About 16 dup(6p) cases have been reported. Common findings include: frontal bossing; hypotelorism; hypoplastic midface; blepharophimosis; low-set and/or malformed ears; cardiovascular defects; small kidneys; sacral dimple; and profound mental retardation. Our subject is the oldest to be described with this syndrome.

Anatomic findings include: arhinencephaly in conjunction with narrow cerebral hemispheres (Fig. 4); right ventricular outflow tract abnormality of the heart; absence of uterus and vagina; hypoplastic ovaries; common mesentery; severe retardation in skeletal development; dolichocephaly consistent with the narrow hemispheres; and a number of abnormalities and deformities of the skull, which are described elsewhere [17].

Muscle variations of interest in the context of this paper include absence of palmaris brevis muscles; absence of left palmaris longus; absence of left peroneus tertius; absence of stylohyoid muscles; variation in extensor indicis muscles; and presence of pectorodorsalis muscles. In addition, there were several other less remarkable variations [17].

DEL(18p)

A fetus with the del(18p) syndrome was dissected to determine the extent of morphologic variation that may occur in this condition. Two rather striking

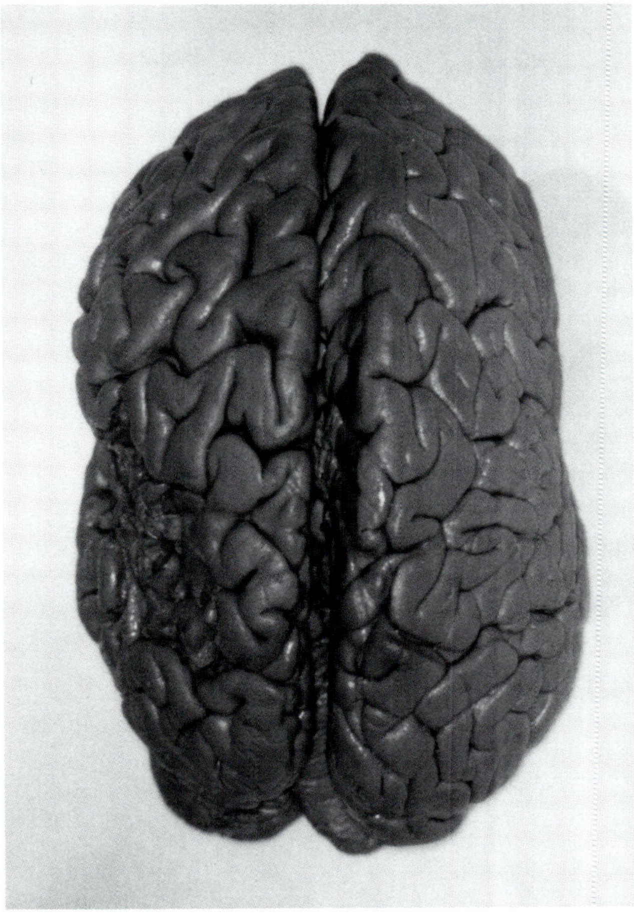

Fig. 4. Photograph of a dorsal view of the brain from a subject with dup(6p). The cerebral hemispheres are very narrow, appear to be relatively elongated and correspond to a dolichocephalic skull.

morphologic defects were observed: 1) the levator palpebrae superioris muscle was absent in 1 orbit and was markedly reduced in the other; 2) there was no indication of the presence of any ligament of the head of the femur or its associated blood vessels bilaterally. It is of interest that ptosis of the eyelids and congenital hip dislocations have been reported in this syndrome [18].

No additional remarkable gross anatomic variations were observed. This appears to represent the first example of a deletion syndrome to be studied anatomically, and it is premature to draw any conclusions.

TRIPLOIDY

Five fetuses with triploidy were studied to determine if they showed anatomic variations similar to those seen associated with trisomy. Three of the fetuses ranged in age from 20 to 26 weeks and were dissectable. The other 2 were at approximately 12 to 14 weeks of gestational age and did not lend themselves to gross anatomic dissection.

Findings of interest from the sample included: 1) bilateral absence of the middle fibers of the trapezius muscle; 2) enlarged anterior thigh muscles with disproportionate enlargement of the short head of biceps femoris in 2 of the 3 dissectable fetuses; and 3) aberrations in the attachments of the extraocular muscles in 1 older fetus and 1 younger fetus. In the latter variation, the 4 rectus muscles attached too far posteriorly and the 2 oblique muscles attached too far anteriorly on the globe.

A number of other muscle variations was observed in the 3 dissectable fetuses but a consistent constellation was not observed. One of the 3 had 15 observable variations; the other 2 had about 9 each. These are discussed elsewhere [19].

MOUSE TRISOMY 1

Breeding schemes for the systematic collection and study of trisomic mouse embryos have been developed by introducing Robertsonian translocation chromosomes from feral mice into laboratory strains [20]. Gropp [21, 22] suggested that the trisomy 1 mouse showed defects similar to those observed in the human alobar-holoprosencephaly spectrum of defects and/or human trisomy 13. He suggested that mouse trisomy might serve as an animal model for studying the effects of human trisomy.

Our laboratory undertook an extensive study of trisomy 1 mouse embryos ranging in age from 9.5 to 12 gestational days to evaluate this system as an animal model [23]. A minimum of 10 trisomic embryos and all euploid littermate controls was studied at each of 6 scheduled times: 9.5 days, 10 days, 10.5 days, 11 days, 11.5 days, and 12 days of gestation. Whole embryos were studied with a dissection microscope, and data were collected for somite numbers, weight, crown-rump length, and external characteristics. Subsequently all embryos were embedded and serially sectioned for microscopic analysis.

It was determined that the eye and the brain showed the most consistent defects. Eye defects were apparent early and included aphakia, enlarged intraretinal space, and dysplasia of the optic cup layers. "Pseudolenses" developed from the optic cup layers in some animals lacking lens placodes. Figure 5 shows 3 cranial to caudal sections of such a "pseudolens" in an 11.5-day trisomy 1 embryo.

The most common brain defect was narrowness of the brain vesicles with folds of the vesicle walls. Neural crest-derived mesoderm in the region of the midface and branchial arches was sometimes deficient, resulting in obvious defects. This was not a consistent finding but 5 severely defective embryos were found from among a total of 89 trisomic embryos studied. Each of these showed deficiencies in the neural crest-derived facial region (frontonasal processes and branchial arches) in addition to the brain and eye defects. Only one embryo showed the characteristics of cyclopia with proboscis (Fig. 6).

The most consistent finding among the trisomic embryos is that their development lagged about one-half day behind the development of normal littermates. Our tentative conclusions are: 1) trisomy 1 mice are characterized by growth and developmental retardation and lag about one-half day behind normal littermates; 2) eye and brain are the most commonly defective structures; 3) severely defective embryos exhibit facial defects in areas derived from neural crest cells; 4) embryos fail to survive beyond 12 days of gestation; 5) trisomy 1 in the mouse is not a good model for human alobar holoprosencephaly-cyclopia or for human trisomy 13 but may serve as an excellent model for studying developmental eye defects.

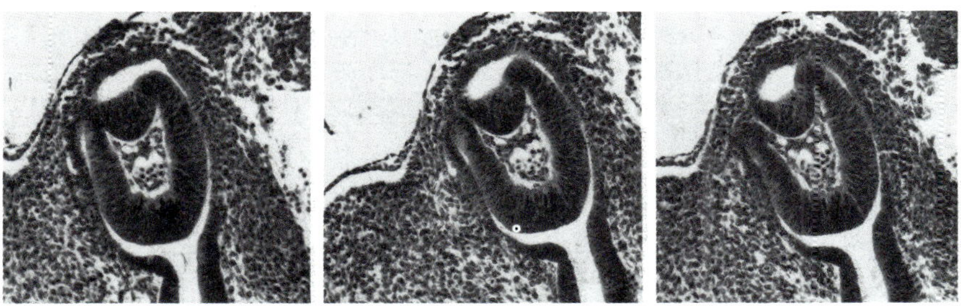

Fig. 5. Cranial to caudal sections, left to right, showing the formation of a "pseudolens" from the optic cup layers in an 11.5-day trisomy 1 mouse embryo. At the right, the "lens" is being pinched off from the optic cup layers (X100).

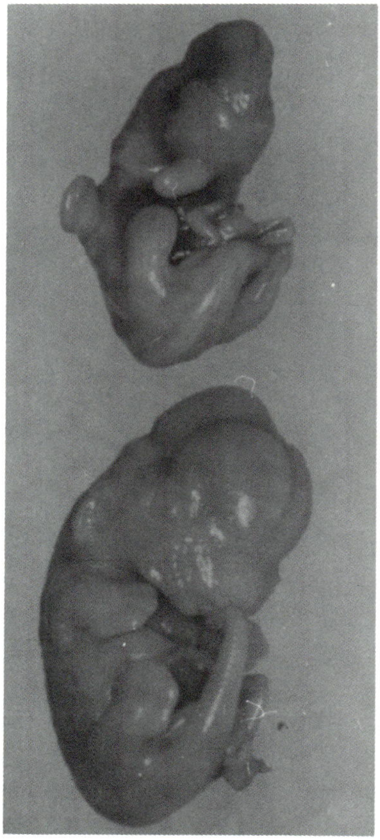

Fig. 6. A 12-day trisomy mouse embryo with proboscis, above, compared to a normal littermate, below. This was the only trisomic embryo from among 89 studied that showed the full characteristics of cyclopia.

MOUSE TRISOMY 19

The observation by Gropp [24] that mice carrying Robertsonian translocation chromosomes could be used to produce trisomic conceptuses was made simultaneously by White et al [25]. They worked with translocations involving chromosome 19. Their early studies focused primarily on the relationship between specific translocation chromosome combinations and the frequency and viability of trisomy 19 conceptuses [26, 27]. An interesting morphologic finding was that a cleft of the secondary palate was associated with a specific combination of translocation chromosomes.

Collaborative studies between Dr. White and our laboratory focused on the developmental aspects of trisomy 19. The only obvious morphologic variation observed so far is a consistent 1-day lag in the affected conceptuses' otherwise normal progression of development (Fig. 7). This lag includes the development of the central nervous system and other organ systems, and parameters such as rate of weight gain, crown-rump length, as well as overall phenotypic appearance. Apart from an occasional severely retarded or dead trisomic conceptus, the degree and nature of this delay is uniform in all trisomic animals [28].

An appealing hypothesis that has been frequently used to explain growth retardation associated with trisomy is that the aneuploid genome disrupts some aspect of cell proliferation. To test this hypothesis, the single-cell DNA content of trisomic and normal littermate thymuses was measured using cell sorting techniques [28, 29]. This procedure allows one to estimate the relative proportions of cells in a proliferating population that are in the different phases of the cell cycle. The results of this analysis, using thymuses from animals from 18 days to term, is shown in Figure 8. Trisomic thymus-cell populations consistently had relatively greater numbers of cells in the synthetic (S) and G_2 phases of the cell cycle than did normal littermates. This pattern is usually indicative of a prolongation of the cell cycle. Thus, it may not be unreasonable to assume that the trisomy 19 genome could be altering cell proliferation, at least in the thymus. However, it should also be noted that the trisomic cell cycle profiles for any given day are not significantly different from profiles of normal animals of the previous gestational day so the difference could simply be another reflection of the overall developmental lag.

MOUSE TRISOMY 16

Of all the mouse trisomies studied to date, the greatest interest has been in trisomy 16, because of anomalies it shares with the Down syndrome. Each shows growth retardation and cardiac defects. However, the most striking similarity between the two conditions is that cells from each show dosage effects for the products of similar genes whose loci are located on human autosome 21 and mouse autosome 16. These shared genes include those coding for superoxide dismutase-1, the α- and β-interferon receptor molecules, and the response of trisomic cells to β-adrenergic agonist stimulation [30, 31]. The last 3 of these 4 genes code for cell surface receptor-linked

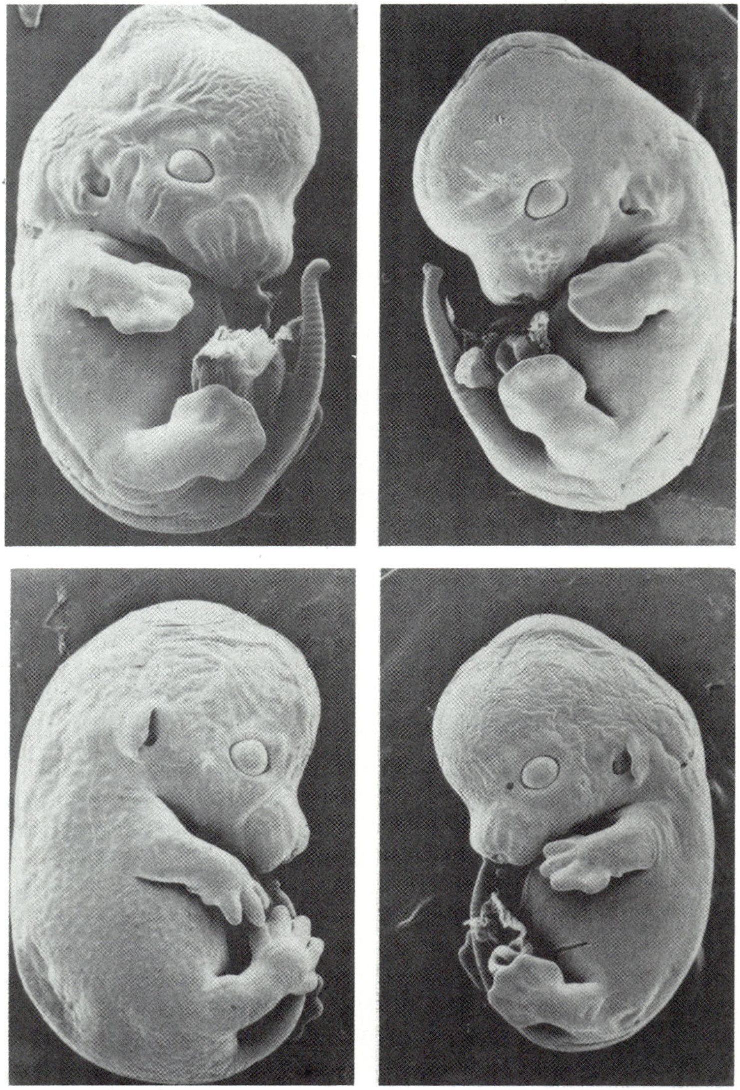

Fig. 7. Scanning electron micrographs of 13-day (top) and 14-day (bottom) mouse fetuses. Trisomy 19 fetuses are on the right. In each case the trisomic fetus is smaller than its normal littermate and shows characteristics similar to those of fetuses of the previous gestational day. All magnifications, ×10.

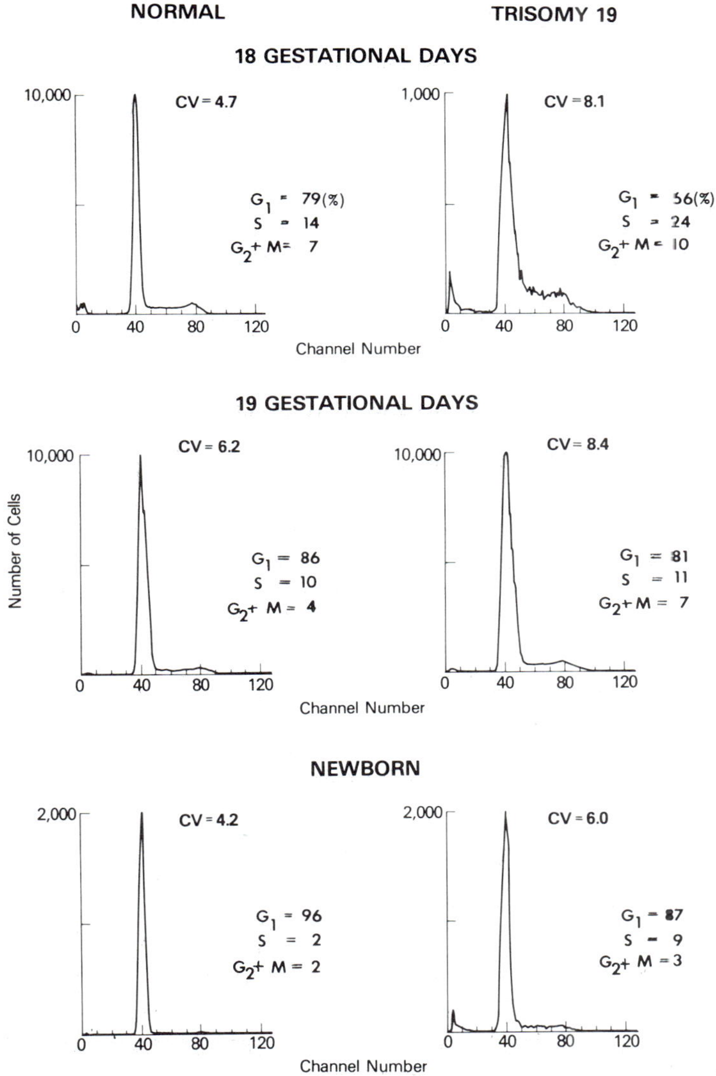

Fig. 8. Representative DNA histograms from normal and trisomy 19 thymic cell suspensions from 18 gestational days to term. Percentages of cells present in the G_1, S and G_2 + M phases of the cell cycle are at the right of each histogram.

systems and it has been shown that these systems, especially the α- and β-interferon receptor systems, have a marked effect on the expression of H-2 cell surface markers [32]. The H-2 markers play an important role in normal cell-cell interactions and it is possible that imbalances in their numbers or distribution caused by the presence of the human trisomy 21 or the mouse trisomy 16 genome could be a factor contributing to the altered development of affected conceptuses. At the present time, studies are being conducted by investigators at the University of Wisconsin-Madison to evaluate the possible relationship of trisomy 16 to altered cell-surface phenomena and altered development [33].

Several efforts completed so far have focused on the nature of the structural alterations due to trisomy 16. Detailed examinations of the brains of affected conceptuses are presented elsewhere in this volume (Kornguth). An evaluation of the progression of development of the overall morphologic phenotype is also currently in progress. In studies to date, the morphologic development of trisomy 16 conceptuses has not shown the consistent and uniform pattern of growth retardation associated with trisomy 19. In trisomy 16, the gross appearance and size of trisomic conceptuses range from near normal to an appearance consistent with a 1-day developmental lag. These observations are in agreement with those of an earlier study of trisomy 16 [34].

The most striking morphologic finding so far, apart from the cardiac defects, is that placental development is markedly affected in conceptuses with trisomy 16. Some of these differences are shown in Figure 9. In addition to being small (as is also the case for trisomy 1 and trisomy 19 placentas) there are greater than normal numbers of small trophoblast cells within the labyrinth of trisomy 16 placentas. These cells form large clusters, which persist to term. Such cells, especially in the form of clusters, are not seen in normal placentas beyond 13 gestational days.

A second difference in the trisomy 16 placenta is that the basal zone persists throughout gestation as a narrow band of giant cells rather than differentiating into a broad band composed of clusters of small trophoblast cells and cells filled with glycogen. These variations are not seen in trisomy 19 placentas.

The manner in which these alterations affect the growth and/or development of trisomy 16 fetuses is not known. However, as with other observations from the trisomic mice, they illustrate that these animals will be useful models for better understanding the relationship between trisomy and altered development.

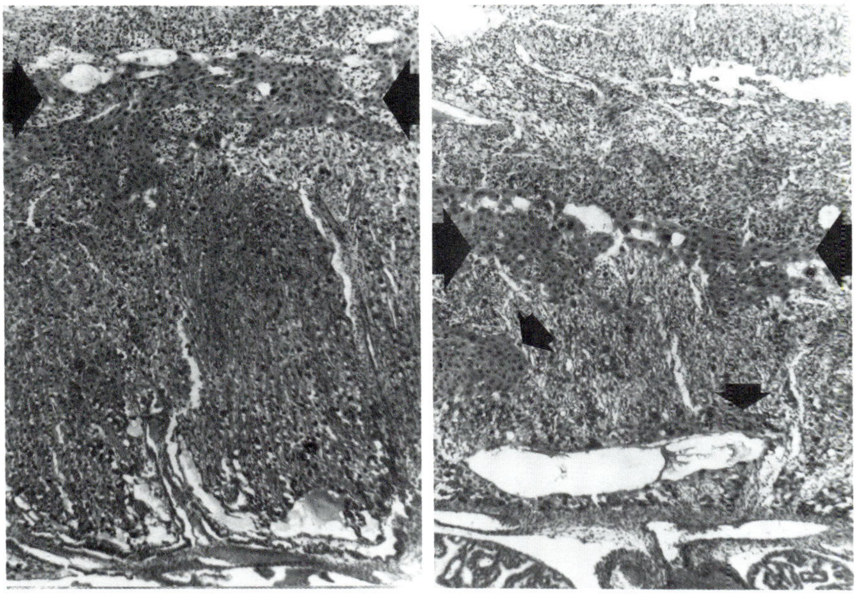

Fig. 9. Sections of placentas from 15-day normal (N) and trisomy 16 (Ts) fetuses cut through the center of the placental disc. The fetal surface is at the bottom of each micrograph. The labyrinth of the normal placenta extends from the bottom to near the top of the micrograph, where the basal zone (horizontal arrows) can be seen to be composed of islands of small trophoblast cells and glycogen cells. The labyrinth of the trisomic placenta extends to near the center of the micrographs (horizontal arrow) and is composed primarily of large giant cells. Arrows within the labyrinth point to islands of small trophoblast cells. Original magnification, ×40. Stained with hematoxylin and eosin.

ACKNOWLEDGMENTS

The authors wish to acknowledge the following former students who worked with them during the past few years: Sharon Colacino, Ph.D., Gregory Mieden, Ph.D., Barbara Smith, Ph.D., Gordon Koltis, M.D., Michael White, M.D., and medical students John Andrews, David Moen, and Bruce Urban. The latter four were supported by Summer Science Research Grants for Medical Students from the Birth Defects Foundation-March of Dimes. Other portions of the work were supported by Public Health Services/NIH Grant GM20130 from the National Institute of Medical Sciences to the Wisconsin Clinical Genetics Center, NIH Grant HD 13952, an NIH General Research Support Sub-Grant from the University of Wisconsin

Medical School Research Committee, and an interim grant from the University of Wisconsin Graduate School.

REFERENCES

1. Colacino SC, Pettersen JC: Analysis of the gross anatomical variations found in 4 cases of trisomy 13. Am J Med Genet 2:31–50, 1978.
2. Pettersen JC, Koltis GG, White MJ: An examination of the spectrum of anatomic defects and variations found in eight cases of trisomy 13. Am J Med Genet 3:183–210, 1979.
3. Bersu ET, Ramirez-Castro JL: Anatomical analysis of the developmental effects of aneuploidy in man - the 18-trisomy syndrome. I. Anomalies of the head and neck. Am J Med Genet 1:173–193, 1977.
4. Ramirez-Castro JL, Bersu ET: Anatomical analysis of the developmental effects of aneuploidy in man - the 18-trisomy syndrome. II. Anomalies of the upper and lower limbs. Am J Med Genet 2:285–306, 1978.
5. Bersu ET: Anatomical analysis of the developmental effects of aneuploidy in man: The Down syndrome. Am J Med Genet 5:399–420, 1980.
6. Aziz MA: Muscular and other abnormalities in a case of Edwards' syndrome (18-trisomy). Teratology 20:303–312, 1979.
7. Aziz MA: Anatomical defects in a case of trisomy 13 with D/D translocation. Teratology 22:217–227, 1980.
8. Barash BA, Freedman L, Opitz JM: Anatomic studies in the 18-trisomy syndrome. White Plains, NY: The National Foundation-March of Dimes BD:OAS VI(4):3–15, 1970.
9. LeDouble AF: Traité des variations du systême musculaire de l'homme. Schleicher Frères (eds), Paris: Librairie C. Reinwald, 1897.
10. Gasser RF: The development of the facial muscles in man. Am J Anat 120:357–376, 1967.
11. Pettersen JC: Anatomical studies of a boy trisomic for the distal portion of 13q. Am J Med Genet 4:383–400, 1979.
12. Francis CC: Peripheral nervous system. In Anson BJ (ed): "Morris' Human Anatomy," 12th Ed., New York: McGraw-Hill, 1966.
13. Weigner K: Beziehungen des nervus accessorius zu den proximalen Spinalnerven. Anatomische Hefte. Arbeiten aus Anatomischen Instituten. Erste Abteilung 17:551–587, 1901.
14. Streeter GL: The development of the cranial and spinal nerves in the occipital region of the human embryo. Am J Anat 4:83–116, 1905.
15. Patten BM: "Human Embryology," 3rd Ed., New York: McGraw-Hill, 1968.
16. Congdon ED: Transformation of the aortic arch system during the development of the human embryo. Contr Embryol Carneg Instn 14:47–110, 1922.
17. Smith BS, Pettersen JC: An anatomical study of a duplication 6p based on two sibs. Am J Med Genet 20:649–663, 1985.
18. Grouchy J de, Turleau C: "Clinical Atlas of Human Chromosomes." New York: John Wiley & Sons, 1977.
19. Moen DW, Werner JK, Bersu ET: Analysis of gross anatomical variations in human triploidy. Am J Med Genet 18:345–356, 1984.
20. Tettenborn U, Gropp A: Meiotic nondisjunction in mice and mouse hybrids. Cytogenetics 9:272–283, 1970.

21. Gropp A: Morphological consequences of trisomy in mammals. In Ciba Foundation Symposium 40 (new series): "Embryogenesis in Mammals." Amsterdam: Elsevier/Excerpta Medica, 1976, pp 155–175.
22. Gropp A: Value of an animal model for trisomy. Virchows Arch 395:117–131, 1982.
23. Smith BS: Development of the embryonic trisomy 1 mouse. PhD. Thesis, University of Wisconsin, 1985.
24. Gropp A: Fetal mortality due to aneuploidy and irregular meiotic segregation in the mouse. In Boué A and Thibault C, (eds): "Les Accidents Chromosomiques de la Reproduction." Paris: INSERM, 1973, pp 255–269.
25. White, BJ, Tjio JH, Van de Water LC, Crandall C: Trisomy for the smallest autosome of the mouse and identification of the T1Wh translocation chromosome. Cytogenetics 11:363–378, 1972.
26. White BJ, Tjio JH, Van de Water LC, Crandall C: Trisomy 19 in the laboratory mouse. I. Frequency in different crosses at specific developmental stages and relationship of trisomy to cleft palate. Cytogenet Cell Genet 13:217–231, 1974.
27. White BJ, Tjio JH, Van de Water LC, Crandall C: Trisomy 19 in the laboratory mouse. II. Intrauterine growth and histological studies of trisomics and their normal littermates. Cytogenet Cell Genet 13:232–245, 1972.
28. Bersu ET: Morphologic development of the fetal trisomy 19 mouse. Teratology 29:117–129, 1984.
29. Bersu ET, Crandall C, White BJ: Growth characteristics of the murine trisomy 19 thymus. Teratology 26:85–94, 1982.
30. Cox DR, Epstein LB, Epstein CJ: Genes coding for sensitivity to interferon (IFREC) and soluble superoxide dismutase (SOD-1) are linked in mouse and man and map to chromosome 16. Proc Natl Acad Sci USA 77:2168–2172, 1980.
31. Reed W, Oster-Granite ML, Fischkoff S, Raab P, Ozand P: Beta-adrenergic markers in cultured cells of human trisomy 21 and murine trisomy 16. Pediatr Res 17:325(abs), 1983.
32. Lampson L, Fisher C: Weak HLA and beta-2M expression of neuronal cell lines can be modulated by interferon. Proc Natl Acad Sci USA 81:6476–6480, 1983.
33. Kornguth SE, Bersu ET, Auerbach R, Sobkowicz HM, Schutta HS, Scott GL: Trisomy 16 mice: Neural, morphologic and immunological studies. Proc NY Acad Sci (in Press).
34. Miyabara S, Gropp A, Winking H: Trisomy 16 in the mouse fetus associated with generalized edema and cardiovascular and urinary tract anomalies. Teratology 25:369–380, 1982.

Triploidy With an Extra Sex Chromosome (70,XXYY) and Elevated Alpha-Fetoprotein Levels

Lorraine F. Meisner, PhD, Ronald R. Louie, MD, Sunita Arya, MD, and Enid F. Gilbert, MD

Cytogenetics Section (LFM), State Laboratory of Hygiene, Departments of Pathology (RRL, SA, EFG) and Pediatrics (RRL, EFG), University of Wisconsin, Madison, Wisconsin 53706

INTRODUCTION

Human triploidy is a common but essentially nonviable condition that occurs in about 1% of human conceptuses [7]. Gestation most frequently ends in spontaneous abortion with a few surviving to premature delivery followed by early postnatal death. Triploidy is second only to autosomal trisomy in frequency of chromosome abnormality found in abortuses [2,3]. Most triploid fetuses surviving past the first trimester have a 69,XXX or 69,XXY sex chromosome constitution. 69,XYY fetuses have been described in first trimester abortions; however, the fact that they are so underrepresented even in early abortions suggests an even more decreased viability [9]. The pathologic anatomy of the fetus and placenta are fairly characteristic and well described [10,11]. However, to our knowledge there have been no reports of a triploid fetus with sex chromosome aneuploidy in addition to triploidy, probably because of the small probability of these 2 events occurring in 1 conceptus. Here we describe a 70,XXYY triploid fetus discovered as a result of elevated levels of alpha-fetoprotein (AFP) in maternal serum.

CLINICAL REPORT

A 33-year-old gravida 2, para 1 caucasian woman developed an acute gastrointestinal illness at 20 weeks' gestation, and this led her to seek medical

Birth Defects: Original Article Series, Volume 23, Number 1, pages 333–339

attention for the first time during her pregnancy. A routine serum specimen was submitted to the State Laboratory of Hygiene for AFP determination. This test, which was done by radioimmunoassay, yielded an AFP level of 242 ng/ml, which was highly elevated compared to the normal cut-off value for 20 weeks (70 ng/ml).

An amniocentesis and repeat serum AFP were performed at 21 weeks. Although the amniotic fluid AFP was somewhat elevated (13,200 ng/ml compared to 10,000 ng/ml, which was the cut-off for 21 weeks), the serum AFP was again found to be highly elevated (234 ng/ml compared to the normal cut-off value of 78 ng/ml). Ultrasonographic examination done at the time of the amniocentesis did not show any evidence of a neural tube defect, but cytogenetic analysis of the amniotic fluid cells showed triploidy with an extra sex chromosome: 70,XXYY.

The amniocentesis and ultrasonographic examination were repeated a week later with amniography, at which time there was no evidence of fetal swallowing or respiratory movements. The amniotic fluid AFP level was then 11,600 ng/ml, which was still slightly elevated for date (the normal limit at 22 weeks being below 10,000 ng/ml). After counseling, the parents decided to terminate the pregnancy.

ANATOMIC FINDINGS

Necropsy documented the anatomic findings recorded in Table I, which included the facial, limb, genital, and placental anomalies characteristically found in triploid fetuses [1,10,11]. The fetus was small for gestational age and weighed 335 gm. Cleft of lip and hard palate were present, but there was no nasal encephalocele. There was no evidence of meningomyelocele, spina bifida occulta, or spinal sinus tracts. However, upon opening the cranium, an arachnoid cyst (1.5 cm dia.) filled with clear fluid was found lying between the 2 hemispheres above the posterior fossa and cerebellum. There was no evidence of a Dandy-Walker or Arnold-Chiari malformation. The esophagus and entire gut were patent, without atresia, duplication, or malformation. There was no omphalocele. The external genitalia were female, but the internal genitalia were male, with testes, epididymis, and vasa deferentia, present in the pelvis.

Histologically, the testes mostly contained solid seminiferous tubules (Fig. 1A), although a few tubules had a small lumen. There were relatively few large round cells with clear or pale staining cytoplasm (spermatogonia) nestled against the thin basement membrane of the tubules (Fig. 1B). Most cells within these tubules were dispersed fairly evenly from one wall of the

TABLE I. Abnormalities Found in a 70,XXYY Triploid Fetus

Face
  Hypertelorism and periorbital creases
  *Congenital cataracts
  Flat nasal bridge
  *Apparently low-set ears
  *Anterior cleft lip and palate, communicating with maxillary sinus, left
  *Micrognathia
Limbs
  *Simian crease, bilateral
  *Syndactyly, 3rd and 4th digits both hands and feet
Genitalia
  *Atrial septal defect, secundum type
  *Ventricular septal defect, membranous septum
Visceral organs
  *Absent gallbladder
  Cleft spleen
  *Hypoplastic adrenal glands
Central nervous system
  *Hydrocephalus with arachnoid cyst
Placenta
  Weight 200 g.
  *Partial hydatidiform mole with cystically dilated villi

*Previously described abnormalities in triploidy [5].

tubule to the other. The developing seminiferous tubules were separated by a thin mesenchymal tissue and contained Leydig cells. The epididymis was characterized by a decreased number of ductules lined by cuboidal epithelium.

The placenta, which weighed 200 g, was partially retained at delivery and was fragmented. Although distorted, many villi were cystically dilated. Microscopically, the cystic villi showed cistern formation with scalloped outlines.

CYTOGENETIC FINDINGS

Fascial tissue taken from the fetus at necropsy demonstrated a 70,XXYY chromosome constitution (Fig. 2). Quinacrine fluorescence confirmed the presence of 2 Y chromosomes. Sex chromosome studies performed on fibroblast cultures showed only 9% of the cells to have Barr bodies, which is less than one-fourth of the expected frequency.

DISCUSSION

This case is unusual in several respects: the presence of an extra sex chromosome in a nonmosaic triploid fetus, female external genitalia despite

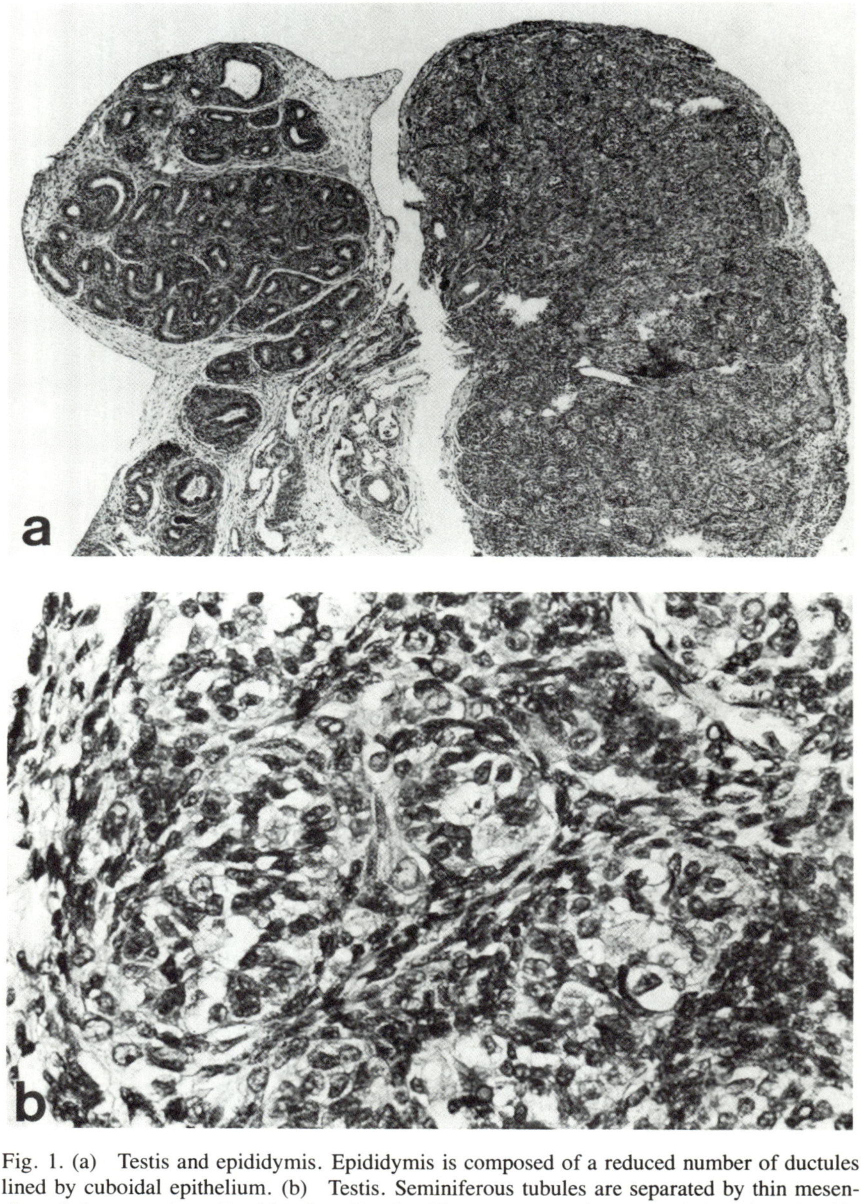

Fig. 1. (a) Testis and epididymis. Epididymis is composed of a reduced number of ductules lined by cuboidal epithelium. (b) Testis. Seminiferous tubules are separated by thin mesenchymal tissue, and are lined by Sertoli cells. The spermatogonia are nestled against the thin basement membrane.

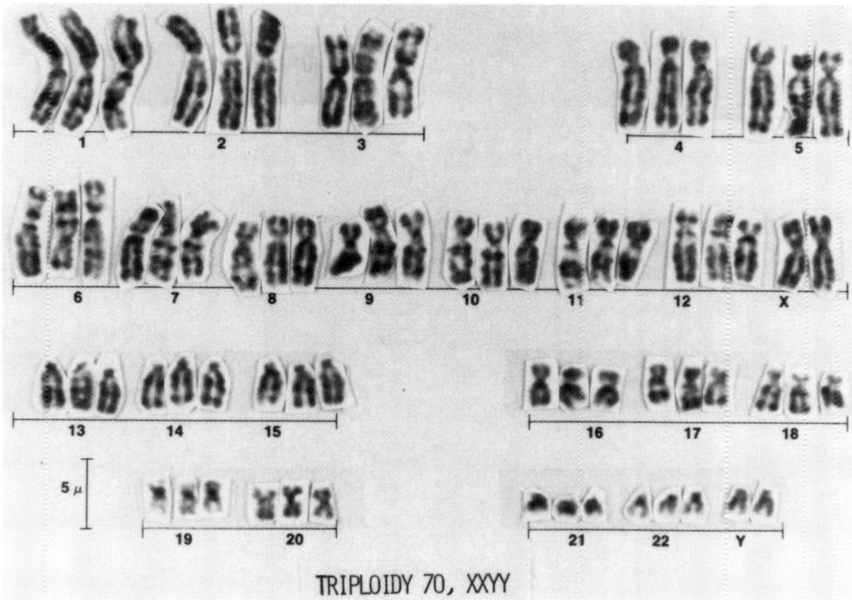

Fig. 2. GTG banded karyotype showing 70,XXYY chromosome pattern.

2 Y chromosomes, elevated AFP levels without open neural tube defect, and highly elevated maternal serum AFP despite only slight AFP elevations in amniotic fluid.

The presence of an extra sex chromosome has, to our knowledge, not been reported previously in nonmosaic triploidy. The origin of triploidy itself seems to be either (1) failure of extrusion of a maternal polar body, (2) dispermic fertilization, or (3) failure of paternal meiosis resulting in a diploid sperm. Triploidy with 70 chromosomes requires 2 abnormal events, one meiotic and the other occurring at the time of fertilization. The first involves nondisjunction during oogenesis or spermatogenesis, leading to a sperm with a 24,YY chromosome constitution or an egg with 24,XX. This would then be followed by a second accident producing triploidy. A recent study of 78 triploid conceptuses and parental chromosomes showed 73% of the cases to be of paternal origin [7]. These authors found that virtually all the triploid conceptuses of paternal origin were associated with partial molar placentae, while placentae of maternally derived triploids tended to be nonmolar. They also found that paternally derived triploids were more likely to survive to the second trimester than triploids due to a maternal accident. Although parental chromosomes were not informative in the present case, the fact that the pregnancy extended well into the second trimester, together with the finding of molar degeneration of the placenta, suggests dispermy as the most likely cause.

A study by Jacobs and Hassold [6] of 39 abortuses in which it was possible to determine the exact mechanism of origin showed that, irrespective of which chromosome was involved in a trisomy, the extra chromosome was almost always maternal in origin, and that 90% of cases were due to an error occurring in the first maternal meiotic division. These findings suggest that the sex chromosome aneuploidy in the present case was due to a maternal error, followed by an error in fertilization leading to triploidy.

Finding a low sex chromatin frequency despite the presence of 2 X chromosomes has been reported in 69,XXY triploidy by Schindler and Mikano [9]. These authors also suggested that the imbalance or deficiency in the amount of heterochromatic X material would lead to abnormal gonadal development, which is characteristic of triploids (eg, tubular hypoplasia, cryptorchidism, etc) [1]; this might also explain the fact that almost half of male triploids have ambiguous genitalia [1]. It is more difficult to explain the finding of female external genitalia in the present case; one might have expected the presence of 2 Y chromosomes to have shifted the balance in the male direction, but such nonspecific effects are not unusual in sex chromosome aneuploidy (eg, gynecomastia being more frequent in 47,XXY than in 46,XX males). Thus, the presence of an additional chromosome, even a Y, might exert nonspecific aneuploidy effects interfering with the normal masculinization of the external genitalia.

The presence of significantly elevated maternal serum AFP despite only slightly elevated amniotic fluid AFP levels may perhaps be explained by placental degeneration facilitating passage of AFP from amniotic fluid to maternal serum. It is more difficult to explain the cause of the mildly elevated amniotic fluid AFP, which might have been still higher were it not entering the maternal circulation so efficiently. An elevated AFP level in maternal serum in the presence of a triploid fetus has been reported once before [8], but the fetus from that report had a meningomyelocele. Although elevated AFP has also been reported in amniotic fluid with a closed cranial anomaly (eg, hydrocephalus), this is rare. It has been suggested that esophageal or duodenal atresia, with limitation of fetal swallowing, could raise the amniotic fluid AFP [4]. In the present case, although the gut was patent, the fetus was not observed to swallow. Since a cerebral anomaly was present, one might speculate that an aberration in the CNS control of swallowing might increase amniotic AFP in the same manner as in duodenal atresia.

In summary, despite the presence of an extra sex chromosome, this fetus shows most of the developmental characteristics of triploidy, including an enlarged placenta [1] with partial molar degeneration, eye and facial abnormalities, apparently low-set ears, and limb and gonadal genital abnormalities. The abnormal conceptus probably arose as a result of 2 unrelated phenomena—a meiotic accident in maternal meiosis, followed by fertilization of the XX egg by 2 sperm.

REFERENCES

1. Blackburn WR, Miller WP, Superneau DW, Cooley NR, Zellweger H: Complete studies of infants with mosaic and complete triploidy: An analysis of 55 cases. New York: Alan R. Liss, Inc., for the March of Dimes Birth Defects Foundation. BD:OAS 18(3B):251–274, 1982.
2. Boué J, Boué A, Lazar D: Retrospective and prospective epidemiological studies of 1500 karyotyped spontaneous human abortions. Teratology 12:11–26, 1975.
3. Carr DH, Gideon M: Population genetics of human abortuses. In Hook EG, Porter IH (eds): "Population Genetics." New York: Academic Press, 1977, pp 1–9.
4. Cruikshank DP: Fetal antigens and prenatal diagnosis. Semin Perinatol 1:135–147, 1977.
5. Gilbert EF, Opitz JM: Developmental and other pathological changes in syndromes caused by chromosomal defect. In Rosenberg HS, Bernstein J (eds): "Perspectives in Pediatric Pathology." New York: Masson Publ USA 7:1–63, 1982.
6. Jacobs PA, Hassold TJ: The origin of chromosome abnormalities in spontaneous abortion. In Porter IH, Hook EB (eds): "Human Embryonic and Fetal Death." New York: Academic Press, 1980, pp 289–298.
7. Jacobs PA, Szulman AE, Funkhauser J, Matsuura JS, Wilson CC: Human triploidy: Relationship between parental origin of the additional haploid complement and development of partial hydatidiform mole. Ann Hum Genet 46:223–231, 1982.
8. Porreco RP, Matson MR, Young PE, Bradshaw C, Leopold G, Jones OW: Diagnosis of a triploid fetus at genetic amniocentesis. Obstet Gynecol 56:115–118, 1980.
9. Schindler A, Mikamo K: Triploidy in man: Report of a case and a discussion on etiology. Cytogenetics 9:116–130, 1970.
10. Szulman AE, Phillippe E, Boué JG, Boué A: Human triploidy: Association with partial hydatidiform moles and nonmolar conceptuses. Hum Pathol 12:1016–1021, 1981.
11. Wertelecki W, Graham JM, Sergovich FR: The clinical syndrome of triploidy. Obstet Gynecol 47:69–75, 1976.

Neural Development of Trisomy 16 Fetal Mice

Steven Kornguth

Departments of Neurology and Physiological Chemistry, University of Wisconsin, Madison, Wisconsin 53706

INTRODUCTION

The presence of additional chromosomes in cells is frequently accompanied by organ dysgenesis and biochemical dysfunction. Down syndrome (DS), trisomy of chromosome 21, is the trisomy condition of most frequent occurrence in the human postnatal population and accounts for 1 in 700 live births. Individuals born with trisomy for autosome 21 have neural dysgenesis, mental retardation, and multiple congenital anomalies [1,2]. Mouse trisomy 16 is considered to be the trisomy most comparable to human DS because mouse chromosome 16 codes for several genes that are also coded by human 21; the gene products include superoxide dismutase, α- and β-interferon receptors, and proteins involved in the response of cells to β-adrenergic agonists [3–7].

The brains of the mouse trisomy 16 fetuses and control littermates were examined to determine the consequences of an additional chromosome 16 on neural development. Earlier studies [5,8,9] documented changes in the ontogeny of the nervous system in the mTs 16. The fetuses were studied because the mTs 16 conceptuses obtained to date do not survive till birth [10,11]. The mTs 16 were bred using sires that were doubly metacentric [Rb(16.17)8Lub/Rb(11.16)2H], and BALB/c dams. We examined the hypothesis that the structures of neural tissues of the mTs 16 conceptuses differed from that of control littermates, and that the differences may be related to the expression of the major histocompatibility complex H-2 Kk and H-2 d on the surfaces of the neural cells. The observation that interferon modulates the expression

Birth Defects: Original Article Series, Volume 23, Number 1, pages 341–350

of histocompatibility antigens on neurons [12] increased our interest in this area of investigation.

RESULTS

Measurements of Nissl stained serial sections of the brains from Ts 16 fetuses and control littermates showed that trisomy 16 tissues were reduced in size in several particular areas. The cerebellum, colliculi, and region of the brain between the parietal cortex (coronal sections containing the developing fornix, anterior commissure) and the occipital cortex (coronal sections containing the developing anterior colliculus and hippocampus) were particularly reduced in size in the trisomic mice at day 18 of gestation. Other regions of the brain appeared similar in the trisomy mice and their control sibs. The brains of over 25 Ts 16 and control fetuses were examined.

Coronal sections of the cerebella of 3 trisomy 16 conceptuses at 18 days of gestation and of 3 of their control sibs were examined in detail (Fig. 1). Sagittal sections of fetuses at the same age of development were also examined. The cerebellum was readily identified in the 15-day trisomy and control fetuses; by day 18 of gestation the dimensions of the cerebella in the trisomic animals were smaller than those of control animals. At day 18, the longest dimension of the cerebellum (one lateral edge to the other) in the normal control fetuses ranged between 2.9 and 3.2 mm while in the trisomy mouse the range was 2.7 to 2.8 mm. The midline dimensions of the cerebella from control and trisomy animals were similar; for one pair the ventral-dorsal thickness was 0.4 mm. In a second pair the midline ventral-dorsal thickness was 0.6 mm in control littermate and 0.5 mm in the trisomic fetus. Other pairs exhibited a similar dimension. In the lateral-most portion, the presumptive flocculus, the dimensions in the coronal plane of the trisomic and of the control cerebella were similar and ranged from 0.8 to 1.0 mm. Sagittal sections of the cerebella documented a larger major dimension of the control cerebella (1.0 mm) than of the trisomic tissue (0.7 mm) at the midline. The minor dimension of the control and trisomic animals was similar (0.5 mm). Because the major axis of the cerebellum is inclined caudally when the base of the brain is used as a reference, the minor axis in the sagittal plane is most similar in orientation to the thickness of the cerebellum in the coronal plane.

Nissl stained coronal sections (Fig.1) show similarities in cellular organization between the control and trisomic cerebella. However, the control littermates have a more distinct molecular layer at the lateral portion of the cerebellum, and the presumptive Purkinje cell layer is more compact than that in the trisomic tissue (Fig.1).

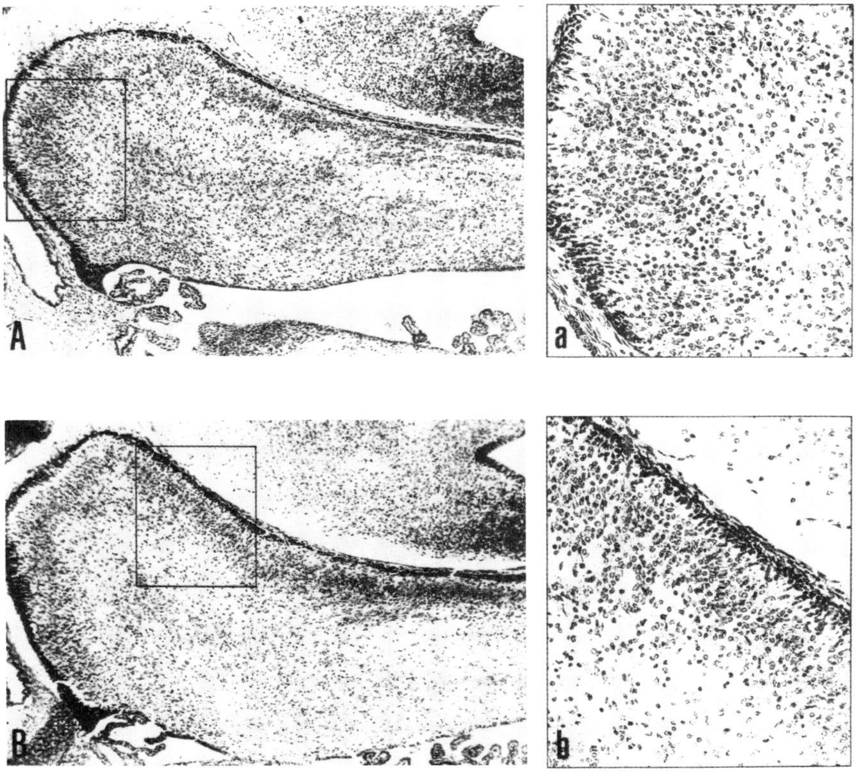

Fig. 1. Light microscopic photographs of Nissl stained coronal sections of cerebella from 18-day-old mouse fetuses. A. Section of cerebellum from a trisomy 16 conceptus. The area enclosed by the rectangle is shown to the right ×100. a. Enlargement of A ×460. B. Section of cerebellum from a control littermate of the trisomic animal ×100. b. Enlargement of B ×460. The presumptive Purkinje cell layer is more discrete and compact in the control conceptus compared with the trisomic animal.

The trisomic brains also had a reduced dimension between the anterior colliculus (Fig. 2A,B) and the fornix/parietal cortex region (Fig. 2C,D) when compared with control sibs at day 18 of gestation. In the coronal sections of the control sibs, the distance separating these sections was in the range of 1150–1200 μ, whereas in the trisomic animals the distance was 900–1000 μ. On sagittal sections of 18-day-old fetuses, the distances in the control brain tissue were 1200 μ and in the trisomic were 900–1000 μ as measured directly on the serial sections. The other brain regions, with the exception of

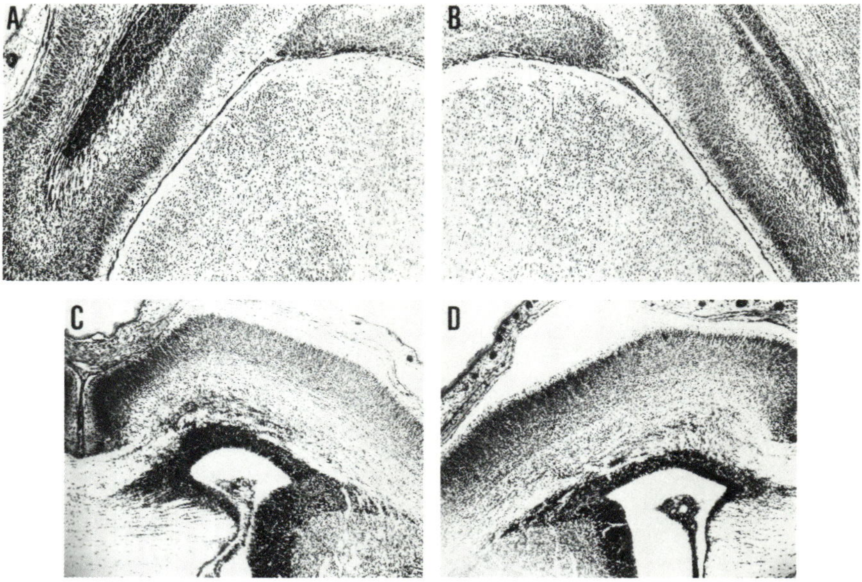

Fig. 2. Light microscopic photographs of Nissl stained coronal sections of colliculi (A,B) and the parietal cortex/fornix region (C,D) from 18-day-old mouse fetuses. A,C—Sections from a trisomy 16 fetus. B,D—Sections from control littermates taken at the same plane as that from the trisomy animal. The distance between the collicular plane (A,B) and the fornix plane (C,D) is smaller in the trisomic animals (900–1000 μ) than in the control (1200 μ). × 100.

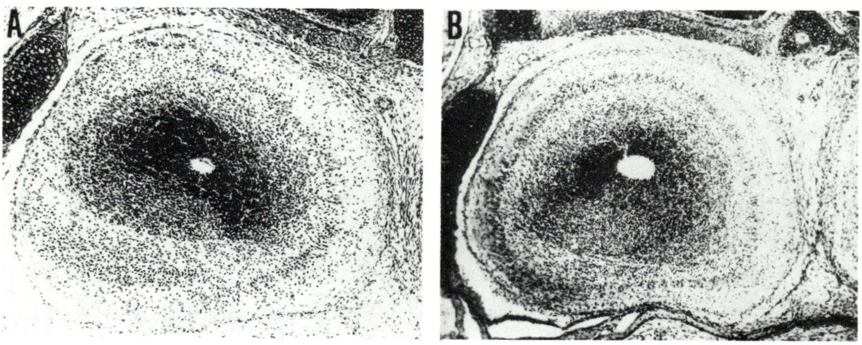

Fig. 3. Light microscopic photographs of Nissl stained sections of olfactory bulb from a trisomy 16 mouse fetus and control littermate (18-day-old conceptus). ×100

the colliculi, were similar in dimension in the trisomy and control brain samples (eg, the olfactory bulb, Fig. 3).

ULTRASTRUCTURE OF THE TRISOMIC AND CONTROL CEREBELLA

From the light microscopic studies we observed that the cerebella of the trisomic animals were smaller than those of control littermates and that the presumptive Purkinje cell layer was less compact in the trisomy than in the control sibs. The developing Purkinje cells were examined in thin sections of 18-day fetal cerebella and the number of synaptic contacts between individual Purkinje cells and other neurons was measured by counting identifiable synaptic contacts per unit area. The Purkinje cells in the control and in the trisomic cerebella appeared similar (Fig. 4) in the electron micrographs. To determine the number of synaptic contacts per unit area, montages were prepared of electron micrographs taken in the developing Purkinje cell layer. Each montage was of an area 1400 square microns. Three trisomic fetuses and two control littermates from two different litters were examined. Synaptic contacts were identified by the presence of vesicles, and pre- and post-synaptic thickenings on appropriate structures. Control cerebella had an average of 18–25 synaptic contacts per 1400 square microns, while trisomic cerebella had an average of 6–8 such contacts. A total area of at least 4200 square microns was examined in the cerebellar sections from each animal.

MAJOR HISTOCOMPATIBILITY COMPLEX ANTIGENS ON NEURAL CELLS IN CONTROL AND TRISOMIC BRAIN SECTIONS

Previous studies done in cooperation with Dr. Chella David, Mayo Clinic, Minnesota, and with Dr. Robert Auerbach, University of Wisconsin-Madison, demonstrated that the double metacentric sires were reactive with immunoglobulins against the murine H-2 Kk marker and were unreactive with immunoglobulins against other H-2 markers. It has been shown in other laboratories that the BALB/c dams are H-2 reactive. The reactivity of ethanol fixed frozen sections (8 μ thick) of brain from 18-day-old trisomy 16 and control littermates with fluorescein-labeled immunoglobulins was examined. Antiallotypic immunoglobulins, reactive with the H-2 Kk, H-2 d, H-2 b, and H-2 q were incubated with the frozen sections. The sections were washed and then incubated with fluorescein-labeled anti-mouse immunoglobulin (B-D). The sections were washed, covered with phosphate-buffered glycerol and then examined in the microscope. The trisomic sections of cerebellum and colliculus bound the anti-H-2 Kk and H-2 d immunoglobulins to a greater

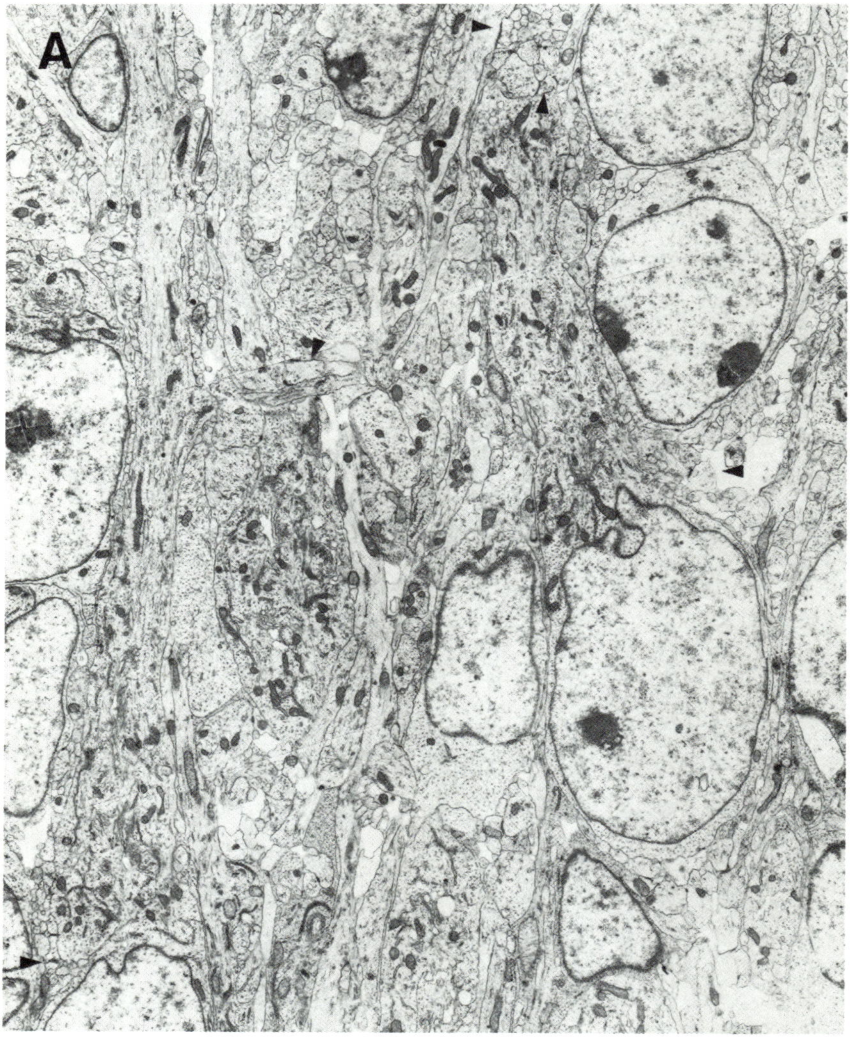

Fig. 4. Electron micrograph of the Purkinje cell layer of cerebellum from 18-day conceptuses. A is from the cerebellum of a trisomy 16 mouse and B is from control littermate. The number of synaptic contacts (ie, postsynaptic thickening and presynaptic vesicles) in the control tissue was greater than that in the trisomic tissues. Arrow head indicates synaptic contacts. ×14,100

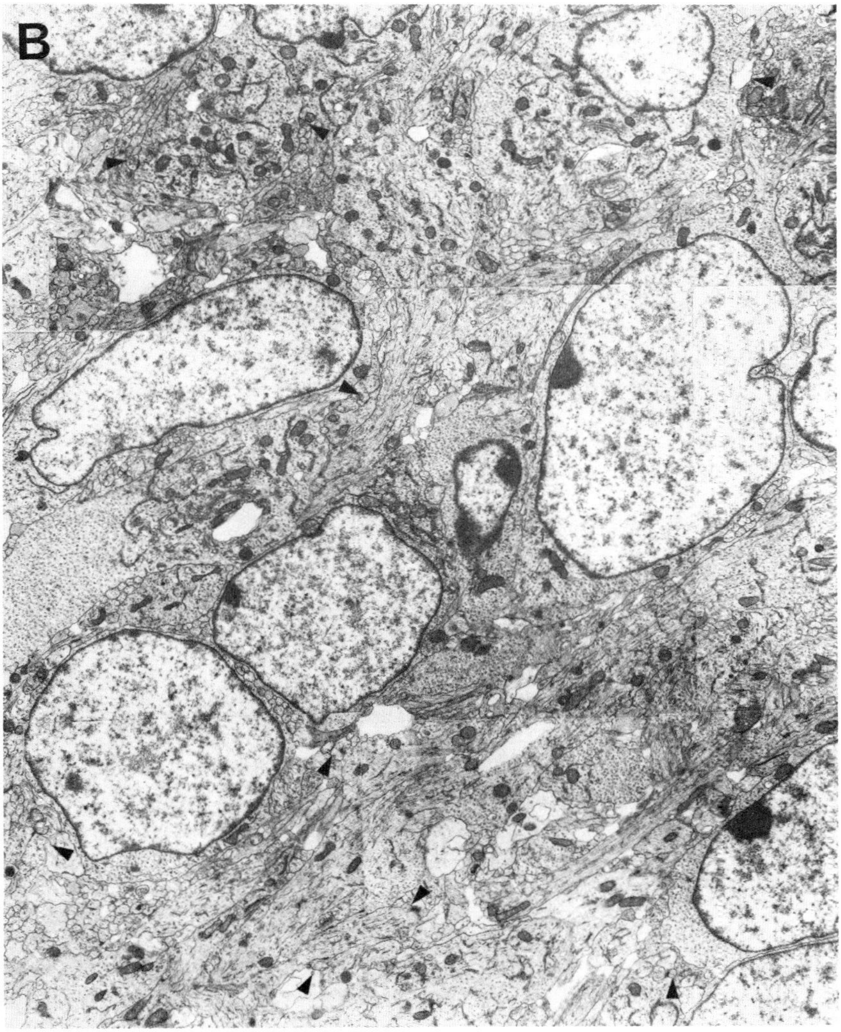
B

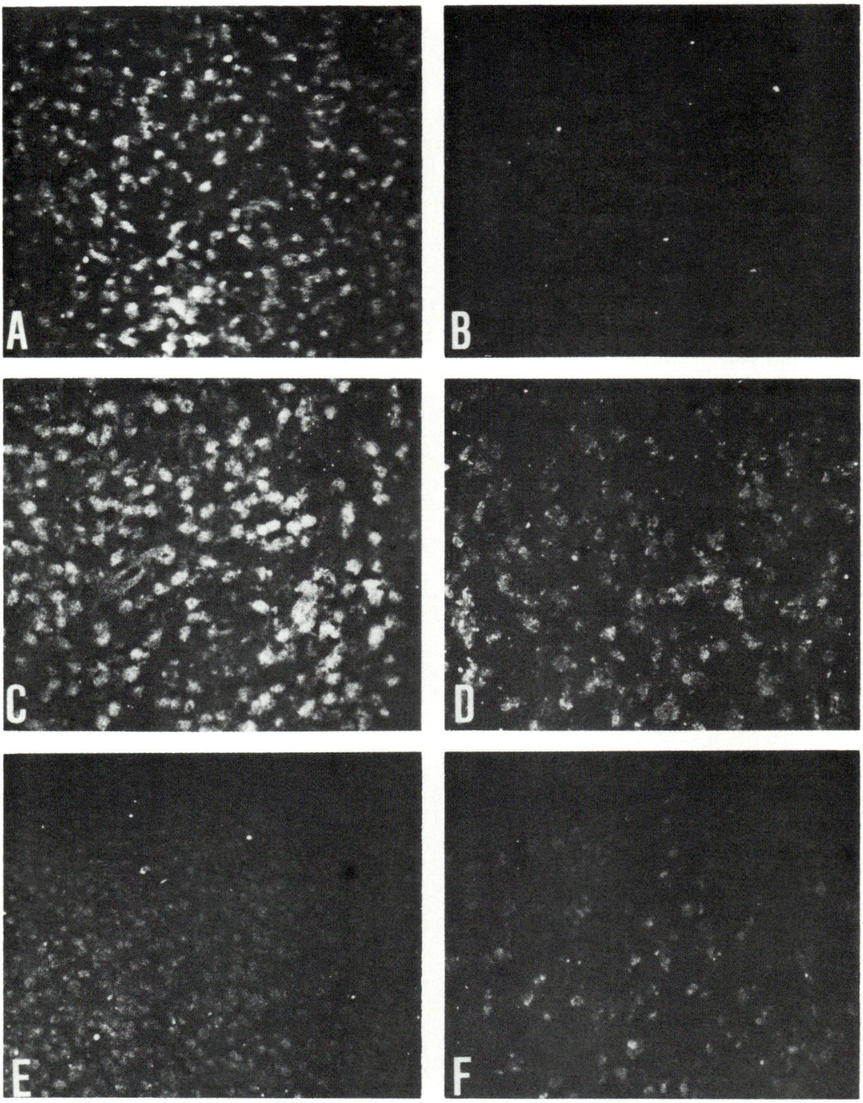

Fig. 5. Fluorescent microscopic photographs of neural tissue from 18-day-old trisomy 16 and control littermates. The colliculi of a trisomy 16 conceptus (A,C,E) and of control (B,D,F) were reacted with fluorescein-labeled immunoglobulins to reveal the distribution of major histocompatibility complex antigens on the neural cells. A,B were treated with antiallotypic H-2 Kk. C,D were treated with anti-H-2 d, while E,F were treated with anti-H-2 q. The H-2 Kk and H-2 d expression of the neural cells was elevated in the trisomy 16 animals.

degree (more fluorescence per cell) than the control cells (Fig. 5). Both the trisomy and control bound the anti-H-2 b and anti-H-2 q to a similar degree.

CONCLUSIONS

1. Mouse trisomy 16 fetuses, at day 18 of gestation, have altered brain growth compared with control sibs.

2. The most severely affected regions include the cerebellum, colliculi, and region between the anterior colliculus and fornix/parietal cortex.

3. Although the ultrastructure of the cerebellar Purkinje cells in the trisomic animals and control sibs appears similar, the number of synaptic contacts per unit area, involving developing Purkinje cells, is reduced in the trisomic animal compared with the control sibs.

4. The colliculi and cerebella of trisomy 16 fetuses, at 18-day gestational age, have a higher level of H-2 Kk and H-2 d antigens on their surface than do control sibs. The increased level of the H-2 markers is consistent with the hypothesis that an imbalance in the level of these markers on neuronal cell surfaces affects the ability of the neurons to form synaptic connections.

REFERENCES

1. Petit TL, LeBoutillier JC, Alfano DP, Becker LE: Synaptic development in the human fetus - a morphometric analysis of normal and Down's syndrome neocortex. Exp Neurol 83:13–23, 1984.
2. Burgio G, Ugazio A, Nespoli L, Maccario R: Down syndrome: A model of immunodeficiency. In "Primary Immunodeficiency Diseases." March of Dimes Birth Defects Foundation BD:OAS 19(3):325–328, 1983.
3. Cox C, Smith S, Epstein L, Epstein C: Mouse trisomy 16 as an animal model of human trisomy 21 (Down's syndrome): Production of viable trisomy 16 diploid mouse chimeras. Dev Biol 101:416–424, 1984.
4. Cox DR, Epstein LB, Epstein CJ: Genes coding for sensitivity to interferon (IFREC) and soluble superoxide dismutase (SOD-1) are linked in mouse and man and map to mouse chromosome 16. Proc Natl Acad Sci USA 77:2168–2172, 1980.
5. Ozand P, Hawkins R, Collins R, Reed W, Raab P, Oster-Granite M: Neurochemical changes in murine trisomy 16: Delay in cholinergic and catecholaminergic systems. J Neurochem 43:401–408, 1984.
6. Reed W, Oster-Granite M, Fischkoff S, Raab P, Ozand P: Beta adrenergic markers in cultured cells of human trisomy 21 and murine trisomy 16. Pediatr Res 17:325 (Abstract), 1983.
7. McSwigan JD, Hanson DR, Lubiniecki A, Heston LL, Sheppard JR: Down syndrome fibroblasts are hyperresponsive to beta adrenergic stimulation. Proc Natl Acad Sci USA 78:7670–7673, 1981.
8. Oster-Granite ML, Hatzidimitriou G: Development of the hippocampal formation in trisomy 16 mice. Pediatr Res 19:328 (Abstract), 1985.

9. Singer H, Tiemeyer JC, Hedreen JC, Gearhart J, Coyle JT: Morphologic and neurochemical studies of embryonic brain development in murine trisomy 16. Dev Brain Res 15:155–166, 1984.
10. Miyabara S, Gropp A, Winking H: Trisomy 16 in the mouse fetus associated with generalized edema and cardiovascular and urinary tract anomalies. Teratology 25:369–380, 1982.
11. Gropp A, Winking H: Robertsonian translocations: Cytology, meiosis, segregation patterns and biological consequences of heterozygosity. Symp Zool Soc Lond 47:141–181, 1981.
12. Lampson L, Fisher C: Weak HLA and beta-2M expression of neuronal cell lines can be modulated by interferon. Proc Natl Acad Sci 81:6476–6480, 1983.

A Multidisciplinary Committee Approach to Prenatal Diagnosis and Management of Fetuses With Congenital Anomalies

G.A. Machin, MD, S.F. Nicholson, MD, and C.A. Nimrod, MD

Departments of Pathology (GAM), Radiology (SFN), and Obstetrics and Gynecology (CAN), Foothills Hospital, Calgary, Alberta, Canada T2N 2T9

INTRODUCTION

The ability to study fetal anatomical details *in utero* by ultrasound has opened up a new era in the management of pregnancies in which the fetuses have congenital anomalies [1]. The benefits of early (sometimes intrauterine) treatment of disorders such as urinary tract obstruction and certain types of hydrocephalus seem obvious, but a note of conservatism is now replacing earlier enthusiasm [2,3]. Furthermore, there are many fetuses in which specific diagnoses cannot be reached by ultrasonography alone, and ancillary techniques are required [4,5]. In other cases, the natural history of the anomaly has never been followed from an early gestational age, and optimal management is not known [6]. In another group, intrauterine findings clearly indicate lethal anomalies. These pregnancies pose particular management problems, and require careful explanations to the parents. In all of these considerations, the current pregnancies must be regarded as increments in knowledge about the early appearances of fetal anomalies, and also as indicators of reproductive potential for the parents concerned.

Because of the gravity of these decisions, a multidisciplinary committee has evolved to meet on an *ad hoc* basis to consider and give advice on the diagnosis and management of pregnancies in which the fetuses have congenital anomalies. The main functions of the committee are (1) to coordinate

Birth Defects: Original Article Series, Volume 23, Number 1, pages 351–366

pre- and postnatal investigations of fetuses to confirm diagnoses and give appropriate genetic counseling regarding future pregnancies; (2) to coordinate pre- and postnatal treatment where appropriate; (3) to advise and support the referring physicians, especially where diagnoses are in doubt or anomalies are considered lethal; (4) to accumulate shared experience in this new field, and to educate residents and the wider community.

MATERIALS AND METHODS

The *ad hoc* committee consists of a core group of ultrasonographers, perinatologists, neonatologists, clinical geneticists, and a pediatric pathologist. According to need, organ system specialists, (eg, cardiologist, neurosurgeon, pediatric surgeon) may also be invited to participate. The group does not have any official status as a hospital committee, and it does not include ethical, theological, or legal experts. It meets at short notice, often within 3 or 4 hours of the detection of a fetal anomaly. It reviews the clinical history, and the ultrasound findings are then demonstrated on video tape by the ultrasonographers. The group discusses the diagnosis, confirmatory diagnostic steps, probable diagnostic outcome, and possibility and timing of pre- or postnatal treatment. Opinions may not be unanimous, and the group has no executive power in the management of the pregnancy. The referring physician makes a brief summary of the committee's discussion, and this is included in the patient's chart. He or she then proceeds to manage the pregnancy in the light of his/her own experience, the views of the committee, and the wishes of the parents. To date, autopsies have been carried out on all lethally affected fetuses, and genetic counseling is offered in all cases.

These functions of the committee are illustrated through 12 consecutive cases reviewed in the last 18 months (Table I). Cases 4, 7 and 8 are reported in detail because they involved particularly difficult problems of diagnosis and management.

CLINICAL HISTORIES

Case 4

A 33-year-old gravida 4, para 2 woman was seen at 16 weeks' gestation for confirmation of dates. A previous ultrasound scan at 10 weeks' gestation was reported as normal. The ultrasound findings at 16 weeks included severe oligohydramnios, a cystic abdominal mass arising out of the pelvis, and an apparently small chest (Fig. 1). The kidneys had an echogenic appearance not indicative of hydronephrosis (Fig. 2). As a result of the discussions of the *ad hoc* committee, the fetus was subjected to 2 urinary bladder decompression procedures utilizing a vesico-amniotic shunt. Success was achieved on both occasions for a period of less than a week. Direct aspiration of the fetal bladder was accomplished on a third occasion.

The fetus continued to grow but the chest size was disproportionately small. Spontaneous rupture of the membranes occurred at 27 weeks' gestation and the patient was delivered by cesarean section at 33 weeks after steroid therapy. The male fetus weighed 1500 g and died at age 3 hours.

Autopsy indicated a male fetus with pulmonary hypoplasia, right pneumothorax, and a distended bladder (Fig. 3); urethral stenosis and multicystic kidneys (Potter type IV) secondary to urinary tract obstruction (Fig. 4) were demonstrated. The fetus was noted to have postural deformities, and amnion nodosum was present. Chromosome evaluation indicated a *de novo* apparently balanced reciprocal translocation, 46,XY,t(3;17)(p14;p11).

Case 7

A 32-year-old primigravid woman was first seen at 14 weeks' gestation with antepartum hemorrhage. Ultrasonography showed a normal fetus with a slight elevation of the amniotic membranes and a blood clot over the internal os. This patient was seen again at 32 weeks and a diagnosis of thoracogastroschisis with ectopia cordis was made (Fig. 5). There was dorsiflexion of the spine in conjunction with a flattened fetal head and ventricular dilation.

At the *ad hoc* group meeting, a provisional diagnosis of amniotic band syndrome was made. A decision to obtain amniotic fluid for chromosomes was taken and amniography was performed (Fig. 6) to outline the amniotic sac and to clarify fetal position and condition. Also, further detailed evaluation of the fetal heart was done. It was seen that the fetal head was in the left upper quadrant and the thoracogastroschisis was the presenting part. This abnormal presentation necessitated a cesarean section for delivery. The head was trapped in the left horn of a bicornuate uterus, and this gave rise to the flattened appearance. The ultrasound findings were confirmed (Fig. 7) and an amniotic band was attached to the right foot (Fig. 8). Chromosomes were apparently normal (46,XY). The infant died at 2 hours.

Case 8

A 27-year-old gravida 3, para 2 woman with a history of a previous cesarean section, was referred with an ultrasound diagnosis of omphalocele. Reevaluation was done ultrasonically at 35 weeks of gestation and this confirmed the omphalocele, but a cardiac abnormality was also noted.

TABLE I. Clinical Summary of the 12 Cases

Case No.	Reason for initial scan	Ultrasound findings	Age at diagnosis (weeks)	Committee recommendations	Age at delivery (weeks)	Mode of delivery	Outcome	Final outcome	Reproductive prognosis
1	Vaginal bleeding	Hydrocephalus, fetal ascites, cystic kidneys, oligohydramnios, intrauterine growth failure	30	Fetal abdominal paracentesis, biochemical studies, lethal malformations, suggest induction of labor	31	Induced vaginal	1,290 g male, Apgar scores 3 & 4. Died age 2 hrs.	Potter type IV cystic kidneys, pulmonary hypoplasia, hydrocephaly, 47,XYY.	Candidate for amniocentesis for chromosomes in subsequent pregnancy
2	Large for dates	Fetal ascites, large placenta	17	Fetal abdominal paracentesis, shunting procedure done. Macrophages demonstrated lethal storage disorder — suggest induction	27	Induced vaginal	1,880 g female, Apgar scores 1 & 1. Died at 1 hr	Lysosomal storage disorder confirmed	Presumed autosomal recessive. Ultrasound and amniocentesis in subsequent pregnancy

3	Vaginal bleeding	Fetal ascites, polyhydramnios	34	Steroid administration and delivery	34	Induced vaginal	2,780 g male, Apgar scores 3 & 10. Survived	Meconium stained ascites, secondary to multiple intestinal atresias requiring multiple gut resections, ventricular septal defect	Rule out cystic fibrosis (subsequently done)
4	Confirmation of dates	Bladder outlet obstruction, pulmonary hypoplasia	16	Chest size evaluation, vesicoamniotic shunt	33	Cesarean section	1,560 g male, Apgar scores 2 & 3. Died at 3 hrs	Urethral stenosis, distended bladder, Potter type IV cystic kidneys, pulmonary hypoplasia, balanced translocation	Low recurrence risk
5	Confirmation of dates	Hydrops fetalis, cystic hygroma	19	Amniocentesis, hemoglobin electrophoresis. Induction	20	Induced vaginal	630 g female, stillbirth	Cystic hygroma, hydrops, 45,X	Candidate for amniocentesis for chromosomes
6	Large for dates	Hydrops	22	Biochemical evaluation. Induction	22	Induced vaginal	940 g female, stillbirth	Idiopathic hydrops	May be familial. Ultrasound in subsequent pregnancy

(continued)

TABLE I. Clinical Summary of the 12 Cases (Continued)

Case No.	Reason for initial scan	Ultrasound findings	Age at diagnosis (weeks)	Committee recommendations	Age at delivery (weeks)	Mode of delivery	Outcome	Final outcome	Reproductive prognosis
7	Polyhydramnios	Thoracogastroschisis with ectopia cordis, amniotic band syndrome	32	Amniocentesis, amniography. No active intervention	32	Cesarean section to facilitate delivery and diagnosis	1,850 g male, Apgar scores 2 & 1. Died at 2 hrs	Amniotic band syndrome, with multiple severe disruptions as per ultrasound	Extremely low risk of recurrence
8	Patient reassurance	Omphalocele, hypoplastic left heart	35	Detailed cardiac evaluation, amniocentesis. No active fetal intervention	39	Repeat cesarean section	2,300 g male, Apgar scores 2 & 6. Died at 3 days	Omphalocele, hypoplastic left heart, hydronephrosis	2–4% recurrence risk for congenital heart disease
9	Vaginal bleeding	Omphalocele	32	Amniocentesis for pulmonary maturity, repeat ultrasound. Planned cesarean section with repair of defect	38	Elective cesarean section and immediate repair	2,830 g male, Apgar scores 5 & 9. Survived.	Omphalocele repaired, ventricular septal defect, required no correction. Alive and well	2–4% for congenital heart defect and omphalocele

10	Confirmation of dates	Omphalocele	26	Repeat ultrasound for bowel evaluation, planned elective cesarean section with repair	35	Elective cesarean section	2,200 g female, Apgar scores 1 & 8. Survived	Omphalocele repaired. Alive and well	2–4% for omphalocele
11	Confirmation of dates	Occipital encephalocele	28	Amniocentesis for chromosomes and α-fetoprotein. Induction	34	Repeat cesarean section for failed induction	2,100 g male, Apgar scores 2 & 1. Died at 4 hrs	Occipital encephalocele, not suitable for repair	As for neural tube defect
12	Small for gestational age	Ventricular dilation, occipital encephalocele, gastroschisis, scoliosis, amniotic band syndrome	23	Amniocentesis for α-feto-protein and chromosomes, lethal anomalies. Induction	26	Induced vaginal	880 g male, stillbirth	Amniotic band syndrome with severe disruptions as per ultrasound	Extremely low risk of recurrence

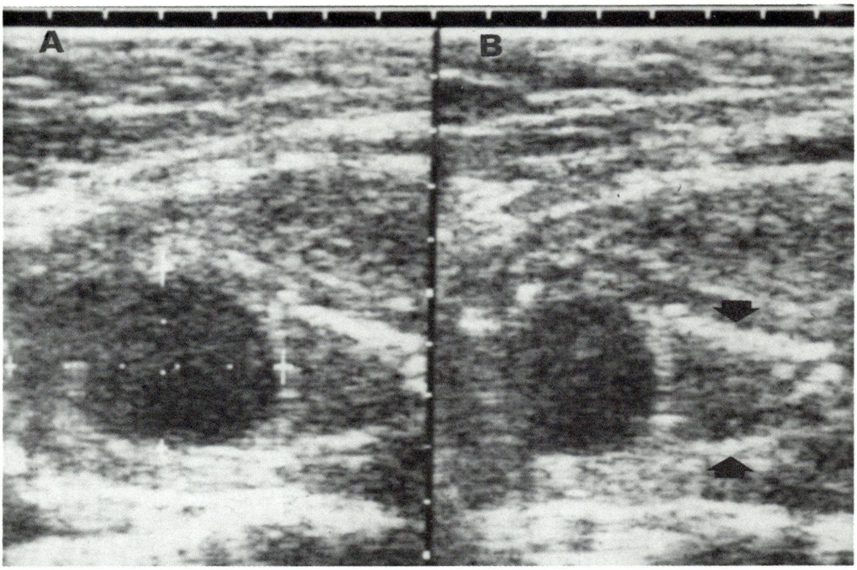

Fig. 1. Case 4. Longitudinal scans (A and B) at 16 weeks show large bladder (+) filling almost entire fetal abdomen. Fetal chest (arrows) is small and there is oligohydramnios.

The left ventricle was hypoplastic with a small ascending aorta and abnormally bright echoes of the interventricular septum (Fig. 9). As a result of the group meeting, it was concluded that the priority of delivery would be to reconfirm the cardiac observations and postpone any decisions on reparative surgery until the full nature of the cardiac lesion was ascertained.

The patient was delivered by a repeat cesarean section at 29 weeks' gestation. The omphalocele was confirmed and a 2-D echocardiogram also confirmed the presence of a hypoplastic left heart syndrome. No active measures were taken and the infant died on day 3. Left heart hypoplasia was confirmed at autopsy (Fig. 10).

DISCUSSION

Prenatal diagnosis by various methods has greatly increased the range of possibilities for managing fetuses with congenital anomalies. Ultrasonic detection of anatomic anomalies offers advantages in the planned delivery of infants known to have apparently simple and correctable malformations such as diaphragmatic hernia and omphalocele [7,8]. There has also been initial

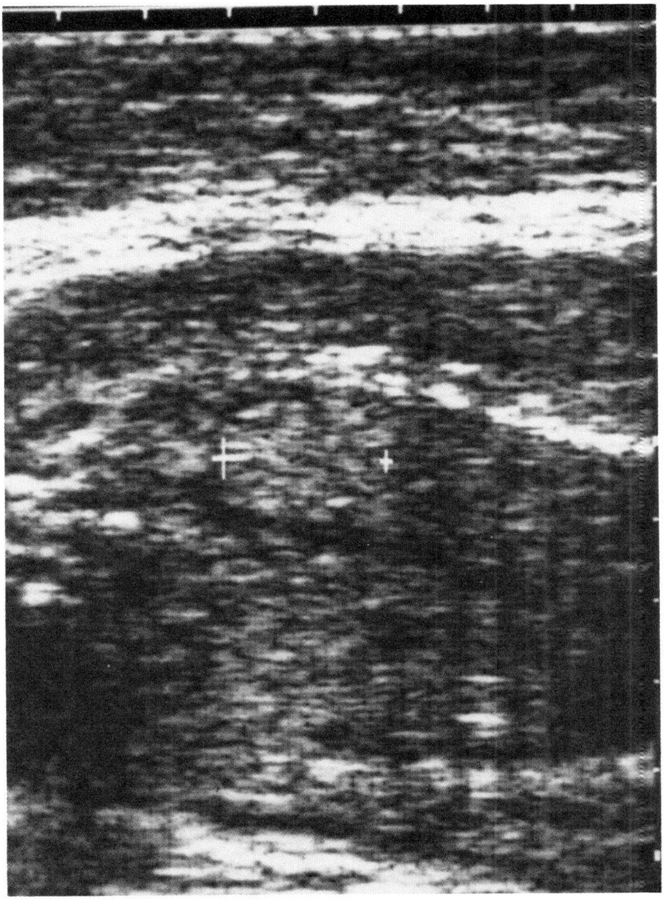

Fig. 2. Case 4. Coronal scan of fetal abdomen at 22 weeks shows an echogenic kidney (+) with no dilatation of the renal pelvis.

enthusiasm for fetal surgery in cases with mechanical/obstructive lesions such as hydrocephalus and obstructive uropathy. This has now been tempered by the realization that the natural history of these diseases is often not known, and that severe parenchymal organ damage may already have occurred before the earliest possible time to diagnosis by ultrasound [6]. However, in addition, ultrasonography can detect fetal anatomic defects that are not easily correctable on simple mechanical principles. Some of these defects are multiple (as in amniotic band syndrome [9]); other fetal disorders are due to

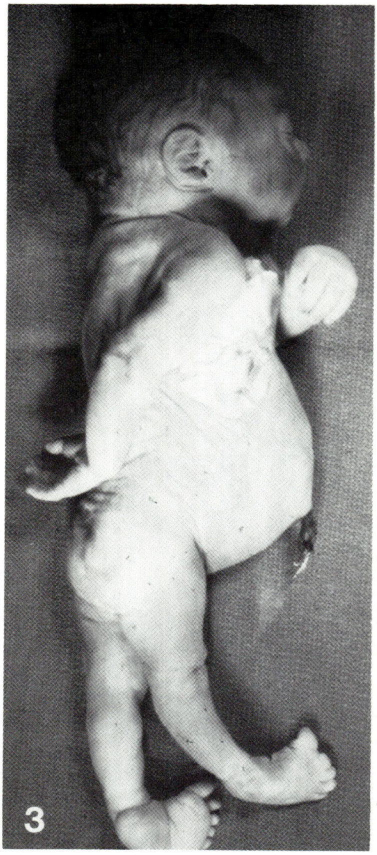

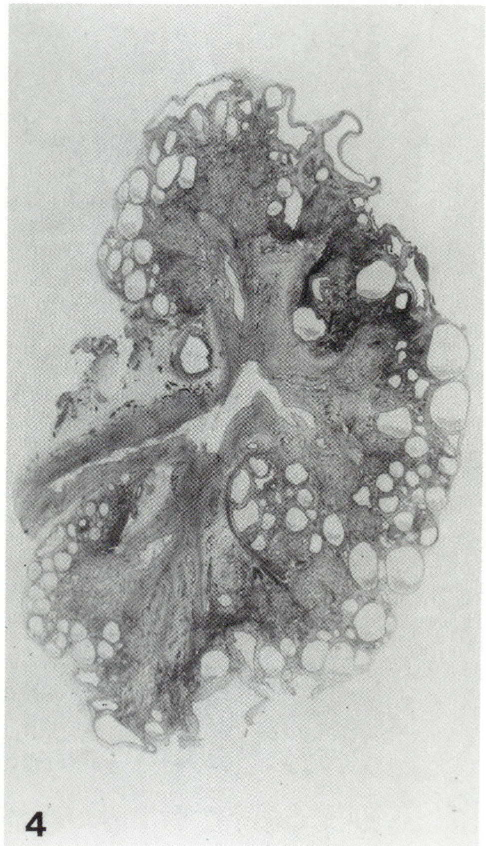

Fig. 3. Case 4. Lateral view shows intercostal tube draining right pneumothorax secondary to pulmonary hypoplasia; there is abdominal distension by megacystis; positional foot deformities are secondary to oligohydramnios.

Fig. 4. Case 4. Coronal section of multicystic left kidney shows dilated ureter, with multiple subcortical cysts secondary to urinary tract obstruction. (H&E, 4× life size.)

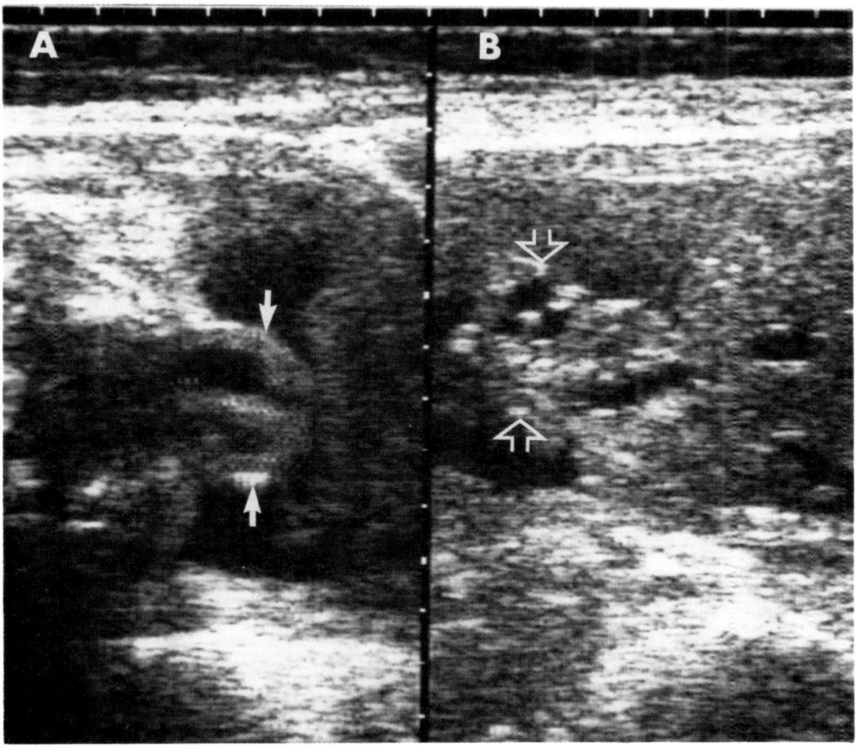

Fig. 5. Case 7. Transverse scan of fetal chest (A) shows the heart (arrows) outside the thorax, surrounded by amniotic fluid. The two ventricles are clearly seen. Transverse scan of fetal abdomen (B) shows bowel (open arrows) free in amniotic cavity. No surrounding membrane could be seen. There was oligohydramnios.

multiple causes (eg, hydramnios, hydrops, ascites [10,11]). The detection of lethal anomalies offers particularly difficult choices in the management of the pregnancy.

It is also clear that some apparently simple anomalies are actually components of syndromes that are associated with considerable morbidity and mortality. For instance, omphalocele frequently is a component of trisomy syndromes [12–14], and amniocentesis for chromosome analysis is indicated, even late in the pregnancy, in order to allow for this consideration in postnatal management. This is illustrated in a series of prenatal diagnoses from Oxford [15] in which a good prognosis was predicted for fetal omphalocele, followed by an elective cesarean delivery of an 18-trisomy fetus (case 5). Full prenatal

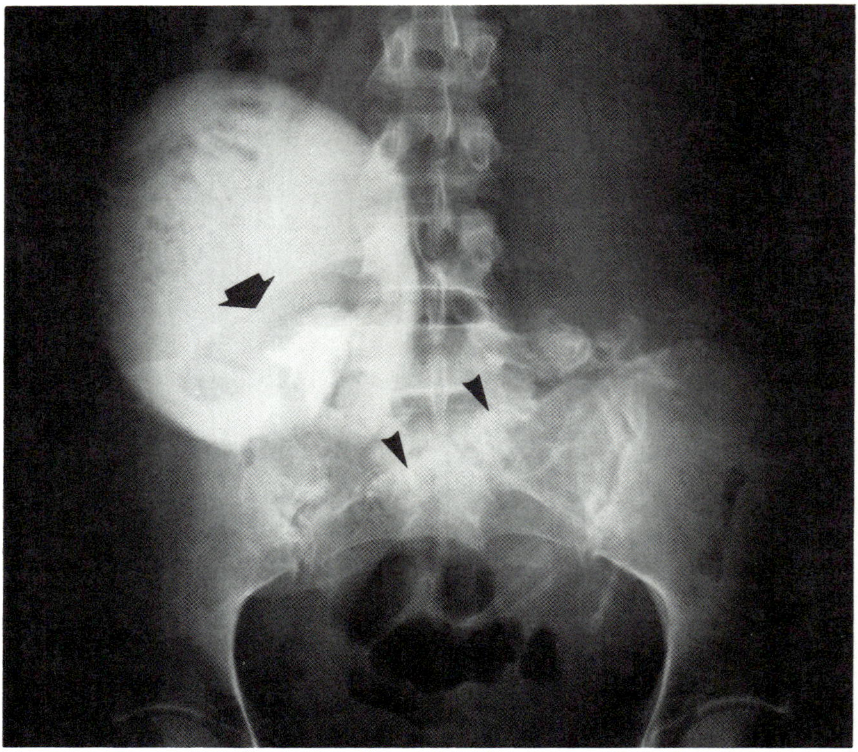

Fig. 6. Case 7. Contrast injection shows only fetal leg (large arrow) in amniotic cavity. Remainder of the fetus is extraamniotic. Fetal spine (arrow heads) is abnormally curved, and the fetal abdomen is the presenting part. Base of fetal skull is seen above left maternal sacroiliac joint.

diagnosis by a multidisciplinary committee could have obviated cesarean delivery in this case, an event which has been documented in the past [16,17].

It is because of the rapid development in the complexity of decisions to be taken in these pregnancies that the *ad hoc* committee evolved. Some diagnoses in this series were relatively straightforward (cases 4,9–11), and the best management of the pregnancy was easily decided on the basis of the available fetal assessment at the time. But our experience also included a high proportion of cases where the diagnosis was not clear (cases 3,7,12), where there were multiple disorders that could cause the observed defects (cases 1,2,5,6), or where treatable and nontreatable defects were both present

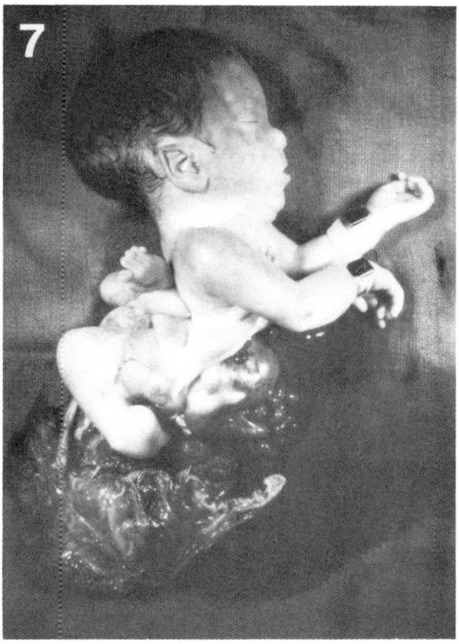

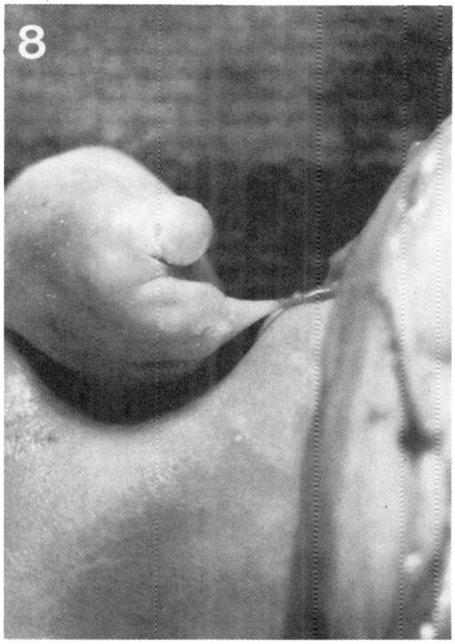

Fig. 7. Case 7. Lateral view corresponding with Fig. 6. There is cephalic deformity secondary to trapping in the left uterine horn. Anterior thoracoabdominal wall shows extensive disruption with dorsal displacement of the legs.

Fig. 8. Case 7. Right foot, showing syndactyly and amputation of toes. Amniotic band joins fused toes to edge of body wall defect.

in the same fetus (case 8). In these situations, a broad spectrum of knowledge and expertise is needed in order to arrive at a consensus for management.

Therefore the *ad hoc* committee has placed priority on accurate diagnosis, and recommends further investigation beyond ultrasonography where indicated. The objective of accurate diagnosis is met for two reasons: so that the natural history and/or effects of intervention may be documented and added to the accumulating body of knowledge on fetal anomalies; in addition, the committee was concerned that intrauterine death of the fetus before full diagnosis of the nature of the disorder greatly lessens the chance of reaching an accurate diagnosis of any genetic disease underlying only partially elucidated anatomic defects. Although it may already be clear that the current pregnancy will result in the birth of a fetus with lethal defects, information must be obtained from the fetus which is sufficient to form the basis of accurate counseling for future pregnancies. This principle underlies the aggressive prenatal diagnosis documented in cases 1,2,4–7, and also the

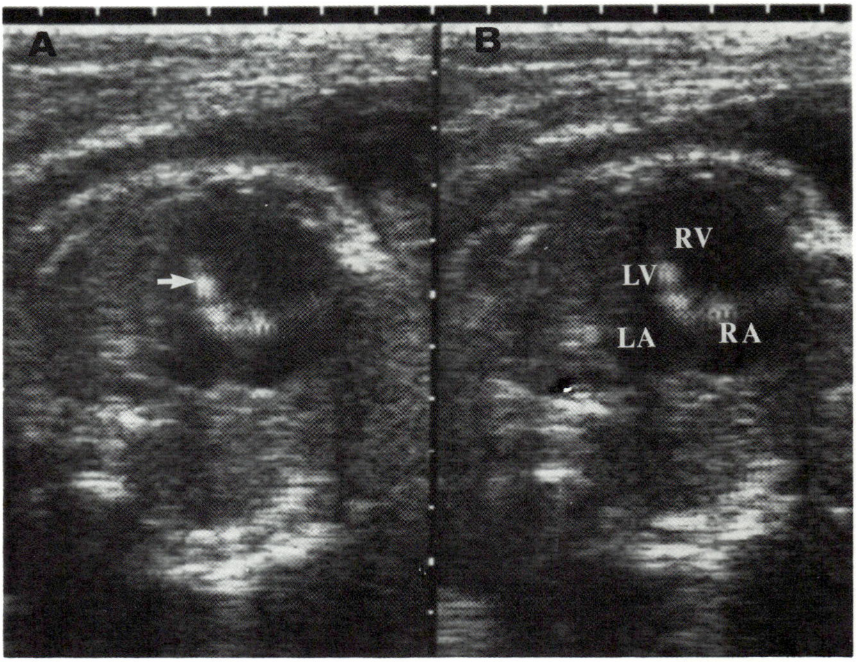

Fig. 9. Case 8. Four-chamber views of the heart (A & B) show small left ventricle. There was no mitral or aortic valve motion. The still frames do not show the absent left ventricle cavity apparent during real time examination. Note bright echoes of left ventricular side of interventricular septum (arrow) shown at autopsy to be areas of obliterating fibrosis.

delivery by cesarean section of fetuses rightly presumed to have lethal anomalies (cases 4,7).

The *ad hoc* committee also acts as support for the referring physician, who is often faced with difficult choices in communicating with parents and managing the malformed fetus. The expertise available from an informed group helps to set priorities for the optimal outcome of the pregnancy, including the prognosis for future pregnancies. In this way, a viable nucleus of physicians from different disciplines is able to add their expertise in this field, and educate residents and support staff. The advantages in terms of litigation are obvious. The committee as a whole is venturing into difficult areas, which may well lay it open to ill-judged litigation; but the primary care physicians can feel secure in having tapped the best available source of information and clinical judgment.

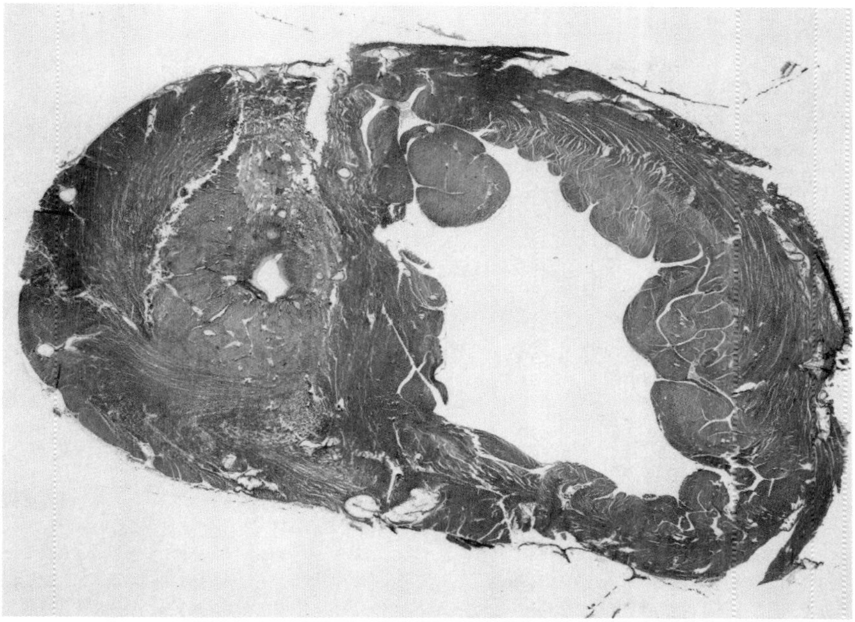

Fig. 10. Case 8. Transverse histologic section of heart, showing a minute left ventricular cavity surrounded by dense fibrovascular tissue. Right ventricular cavity is normal size. (H&E, 4× life size).

This series of fetal anomalies is representative of our continuing experience in this hospital. It includes only a small proportion of cases that are readily correctable by prenatal manipulation to relieve obstruction, or by planned postnatal surgical correction. Only 3 of the 12 fetuses survived, and only 2 (the omphalocele cases) are well. The dismal outcome is due to the severity of the anomalies, which are of diverse cause and pathogenesis. However, the diagnosis was clear in all cases, and accurate information is therefore available for reproductive prognosis. While progress is being made in the treatment of malformed fetuses, we have experienced a high proportion in which treatment is not readily available. In some cases, eg, amniotic band syndrome, the severity and multiplicity of the defects make the likelihood of corrective treatment remote. While the relative lack of successful outcome in this series is a depressing fact, we wish to emphasize the importance of aggressive diagnosis in the management and counseling for future pregnancies. Also required is a follow-up program to assess the ability of parents to respond to perinatal grief under these new circumstances of interventive obstetric management of seriously malformed fetuses [18].

REFERENCES

1. Harrison MR, Golbus MS, Filley RA: Management of the fetus with a correctable congenital defect. JAMA 246:774, 1981.
2. Harrison MR, Golbus MS, Filley RA: Management of the fetus with congenital hydronephrosis. J. Pediatr Surg 17:728, 1982.
3. Clewell WH, Johnson ML, Meier PR, et al: A surgical approach to the treatment of fetal hydrocephalus. N Engl J Med 306:1320, 1982.
4. Kleinman CS, Donnerstein RL, De Vore CTR, et al: Fetal echocardiography for evaluation of in utero congestive cardiac failure. N Engl J Med 306:568, 1982.
5. Schneider AS, Menutti MT, Zackai EH: High cesarian section rate in trisomy 18 births: A potential indication for late prenatal diagnosis. Am J Obstet Gynecol 140:367, 1981.
6. Harrison MR, Filley RA, Golbus MS, et al: Fetal treatment 1982. N Engl J Med 307:1651, 1982.
7. Marwood RP, Davison OW: Antenatal diagnosis of diaphragmatic hernia. Case Report. Br J Obstet Gynecol 88:71, 1981.
8. Didolkar SM, Hall J, Phelan J, et al: The prenatal diagnosis and management of a hepatoomphalocele. Am J Obstet Gynecol 141:221, 1981.
9. Northern NJ, Lawrence D, Bustillo M: Amniotic band syndrome: Antepartum ultrasound diagnosis of discordant anencephaly. JCU 8:453, 1980.
10. Hansmann M, Redel DA: Prenatal symptoms and clinical management of heart disease. In Proceedings, Ier Symposium International d'Echocardiologie Fetal, Strasbourg, 1982, p 137.
11. Quinlan RW, Cruz AC, Martin M: Hydramnios: Ultrasound diagnosis and its impact on perinatal management and pregnancy outcome. Am J Obstet Gynecol 145:306, 1983.
12. Hauge M, Bugge M, Nielson J: Early prenatal diagnosis of omphalocele constitutes indication for amniocentesis. Lancet 2:507, 1983.
13. Clementi M, Ten R, Turolla L: Further investigations when abdominal wall defects are diagnosed in utero. Lancet 2:1083, 1983.
14. Rodeck CH: Fetal therapy. In Rodeck CH, Nicolaides KH (eds.): Proceedings of the Eleventh Study Group of the Royal College of Obstetricians and Gynaecologists. Chichester: John Wiley and Sons, 1984, pp 331–341.
15. Griffiths DM, Gough MH: Dilemmas after ultrasonic diagnosis of fetal abnormality. Lancet 1:623, 1985.
16. Schneider AS, Zackai EH, Menutti MT: High caesarian section rate in trisomy 18 births: An indication for late prenatal diagnosis. Am J Hum Genet 31:109A, 1979.
17. David TJ, Glew S: Morbidity of trisomy 18 includes delivery by caesarian section. Lancet 2:1295, 1980.
18. Machin GA, Popkin JS, Styles S: Termination of pregnancy during the third trimester (letter). N Engl J Med 311:264, 1984.

Antenatal Diagnosis of Skeletal Dysplasia Using Ultrasound

J. McGuire, MB, BS, F. Manning, MD, FRCS(C), I. Lange, MD, FRCS(C), E. Lyons, MD, FRCP(C), and D.J. deSa, MB, DPHiL, FRC PaTH

Departments of Obstetrics and Gynecology (JM, FM, IL), Ultrasound (EL), and Pathology (DJdS), University of Manitoba, Winnipeg, Canada

INTRODUCTION

Ultrasound plays an increasingly important role in the antenatal assessment of the developing fetus. Congenital anomalies can be diagnosed with a high degree of accuracy by real-time and static ultrasonography. We present 8 previously unreported cases of major skeletal dysplasias diagnosed antenatally, together with the salient ultrasonic findings of 7 of these.

The fetuses had thanatophoric dwarfism with cloverleaf skull, osteogenesis imperfecta, hypophosphatasia (n=2), twins with achondrogenesis type II, and a pair of sibs with an unclassified chondrodysplasia. These cases were detected by the obvious abnormalities in the skeletal measurements and the discrepancy between the head and abdominal circumferences. Several of the fetuses were associated with polyhydramnios.

CLINICAL REPORTS

The femoral lengths (Fig. 1), head and abdominal circumferences (Figs. 2 and 3), and head/abdominal circumference ratio are shown for those fetuses where they were calculated or measured. In some fetuses (eg, patients 1 and 4) more than 1 measurement was made, either on repeated visits (patient 1) or at the same visit.

Birth Defects: Original Article Series, Volume 23, Number 1, pages 367–384

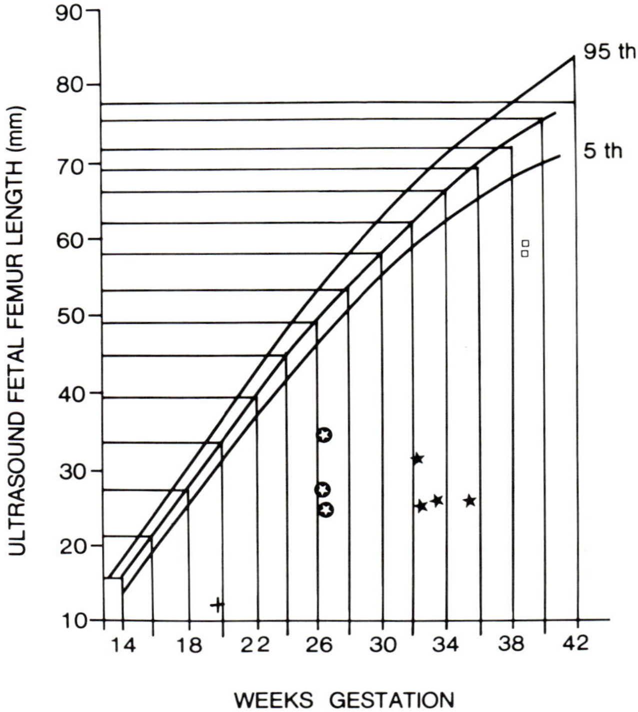

Fig. 1. Ultrasound assessment of fetal femur length and gestational age in 6 infants with skeletal dysplasia. The mean, 5th, and 95th centiles are shown. In this Figure and in Figures 2 and 3: + = unclassified chondrodysplasia (patient 6); ✪ = twins with achondrogenesis II (patients 5, 6), 1 twin having had 2 measurements; ★ = thanatophoric dwarfism (patient 1), multiple measurements at different visits; □ = hypophosphatasia (patients 3, 4).

Patient 1: Thanatophoric Dysplasia I With Cloverleaf Skull Deformity

This infant was born to a 27-year-old, gravida V, para IV mother. She was noted to be "large for dates" at 32 weeks gestation and was referred to the Fetal Assessment Unit at the Health Sciences Centre in Winnipeg. Real-time ultrasonic assessment confirmed marked polyhydramnios and showed a single fetus with short, thick limbs. The skull was noted to be cloverleaf in shape with significant ventricular dilation (Fig. 4a,b). Facial structures were well visualized showing hypertelorism, a saddle nose with anteverted nares, and triangular shape of mouth with an unusually mobile tongue. The neck was short and the chest appeared relatively small with shallow breathing movements. The abdomen appeared protuberant but no abnormality of the

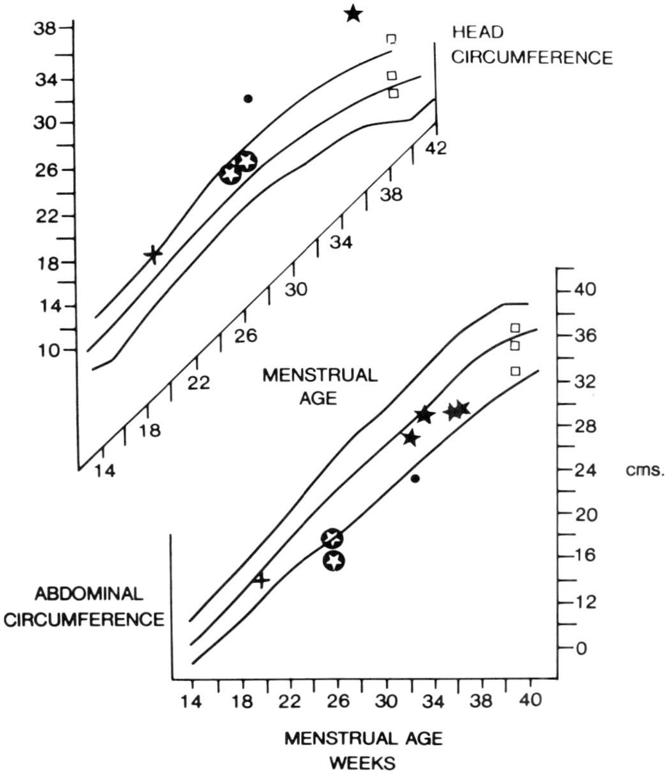

Fig. 2. Head and abdominal circumferences, as assessed by ultrasound, compared with menstrual age. The mean, 5th, and 95th centiles are shown. Legend for measurements as in Figure 1, with the addition of ● = osteogenesis imperfecta (patient 2).

intraabdominal organs was identified. The patient was followed with ultrasound on subsequent visits until she developed spontaneous rupture of membranes at 37 weeks; shortly thereafter she delivered a stillborn male infant with cloverleaf skull deformity (Fig. 4c) and the typical radiologic skeletal changes of thanatophoric dysplasia (Fig. 5a,b).

Patient 2: Osteogenesis Imperfecta

This child was born to a 33-year-old, gravida IV, para III mother, who 3 years previously had delivered a "hydrocephalic" male infant who had died neonatally. At approximately 30 weeks during the present pregnancy she developed a sudden increase in abdominal girth; there had been minor

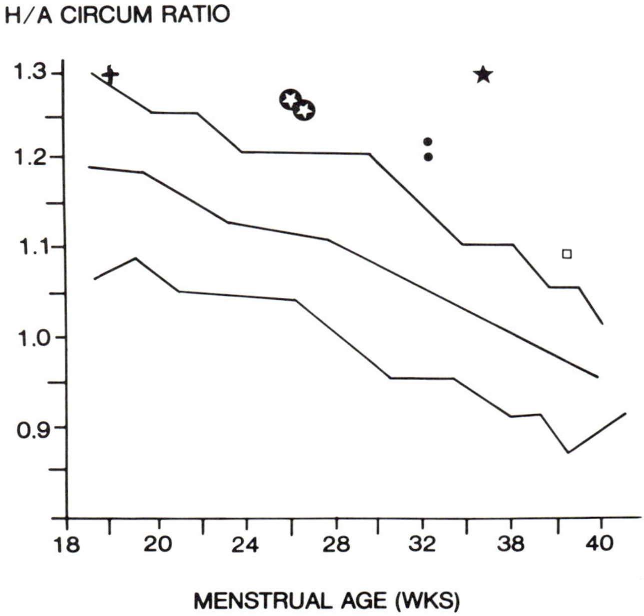

Fig. 3. Head/abdominal circumference ratio as assessed by ultrasound measurement. Legends as in Figures 1 and 2.

episodes of vaginal bleeding at about 12 weeks of gestation. At ultrasonic assessment the skull was identified but was seen to be easily deformed with decreased echogenicity (Fig. 6a). The orbits were unusually clearly visualized and the thorax appeared narrow with multiple irregular echoes from the ribs, suggesting healing fractures (Fig. 6b). No abnormality of the abdomen was identified but the limbs appeared short and irregular. Radiologically there was evidence of decreased mineralization with multiple fractured ribs and the findings were interpreted as strongly suggestive of osteogenesis imperfecta, but the possibility of hypophosphatasia was also considered in the differential diagnosis. Spontaneous rupture of membranes occurred at 31 weeks gestation; induction of labor was required at 33 weeks. The infant, who weighed 960 gm, died neonatally. The postmortem radiologic findings were consistent with osteogenesis imperfecta showing multiple rib fractures, numerous wormian bones in the skull, and several fractures of the extremities in various stages of healing. Histologically the presence of poorly formed bony trabeculae, predominantly of woven bone, with abundant callus forma-

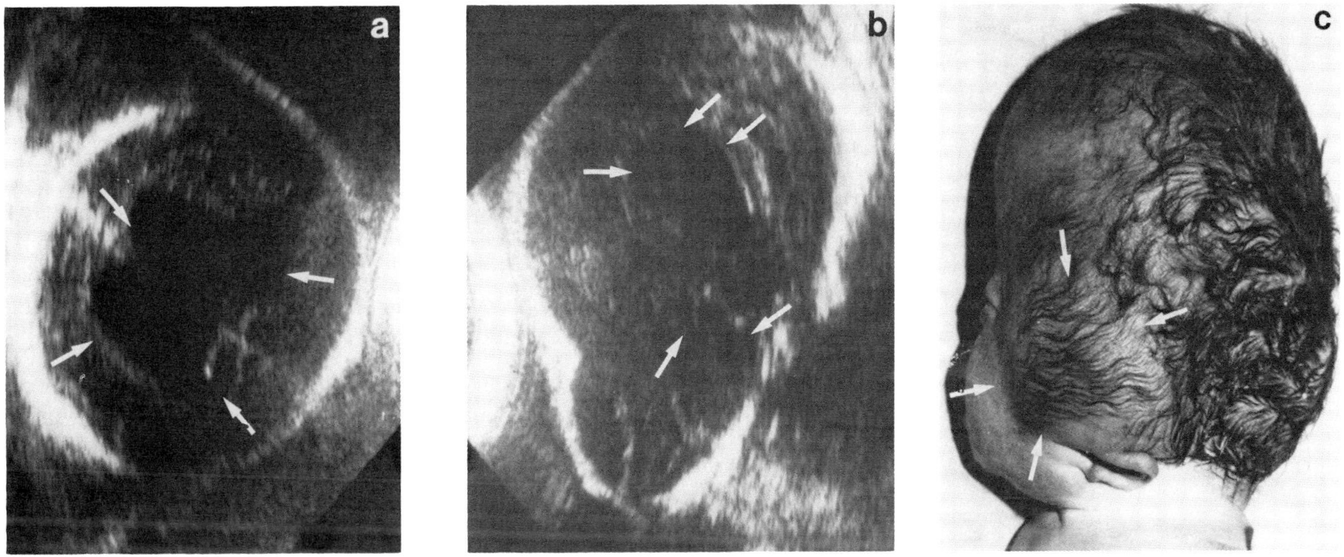

Fig. 4. Ultrasound demonstration of ventricular dilatation (arrow) in patient 1, (a) coronal plane view, (b) parasagittal view, (c) comparable view to (b) of infant's skull showing distortion of pinna due to left lateral projection of dilated ventricle.

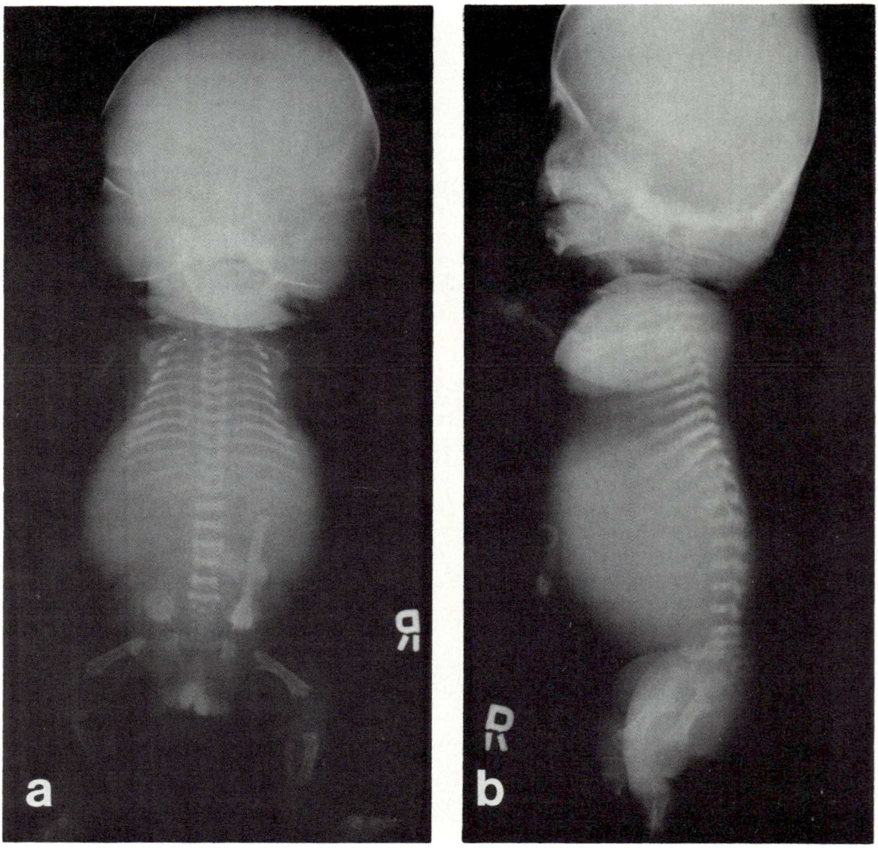

Fig. 5. Anterio-posterior (a) and lateral (b) views at autopsy of patient 1 showing cloverleaf-skull deformity and classic radiologic indications of thanatophoric dysplasia.

tion at the site of the fractures confirmed the diagnosis of osteogenesis imperfecta.

Patient 3: Hypophosphatasia

This child was born to a 16-year-old primigravida who had an uncomplicated pregnancy until she went into spontaneous labor at 39 weeks. Since the presentation was uncertain, antepartum x-ray examination was carried out and showed a footling breech presentation with severe skeletal hypomineralization (Fig. 7). A diagnosis of hypophosphatasia was suggested. Shortly afterward, she delivered a male from a footling breech position with Apgar

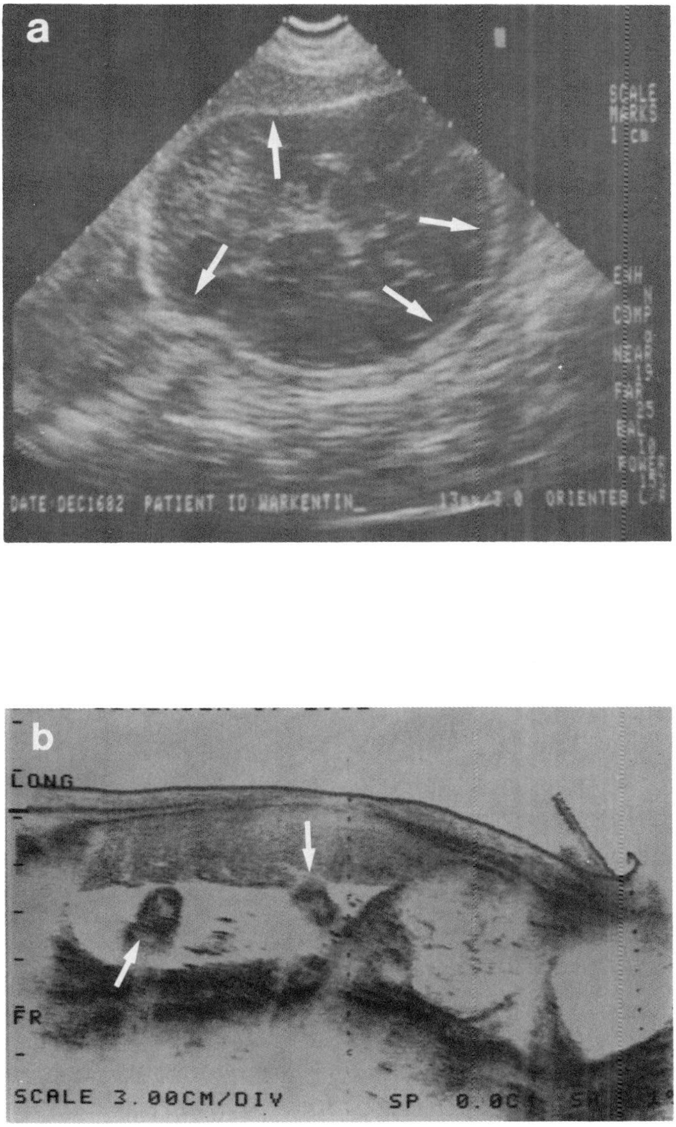

Fig. 6. Patient 2 (osteogenesis imperfecta) showing (a) the easily deformed cranial vault (arrows); (b) longitudinal view showing short deformed limbs (arrows), and reduced skeletal mineralization.

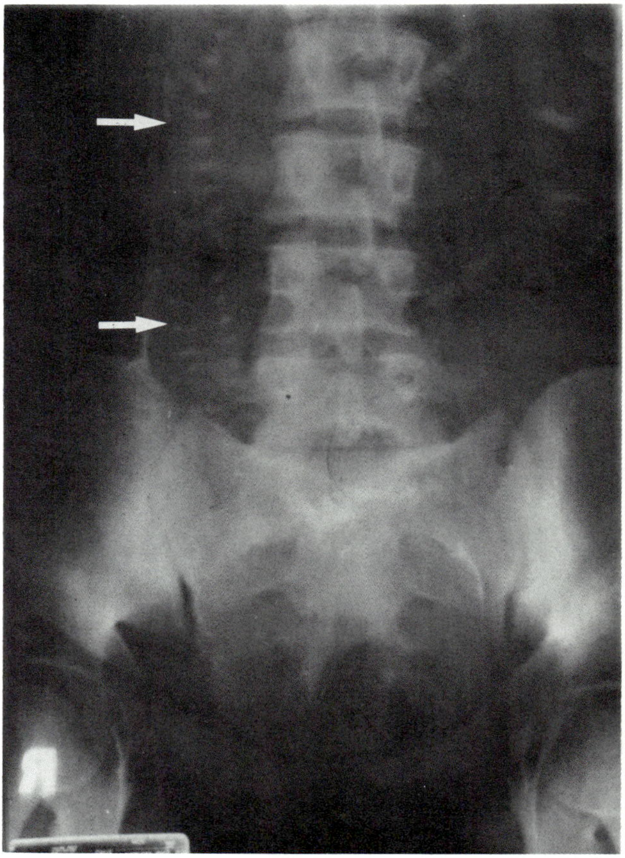

Fig. 7. Antenatal x-ray of mother of patient 3 (hypophosphatasia) showing extreme undermineralization of the infant's skeleton. The vertebrae and ribs are visible (arrows), and the head fills the pelvis. (Courtesy of Dr. R. Lloyd, Bethel Hospital, Winkler, Manitoba.)

scores of 4 at 1 and 5 minutes. The infant had sustained bradycardia (a fetal heart rate of less than 60) and died shortly after delivery. At autopsy the skull was extremely underossified and globular in shape. The chest was flat, the lungs were small, and the skeleton was extremely hypominerlized with flared long bone metaphyses. The ribs showed multiple irregularities, suggesting organized fractures with callus. Microscopic examination showed the presence of abundant osteoid in the medullary regions of the long bones with hypertrophied chondroid columns at the lines of ossification. No alkaline phosphatase could be identified in histochemical studies of the kidney and liver and no alkaline phosphatase could be identified in the baby's serum. Insufficient amounts of urine were available for analysis. The diagnosis of hypophosphatasia was confirmed.

Patient 4: Hypophosphatasia

This infant was born to a 25-year-old, gravida II, para I mother, who had an uncomplicated pregnancy until the 30th week, when she developed a sudden increase in abdominal girth. Ultrasound examination confirmed the presence of marked polyhydramnios, with a single fetus with marked skeletal abnormalities characterized by hypomineralization. The long bones had a dumb-bell shaped appearance with marked flare of the metaphyses (Fig. 8). Hypophosphatasia was suspected but osteogenesis imperfecta was considered in the differential diagnosis.

Labor was induced at 39 weeks and she delivered a male child weighing 3.6 kg; the infant died within 24 hours. A postmortem radiograph showed flat undermineralized vertebrae, flared long bone metaphyses (Fig. 9a) and a hypomineralized calvaria (9c). The ribs had multiple nodular densities (Fig. 9b). Autopsy examination confirmed the presence of multiple irregularities of the ribs with excess callus formation, abundant osteoid, and moderate

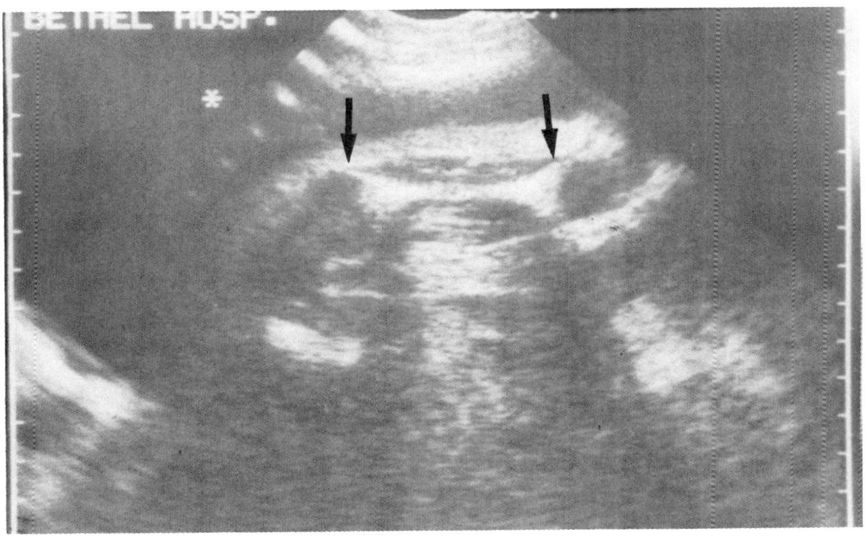

Fig. 8. Patient 4 (hypophosphatasia) showing an irregularly flared femoral metaphysis (arrows). (Courtesy of Dr. R. Lloyd, Bethel Hospital, Winkler, Manitoba.)

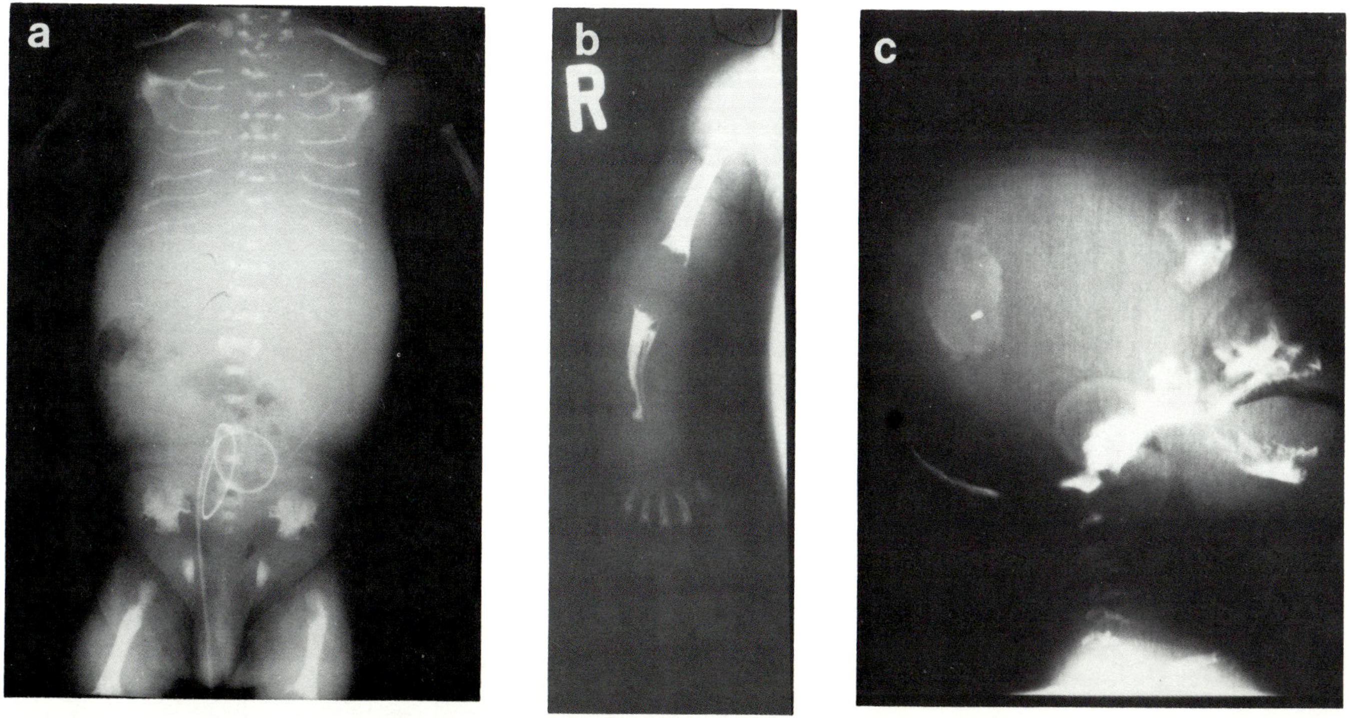

Fig. 9. Patient 4, showing (a) generalized skeletal undermineralization and thin ribs, (b) flared metaphyses of right humerus, radius, and ulna, and (c) exceptionally low mineralization of cranial vault.

hypertrophy of cartilaginous columns at the lines of ossification. Irregular foci of chondroid matrix were identified in the long bones and were scattered irregularly throughout the metaphysis. Stainable alkaline phosphatase could not be demonstrated in the kidney or liver and the phosphorylethanolamine levels were greatly increased in urine. No alkaline phosphatase could be demonstrated in the serum. The diagnosis of hypophosphatasia was confirmed.

Patients 5 and 6: Sibs With an Unclassified Chondrodysplasia

The first infant was born to a 22-year-old primigravid mother, who had an uncomplicated pregnancy until the 29th week, when she developed polyhydramnios and severe toxemia of pregnancy of 4 days duration. It was noted that her hemoglobin level had fallen from 122 to 77 g/L over a period of 48 hours. The anemia was microcytic, hypochromic in nature, with no evidence of hemolysis. Ultrasound showed the presence of a single pregnancy with polyhydramnios, severe fetal hydrops and evidence of severe reduction in limb length (Fig. 10). An intrauterine transfusion was considered, but, in view of the skeletal abnormalities, the possibility of a chondrodysplasia was

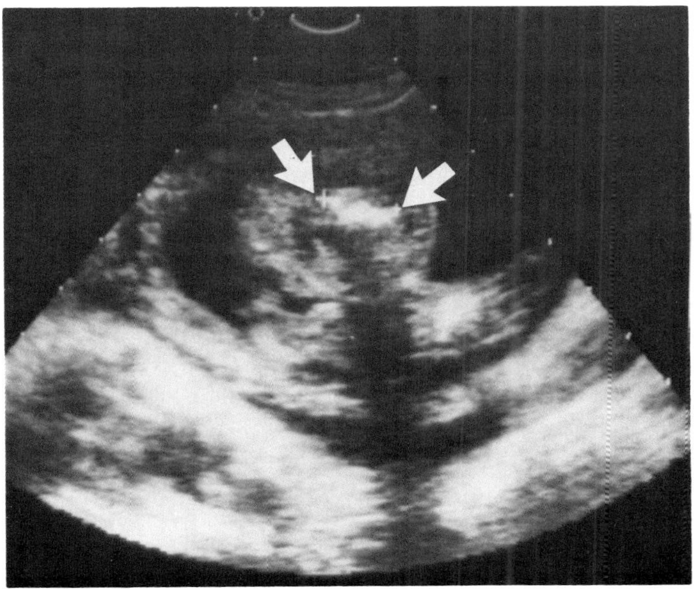

Fig. 10. Patient 5 (currently unclassified chondrodysplasia). Ultrasound demonstrates an extremely short, thick humerus (arrows).

considered and a fetal paracentesis was performed instead. Labor was induced; there was a breech presentation and cord prolapse resulted in intrauterine death. During delivery accidental decapitation of the extremely fragile head occurred. The infant was grossly deformed, and weighed 2000 gm. Radiographic examination at autopsy showed reduced mineralization of the skull, including the petrous temporal bone. The vertebral bodies were underossified and the limbs showed grossly distorted long bones with a suggestion of calcification occurring in focal nodular deposits (Fig. 11a). There was no clear definition of any epiphysial plates and the vertebrae showed mottled calcification within the cartilage. Sternum and costochondral junctions were abnormal (Fig. 11b). Histologically there was fibrous replacement of the marrow spaces, and abundant osteoid bony trabeculae obscured much of the

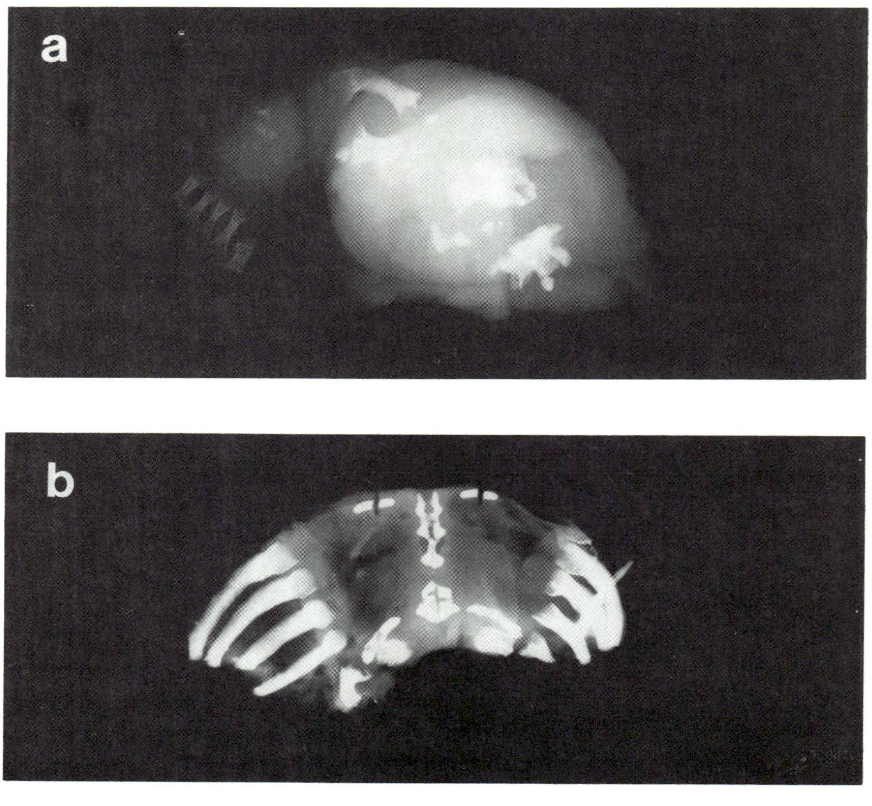

Fig. 11. Radiographs of (a) dissected right lower limb and right hemipelvis at autopsy, (b) dissected ribs and vertebrae, in patient 5.

medullary cavity. Marked extramedullary erythropoiesis was seen in the liver.

The second sib was born 3 years later. In view of the previous history, ultrasound examination was undertaken at 19 weeks of gestation. Real-time ultrasonography confirmed the presence of a single fetus with marked rhizomelic shortness of the limbs, and reduced calcification of the vertebral bodies. She elected to terminate and was delivered at 20 weeks gestation; the infant weighed 290 g and had severe rhizomelic shortness of the limbs, underossification of the cranium; short, narrow, thin ribs, and similar long bone abnormalities to those seen in the first sib (Fig. 12a,b).

These sibs were born to parents who were distantly related. Currently this chondrodysplasia is unclassified, with some changes suggesting chondrodysplasia punctata and others an unusual form of osteopetrosis.

Patients 7 and 8: Achondrogenesis Type II

These twins were born to a 19-year-old gravida II mother, who was referred to the Fetal Assessment Unit at 27 weeks of gestation because the abdominal size was greater than expected. Two years previously she had had a spontaneous abortion of twins at 18 weeks. Details of that pregnancy and of those embryos are not known. During this pregnancy assessment with real-time ultrasound confirmed a twin pregnancy with fetuses with very short limbs and decreased mineralization of the spine. Both twins showed moderate hydronephrosis with bilateral pelviureteric stenosis. The hydronephrosis was more marked in twin B, and was sufficiently prominent to suggest the "double-bubble sign" indicative of duodenal atresia (Fig. 13a,b).

The patient went into labor at 28 weeks of gestation and delivered twins weighing 560 and 500 g with monochorionic, diamniotic placentation. Both were in a footling breech position. Both twins had essentially similar anomalies with shallow orbits, anteverted nares, cleft palate, and micrognathia. The ribs and vertebrae were thin and hypoplastic and there was reduced ossification of the ischia but relatively normal ossification of the calvaria (Fig. 14). Examination of epiphysial regions of long bones and cartilaginous bones in general showed bulky, myxoid-appearing cartilage which histologically consisted largely of loose immature chondrocytes with inadequate amounts of chondroid matrix. No inclusions were identified within the cells. A diagnosis of achondrogenesis type II was made.

DISCUSSION

A review of the literature suggests that the real-time scanner may be of greater value than the static scanner in the antenatal assessment of fetal

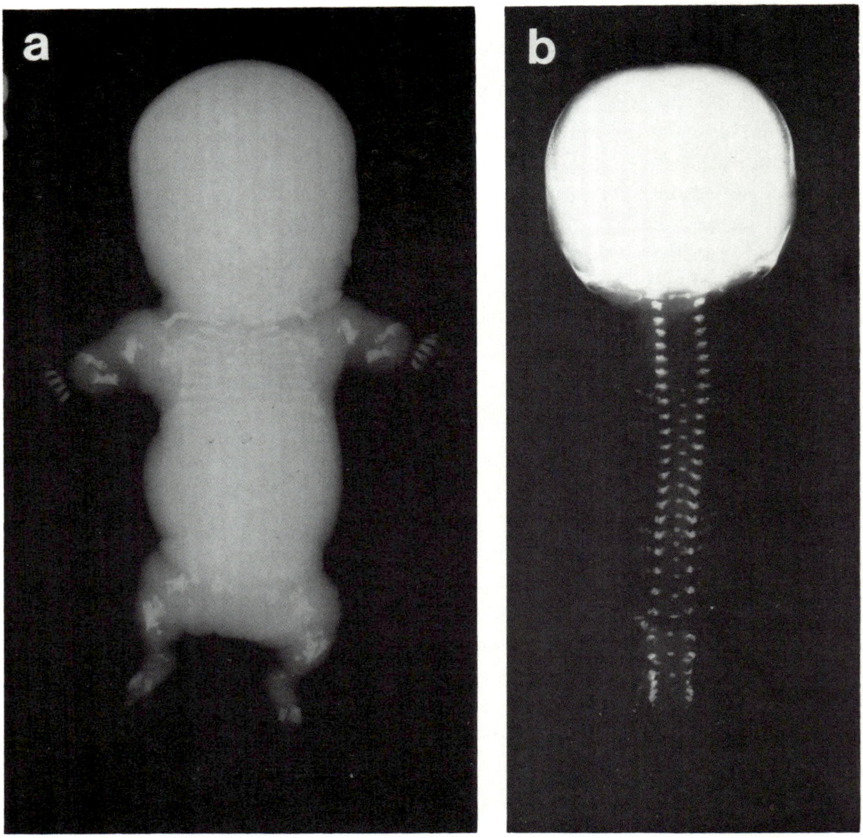

Fig. 12. Postmortem radiographs of patient 6, younger sib of patient 5, (a) showing the grossly abnormal pattern of skeletal mineralization and (b) showing the dissected axial skeleton.

anomalies [4–6]. Our experience suggests that both are required for accurate diagnosis. Initially, our second case was not diagnosed with real-time ultrasound, and it was only when the case was reviewed with the static scanner (when the skull was noted to be easily deformable), that osteogenesis imperfecta or hypophosphatasia was suspected.

The 2 cases of hypophosphatasia and the case of osteogenesis imperfecta illustrate the difficulties encountered in the ultrasonic assessment of the fetus with generalized skeletal undermineralization. Hypophosphastasia tends to be associated with more demineralization of the calvaria than in osteogenesis

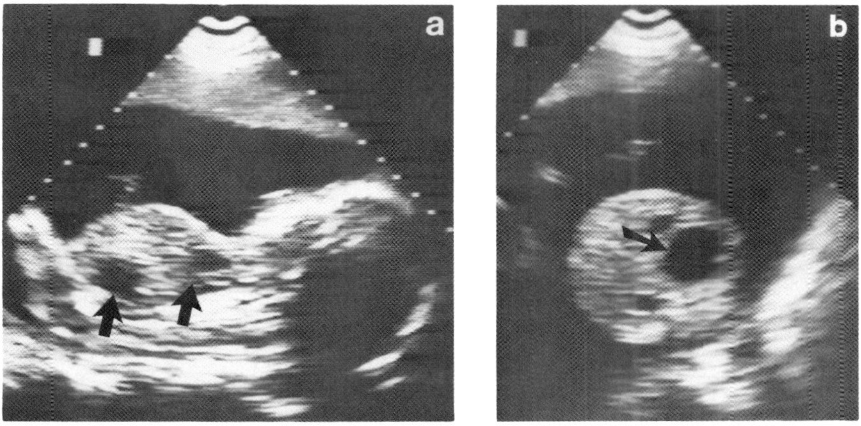

Fig. 13. Longitudinal (a) and transverse (b) views of patient 8 (achondrogenesis II) showing marked hydronephrotic dilatation (arrows) mimicking duodenal atresia (especially in the longitudinal views). In the longitudinal view, (a), distal to the hydronephrosis the lower limb appears short. The skeleton is identified only with considerable difficulty, indicative of reduced mineralization.

imperfecta, whereas the latter is associated with thicker and shorter limbs than the thinner tubular appearance seen in hypophosphatasia [4,5]. However, if generalized demineralization is readily detected antenatally, using both ultrasonic and radiologic examination, it is highly likely that one is dealing with a severe expression of one or other of these disorders, which tends to be lethal in early life in both instances [1,2,7–9,18]. Therefore, we suggest that the antenatal differentiation between these 2 conditions may not be essential, since a more precise diagnosis will not alter either the management of the pregnancy, or the eventual outcome. However, it is obvious that an accurate postmortem diagnosis is essential for parental counseling.

The ultrasonic and radiologic changes of thanatophoric dysplasia are well documented [13–17], and our case was diagnosed without difficulty. The cloverleaf skull deformity, saddle nose, anteverted nares, narrow chest, protuberant abdomen, short thick limbs, and polyhydramnios were characteristic. With this information we were able to prepare the patient psychologically and offer early counseling to both parents [1].

The mother of patients 5 and 6 developed severe toxemia of pregnancy in her first pregnancy at 29 weeks, and there was an absolute indication for induction. While the detection of severe fetal anomalies by ultrasound would not have influenced management of the pregnancy (since a severe anomaly was known to be present), intrauterine fetal treatment was modified. Despite

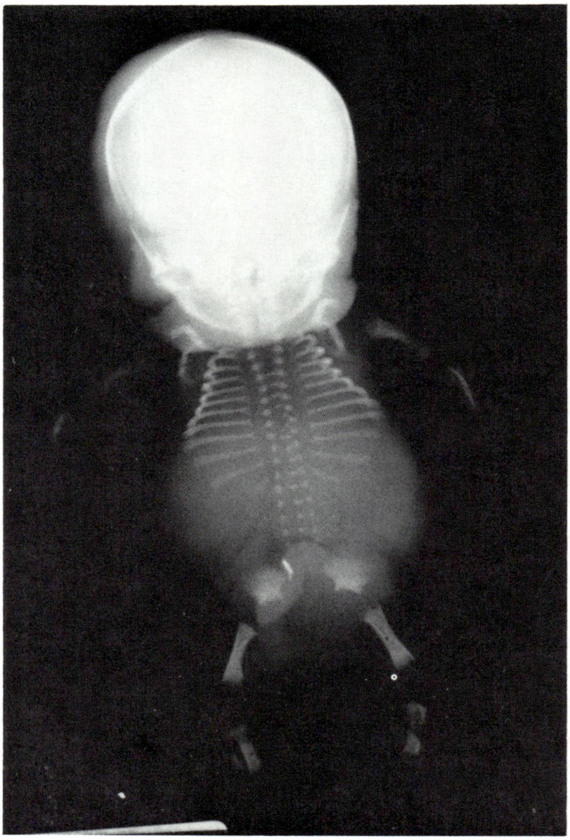

Fig. 14. Postmortem radiograph of patient 7 (identical twin of patient 8) showing classic changes of achondrogenesis II.

detailed radiographic and pathologic studies—including referral of our material to external authorities—no adequate classification of the chondrodysplasia in these sibs has been made.

Our experience with 6 of the 8 cases who presented with polyhydramnios is in keeping with the known association of polyhydramnios and skeletal dysplasia [3–5]. The ratio of head circumference to the abdominal circumference (H/A ratio) is of value in detecting relative disproportion of head and trunk growth [3–5]. In the skeletal dysplasias the H/A ratio is often markedly abnormal, with head size exceeding the 95th centile of normal for gestation in many cases. Therefore, the H/A ratio is of value in suggesting skeletal dysplasia, especially when associated with short limbs, narrow chest, and polyhydramnios.

Although skeletal dysplasias are rare, it is possible to diagnose the presence of a skeletal dysplasia such as Jeune syndrome [19] Meyer's oligodactyly [20], achondroplasia [21], diastrophic dysplasia [22], and Ellis van Creveld syndrome [4] with antenatal ultrasonography. However, more data have to be collected in order to establish the ultrasonic characteristics of many of the skeletal dysplasias. In turn, and in every case, the ultrasonic changes leading to a diagnosis of skeletal dysplasia must be confirmed by adequate radiologic and pathologic examination.

ACKNOWLEDGMENTS

We wish to thank Dr. R. Lloyd of Bethel Hospital, Winkler, Manitoba for information and ultrasound data on 2 cases. We also appreciate the help of our colleagues in Winnipeg and especially wish to thank Drs. G.R. Askew, C.S. Levi, and J. Schollenberg.

REFERENCES

1. Smith DW: "Recognizable Patterns of Human Malformation," 3rd ed. Philadelphia: W.B. Saunders, 1982.
2. Lamy ME: Hereditary disorders of bones: An overview. In Bergsma D (ed): The Clinical Delineation of Birth Defects," Part IV: "Skeletal Dysplasias." March of Dimes-Birth Defects Foundation BD:OAS 5(4):8, 1969.
3. Hobbins JC, Mahoney MJ: Diagnosis of fetal skeletal dysplasia with ultrasound. Am J Obstet Gynecol 142:306–312, 1982.
4. Hobbins JC, Mahoney MJ: In Sanders RC, James AE (eds): "Principles and Practice of Ultrasonography in Obstetrics and Gynaecology," 3rd ed. New York: Appleton-Century-Crofts, 1983.
5. Grannum PA, Hobbins JC: Prenatal diagnosis of fetal skeletal dysplasias. Semin Perinatol 7:127–137, 1983.
6. Wladimoroff JW, Stewart PA: Prenatal diagnosis of skeletal dysplasia by real-time ultrasound. Obstet Gynecol 63:360, 1980.
7. Chervenak FA, Hobbins JC: Antenatal sonographic findings of osteogenesis imperfecta. Am J Obstet Gynecol 143:228–230, 1982.
8. Brown BSJ: The prenatal ultrasonographic diagnosis of osteogenesis imperfecta lethalis. J Can Assoc Radiol 35:63–66, 1984.
9. Zervoudakis IA, Hawks GG: Diagnosis and management of osteogenesis imperfecta congenita in labor. Am J Obstet Gynecol 131:116–117, 1978.
10. Munsick RA: Human fetal extremity lengths in the interval from 9 to 21 menstrual weeks of pregnancy. Am J Obstet Gynecol 149:883–887, 1984.
11. Graham D, Sanders RC: Early second trimester sonographic diagnosis of achondrogenesis. J Clin Ultrasound 11:336–338, 1983.

12. Smith WL, Dinno N: In utero diagnosis of achondrogenesis, type I. Clin Genet 19:51–54, 1981.
13. Campbell RE: Thanatophoric dwarfism in utero. Am J Roentgenol 112:198–200, 1971.
14. Houston CS, Awen CF, Kent HP: Fatal neonatal dwarfism. J Can Assoc Radiol 23:45–61, 1972.
15. Thompson BH, Parmley TH: Obstetric features of thanatophoric dwarfism. Am J Obstet Gynecol 109:396–401, 1971.
16. Cremin BJ, Shaff MI: Ultrasonic diagnosis of thanatophoric dwarfism in utero. Radiology 124:479–480, 1977.
17. Burrows PE, Baker ML: Early antenatal sonographic recognition of thanatophoric dysplasia with cloverleaf skull deformity. Am J Roentgenol 143:841–843, 1984.
18. Mullivor RA, Zackai EH: Prenatal diagnosis of hypophosphatasia: Genetic biochemical and clinical studies. Am J Hum Genet 30:271, 1975.
19. Elejalde BR, de Elejalde MM, Pansch D: Prenatal diagnosis of Jeune syndrome. Am J Med Genet 21:443–438, 1985.
20. Elejalde BR, de Elejalde MM, Booth C, Kaye C, Hollison L: Prenatal diagnosis of Weyers Syndrome (deficient ulnar and fibular rays with bilateral hydronephrosis). Am J Med Genet 21:439–444, 1985.
21. Filly RA, Golbus MS, Carey JC, Hall JG: Short limbed dwarfism: Ultrasonographic diagnosis by measurement of fetal femoral length. Radiology 138:653–656, 1981.
22. Mantagos S, Weiss RR, Mahoney M, Hobbins JC: Prenatal diagnosis of diastrophic dwarfism. Am J Obstet Gynecol 139:111–113, 1981.

Management of the Fetus With Urinary Tract Dilatation

Renata Laxova, Leslie E. Biesecker, Richard O. Friday, Jr., Glen Snyder, Ronald W. Olson, Natalie Krassikoff, and Enid F. Gilbert

Departments of Pediatrics (RL, LEB, GS, NK), Medical Genetics (RL, NK), Radiology (ROF), Obstetrics and Gynecology (RWO), and Pathology and Laboratory Medicine (EFG), University of Wisconsin, Madison, Wisconsin 53792

INTRODUCTION

Recent developments in the frequency and quality of prenatal ultrasound evaluation have led to the detection of increasing numbers of fetuses with various types of urinary tract obstruction. No definitive guidelines are available for the obstetrician, geneticist, urologist, or family, all of whom are faced with the dilemma of a frequently ill-defined fetal abnormality, the implications of which are uncertain. A recent review by Adzick et al [1] focuses on the treatment of the fetus with bilateral hydronephrosis and presents an algorithm for the management of such patients.

Here we summarize our experience with 18 fetuses studied because a previous ultrasound examination suggested a urinary tract anomaly. In addition, in this study we present an algorithm for physicians and their patients that could aid in the management of fetal urinary tract obstruction.

METHODS

Patients were referred to either the high-risk obstetric service or the genetics center at the University of Wisconsin, Madison, between August 1981 and May 1986. Seventeen of the 18 patients were seen between 1983

Birth Defects: Original Article Series, Volume 23, Number 1, pages 385–399

and 1986. All patients had prenatal evidence of fetal urinary tract dilatation on initial ultrasound examination. The age range of the mothers was 21 to 36 years with a mean of 28.5 years. The gestational age at the time of the initial ultrasound examination ranged from 14 to 39 weeks with a mean of 25 weeks. Indications for the initial ultrasound studies included (1) dating in 6 patients; (2) amniocentesis for advanced maternal age in 4; (3) disproportionate uterine size in 3; (4) elevated maternal serum alpha fetoprotein level in 2; (5) premature labor in 1; (6) "routine" ultrasonography in 1; (7) unknown in 1 case. Ultrasound examinations at our center were performed by one of us (R.O.F.) on a Philips model 3000, 100 degree sector ultrasound scanner. Most women underwent more than 1 examination. Each patient was evaluated comprehensively and all results were discussed in detail with consulting physicians and the family. Additional investigations in some patients (where appropriate and possible) included amniocentesis, chromosome analysis, and 1 fetal cystocentesis. Each pregnancy was followed to its conclusion, and all outcomes were documented and followed. Autopsies were performed on all infants where pregnancies ended in termination, stillbirth, or neonatal death. Follow-up information was obtained about surviving infants from the University of Wisconsin pediatric renal clinic, urology clinic, or outside physicians.

For the purposes of this study, the patients were divided into 4 groups (Table I) based on our prenatal ultrasonographic findings. Group I included 4 patients with evidence of unilateral fetal urinary tract dilatation and normal amounts of amniotic fluid. Group II included 6 patients with bilateral fetal urinary tract dilatation and normal amniotic fluid volume. Group III (5 patients) also had bilateral fetal urinary tract dilatation but absent or decreased volume of amniotic fluid. Group IV, the remaining 3 patients, had prenatal ultrasonographic evidence of additional fetal (nonurinary tract) malformations. No additional fetal malformations were detected prenatally in groups I–III. There were no patients who had unilateral urinary fetal tract dilatation and oligohydramnios.

RESULTS

Detailed information on all 18 patients is provided in Table II. Eleven infants survived. The 3 with unilateral dilatation (patients A, B, C in group I) were alive and doing well at last follow-up. One infant (E) in group II, who was suspected prenatally of bilateral involvement, was found postnatally to have only unilateral involvement and was also doing well. The 5 other patients in group II (patients F,G,H,I,J) with normal amniotic fluid volume

TABLE I. Classification of Patients Into Groups*

Patient	Group†	Prenatal Dx	Management	Postnatal Dx
A	I	R. UPJ	No intervention	R. DUPL
B	I	L. UPJ	No intervention	L. UPJ
C	I	L. UPJ	No intervention	L. UPJ
D	I	R. UPJ	Termination	R.L. UVO
E	II	PUV	No intervention	L. UPJ
F	II	PUV	Early delivery	R. DUPL + B. reflux
G	II	PUV	No intervention	B. reflux
H	II	B. UPJ	No intervention	R. DUPL + L. reflux
I	II	B. UPJ	Early delivery	R. DUPL + B. reflux
J	II	B. UPJ	Early delivery	B. reflux
K	III	B. UPJ	No intervention	B. UPJ + mult. malf. 7p+
L	III	PUV	Termination	PUV (familial)
M	III	PUV	Termination	PUV
N	III	IPCKD	No intervention	IPCKD
O	III	PUV	Cystocentesis, no intervention	L. agenesis R. hydronephrosis
P	IV	Megacystis + Omphalocele	Termination	Urethral atresia + megacystis
Q	IV	Meckel syndrome	Termination	Meckel syndrome
R	IV	B. UPJ, Trisomy 13	Termination	Trisomy 13

*According to prenatal diagnosis of uni- or bilaterality of obstruction, amount of amniotic fluid, and presence of additional malformations.
†Group I—Unilateral dilatation, appropriate amt. of amniotic fluid.
Group II—Bilateral dilatation, appropriate amt. of amniotic fluid.
Group III—Bilateral dilatation, oligohydramnios.
Group IV—Uni/bilateral dilatation + additional malformations.

were followed without intervention during pregnancy. All 5 had bilateral involvement (not necessarily obstruction) confirmed on postnatal examination. The remaining 2 survivors were less fortunate. Infant K (in group III) was liveborn with multiple serious malformations, and chromosome analysis showed a *de novo* tandem duplication of 7pter→p22.1. This was not detected prenatally because oligohydramnios precluded amniocentesis. Finally, infant R in group IV was liveborn at another hospital, said to have "prune belly syndrome," and was unavailable for postnatal follow-up. We had followed this infant's mother prenatally from 17 weeks of gestational age when oligohydramnios, large fetal bladder and ascites, and a maternal ovarian cyst were diagnosed. Diagnostic fetal cystocentesis was performed at 20 weeks of gestational age and was followed by an increase in amniotic fluid volume and decreased ascites on subsequent examinations.

TABLE II. Pre- and Postnatal Findings on 18 Patients With Fetal Urinary Tract Dilatation

PATIENT DATE OF DELIV.	REASON FOR AND G.A. AT INITIAL U/S	PRENATAL FINDINGS/ DX.	GRP	PRE-NAT. MGT.	POST NAT. DX.	SEX	R.D.	AGE AT LAST F/U	RE-FLUX	UTI	ABN. RENAL FXN	HTN	GROWTH FAILURE	COMMENTS
A 21 y.o. G_1 P_1* 1-7-86	dating 39 wks	R. Hydron. unilat. (R) UPJ obstruct.	I	0	Unilat. (R) duplicated collecting system								-	
B 27 y.o. G_3 P_1 Ab_2 5-21-84	previous pregnancy loss 27 weeks	L. Hydron. Unilat. L. UPJ obstruct.	I	0	Unilat. (L) UPJ obstruct.	M	-	7/12	nk	nk	nk	-	-	pyelo-plasty at 7 mo-doing well
C 29 y.o. G_1 P_1 1-23-84	routine 31 weeks	L. Hydron. Unilat. L. UPJ obstruct.	I	0	Unilat. (L) UPJ obstruct.	M	-	11/12					-	pyelo-plasty at 11 mo-doing well
D 29 y.o. G_3 P_2 Ab_1 7-4-84	dysproportionate uterine size 23 weeks	R. Hydron. Unilat. R. UPJ obstruct.	I	termin-ation at 23 wks.	Bilat. (R>L) ureterovesical obstruct.									see text for dis-cussion of term-ination
E 8-21-84	Premature labor 32 weeks	Bilat Hydro-nephrosis posterior urethral valves	II	0	Unilat. (L) ureteropelvic junction obstruction					+		+	-	pyelo-plasty at 6 mo.
F 27 y.o. G_6 P_1 Ab_5 8-15-81	dating 32 weeks	Bilat Hydron. R. Hydroureter large bladder post. urethral valves	II	early deliv-ery at 36 wks.	Duplicated collecting system. R. ureterocele		+	3 yr	+	+	-		-	est. fetal maturity at delivery 32 wks by Ballard exam. Ureterocele unroofing at 2 days & re-section of nonfunct. R. upper renal pole & reim-plantation of lower pole ureter at 3 years
G 32 y.o. G_3 P_1 Ab_2 8-6-84	increased mat. serum AFP 21 weeks	Bilat Hydro-neph., hydro-ureter, large bladder post. urethral valves	II	0	Bilat primary reflux	M	-	21 mo	+	+	+	-	-	Vesicostomy at 7 mos, bilat ureteral reimplantation at 15 mos.
H 33 y.o. G_2 P^1 Ab_1 6-13-84	dating 32 weeks	Unilat Hydro-nephrosis, then later bilateral. Bilat. UPJ obstruct.	II	0	Unilat (R) duplicated collecting system. Unilat (L) vesico-ureteral reflux	F	-	4 1/2 mo	+	+	-	nk	-	R. hemi-nephrectomy at 4 mos.
I 24 y.o. G_1 P_1 12-9-84	dating 29 weeks	Bilat Hydro-nephrosis & hydroureter Bilat UPJ obstruct.	II	early in-duc-tion at 36 weeks due to increasing hydro-nephrosis	Unilat (R) collecting system dupl., Bilat vesico-ureteral reflux	F	-	2 mo	+	+	-	-	-	R. hemi-nephrectomy

*parity includes the fetus/infant reported here in all cases

(continued)

TABLE II. Pre- and Postnatal Findings on 18 Patients With Fetal Urinary Tract Dilatation (continued)

PATIENT DATE OF DELIV.	REASON FOR AND G.A. AT INITIAL U/S	PRENATAL FINDINGS/ DX.	GRP	PRE-NAT. MGT.	POST NAT. DX.	SEX	R.D.	AGE AT LAST F/U	RE-FLUX	UTI	ABN. RENAL FXN	HTN	GROWTH FAILURE	COMMENTS
J 36 y.o. G_4 P_3 Ab_1 5-24-85	advanced mat. age 15 weeks	Unilat hydroureter, later bilat hydroureter/possible bilat ureteropelvic junct. obstruct.	II	early induction at 37 weeks	Bilat vesicoureteral reflux					+	+		+	Developed oligohydramnios at 32 weeks. Renal biopsy shows cystic dysplasia
K 22 y.o. G_3 P_1 Ab_2 mat. drug & alcohol abuse 7-14-85	uterine dysproportion 28 weeks	Bilat hydronephrosis decreasing amniotic fl. Bilat UPJ obstruct.	III	0	Bilat ureteropelvic junction obstruction	F	–	1 yr	+	+	+	–	+	Multiple congenital anom. 46XX 7p+ Multiple urol procedures.
L 35 y.o. G_3 P_1 Ab_2 4-20-85	advanced mat. age 14 weeks	Bilat hydroureter, large bladder, dilated proximal urethra/ posterior urethral valves	III	termination at 18 wks	Posterior urethral valves, hypoplastic lungs	M								
M 30 y.o. G_2 P_0 Ab_{v2} 10-8-83	previous child with posterior urethral valves 19 weeks	Bilat hydronephrosis & hydroureter. No amniotic fluid, large bladder/post. urethral valves	III	termination at 22 weeks	Posterior urethral valves, pulmonary hypoplasia	M								Subsequent child normal (female)
N 30 y.o. G_1 P_1 12-20-84	uterine dysproportion 34 weeks	Large cystic kidneys, oligohydramnios IPCKD	III	premature labor at 34 wks	Infantile polycystic kidney disease, Potter sequence with pulmonary hypoplasia	M	+							Died several hours after birth
O 24 y.o. G_3 P_2 Ab_1 mat. dilantin usage 11-85	increased mat.serum AFP 17 weeks	large cystic abdominal mass, hydroureter bilat, R. hydronephrosis, Posterior urethral valves	III	fetal cystocentesis, Na 99 mmol/liter Cl 80 mmol/liter, BUN 13 mg/dl	Prune belly sequence R. hydronephrosis and hydroureter L. renal agenesis	M	–	9/12	–	–	–	nk	+	L. congenital dislocated hips Equinovarus
P 27 y.o. G_1 Ab_1 mat. phenobarbitol 1-8/83	dating 19 1/2 wks.	large cystic structure in abdomen, omphalocele	IV	termination at 23 wks	Omphalocele urethral atresia, bilat renal hypoplasia, pulmonary hypoplasia	M								Subsequent child normal
Q 23 y.o. G_3 P_2 Ab_1 1-26-83	previous child with Meckel's syndrome	multicystic kidneys Meckel's syndrome	IV	termination at 26 weeks	Meckel's syndrome	F								
R 33 y.o. G_2 P_{v1} Ab_1 2-24-83	nk 24.4 wks	L. hydronephrosis, hydrops, microcephaly, Trisomy 13, L. UPJ obstruct	IV	termination at 26 weeks	Trisomy 13 L. Ureterovesical junct. obstruct., pulmonary hypoplasia	M								

Seven of the 18 pregnancies resulted in termination in 6 patients and neonatal death in 1. Five of the 6 terminated pregnancies had fetal disorders that were incompatible with life. They included 2 with posterior urethral valves (PUV) with early oligohydramnios (patient L [Fig. 2] and patient M), urethral atresia (patient P [Fig. 3A,B], Meckel syndrome (patient Q), and trisomy 13 (patient R). The sixth family had a prenatal diagnosis of unilateral fetal ureteropelvic junction (UPJ) obstruction but elected to terminate the pregnancy. One neonatal death occurred in an infant (patient N) with infantile polycystic kidney disease (IPCKD).

DISCUSSION

The patients in this study were retrospectively divided into 4 groups (Table I) based on prenatal ultrasonographic findings. The groups were defined simply (see above) and should be universally applicable. The experience at our center indicated that they were of prognostic value. We are aware of no other studies that have defined such groups for this purpose.

The first group consisted of patients with unilateral dilatation and normal amniotic fluid volume. Several authors have stressed that intervention is not indicated in this situation [2,3] and our experience with the favorable outcome in group I substantiates that view. Our management of this group of patients consisted of close follow-up with repeated ultrasound examinations at 2–4-week intervals. The scans were performed to detect progression of dilatation, development of contralateral involvement, or appearance of previously unidentified malformations. It is important to identify such complications because later intervention may be indicated. For example, massive dilatation may be an indication for prenatal decompression to facilitate delivery or interrupt premature labor [4]. A change in amniotic fluid volume or a change from uni- to bilateral pathology might alter management. Patient D and her husband (group I) were informed that the outlook for their fetus was favorable but elected to terminate the pregnancy for what we suspect were additional (possibly social) reasons. It was interesting to note that on autopsy this fetus had bilateral involvement; the undiagnosed side was less severely affected.

No special group was proposed for patients with unilateral dilatation, normal contralateral kidney, and oligohydramnios since in most cases extrarenal causes would account for the oligohydramnios in potential patients with this combination of findings. Patient O (group III), in whom unilateral hydronephrosis with contralateral agenesis was found postnatally, may have been mistaken for unilateral involvement and oligohydramnios. Prenatally, a diagnosis of PUV had been established (hence classification in group III) but postnatal attempts to identify an obstruction were unsuccessful.

Group II patients had bilateral dilatation with normal amniotic fluid volume. This was our largest group of patients, the prenatal diagnosis was frequently different from that determined postnatally, and all infants survived. There were 3 instances of an incorrect prenatal diagnosis of PUV. Two of these infants (F,G) were subsequently found to have bilateral vesicoureteral reflux (VUR) (Fig. 1A, B, C), and in addition 1 of them (patient F) had unilateral ureteral duplication. The third infant (E) had only a unilateral UPJ obstruction. The prenatal diagnoses in the remaining 3 fetuses in group II, namely, bilateral UPJ obstruction, were also incorrect. Various combinations of reflux and duplication were found postnatally. We do not know if this diagnostic error has occurred at other centers or if the prenatal diagnosis of VUR or ureteral duplication is feasible. Bilateral UPJ obstruction has been estimated to occur in 1/3 of patients with UPJ obstruction. The prenatal diagnostic error of bilateral UPJ obstruction with postnatal diagnosis of reflux has been noted [5]. As the outcome in group II was uniformly good, it would be difficult to recommend intrauterine intervention in future similar situations until more information is available about its risks and benefits. Previous reports have been in agreement with a conservative approach [6]. However, induced delivery may be justified for this type of patient when amniotic fluid testing and dating suggest pulmonary maturity. The risk of delivery is relatively low and there is a possibility that some renal parenchymal damage could be averted.

The 5 patients in group III (bilateral urinary tract dilatation and oligohydramnios) had a uniformly poor outcome including termination with subsequent diagnosis of fetal pulmonary hypoplasia in patients L (Fig. 2) and M, multiple malformations (patient K), neonatal death (patient N), and prune belly sequence (patient O). This experience is reflected in the current literature, which describes a poor outcome for all patients with early oligohydramnios regardless of cause [7]. Although there is uncertainty about the specific time at which pulmonary development occurs, it is agreed that there is a critical time period of unknown duration, during the late second and early third trimesters, when the presence of amniotic fluid is required for proper pulmonary development. It is our view that repeated demonstrations of oligohydramnios prior to or during the 18th through 24th weeks of gestation suggest a very poor prognosis for adequate pulmonary development. However, early demonstration of oligohydramnios must be considered carefully because a few patients, like patient O in this series, may develop amniotic fluid later in the pregnancy, which may markedly improve their prognosis

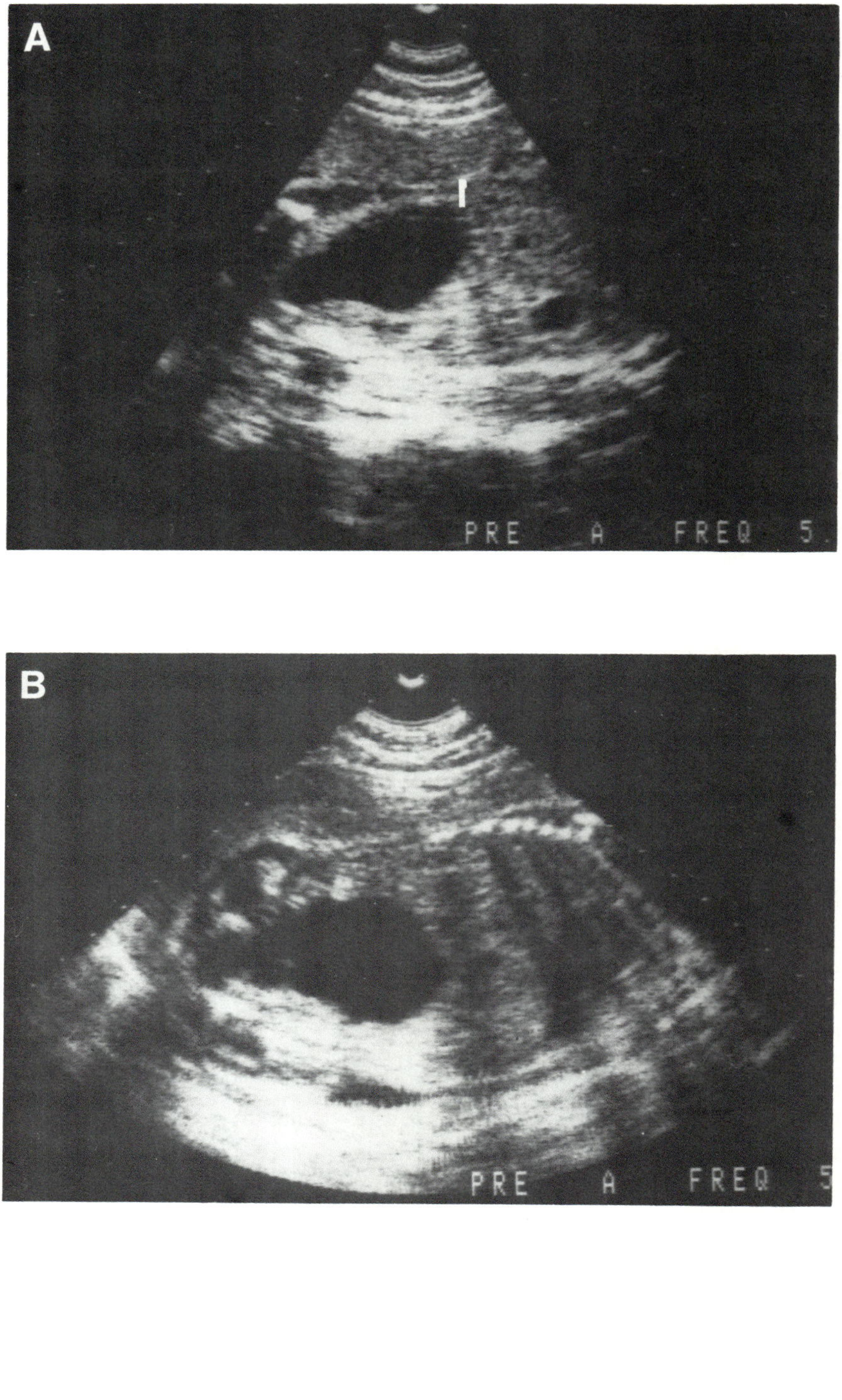
A
PRE A FREQ 5.
B
PRE A FREQ 5

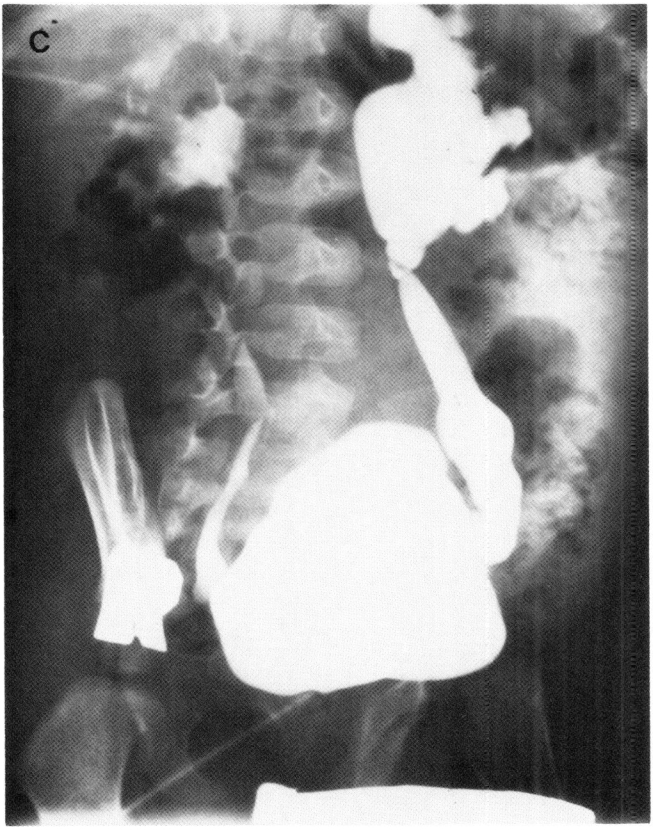

Fig. 1. (A) Fetus G: ultrasound 19 weeks, increased bladder size, susp. PUV; (B) Fetus G: ultrasound 23 weeks, increased bladder size, susp. PUV; (C) Infant G: Age 14 months, voiding cystourethrogram showing bilateral reflux.

for pulmonary development. Two or 3 ultrasound examinations that consistently demonstrate early oligohydramnios are sufficient to justify a prenatal diagnosis of pulmonary hypoplasia. Conversely, demonstration of sufficient amniotic fluid at >30 weeks probably suggests adequate pulmonary development. The prognosis is intermediate for gestations between 24 and 30 weeks that demonstrate oligohydramnios and probably depends on its duration. Present understanding of urinary tract development does not allow accurate predictions of renal function on the basis of amniotic fluid volume

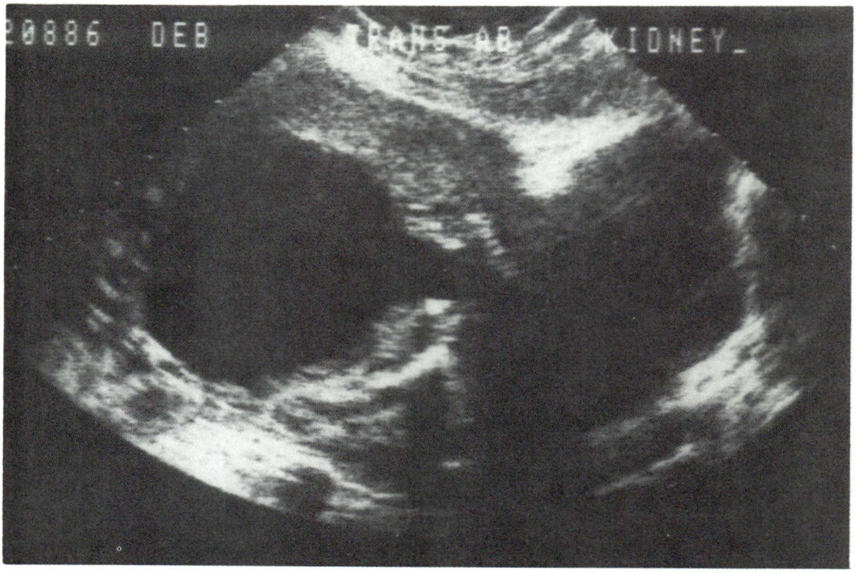

Fig. 2. Fetus L: ultrasound 19 weeks, massive bladder dilatation, oligohydramnios, susp. PUV confirmed, with severe pulmonary hypoplasia on autopsy after termination.

or bladder dynamics. Fetal urine analysis has been suggested to be helpful, as it was in patient O, but insufficient information is available. Because of this uncertainty, we cannot confidently predict renal functional outcome and therefore our counseling was based on considerations of pulmonary function.

The issue of intrauterine therapy in patients with oligohydramnios is a complicated one. Decompression of the fetal bladder with diversion to the amniotic space with double pig-tail shunts is difficult to perform in patients with oligohydramnios, and such catheters are prone to displacement [8, 9]. External catheter drainage is cumbersome [10, 11] and carries a risk of infection. Neither the double pig-tail nor the external drainage technique have been proven effective in rigorous studies in patients with oligohydramnios. Episodic instillation of aspirated fetal urine into the amniotic space has been shown to be ineffective in promoting pulmonary development. Fetal surgery by hysterotomy has been demonstrated in a 21-week fetus [7] with oligohydramnios and bilateral dilatation. The procedure clearly produced decompression of the urinary tract but did not increase amniotic fluid volume, and the infant died soon after delivery at 35 weeks gestational age. The failure to correct oligohydramnios and thus pulmonary outcome in this patient causes us to be pessimistic about *in utero* therapy for any patient with oligohydramnios beyond 20 weeks.

Two patients in group III deserve further comment. Patient N presented to us with oligohydramnios and bilateral dilatation of the fetal collecting system with large renal cysts and an irregular cortical contour. Although the final diagnosis in this infant was IPCKD, this patient was included in the present study because the differential diagnosis included urinary tract obstruction. Patient O was the only patient in this study in whom intrauterine intervention was attempted. Cystocentesis was performed to determine fetal renal function, and consultation was obtained with Dr. M. Golbus of the University of San Francisco Medical Center. The finding of hypotonic urine suggested normal renal function and was helpful in making recommendations for this patient. The subsequent ultrasound examinations demonstrated continued bladder decompression and increased amniotic fluid volume. It is difficult to ascribe this improvement to a single cystocentesis, as it has been shown that such therapy is generally ineffective. Nevertheless, it is reasonable to assume that, irrespective of the mechanism, the increase in amniotic fluid was responsible for the development of adequate pulmonary function and survival of the patient.

The 3 patients in group IV, all of whom had additional malformations, had a poor outcome. Obstructive uropathies may be isolated or part of a multiple malformation syndrome. For this reason it is advisable to perform chromosome analysis (when possible) on all patients who present with fetal urinary tract dilatation. An initial suspicion of urologic abnormalities on ultrasonographic examination led to the detection of (nonurologic) birth defects in patients Q and R. The mother of patient Q had a previous stillbirth with Meckel syndrome and was aware of the 25% risk when the initial ultrasound was performed. The recurrence of Meckel syndrome was confirmed on autopsy. Patient R (who had trisomy 13) had no family history suggestive of either aneuploidy or urologic obstruction. The initial scan was performed for reasons unknown to us. Patient P presented with an abdominal mass that was thought to be either an omphalocele or megacystis (Fig. 3A) and was classified in group IV because of the suspicion of a major nonurologic malformation. This family elected to terminate the pregnancy. Diagnoses at autopsy included megacystis with urethral atresia and a small omphalocele (Fig. 3B). It was difficult to explain the presence of polyhydramnios in this fetus with urethral atresia.

In situations where early ultrasound findings indicate additional nonurologic malformations and a potentially poor pregnancy outcome, it is important to discuss the option of termination with the family and their physicians.

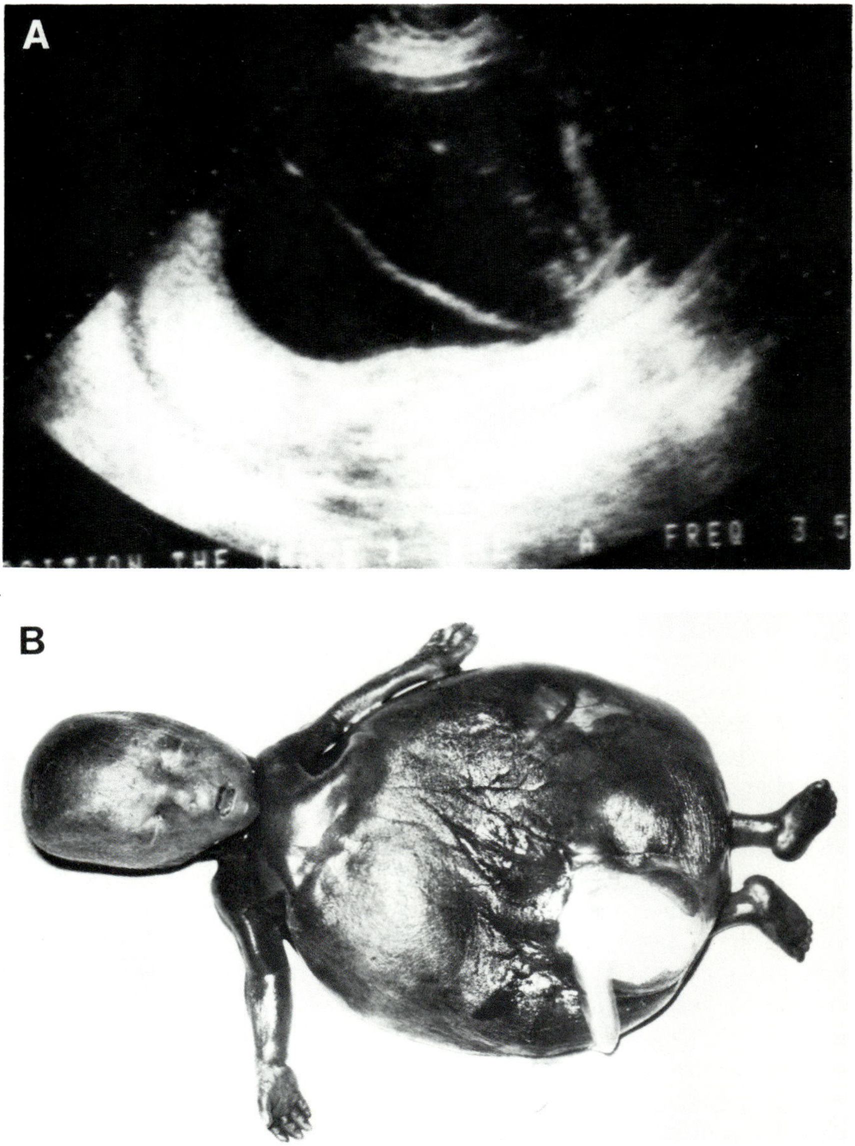

Fig. 3. (A) Fetus P: ultrasound 19 weeks, massive bladder dilatation; (B) Fetus P: after pregnancy termination: omphalocele, megacystis with urethral atresia.

All 3 families in group IV elected to terminate their pregnancies. In reviewing the 3 patients in this group, we found that the urologic abnormalities were not the primary determinant for pregnancy termination. Had they elected to continue their pregnancies, then the same criteria for management as those used for groups I–III would have applied. Figure 4 is an algorithm representing our experience with patients in all groups and our understanding of the literature on the subject. The major branching points of the algorithm were determined by considerations of family history, chromosome constitution, presence of additional malformations, volume of amniotic fluid, and the location of urinary tract dilatation. The algorithm corresponded to a reasonable sequence of information collection and should prove useful in actual patient care situations. Because of the uncertainty surrounding predictions of renal function in fetuses with uropathy, we based our counseling on considerations of pulmonary outcome. This agrees with those who argue that there

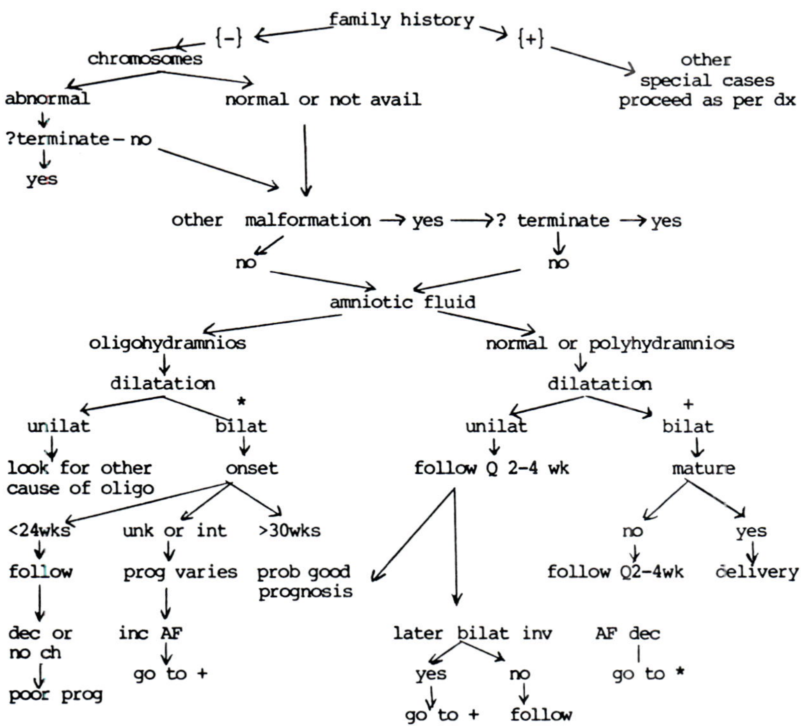

Fig. 4. Obstructive Uropathy Algorithm. unk=unknown; inc=increased, int=intermediate, inv=involvement, no ch=no change, dec=decreased.

are no real indications for *in utero* intervention and that the major justification for prenatal diagnosis is to allow early postnatal diagnosis and therapy.

SUMMARY

This report describes our experience with 18 pregnant women who presented to our center with suspected fetal urinary tract dilatation. The patients were divided into 4 groups: group I had unilateral fetal urinary tract dilatation and normal amniotic fluid volume, group II had bilateral dilatation and normal amniotic fluid volume, group III had bilateral dilatation and oligohydramnios, group IV had nonurinary tract malformations in addition to urinary tract dilatation. Patients with normal amniotic fluid volume and either unilateral or bilateral fetal dilatation (groups I and II) had a good pregnancy outcome. Patients with oligohydramnios and bilateral dilatation had a poor pregnancy outcome. No intrauterine surgery or shunting was performed in any of the patients. The initial diagnosis of urinary tract dilatation led to the prenatal diagnosis of major nonurologic malformations (group IV) in 3 patients who also had a poor outcome. An algorithm is presented that reflects our experience with the management of these patients and could serve as a guide for others caring for similar patients.

REFERENCES

1. Adzick NS, Flake AW, Harrison MR: Recent advances in prenatal diagnosis and treatment. Pediatr Clin North Am 32:1103–1116, 1985.
2. Harrison MR, Filly RA, Parer JT, Fraer MJ, Jacobson JB, de Lorimier AA: Management of the fetus with a urinary tract malformation. JAMA 246:635–639, 1981.
3. McFadyen IR: Obstruction of the fetal urinary tract: A role for surgical intervention in utero? Br Med J 288:459–462, 1984.
4. Kirkinen P, Jouppila P, Tuononen S, Paavilainen T: Repeated transabdominal renocentesis in a case of fetal hydronephrotic kidney. Am J Obstet Gynecol 142:1049–1052, 1982.
5. Turnock RR, Shawis R, Rickwood AMK: Obstruction of the fetal urinary tract: A role for surgical intervention in utero? Br Med J 288:1453 (letter), 1984.
6. Diament MJ, Fine RN, Ehrlich R, Kangarloo H: Fetal hydronephrosis: Problems in diagnosis and management. J Pediatr 103:435–440, 1983.
7. Harrison MR, Golbus MS, Filly RA, Callen PW, Katz M, de Lorimier AA, Rosen M, Jonsen AR: Fetal surgery for congenital hydronephrosis. N Engl J Med 306:10:591–593, 1982.
8. Golbus MS, Harrison MR, Filly RA, Callen PW, Katz M: In utero treatment of urinary tract obstruction. Am J Obstet Gynecol 142:383–388, 1982.
9. Manning FA, Harman CR, Lange IR, Brown R, Decter A, MacDonald M: Antepartum chronic fetal vesicoamniotic shunts for obstructive uropathy: A report of two cases. Am J Obstet Gynecol 145:819–822, 1983.

10. Shalev E, Weiner E, Feldman E, Sudarsky M, Shmilowitz L, Zuckerman H: External bladder-amniotic fluid shunt for fetal urinary tract obstruction. Obstet Gynecol 63:3 (suppl.), 31S–34S, 1984.
11. McFadyen IR, Wigglesworth JS, Dillon MJ: Fetal urinary tract obstruction: Is active intervention before delivery indicated? Br J Obstet Gynaecol 90:342–349, 1983.

Femoral Cylinder Index in the Diagnosis of the Ullrich-Turner Syndrome

C. Kaplan, MD, M. Heneghan, MD, C. Trunca, PhD, and B. Rochelson, MD

Departments of Pathology (CK), Radiology (MH), Obstetrics and Gynecology (CT,BR), Health Sciences Center, SUNY Stony Brook, Stony Brook, New York 11794

INTRODUCTION

The Ullrich-Turner syndrome (UTS), (45,X) is the most common chromosome abnormality in spontaneously aborted embryos and fetuses. Studies from early abortions indicate that about 16% of chromosomally abnormal abortuses show this karyotype. Loss continues throughout pregnancy leading to a death rate of over 95% of conceptions with monosomy X with an incidence at birth of individuals with UTS estimated at only 1 in 2500 females [1].

Diagnosis of this cause of fetal loss is important for genetic counseling, as UTS, compared with other malformation complexes, has little risk for recurrence in future pregnancies. Making this diagnosis in early fetuses may be difficult due to incompletely developed phenotype or severe maceration. Cytogenetic confirmation may only be obtainable on placental tissue culture.

We recently observed a typical UTS fetus, cytogenetically proven to be 45,X, who appeared to have unusually short limbs (Fig. 1). Although actual limb lengths were not significantly reduced [2], a radiographic measure of limb morphology, the femoral cylinder index (FCI) of Whitley and Gorlin [3], suggested growth retardation. Retrospective analysis of other UTS and control fetuses was undertaken to evaluate whether decreased FCI was diagnostically useful in 45,X fetuses.

Birth Defects: Original Article Series, Volume 23, Number 1, pages 401–410

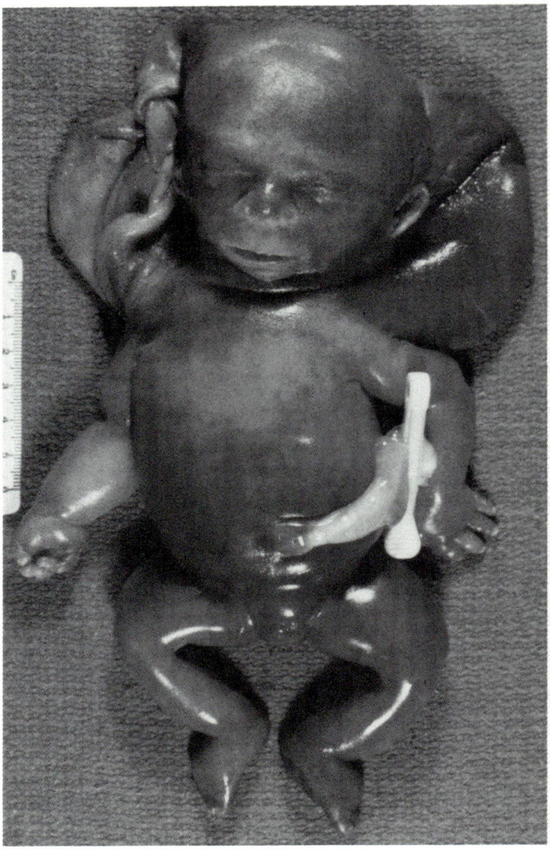

Fig. 1. Fetus 1, the 45,X index fetus shows typical external UTS phenotype including nuchal hygroma and severe peripheral edema. The limbs appear slightly short.

MATERIALS AND METHODS

The study population consisted of all spontaneously and therapeutically aborted fetuses with the diagnosis of UTS during 1981–85. One published radiograph of an UTS fetus [4] was similarly analyzed. Fetuses thought to have UTS were identified either postnatally from gross appearance or prenatally by identification of a nuchal hygroma. The control population consisted of normal fetuses, ones with chromosome abnormalities other than UTS, and a variety of malformations and abnormalities.

Radiographic examination was performed in each case of the study and control populations. These were done in a Faxitron, using X-omat TL film, which was processed routinely. The fetus was positioned directly on the film as flat as possible. The femoral cylinder index (FCI) [3] was measured directly on the radiograph by taking the ratio of femoral length to midshaft femoral width, both to the nearest millimeter (Fig. 2).

Cytogenetic studies were performed on cultured fetal tissues if possible. In cases in which the fetus was macerated, placental tissue was used.

All fetuses were dissected using usual autopsy procedures, including complete examination of the heart and genitourinary system. Gestational age was assessed by crown-rump and foot length measurements and by ultrasound data, when available. Histologic sections of the fetus and placenta, including decalcified bone sections, were also examined.

Measurement data were analyzed using Student's *t* test. The Pearson "product moment" correlation (*r*) was calculated for the FCI versus gestational age.

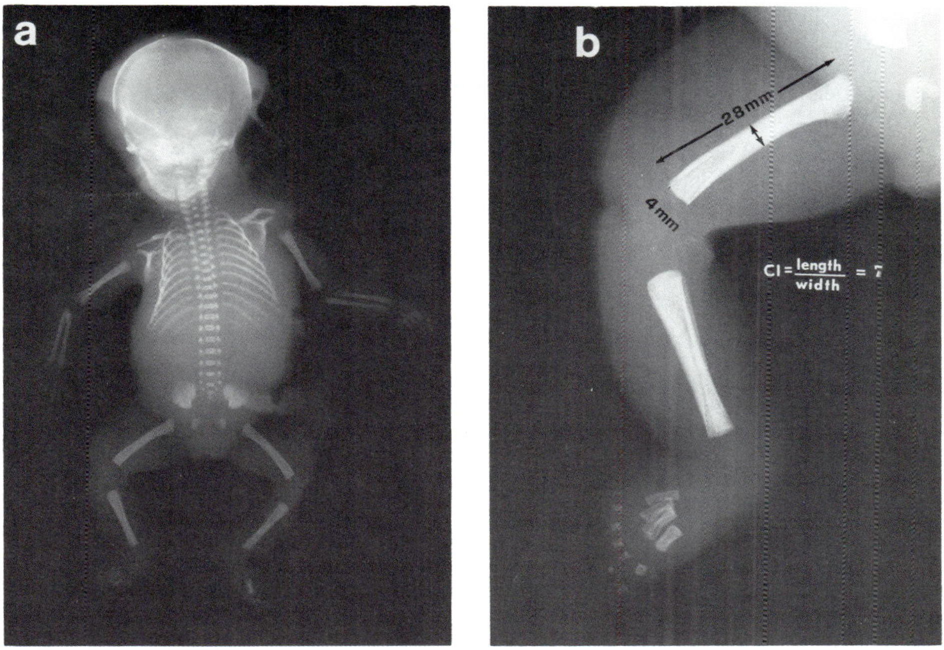

Fig. 2a. Whole body radiograph of fetus #1. Overall bone structure is normal, and femoral length is within normal limits for gestational age. 2b. Detail of right femur showing measurement data for deriving the femoral cylinder index.

RESULTS

The study population included 8 fetuses with cytogenetic and/or morphologic diagnosis of UTS (Table I). The mean gestational age was 16 weeks (range 12–22 weeks). Two additional 18-week fetuses were also evaluated as described, although not included in the statistical analysis. One of these (#9) showed 45 chromosomes with a 22/X translocation, resulting in a partial deletion of the distal short arm of the X {45,X,-X,-22,+t(X;22)(p22;q11)} (Fig. 3). The other (#10) was a 47,XY +21/46,X,+21 mosaic. Twenty-four control fetuses were similarly studied (Table II). The 7 normal appearing, non-growth-retarded fetuses were from very early premature deliveries, associated with chorioamnionitis or placental hemorrhage. The mean age in the control group was 22 weeks (range 14–36 weeks).

Distributions of femoral cylinder index measurements in the 8 UTS and 24 control fetuses are shown in Figure 4. The mean of the control fetuses was 10.85 (range 8–13), while that of the UTS fetuses was 8.38 (range 7–9). The mean FCI in the 45,X group was significantly lower ($p < .001$) from that of the normal and abnormal control fetuses. The chromosomally abnormal fetus with the partial X short arm deletion had an FCI of 7.4, while the mosaic fetus had a FCI value of 10. FCI values were similar in normal and abnormal control fetuses. Three control fetuses were found to have FCI values clearly in the range of UTS fetuses. These were all abnormal, one with a pattern of deformation seen with oligohydramnios (46,XX), one with homozygous beta-thalassemia, and a third fetus with a 46,XX,10q- chromosome complement.

FCI measurement remained relatively constant across gestational age in the control fetuses (Fig. 5a). However, in the 45,X fetuses there seemed to be a tendency for the femoral cylinder index to decrease with increasing gestational age (Fig. 5b).

Histologic examination of bone sections from the UTS fetuses showed no significant alteration from a normal ossification pattern, nor was spicule size altered.

DISCUSSION

There is an increasing interest in mechanisms of fetal wastage and a greater desire by parents for a complete answer when they have had such an experience. Thus, evaluation of useful procedures in this area is relevant. The ideal investigation into a fetal loss would include gross and microscopic studies, microbiologic techniques, cytogenetic analysis, and radiographs [5]. The nature of material received, cost, and facilities available limit the possi-

TABLE I. Morphologic Abnormalities of UTS Fetuses

Case	Karyotype	Gestation	FCI	Hygroma	Edema	Effusions	Anomalies: Coarct	Anomalies: Renal	Anomalies: Other	Maceration	Femur length (cm)
1	45,X	22	7.0	+	+	+	+	−	−	+/−	2.8
2	45,X	18	7.3	+	+	−	−	−	−	+/−	2.3
3	—	16	8.2	+	+	+	−	−	+*	+	2.2
4	45,X	14	8.0	+	−	−	−	−	+†	+	1.4
5	45,X	12	9.0	+	+/−	+	−	−	−	+	1.4
6	45,X	16	9.0	+	+	+	+	−	+†	−	1.9
7	—	15	9.5	+	+	+	+	−	−	+	1.8
8	45,X‡	17	9.0	+	+	NA	NA	NA	NA	NA	NA
9	**	18	7.4	−	−	−	−	+	+	−	3.0
10	45,X/46,XY	18	10.0	−	−	−	+	−	+	−	3.1

†Single umbilical artery.
*Diaphragmatic hernia.
**22/X translocation.
‡Graham et al (1984) [4].

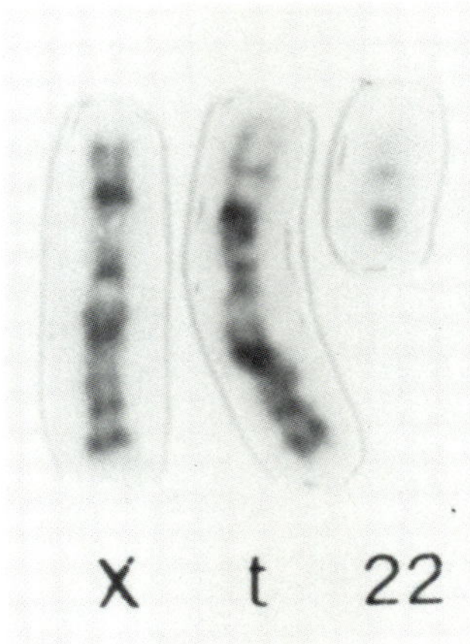

Fig. 3. Partial karyotype of fetus #9 with 45,X,-X,-22,+t(X;22)(p22;q11). FCI was 7.4 in this fetus. Deletion of the distal short arm of the X is associated with short stature.

TABLE II. Control Fetuses

Diagnosis	No. cases	Average FCI	Range FCI	Gestation (weeks)
Normal	7	10.8	10.0–11.8	12–25
Growth retardation	1	11.5	—	32
Infant of diabetic mother	1	10.0	—	36
Oligohydramnios sequence	1	8.0	—	18
VATER	1	12.8	—	24
Renal anomalies	2	12.1	11.4–12.8	24,32
Arthrogryposis	1	10.6	—	32
Acardiac twin	1	13.0	—	20
Neural tube defect	2	10.9	10.0–11.9	20,22
Dandy-Walker malformation	1	10.0	—	18
β-thalassemia	1	9.0	—	21
Trisomy 21	2	11.8	11.3–12.3	20,23
Triploidy	1	12.0	—	13
Other chromosome defect	2	9.4	7.8–11.0	20,21

bility of performing many of these, but a thorough morphologic evaluation and radiographs can be done on fixed material and, thus, in virtually all cases. When more extended study possibilities exist, these evaluations serve as preliminary studies. Since monosomy X is known to occur frequently among cytogenetically studied spontaneous abortions [1], it may be underdiagnosed by routine evaluations at present.

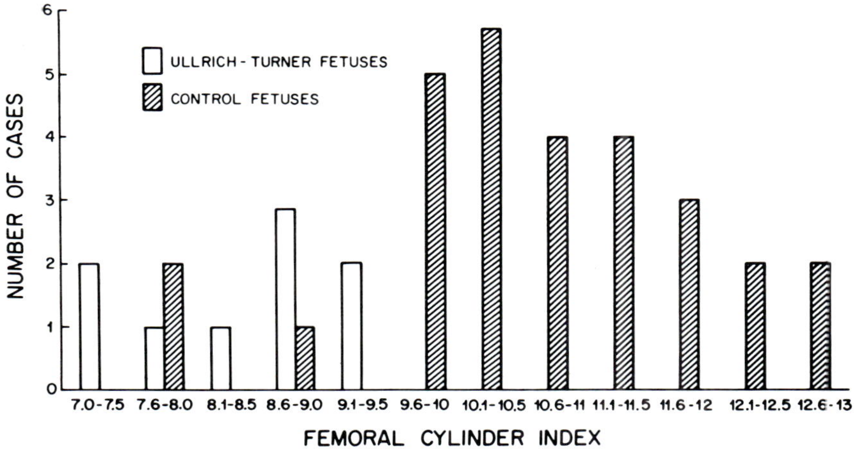

Fig. 4. Distribution of FCI measurements in 8 UTS and 24 control fetuses. Mean value in control fetuses is 10.85 while that of UTS fetuses is 8.38. Mean FCI in the 45,X group is significantly lower ($p < .001$) than in control fetuses.

The prenatal phenotype of the UTS has been described [6–9]. Early embryos may be intact but empty sacs. The later embryo or fetus may appear normal, but many show a spectrum of abnormalities including limb and trunk edema with nuchal accentuation ("cystic hygroma"), and cardiac and renal anomalies. Internal and external genitalia are female. Growth retardation is common in the UTS; this phenomenon appears to have its onset before birth. Newborn girls with monosomy X are of low birth weight and their total length is reduced. The stature of adolescents and adults with UTS is also well below average [10,11]. In these individuals long bone length is reduced, but the diameter is relatively unaffected [12]. In the femur these changes are manifest radiographically as a low FCI. Unlike older patients, 45,X fetuses do not show significant femoral length reductions measured radiographically or sonographically at any gestational age. Nevertheless, FCI in UTS fetuses is lower than that of control fetuses, indicating that growth disturbances are present *in utero*.

The FCI appears to be a reliable, reproducible, and sensitive indicator of developmental growth alterations. Since this value is a ratio, it is independent of technical factors such as magnification.

Control values for FCI in infants have not been described previously [3]. Fetuses with an FCI greater than 10 are unlikely to have a 45,X chromosome constitution. Conversely, FCI less than 10 appears to be highly suggestive

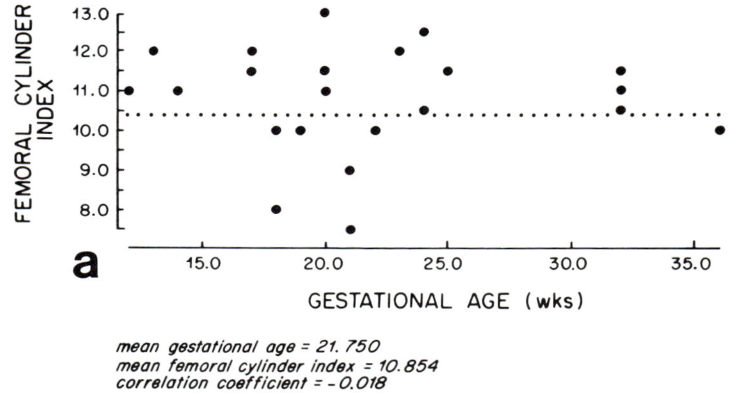

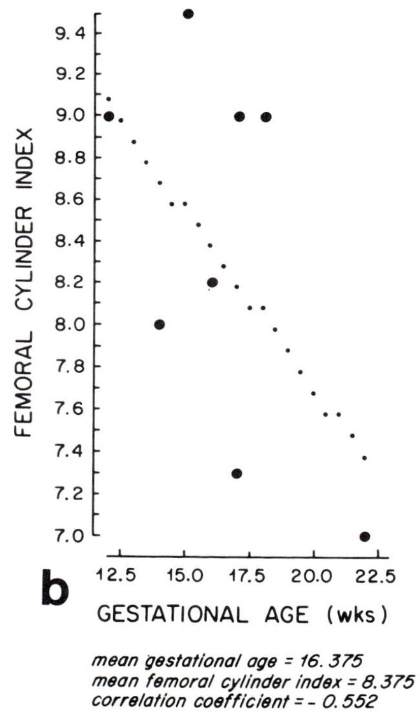

Fig. 5a. FCI measurement remained constant across gestational age in the control fetuses (r=-0.018). 5b: In UTS fetuses there was a tendency for the femoral cylinder index to decrease with increasing gestational age (r=-0.552).

although not diagnostic of UTS. Reduced FCI is highly associated with chromosome abnormalities. Overall, of all fetuses in our series with values less than 10, 82% (9/11) were chromosomally abnormal.

Three of the abnormal control fetuses had values less than 10. Other abnormalities of these fetuses were not suggestive of UTS. It is unclear whether these should be considered false positives. The particular chromosome 10 long arm deletion observed is extremely unusual, and although the exact phenotype is not established, it has been associated with short stature in some cases [13]. Prenatal growth disturbance may be a characteristic of this and β-thalassemia. While several control fetuses had deformations related to oligohydramnios, FCI was reduced in only one case.

"Cystic hygromas" are frequently the most obvious external anomaly at pathologic exam and on ultrasonography. It has been well documented that all cystic hygromas are not due to UTS and they may be a component of several other syndromes [14–17]. As all our fetuses with cystic hygromas were proven to have UTS, we have been unable to evaluate the FCI in isolated cystic hygroma. It may well prove to be a further differentiating trait.

The two chromosomally abnormal fetuses without classic UTS illustrate the differential diagnostic value of the FCI. The particular deletion in the short arm of the X chromosome of fetus 9 is known to be associated with short stature [13,18]. The FCI of 7.4 reflects this morphologic abnormality and supports the specificity of this ratio for the growth retardation in UTS. The X/XY mosaic fetus (10) had a value of 10, at the lower limit of normal. Phenotypic effects of mosaicism are variable and difficult to predict.

We conclude that the femoral cylinder index is a very sensitive and reasonably specific diagnostic parameter for monosomy X. A value of less than 10 is highly suggestive of chromosome abnormality and is an indication for chromosome evaluation. The FCI can be useful to pathologic examination and possibly postnatally. Presently it seems of little use in ultrasound diagnosis because of the difficulty of precise femoral width measurement.

REFERENCES

1. Carr DH: Cytogenetics of human reproductive wastage. In Kalter H (ed): "Issues and Reviews in Teratology," Vol 1. New York: Plenum, 1983.
2. Hadlock FP, Harrist RB, Deter RL, Park SK: Fetal femur length as a predictor of menstrual age: Sonographically measured. AJR 138:875–878, 1982.
3. Whitley CB, Gorlin RJ: Achondrogenesis: New nosology with evidence of genetic heterogeneity. Radiology 148:693–698, 1983.

4. Graham JM, Crow HC, Rawnsley EF, Simmons GM Jr, Hoefnagel D: Enhanced visualization of soft tissues in the study of aborted fetuses through the use of xeroradiography. Teratology 30:11–24, 1984.
5. Baldwin VJ, Kalousek DK, Dimmick JE, Applegarth DA, Hardick DF: Diagnostic pathologic investigation of the malformed conceptus. In Rosenberg HS, Bernstein J (eds): "Perspectives in Pediatric Pathology." New York: Masson (7): 1982.
6. Singh RP, Carr DH: The anatomy and histology of XO human embryos and fetuses. Anat Rec 155:369–384, 1966.
7. Gilbert EF, Opitz JM: Developmental and other pathological changes in syndromes due to chromosome abnormalities. In Rosenberg HS, Bernstein J (eds): "Perspectives in Pediatric Pathology" New York: Masson (7):1982.
8. Poland BJ, Dill F, Paradice B: A Turner-like phenotype in the aborted fetus. Teratology 21:361–365, 1980.
9. Byrne J, Blanc WA, Warburton D, Wigger J: The significance of cystic hygroma in fetuses. Hum Pathol 15:61–67, 1984.
10. Brook CGD, Murse G, Zachmann M, Prader A: Growth in children with 45,XO Turner's syndrome. Arch Dis Child 49:789–795, 1974.
11. Finby N, Archibald RM: Skeletal abnormalities associated with gonadal dysgenesis. Am J Roent 89:1222–1234, 1963.
12. Varrela J, Vinkka H, Alvesalo L: The phenotype of 45,X females: An anthropometric quantification. Ann Hum Biol 11:53–66, 1984.
13. Schinzel A: "Catalogue of Unbalanced Chromosome Alterations in Man." New York: de Gruyter, 1984.
14. Cowchock FS, Wapner RJ, Kurtz A, Chatzkel S, Barnhart JS, Lesnick DC: Not all cystic hygromas occur in the Ullrich-Turner Syndrome. Am J Med Genet 12:327–331, 1982.
15. Bieber FR: Comments on "A Turner-like phenotype in the aborted fetus." Teratology 21:418, 1980.
16. Poland BJ, Dill F, Paradice B: Response to comments on "A Turner-like phenotype in the aborted fetus." Teratology 21:419, 1980.
17. Chervenak FA, Isaacson G, Blakemore KJ, Breg R, Hobbins JC, Berkowitz RL, Tortora M, Mayden K, Mahoney MJ: Fetal cystic hygroma: Cause and natural history. N Engl J Med 309:822–825, 1983.
18. Therman E, Denniston C, Sarto GE: X chromosome constitution and the human female phenotype. Hum Genet 54:113–143, 1980.

The Hydrolethalus Syndrome

Natalie Krassikoff, MD, Larry Konick, MD, and Enid F. Gilbert, MD

Departments of Medical Genetics, Pediatrics, and Pathology, University of Wisconsin-Madison, Madison, Wisconsin 53706

INTRODUCTION

In 1981, Salonen et al [1] described a lethal syndrome in 18 families associated with hydrocephalus, "keyhole" foramen magnum, polydactyly, polyhydramnios, and craniofacial anomalies. Autosomal recessive inheritance was postulated based on one case of consanguinity and 8 families in which there were sib recurrences. One additional case has been reported [2] in a family of non-Finnish ancestry.

Although the abnormalities in the patient we examined are best described by the syndrome of hydrolethalus, a number of the individual traits suggest an overlap with other disorders. This will be summarized in the discussion.

Consanguinity in this family supports the likelihood of autosomal recessive inheritance.

CLINICAL HISTORY

A 24-year-old G_3P_O woman was referred to the Prenatal Diagnostic Clinic at 37 weeks of gestation because of fetal anomalies detected by ultrasound. Twins had been suspected before ultrasonography although only a single fetal heartbeat had been detected. The parents were first cousins once removed who had had two previous miscarriages at 2½ to 3 months. The pregnancy was uncomplicated except for suppuration of a wisdom tooth. In retrospect, the mother did not recall that the fetus had ever completely changed position. The only medication taken was a prescribed prenatal vitamin. A repeat

Birth Defects: Original Article Series, Volume 23, Number 1, pages 411–419 ultrasound exam confirmed marked polyhydramnios and a singleton in breech position with massive hydrocephalus and what was interpreted as holoprosencephaly (Fig. 1). The BPD and AP diameter of the head were estimated to be approximately 20 cm. Facial parts were not clearly visible. There was widening of the posterior cervical spinal processes with a protruding sac suggesting a cervical meningocele. No other internal anomalies were detected. The mother was admitted within a week after a discussion of the implications of the ultrasound findings because of cervical dilatation and projected difficult delivery. Induced vaginal delivery, after transabdominal decompression of the hydrocephalus yielded approximately 3 liters of cerebrospinal fluid, and resulted in a female infant with multiple congenital anomalies. Apgar scores were 2 and 1 and the infant expired approximately 1 hour after delivery.

Review of the family history showed that the mother's maternal grandmother (the father's maternal aunt) had had 13 miscarriages and lost an infant because of Rh incompatibility. Also there was a history of infants with anomalies born to relatives in both families but detailed records were not available. None of the latter individuals were related to both parents. On examination, both parents were eumorphic.

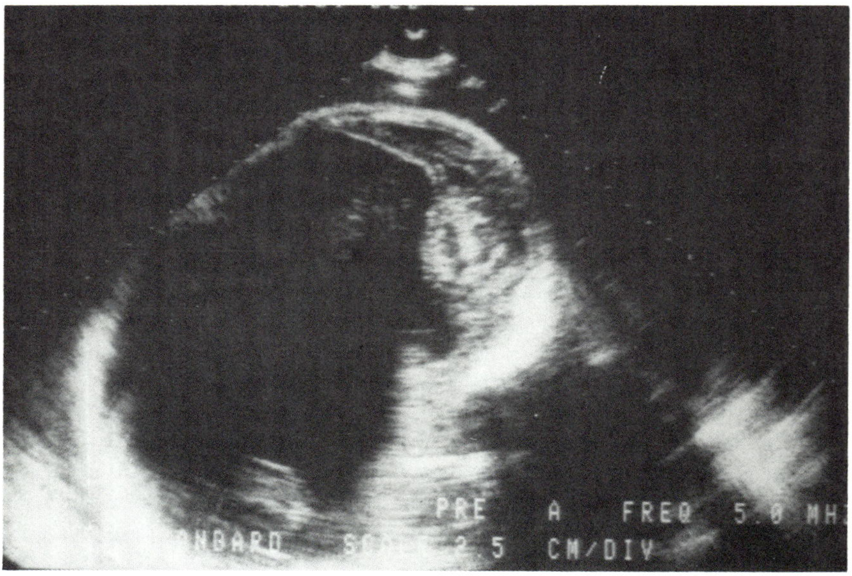

Fig. 1. Sagittal view of the head by ultrasonography at 36 weeks' gestation.

PATHOLOGIC FINDINGS

At postmortem examination, the 1300 gm female infant was 57 cm long. There was severe hydrocephalus resulting in a globular skull with an apical posterior midline hair whorl and long tongues of hair extending over the cheeks (Fig. 2). The facial structures were flattened with prominent zygomatic arches. Palpebral fissures were short, apparently "low-set" and downslanting. There was anophthalmia and hypertelorism. The most striking facial anomaly was the large midline defect produced by the absent nasal bone and cartilages associated with cleft lip and palate. The nasopharynx was small and sharply angulated downward. The ears were small (3 cm), very low-set and "faunlike" with overfolded superior helices. External auditory canals were present but abnormally angulated. The neck was webbed anteriorly with limited extension and there was micrognathia. Although cervical spinal processes appeared widened and there was an area of skin redundancy at the base of the skull, spina bifida was not present. There was a 3-vessel cord. There was bilateral postaxial hexadactyly of the hands (but not feet) with mildly short fifth digits and no cortical thumbs. Major creases were normal,

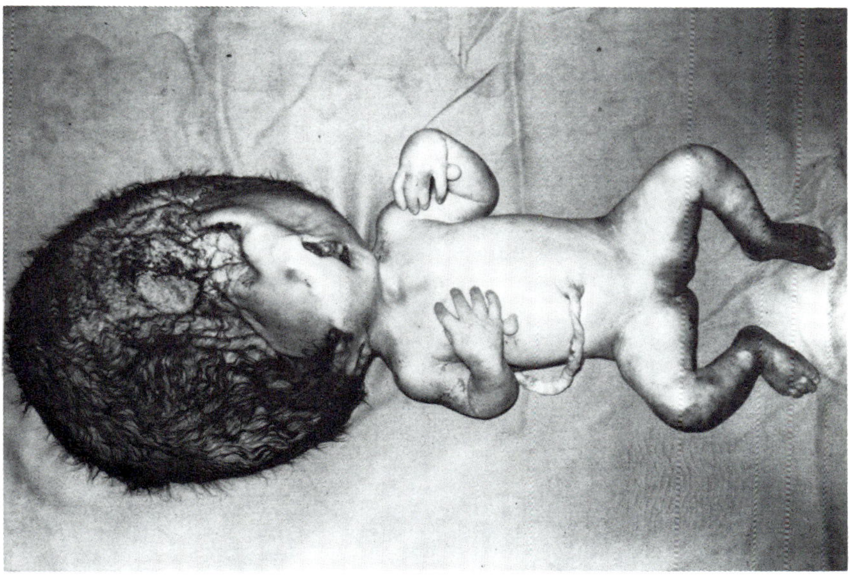

Fig. 2. Postmortem photograph showing craniofacial abnormalities, hydrocephalus, and hexadactyly of hands. (Reprinted by permission of Little, Brown.)

and dermatoglyphics of the 10 normal digits showed 6 whorls, 3 ulnar loops, and an arch. Otherwise the examination of the infant was unremarkable.

Three defects were noted in the base of the occipital bone, and there were widely spaced islands of markedly thinned bone throughout the calvaria. The largest was a midline "keyhole-shaped" defect extending dorsally from the relatively stenotic foramen magnum, which was covered by redundant skin. Two other occipital bone defects were circular at the left base and covered by skin.

Intracranially, the falx cerebri was present. The cerebral hemispheres were widely separated at the base of the skull (Fig. 3). The pituitary, corpus callosum, and septum pellucidum were absent. The lateral ventricles communicated directly with the subdural space resulting in the apparent holoprosencephaly noted on ultrasonography. The cerebral mantles were less than 1 cm thick. The fourth ventricle was dilated. Hypoplastic optic nerves were attached to dysplastic eyes. The cerebellum was small, but there were no gross abnormalities of the brain stem. Postmortem radiographs did not detect vertebral abnormalities.

There were no abnormalities of the heart, great vessels, reproductive organs, or gastrointestinal tract. The liver and spleen were composed of sev-

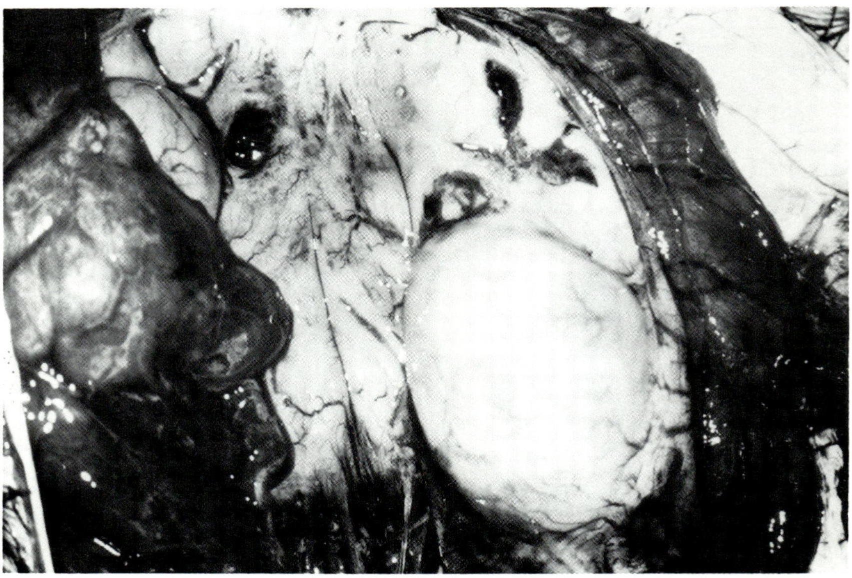

Fig. 3. In situ appearance of the brain after cranial decompression.

eral lobules and had accessory fissures. The right lung was bilobed. There was no renal anomaly except for hydroureters, and the adrenal glands could not be detected grossly although microscopic examination disclosed tiny remnants of intraabdominal dysplastic adrenal tissue.

DISCUSSION

The findings noted in this infant are consistent with the diagnosis of hydrolethalus as summarized in Table I. One unusual anomaly noted in our patient was the presence of hydroureters. No site of obstruction was found and it is postulated that the ureteral dilatation was on the basis of neurogenic dysfunction.

TABLE I. Manifestations of Hydrolethalus

	Case	
Manifestation	Previous	Present
Breech presentation	18/28	+
Polyhydramnios	24/26	+
Stillborn	28/29	+
Hydrocephalus	27/28	+
Absent pituitary	4/29	+
Absent corpus callosum, septum pellucidum	8/27	+
Defect in occipital bone	8/11	+
Small mandible	23/23	+
Cleft lip/palate	16/27	+
Small tongue	10/13	+
Eyes deeply set, micro/anophthalmia	14/15	+
Anomalous nose	10/10	+
Ears apparently low-set, malformed	14/15	+
Abnormal larynx, trachea, or bronchi	18/25	−
Lungs, defective lobation	14/24	+
Cardiovascular defect*	16/27	−
Hydronephrosis	2/25	−
Hydroureters	?	+
Abnormal genitalia	16/23	−
Uterus duplex/bicornuate	5/13	−
Adrenal hypoplasia or dysplasia	9/27	+
Malrotation of gut	6/27	−
Accessory spleens	4/27	−
Polydactyly	22/27	
of fingers	15/27	+
of toes	20/27	−
Clubfoot	15/20	−

*Vessels or septal defects.

Some of the components of hydrolethalus may be found in other disorders such as trisomy 13 [3], Meckel syndrome [4,5,7], Smith-Lemli-Opitz (or RSH) syndrome [6,7], septo-optic "dysplasia" [8,9], Warburg syndrome (HARD±E) [10,11], oculo-auriculo-vertebral dysplasia [12–14], Fryns syndrome [15] and asplenia/polysplenia [16–19] (Table II). However, the differentiating characteristics noted in Table III distinguish hydrolethalus from these other disorders.

It has been proposed by Opitz and Gilbert [20] that the hydrolethalus syndrome is an example of a midline developmental field susceptibility resulting in clefting and midline CNS defects. This has been expanded upon by Toriello and Bauserman [2] who have suggested that the abnormal pulmonary development is an extension of the developmental field defect. The association of optic dysplasia with hydrolethalus suggests that the effects of the gene disorder may occur as early as the 24th day of embryonic development. The particularly severe craniofacial manifestations noted in this infant suggest a sequence of secondary malformations in which the rapidly expanding hydrocephalus outpaces the growth of the cranial and facial structures.

Cranial decompression is often a necessity for vaginal delivery. Brainstem and cord compression at the level of the stenotic foramen magnum or anomalous respiratory tract development are contributory causes of death in individuals with the disorder.

Prenatal diagnosis by ultrasound as early as 16–18 weeks should be possible; one of the original patients described by Salonen et al [1] was detected at 18 weeks' gestation. Two others did not show definite hydrocephalus until 25 weeks. However, the likelihood of such early prenatal diagnosis is complicated by the occurrence of a more typical hydrocephalus noted in some of the patients of Salonen et al. Such hydrocephalus may develop at any time during late second and third trimesters, so ultrasonic confirmation of an affected fetus may not always be possible before 24 weeks. In addition, two sibs of affected individuals did not have hydrocephalus by physical examination but were thought to have hydrolethalus. One was described as a "classic" anencephalic with multiple other anomalies and atypically small, recessed eyes. This could have been a coincidental occurrence in a family of both a complex anencephaly and hydrolethalus; alternatively, anencephaly may be another manifestation of the developmental field defect resulting in hydrolethalus. The description of the eyes supports the latter explanation. The other patient with two sibs with hydrolethalus had no apparent hydrocephalus at birth, but did have a small mandible and an anomalous tongue. No postmortem examination was done and no comment was made about parental facial characteristics. It is difficult to be certain of the implications of this particular individual's abnormalities for prenatal diagnosis.

TABLE II. List of Differential Diagnoses of Hydrolethalus (HL) and Common Manifestations

Features	HL	T13	Meckel	RSH	SOD	Warburg	OAVD	Fryns	A/Poly-splenia
Polyhydramnios	++++	+	−	±	−	±	−	++	±
Prenatal growth retardation	−	+	+	+	−	−	+	−	−
Neonatal death	++++	++	++++	±	−	++	±	++++	+
Central nervous system									
Hydrocephalus	++++	+	+	++	±	++++	++	−	±
Midline defects	++++	++++	++++	++	++	+++	++	+	±
Craniofacial									
Micrognathia	++++	+++	++	++++	−	−	++	++++	−
CL/P	++	+++	++/+	++/	−	−	++	++++/+	±
Low malformed ears	+++	++++	++++	+++	−	+	++++	++	−
Micro/anophthalmia	++++	+++	+++	−	−	++	++	+	−
Optic nerve hypoplasia	+	+	++	−	++++	+	?	−	−
Unusual face	+++	++++	+++	++++	−	+++	+++	+++	−
Cardiac and respiratory									
Septal/vessel defects	++	+++	+	++	−	−	++	−	+++
Respiratory tract anomalies other than hypoplastic lung	+++	+	+	±	−	−	+	+++	+++
Gastrointestinal	+	+++	+	±	−	±	−	++	++++
Genitourinary									
Hydronephrosis/ureter	+	+	+	+	−	−	+	+	±
Abnormality of external genitalia	+	++++	++++	++	−	−	−	+	−
Skeletal									
Polydactyly	++++	++++	++	+	−	−	−	−	−

Key: HL = hydrolethalus; T13 = Trisomy 13; Meckel syndrome; RSH = Smith Lemli-Opitz syndrome; SOD = septo-optic "dysplasia"; Warburg syndrome; OAVD = oculo-auriculo-vertebral dysplasia; Fryns syndrome; A/polysplenia = asplenia/polysplenia syndromes.
Interpretation by the authors of the frequency of anomalies is as follows: ++++ greater than 75%; +++ roughly 75%; ++roughly 50%; + roughly 25%; ± roughly 1–15%; − virtually 0.

TABLE III. Major Differentiating Characteristics

Trait	Likely Diagnoses
Chromosomal abnormality	Trisomy 13, others
Interhemispheric cerebral cyst	Hydrolethalus
Encephalocele	Warburg, OAVD
Agyria	Warburg
"Keyhole" foramen magnum	Hydrolethalus
Anterior chamber defects/retinal dysplasia	Trisomy 13, Warburg
Situs inversus	Asplenia/polysplenia, trisomy 13
Diaphragmatic hernia	Trisomy 13, Fryns syndrome
Pancreatic giant cells	RSH syndrome
Renal cysts	Trisomy 13, Meckel, RSH, Fryns syndrome
Polydactyly	Hydrolethalus, trisomy 13, Meckel, RSH syndrome
Hemivertebrae	OAVD

The mother, at the time of this report, is pregnant without evidence of hydrolethalus in the fetus by ultrasound at 15 or 19 weeks' gestation.

ACKNOWLEDGMENTS

We are grateful to Dr. Richard Pauli for his helpful discussion, Sandy Keller for her drawing and secretarial assistance, Jeannie Olson for secretarial assistance, and Jim Olson for photography. Our thanks to Dr. Meghan Landauer for referring this family to us.

REFERENCES

1. Salonen R, Herva R, Norio R: The hydrolethalus syndrome: Delineation of a "new," lethal malformation syndrome based on 28 patients. Clin Genet 19:321–330, 1981.
2. Toriello HV, Bauserman SC: Bilateral pulmonary agenesis: Association with the hydrolethalus syndrome and review of the literature from a developmental field perspective. Am J Med Genet 21:93–104, 1985.
3. Magenis E, Hecht F: Chromosome thirteen trisomy syndrome. In *Birth Defects Compendium*, 2nd Ed. New York: Alan R. Liss, 1979, pp 212–213.
4. Fraser FC, Lytwyn A: Spectrum of anomalies in the Meckel syndrome, or: "Maybe there is a syndrome with at least one constant anomaly." Am J Med Genet 9:67–73, 1981.
5. Mecke S, Passarge E: Encephalocoele, polycystic kidneys and polydactyly as an autosomal recessive trait simulating certain other disorders: The Meckel syndrome. Ann Génét 14:97–103, 1971.

6. Johnson VP: Smith-Lemli-Opitz syndrome: Review and report of 2 affected siblings. Z Kinderheilk 119:221–234, 1975.
7. Lowry RB: Editorial comment: Variability in the Smith-Lemli-Opitz syndrome: Overlap with the Meckel syndrome. Am J Med Genet 14:429–433, 1983.
8. Acers TE: Optic nerve hypoplasia: Septo-optic-pituitary dysplasia syndrome. Trans Am Ophthalmol Soc 79:425–457, 1981.
9. Margalith D, Jan JJ, McCormick AQ, Tze WJ, Lapointe J: Clinical spectrum of congenital optic nerve hypoplasia: Review of 51 patients. Dev Med Child Neurol 26:311–322, 1984.
10. Aymé S, Mattei JF: HARD (±E) syndrome: Report of a sixth family with support for autosomal recessive inheritance. Am J Med Genet 14:759–766, 1983.
11. Bordarier C, Aicardi J, Goutières F: Congenital hydrocephalus and eye abnormalities with severe developmental brain defects: Warburg's syndrome. Ann Neurol 16:60–65, 1984.
12. Feingold M, Baum J: Goldenhar's syndrome. Am J Dis Child 132:136–138, 1978.
13. Pauli RM, Jung JH, McPherson EW: Letter to the Editor: Goldenhar association and cranial defects. Am J Med Genet 15:177–179, 1983.
14. Wilson G: Cranial defects in the Goldenhar syndrome. Am J Med Genet 14:435–43, 1983.
15. Lubinsky M, Severn C, Rapoport JM: Fryns syndrome: A new variable, multiple congenital anomaly (MCA) syndrome. Am J Med Genet 14:461–466, 1983.
16. Freedom RM: The asplenia syndrome: A review of significant extra-cardiac structural abnormalities in 29 necropsied patients. J Pediatr 81:1130–1133, 1972.
17. Mishalany H, Mahnovski V, Woolley M: Congenital asplenia and anomalies of the gastrointestinal tract. Surgery 91:38–41, 1982.
18. Peoples WM, Moller JH, Edwards JE: Polysplenia: A review of 146 cases. Pediatr Cardiol 4:129–137, 1983.
19. Rose V, Izukawa T, Moes CAF: Syndromes of asplenia and polysplenia. A review of cardiac and non-cardiac malformations in 60 cases with special reference to diagnosis and prognosis. Br Heart J 37:840–852, 1975.
20. Opitz JM, Gilbert EF: Editorial comment - CNS anomalies and the midline as a developmental field. Am J Med Genet 12:443–455, 1982.

NOTED ADDED IN PROOF: Serial ultrasounds during pregnancy did not detect hydrolethalus and the pregnancy resulted in a normal, full term infant.

Congenital Tumors

Jorge Las Heras, MD, PhD, and Hart Isaacs, MD

Instituto de Investigaciones Clinicas, University of Chile, Hospital Paula Jaraquemada, Casilla 5370-Correo 3, Santiago, Chile (JLH) and Department of Pathology, Children's Hospital of Los Angeles, Los Angeles, California 90024 (HI)

INTRODUCTION

Since the classic review of neonatal tumors by Wells in 1940 [1], only a few large series describing tumors in early life have appeared in the literature [2–5]. It has been suggested that tumors that manifest at birth or shortly thereafter have a more favorable prognosis than similar tumors occurring in later life. On this basis some authors [6] have postulated an "oncogenic grace period," beginning in utero and extending into the perinatal period, during which tumors rarely metastasize and even tend to regress. However, some neoplasms initially appearing benign may undergo malignant transformation in later life. Therefore, early diagnosis and proper management of this group are essential for a favorable outcome.

This study reviews the clinical and pathologic characteristics and clinical evolution in newborn infants with tumors seen at the Children's Hospital of Los Angeles during a 15-year period.

MATERIALS AND METHODS

All cases of tumors in children under 1 month of age diagnosed by biopsy or autopsy at Children's Hospital of Los Angeles (CHLA) during the period

Birth Defects: Original Article Series, Volume 23, Number 1, pages 421–431

from 1964 through 1978 were reviewed. Clinical records and follow-up data of the patients were obtained from the Tumor Registry files of CHLA.

Biopsy and autopsy protocols and microscopic sections of the tumors were available for review in all cases, and in many instances tissue was available for more detailed study. Lymphangiomas, hemangiomas, and nevi were excluded from the study.

RESULTS

During the period from 1964 through 1978, 42 neonatal tumors were registered in the Tumor Registry of CHLA (Table I). These neonatal tumors comprised 2% of all pediatric neoplasms recorded over the same period of time (leukemia recorded for autopsies only; all other tumors for biopsy or autopsy). The frequency of tumors in both sexes was the same.

Teratomas

Teratomas occurred in 17 patients (40.5%) (Table II). Nine occurred in females and 8 in males; 14 teratomas were from the sacrococcygeal area and 1 each in the soft palate, thyroid, and nasopharynx (Fig. 1).

In 6 patients the teratoma contained benign, mature tissue only. Mature and immature tissues were found in 7 tumors, and 3 patients had teratomas with histologic malignancy (Table III). The malignant components were all

TABLE I. Congenital Tumors (CHLA, 1964–1978)

Type	Male	Female	No.	%
Teratoma	8	9	17	40.5
Leukemia*	3	2	5	11.8
Neuroblastoma	1	4	5	11.8
Fibrosarcoma-like fibromatosis	2	2	4	9.5
Histiocytosis X	2	—	2	4.8
Mesoblastic nephroma	1	1	2	4.8
Lipoblastoma	1	—	1	2.4
Hepatoblastoma	1	—	1	2.4
Embryonal carcinoma	1	—	1	2.4
Fibrous histiocytoma	—	1	1	2.4
Rhabdomyosarcoma	—	1	1	2.4
Astrocytoma	—	1	1	2.4
Rhabdomyoma	1	—	1	2.4
Total	21 (50%)	21 (50%)	42	100.0

*Only autopsy cases.

TABLE II. Teratoma: Anatomic Location

Location	Male	Female	No.	%
Sacrococcygeal	6	8	14	82.3
Palate	1	—	1	5.9
Thyroid	1	—	1	5.9
Nasopharynx	—	1	1	5.9
Total	8 (47%)	9 (53%)	17	100.0

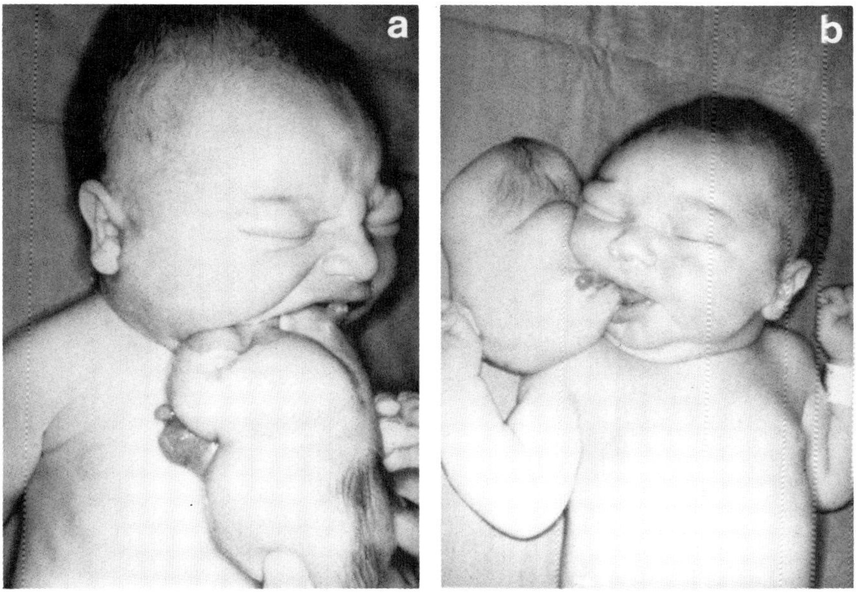

Fig. 1. Nasopharyngeal teratoma presenting in the neonatal period.

embryonal carcinomas. Of the 17 patients, 16 are living without known residual tumor, and 1 patient with sacrococcygeal teratoma containing malignant tissue died at 2 10/12 years with metastases to lung and liver.

Leukemia

Leukemia occurred in 5 patients (11.8%) (Table IV). Three had acute myelogenous leukemia; in 2 the type of acute leukemia was not specified. All 5 infants with leukemia died within 5 months after diagnosis. One was treated with prednisone and died within the first week of treatment. The

TABLE III. Teratoma: Histologic Classification

Location	Benign "Adult" Components		Embryonic Components		Malignant Components		Total
	No.	%	No.	%	No.	%	
Sacrococcygeal	5		6		3*†		14
Palate	1		0		0		1
Thyroid	0		1		0		1
Nasopharynx	1		0		0		1
Total	7	41.2	7	41.2	3	17.6	17

*All embryonal carcinomas.
†One died at 2 10/12 years (metastases to lung and liver).

TABLE IV. Leukemia Tumors*

Case No.	Type	Age at Diagnosis (days)	Sex	Clinical Presentation	Treatment	Follow-up
1.	Acute myelogenous	26	F	Splenomegaly, lymphadenomegaly, cutaneous bruising, leukemia cutis	Steroids	Died at 1 mo. 6 d. I.V. hemorrhage
2.	Acute myelogenous	14		Papular rash, GI bleeding	Chemotherapy	Died at 5 mo. pneumoc. pneum.
3.	Acute myelogenous	1	F	Petechiae, hepatomegaly	None	Died at 21 days viral pneumonitis
4.	Acute, not specified	7	M	Jaundice	None	Died at 1 mo. sepsis
5.	Acute, not specified	28	M	Papular rash, bleeding, fever	None	Died at 1 mo. 9 d. sepsis

*All autopsy cases.

infant who survived for 5 months received chemotherapy and died of pneumonia. The other 3 died within the first month of life without specific treatment.

Neuroblastoma

Neuroblastoma was detected in 5 patients (11.8%) (Table V). There was a preponderance of females (4 to 1). One infant died a few hours after birth and the autopsy showed a neuroblastoma in the neck and metastases to the liver and bone marrow.

Another infant had a neuroblastoma in the posterior mediastinum as a solitary lesion. This patient was treated with chemotherapy and was disease-free 7 years after diagnosis.

TABLE V. Neuroblastoma Tumors

Case No.	Sex	Age at Diagnosis	Site of Tumor	Treatment	Metastasis	Follow-up
1.	M	11 days	Posterior mediastinum	Chemotherapy	None	7 years no recurrence
2.	F	2 days	Retroperitoneum	Chemotherapy	Liver, BM Stage IV-S	3 years no recurrence
3.	F	4 days	Retroperitoneum	Chemotherapy	Iris, bilateral	1½ years no recurrence
4.	F	6 days	Retroperitoneum	Chemotherapy	Liver, periaortic LN Stage IV-S	9 years no recurrence
5.	F	14 hrs	Neck	None	Liver, EM	Died at 14 hrs

TABLE VI. Fibrosarcoma-like Fibromatosis

Case No.	Sex	Age at Diagnosis	Site of Tumor	Treatment	Recurrence or Metastases	Follow-up
1.	F	At birth	Face	Surgery	No	13 years
2.	M	At birth	Neck	Surgery	No	10 years
3.	F	2 weeks	Chest	Surgery	No	10 years
4.	M	At birth	Left flank	Surgery	No	12 years

A third infant had an abdominal neuroblastoma and metastases in both ocular regions. She received chemotherapy and had no recurrences 1½ years after diagnosis.

The other 2 patients had Stage IV-S neuroblastoma. Both received chemotherapy and were disease-free 3 and 9 years, respectively, after diagnosis.

Congenital Fibrosarcoma-like Fibromatosis (CF-LF)

CF-LF occurred in 4 infants (9.5%) (Table VI). In all but one, the tumor was detected at birth as a solitary mass and affected the face, neck, chest, or left flank. The four infants were treated solely with excision of the tumor and were alive without recurrence some 13, 12, 10 and 10 years of follow-up.

Histiocytosis X

Histiocytosis X occurred in 2 infants (4.8%) (Table VII). One was treated with chemotherapy and died at home 3 months after diagnosis. No autopsy was performed. The other, who survived 4 months, was taken out of the hospital by the family who refused treatment. He was readmitted the day of his death. The autopsy showed widespread disease.

TABLE VII. Histiocytosis X

Case No.	Sex	Mode of Presentation	Organs Involved	Treatment	Follow-up
1.	M	Since 1 week: petechial rash, lymphadenopathy, hepatosplenomegaly, anemia, thrombocytopenia	LN, skin	Chemotherapy	Died at 3 months Sepsis, no autopsy
2.	M	Since 2 weeks: petechial rash, hepatosplenomegaly	Liver, lungs, spleen, brain, kidney, testis, LN, bones, muscle	—	Died at 4 months

TABLE VIII. Congenital Mesoblastic Nephroma

Case No.	Sex	Age at Diagnosis	Site of tumor	Treatment	Follow-up
1.	M	3 days	Right	Nephrectomy	11 years, no metast.
2.	F	At birth	Right	Nephrectomy	3 years, no metast.

Congenital Mesoblastic Nephroma

Mesoblastic nephroma was detected in the right kidney of 2 patients (4.8%) (Table VIII). Nephrectomy was performed. Both patients are disease-free 11 and 3 years, respectively, after diagnosis.

Miscellaneous

This heterogeneous group included an embryonal carcinoma, a fibrous histiocytoma, a hepatoblastoma, a case of lipoblastomatosis, an astrocytoma, a rhabdomyosarcoma, and a rhabdomyoma (Table IX). The infant with the embryonal carcinoma died of a respiratory distress syndrome on the first day of life; autopsy showed a left cervical tumor with metastases to the lymph nodes and both adrenals. The fibrous histiocytoma was in the posterior and medial portions of the nasal cavity. The only treatment was surgery; the tumor recurred locally 5 years after diagnosis. After additional surgery the patient was tumor-free 10 years after the initial operation.

The hepatoblastoma occurred as a single mass in the right lobe of the liver. The patient was treated solely with surgery and was without recurrence or metastasis 1 year after diagnosis. The patient with lipoblastomatosis had a large mass in the left buttock and was treated with surgery. The patient was lost to follow-up after 14 years of disease-free survival.

TABLE IX. Miscellaneous Tumors

Case No.	Type of Tumor	Sex	Mode of Presentation	Site of Tumor	Treatment	Recurrence or Metastasis	Follow-up
1.	Embryonal carcinoma	M	Respiratory distress, deviation of trachea, at birth	Left cervical, involving pharynx, larynx, esophagus	—	Adrenals, LN	Died at 1 day HMD
2.	Fibrous histiocytoma	F	Respiratory diffic. and persistent drainage left nostril, 5 days	Posterior and medial portions of the nasal cavity	Surgery	Recurrence at 5 years	10 years, no recurrence
3.	Hepatoblastoma	M	Large hepatomegaly, at birth	Right lobe of liver	Surgery	No	1 year, no recurrence
4.	Lipoblastoma	M	Large mass, at birth	Left buttocks	Surgery	No	14 years, no recurrence
5.	Astrocytoma	F	Progressive hydrocephaly from birth	Right hemisphere	Surgery	—	Died at 1 year 3 mos.
6.	Rhabdomyosarcoma	M	Mass at birth	Right orbit	Radiation chemotherapy	Cervical LN recurrence at 2 months	2 years, no reccurrence
7.	Rhabdomyoma	M	Unusual ECG pattern on routine examination	Posterior wall of left ventricle	Surgery	—	Died at 6 weeks

The infant with an astrocytoma was operated on at age 1 month and received no additional treatment. She died of pneumonia at 1 3/12 years. Autopsy was not performed. The infant with rhabdomyosarcoma had a mass in the right orbit. He received radiotherapy and chemotherapy; 2 months later the tumor recurred in cervical lymph nodes. He continued receiving chemotherapy and was doing well 2 years after the initial diagnosis.

The rhabdomyoma involved the posterior wall of the left ventricle of the heart. The patient was operated on at 6 weeks and died during the procedure.

Developmental Anomalies and Associated Congenital Tumors

Associated congenital defects were present in 4 of the cases with congenital tumors (Table X). Two patients with leukemia had trisomy 21. One of the infants with a sacrococcygeal teratoma had an imperforate anus. The patient with the rhabdomyoma had tuberous sclerosis.

DISCUSSION

A considerable amount of data have been published on the epidemiology of neoplasms in childhood, but references about the frequency of either benign or malignant congenital tumors are scarce. However, as pointed out by Gale et al [5], the occurrence of cancer in the first month of life is probably on the same order as any other 4-week period of childhood.

The death rate from malignancies in children less than 28 old days has been reported as 6.24 per 10^6 live births [2–7]; over 50% of these deaths occurred in the first week of life.

The study by Wells [1] on congenital tumors remains a classic. He collected 255 cases of congenital tumors from the literature, including his own cases, and discussed the significance of congenital malignant growths. Andersen [7] also reported on a large series of neonatal tumors during a 15-year period. Other series of congenital tumors were reported from the Pediatric Pathology Society [3], the National Cancer Institute's Third National Cancer Survey (TNCS) [4], and from the Children's Hospital of Philadelphia [5]. Recently, Dehner [8] completed a comprehensive review of

TABLE X. Developmental Anomalies and Associated Neonatal Tumors

Type of Tumor	No. of Cases	Anomaly
Leukemia	2	Down syndrome (trisomy 21)
Rhabdomyoma	1	Tuberous sclerosis
Sacrococcygeal teratoma	1	Imperforate anus

neoplasms of the fetus and newborn infant, and discussed some of the clinical and pathologic problems posed by congenital tumors.

In the present study, teratomas were the numerically most important group, accounting for 40.5% of the tumors in this series. Teratomas of the sacrococcygeal region are by far the commonest germ cell tumors in the neonatal period [8,9]. In our study, they represented 82.3% of the teratoma group. The 3 cases with malignant components (embryonal carcinoma) belonged to this group. The malignancy rate of 17.6% was similar to that reported by other workers [10]. Other investigators have described a higher incidence of teratomas in females [11]; however, our study showed no relationship between racial, social class, or sex.

Congenital leukemia occurred in 11.8% of the series. This is an uncommon and controversial disorder and according to some workers [4], is the most frequent cause of tumor death in the first month of life. In our series 3 of the cases were fatal examples of acute myelogenous leukemia,and in 2 the primary neoplasm was not highly differentiated. Nevertheless, all of them fulfilled some of the criteria for the diagnosis of congenital leukemia [12]. All the infants died within a period of 5 months regardless of treatment.

Neuroblastoma also represented an important group (11.8%) of neoplasms in this series. Among the retroperitoneal tumors in the newborn infant, approximately ⅔ are neuroblastomas [8]. This was the commonest site of origin in our group. The 3 infants with abdominal tumor had evidence of metastases at the time of diagnosis (Stage IV-s). However, regardless of the extent of the metastases, the clinical evolution and response to chemotherapy was excellent. This finding was in agreement with most reports suggesting that the survival rate for stage IV-s neuroblastoma is 60–70% compared to 30–40% survival for all ages of neuroblastoma [13].

Congenital fibrosarcoma-like fibromatosis (CL-LF) is a term that was coined by Dehner to replace the more ominous-sounding term congenital fibrosarcoma [8]. In fact, despite the morphologic similarities with adult fibrosarcoma, these tumors rarely metastasize or recur following adequate surgical excision. In our series we had 4 cases of CF-LF that were treated successfully with simple surgical resection and were free of disease after several years of follow-up.

Neoplastic disorders of the monocyte-macrophage system in the neonate are represented almost exclusively by histiocytosis X [14]. In our series there were 2 infants who died during the first 4 months of life. The rapidly progressive and lethal course of this disorder is reflected by a survival rate of only 18.9% at 2 years [15].

Congenital mesoblastic nephroma occurred in two cases. This is the commonest renal neoplasm in the newborn infant and rarely presents beyond the first year of life. The right kidney is affected more often than the left, as it happened in our patients, and all cases to date have been unilateral [8]. The prognosis of this tumor seems to be excellent after simple nephrectomy.

In the miscellaneous group we had 1 case of rhabdomyosarcoma. This tumor was found in the orbit and showed an excellent response to treatment in spite of early recurrence at age 2 months. These tumors in the neonatal period are usually, as in our case, very undifferentiated.

Two of the patients died due to surgical complications (astrocytoma and rhabdomyoma) and 1 died of respiratory distress at 1 day of age (cervical embryonal carcinoma). The infant with the rhabdomyoma also had tuberous sclerosis. The association between the rhabdomyoma and the latter disease has been widely reported in the literature [16].

The patient with the hepatoblastoma underwent surgery and had a favorable evolution without additional treatment.

The remaining patients in this series (a fibrous histiocytoma and a lipoblastoma) were treated with local surgery. The infant with a fibrous histiocytoma had a recurrence at age 5 years; after surgery her follow-up was uneventful.

It has been reported that congenital defects are more often present among children with malignant tumors than among control children [17]. The findings in our series do not reflect this incidence and are consistent with the view of Wells [1] and other authors [2] who found no evidence of inheritance in congenital malignancies except for a few specific tumors (retinoblastoma, Wilms tumor, leukemia). Nonetheless, the apparently increased risk of neonatal leukemia in Down syndrome, as present in our series, is consistent with the concept that prenatal, and possibly prezygotic, factors are critical in some cancers developing soon after birth [2].

Congenital tumors remain a rarity, so any conclusion about their origin and biologic behavior must be obtained from epidemiologic studies and larger series of cases. The available evidence suggests that most congenital tumors are caused by factors qualitatively similar to those causing corresponding tumors of later childhood. The collaboration between oncologists, cytogeneticists, virologists, pathologists, and other scientists may help to disclose the probable causal factors in these tumors.

REFERENCES

1. Wells HG: Occurrence and significance of congenital malignant neoplasms. Arch Pathol 30:535–601, 1940.
2. Fraumeni JF, Miller RW: Cancer deaths in the newborn. Am J Dis Child 117:186–189, 1969.

3. Barson AJ: Congenital neoplasia: The Society's experience. Arch Dis Child 53:436, 1978.
4. Bader JL, Miller RW: U.S. cancer incidence and mortality in the first year of life. Am J Dis Child 133:157–159, 1979.
5. Gale GB, D'Angio GJ, Uri A, Chatten J, Koop CE: Cancer in neonates: The experience at the Children's Hospital of Philadelphia. Pediatrics 70:409–413, 1982.
6. Bolande RP: Neoplasia of early life and its relationship to teratogenesis. Perspect Pediatr Pathol 3:145–183, 1976.
7. Andersen DH: Tumors of infancy and childhood. I. A survey of those seen in the pathology laboratory of the Babies Hospital during the years 1935–1950. Cancer 4:890–906, 1952.
8. Dehner LP: Neoplasms of the fetus and neonate. In Naeye RL, Kissane J (eds): "Perinatal Diseases." Baltimore: Williams & Wilkins, 1981, pp 286–345.
9. Mahour GH, Woolley MM, Trivedi SN, Landing BH: Teratomas in infancy and childhood: Experience with 81 cases. Surgery 76:309–318, 1974.
10. Lawson DN, Steward JK: Facilities for paediatric cancer cases and children's tumour registration. In Bloom HJG, Lemerle J, Weidhardt MK, Voute PA (eds): "Cancer in Children." New York: Springer-Verlag, 1975, pp 85–89.
11. Berry CL, Keeling J, Hilton C: Teratoma in infancy and childhood: A review of 91 cases. J Pathol 98:241–252, 1969.
12. Pochedly C: Thrombocytopenic purpura of the newborn. Obstet Gynecol Surv 26:63–103, 1971.
13. Kinnier Wilson LM, Draper GJ: Neuroblastoma, its natural history and prognosis: A study of 487 cases. Br Med J 3:301–307, 1974.
14. Newton WA, Hamoudi AB: Histiocytosis: A histologic classification with clinical correlation. Perspect Pediatr Pathol 1:251–283, 1973.
15. Doede KG, Rappaport H: Long-term survival of patients with acute differentiated histiocytosis (Letterer-Siwe disease). Cancer 20:1782–1795, 1967.
16. Fenoglio JJ Jr, McAllister JA Jr, Ferrans VJ: Cardiac rhabdomyoma: A clinico-pathologic and electron microscopic study. Am J Cardiol 38:241–251, 1976.
17. Miller RW: Relation between cancer and congenital defects in man. N Engl J Med 275:87–93, 1966.

Nonimmunologic Hydrops Fetalis Due to Intrauterine Closure of Fetal Foramen Ovale

Ronald W. Olson, MD, Makoto Nishibatake, MD, Sunita Arya, MD, and Enid F. Gilbert, MD

Departments of Obstetrics and Gynecology (RWO) and Pathology (MN, SA, EFG), University of Wisconsin, Madison, Wisconsin 53792

INTRODUCTION

With the marked reduction of Rh-isoimmunization since the introduction of Rh immunoglobulin in 1968, nonimmunologic fetal hydrops has assumed increased importance. Anderson [1] found a 30-fold increase in the percent of fetal deaths due to nonimmune hydrops from 1970 to 1979, and in 1979, 3 fetal deaths due to nonimmune causes for every 1 due to immune disease.

Ultrasound has made easier the prenatal diagnosis of fetal hydrops [2], but, since most of the nonimmune causes are amenable neither to prevention nor to treatment, the mortality rates have remained high [3,4].

Congenital fetal cardiac disease, with the exception of severe arrythmia, rarely results in hydrops or antenatal death, unless accompanied by other fetal anomalies [3]. Exceptions are conditions that significantly impair the usual right-to-left shunting in the fetal heart. We present an instance of *in utero* closure of the foramen ovale with resulting fetal hydrops and death.

CLINICAL REPORT

The patient, a 31-year-old primigravida, was referred at 27 weeks of gestation because of sonographic evidence of fetal hydrops. Her pregnancy had been uncomplicated until the 24th week when excessive uterine size was noted, prompting ultrasonic examination and referral at 27 weeks. Her past

Birth Defects: Original Article Series, Volume 23, Number 1, pages 433–442

medical history was unremarkable and her family history significant only for adult-onset diabetes.

Her general exam showed no abnormality except for a fundal height of 36 cm. Fetal heart tones were regular at 136/minute. She was blood type "O" Rh positive, with an unreactive antibody screen. Glucose levels were normal. VDRL was nonreactive and she was rubella-immune. Maternal blood did not contain fetal cells.

Ultrasound examination (Figs. 1,2) showed a large homogeneous placenta and mild polyhydramnios. The fetus presented as a breech and there was little movement. Gross fetal ascites was noted. A "cystic mass" measuring 29 × 34 mm was noted in the fetal thorax, thought to represent an enlarged left atrium. Congenital structural heart disease was suspected. After discussion with the patient, a conservative course of action was considered most appropriate.

The patient returned in 1 week. Fundal height was 36 cm and fetal heart tones 132/minute. Fetal movement, though present, was reduced. Repeat ultrasound examination showed no significant interval change; conservative management was continued. One week later the fundal height had increased to 38 cm and the patient noted scant fetal movement. Ultrasonography showed fetal abdominal wall edema and a significant increase in placental size. The fetal heart rate was irregular and the dilated atrium was unchanged (Fig. 3).

A week later the patient returned with absent fetal heart tones. After fetal death was confirmed, labor was induced successfully and the patient delivered a macerated male infant weighing 1425 g, compatible with a 30-week gestational age (Fig. 4).

Significant postmortem findings included (1) Severe hydrops with fluid in the pericardial, pleural, and abdominal cavities; (2) Enlargement of the left and right atria with left ventricular hypertrophy; (3) Severe aortic stenosis, (4) An incompetent mitral valve (Fig. 5); (5) A minute, barely probe-patent foramen ovale (Figs. 5,6); (6) A placenta weighing 680 g—fetal/placental ratio 2.1/1.

DISCUSSION

Normal fetal circulation is shown schematically in Fig. 7. Forty percent of the venous blood from the inferior vena cava, which contains oxygenated blood from the placenta, flows from the right atrium to the left atrium through the foramen ovale. Only 10% of the right ventricular output enters the pulmonary circulation. The rest enters the systemic arterial circulation through

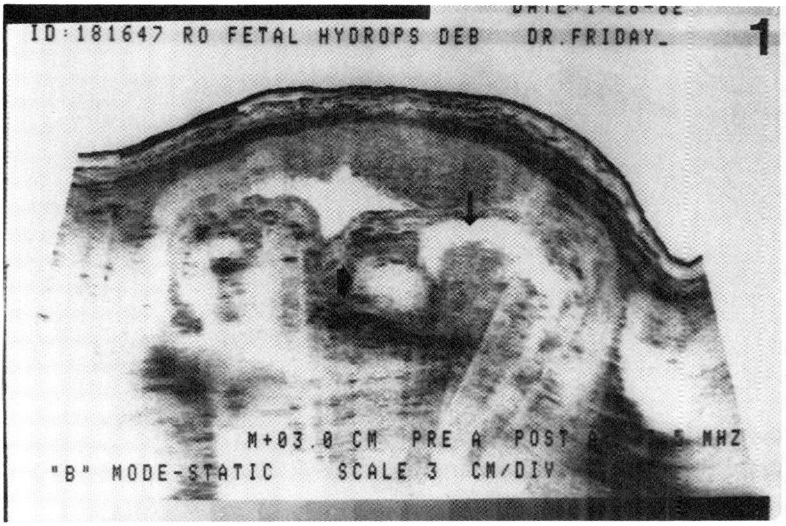

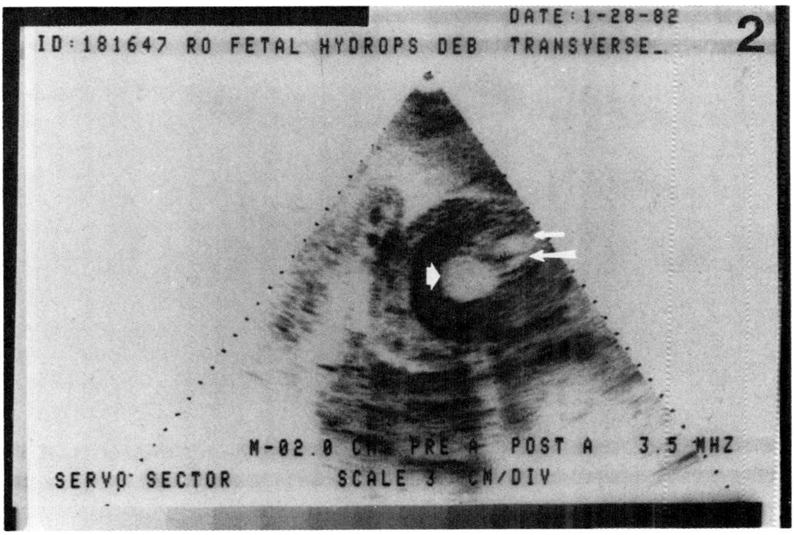

Fig. 1. Sonogram at 27 weeks. Longitudinal scan showing enlarged "left atrium" (arrow head) and massive ascites (arrow).

Fig. 2. Sonogram at 27 weeks. Transverse scan through fetal thorax showing enlarged left atrium (arrow head), right ventricle (large arrow), and left ventricle (small arrow).

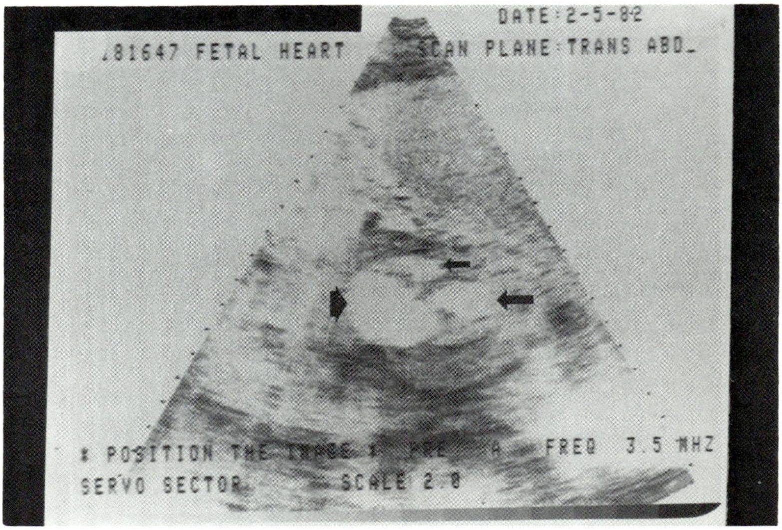

Fig. 3. Sonogram at 29 weeks. Transverse scan through fetal thorax showing enlarged left atrium (arrow head), right ventricle (large arrow), and left ventricle (small arrow).

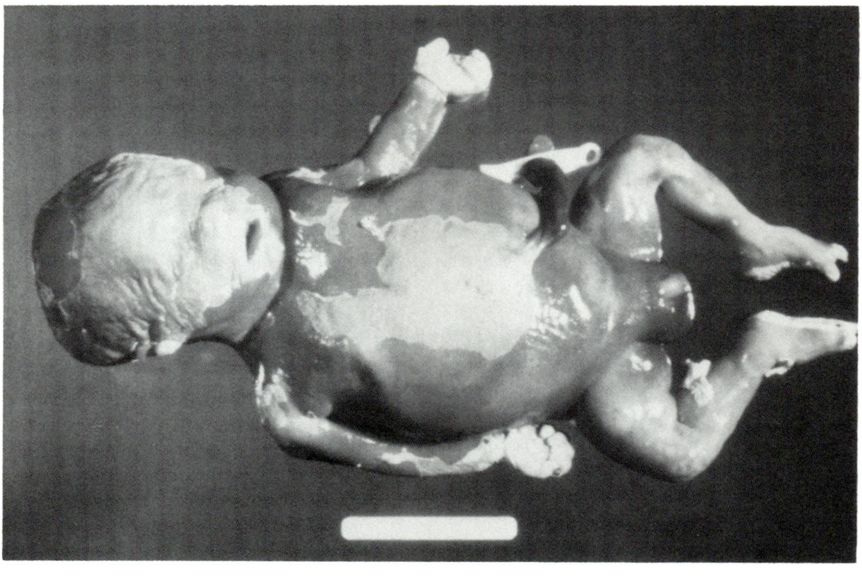

Fig. 4. Severely hydropic fetus stillborn at 30 weeks.

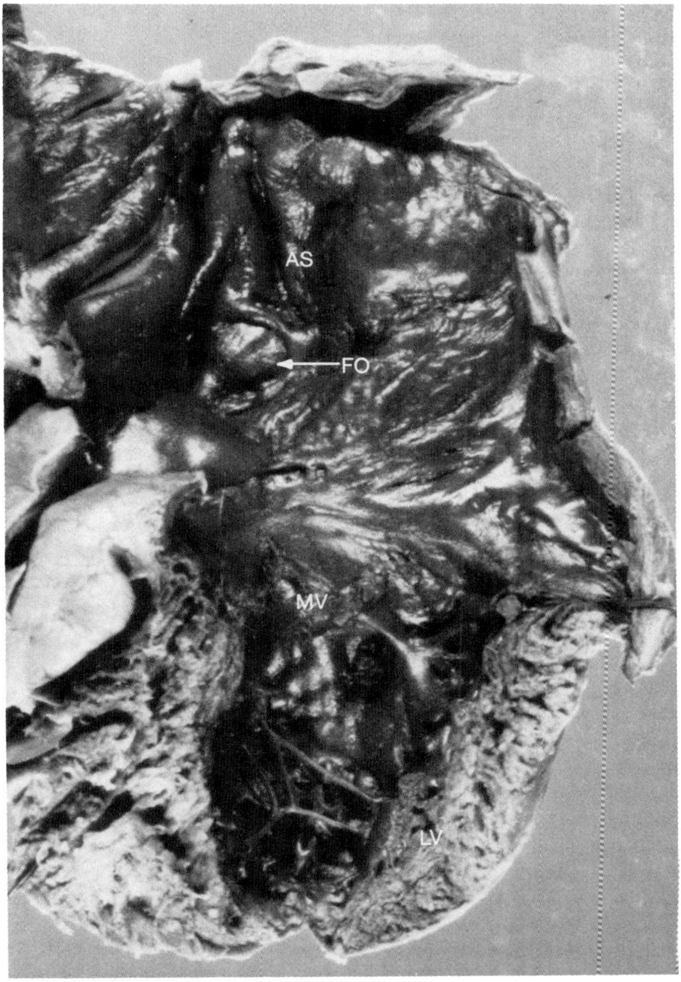

Fig. 5. Atrial septum (A.S.) as seen from the left atrial cavity. The foramen ovale (F.O.) is closed and barely probe-patent. Mitral valve (M.V.) and left ventricle (L.V.).

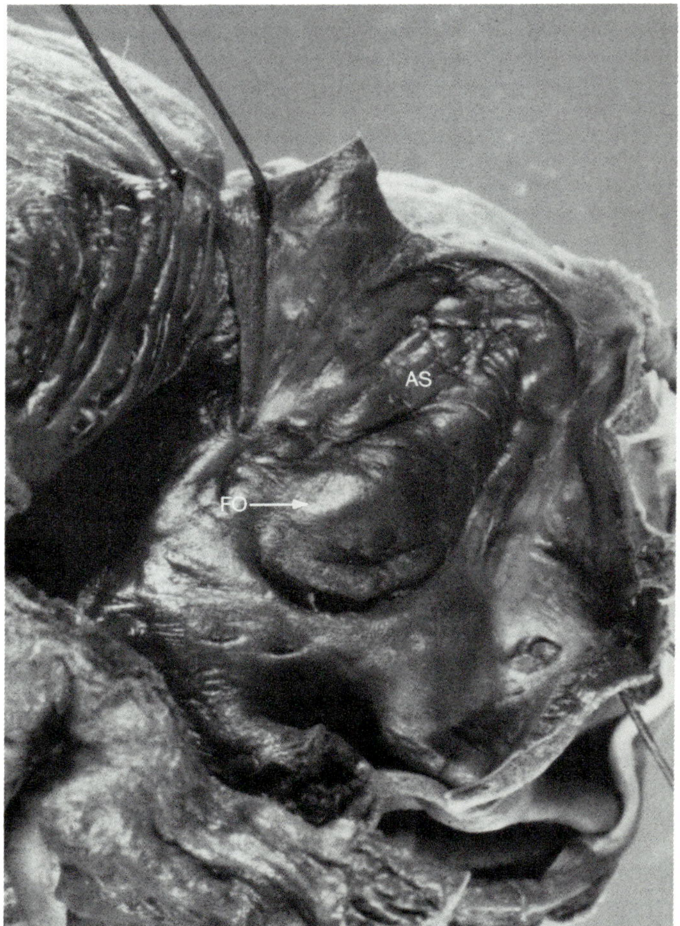

Fig. 6. Atrial septum (A.S.) as seen from the right atrial cavity. Closed foramen ovale (F.O.).

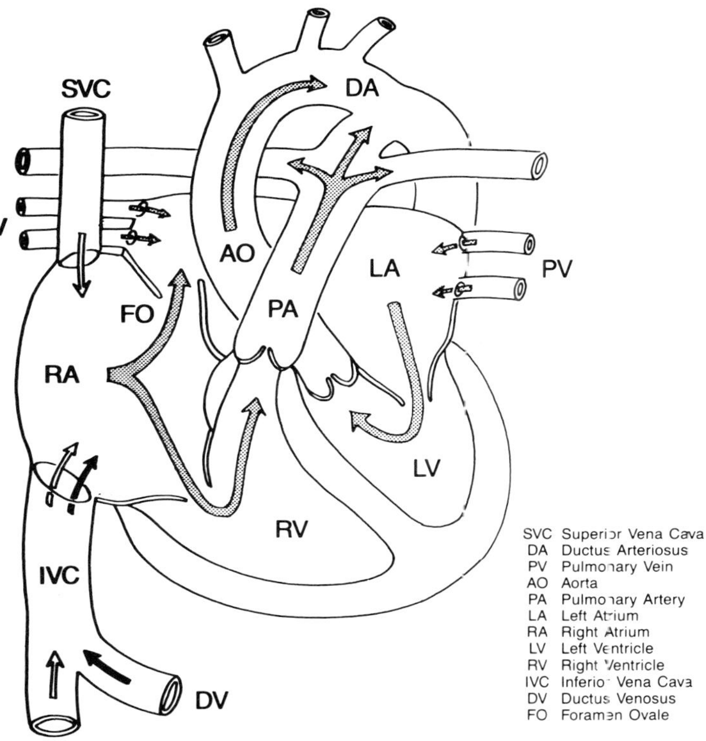

Fig. 7. Normal fetal circulation.

the ductus arteriosus. In the fetal circulation, the right ventricle ejects twice as much blood as the left ventricle. However, the coronary blood supply depends on the output from the left ventricle.

The probable fetal circulation in the case presented is shown in Figure 8 and the probable pathogenesis of congestive heart failure and hydrops illustrated in Figure 9.

Aortic stenosis resulted in increased left ventricular end diastolic pressure. Coupled with mitral regurgitation, this produced increased left atrial pressure which forced the septum primum to close the foramen ovale and resulted in pulmonary edema. Functional closure of the foramen ovale produced right heart volume overload leading to congestive heart failure.

Also, coronary hypoperfusion due to aortic stenosis, probably resulted in inadequate subendocardial perfusion and hypoplasia of the aortic isthmus

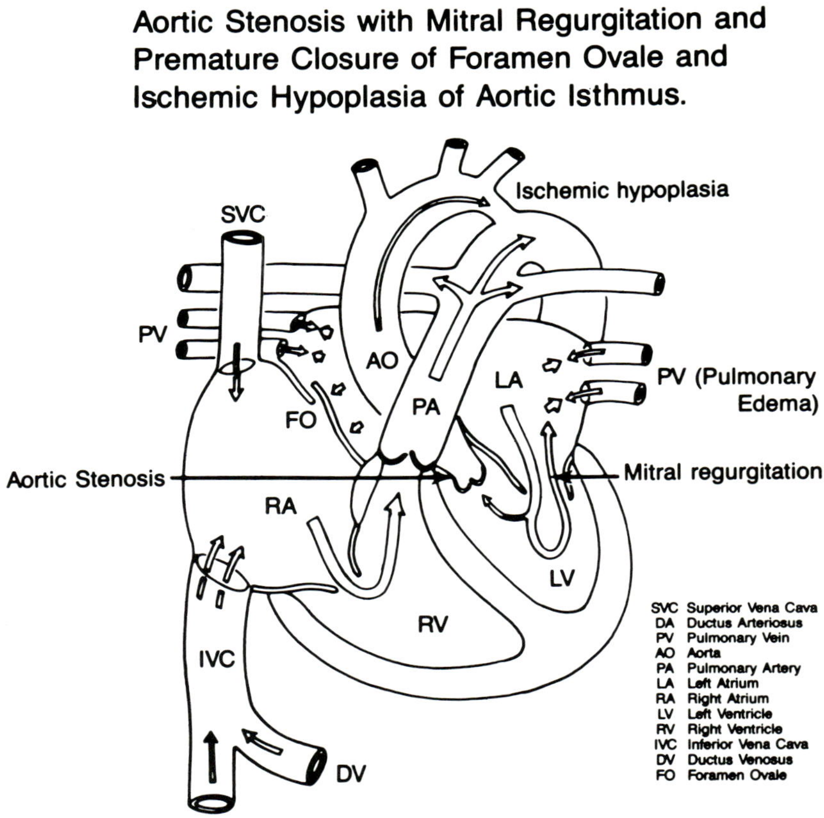

Fig. 8. Postulated abnormality of circulation in this fetus.

with possible decrease in ductus arteriosus flow and further overload of the right heart. Congestive heart failure due to this series of events resulted in increased systemic venous pressure and fetal hydrops.

Prenatal closure or narrowing of the foramen ovale was reported in 12 cases by Naeye [5]. Ten of his subjects were liveborn, neonatal death occurring from 4 hours to 3 weeks after birth. Both stillbirths in his series were at term and none of the 12 demonstrated classic hydrops, though some edema was noted in 6 infants including those stillborn. None of his fetuses demonstrated abnormalities of the aortal or mitral valve. The fetus presented here appeared to have, as the primary pathologic lesions, aortic stenosis and mitral insufficiency with secondary closure, probably in the late second

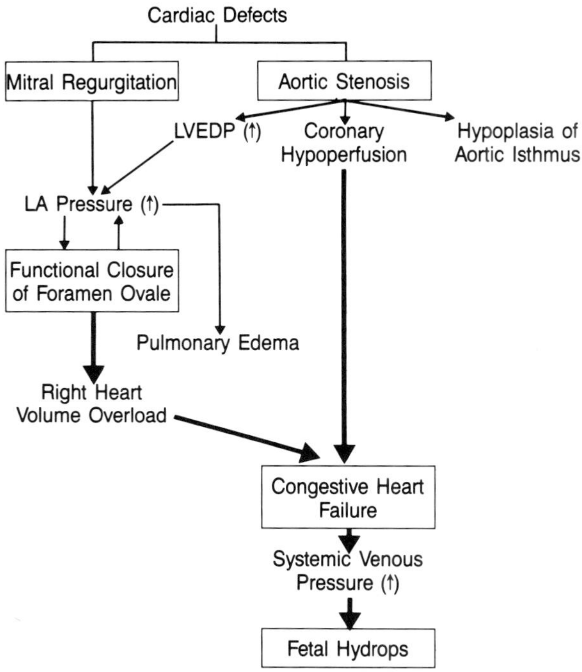

Fig. 9. Pathogenesis of congestive heart failure and fetal hydrops in this fetus.

trimester, of the foramen ovale. Decreased coronary perfusion may also have contributed to heart failure.

CONCLUSION

Nonimmune causes of fetal hydrops are assuming greater relative importance and will be diagnosed more frequently and earlier with increasing use of prenatal ultrasonography. Anatomic fetal cardiac anomalies rarely lead to severe hydrops and fetal death. An exceptional case has been presented. It is debatable whether intervention in the form of early delivery would have altered the final outcome.

REFERENCES

1. Anderson HM, Hutchinson AA, Fortune DW: Nonimmune hydrops fetalis: Changing contribution to perinatal mortality. Br J Obstet Gynecol 90:636–639, 1983.

2. Mahony BS, Filly RA, Callen PW, Chinn DH, Golbus MS: Severe nonimmune hydrops fetalis: Sonographic evaluation. Radiology 151:757–761, 1984.
3. Beischer NA, Fortune DW, Macafee J: Nonimmunologic hydrops fetalis and congenital abnormalities. Obstet Gynecol 38:86–95, 1971.
4. Hutchinson AA, Drew JH, Yu VYH, Williams ML, Fortune DW, Beischer NA: Nonimmunologic hydrops fetalis: A review of 61 cases. Obstet Gynecol 59:347–352, 1982.
5. Naeye RL, Blanc WA: Prenatal narrowing or closure of the foramen ovale. Circulation 30:736–742, 1964.

Experimentally Induced Cardiovascular Malformations in the Chick Embryo. Part I. Morphologic and Physiologic Changes in the Embryonic Chick Heart After Caffeine Administration

Harold J. Bruyere, Jr, PhD, Toshio Nishikawa, MD, Hideo Uno, MD, PhD, Jennifer E. Gilbert, and Enid F. Gilbert, MD

Department of Pathology, University of Wisconsin, School of Medicine, (HJB, TN, JEG, EFG), Madison, Wisconsin 53792, and Wisconsin Regional Primate Research Center (HU), Madison, Wisconsin 53706

Caffeine may be the most widely consumed drug in our society and is especially ubiquitous in Western diets, with intake from foods, over-the-counter drugs, and predominantly, beverages such as coffee, tea, and cola "soft" drinks. It has been suggested that the risk from caffeine to human pregnancy is low and that conservative consumption should not be a cause for concern [1]. However, the safety of caffeine ingestion remains unanswered.

External malformations have been observed in experimental animals following maternal caffeine administration during pregnancy. The effects of the drug on the morphogenesis of major organ systems [2] have not been fully studied. Fujii and Nishimura [3] reported a significant increase in the frequency of cardiac anomalies, relative to offspring from control rats, in offspring from pregnant female rats fed a caffeine-containing diet.

Caffeine administration to Hamburger-Hamilton stage 19 chick embryos (3 days of incubation) had an effect on cardiogenesis with a dose-related production of malformations. A maximum frequency of 70.6% was observed after the administration of 4.7 mg caffeine. Major malformations included

Birth Defects: Original Article Series, Volume 23, Number 1, pages 443–448

common aorticopulmonary trunk and dextroposition of the aorta accompanied by ventricular septal defect with or without pulmonary stenosis.

Dose-response curves showing the effects of caffeine administration on survival rate and frequency of malformations are shown in Figure 1. Survival rate of embryos to day 14 was not affected until caffeine doses reached 2.7 mg/egg. Survival rate was dose-dependent. Furthermore, only at doses 3.5 mg/egg were frequencies of caffeine-treated embryos with a cardiac malformation significantly different from those in control animals. A distribution of specific caffeine-induced cardiac malformations is shown in Table I. Malformations included VSD with an aortic valve that was morphologically normal but more than 50% displaced into the right ventricle, pulmonary stenosis (Fig. 2A) with dextroposition of the aorta and VSD, and common aorticopulmonary trunk with VSD (Fig. 2 B,C).

Effects of caffeine on embryonic heart function were also studied. Qualitative analysis of cinegraphs following administration of 1.0 ml chick Ring-

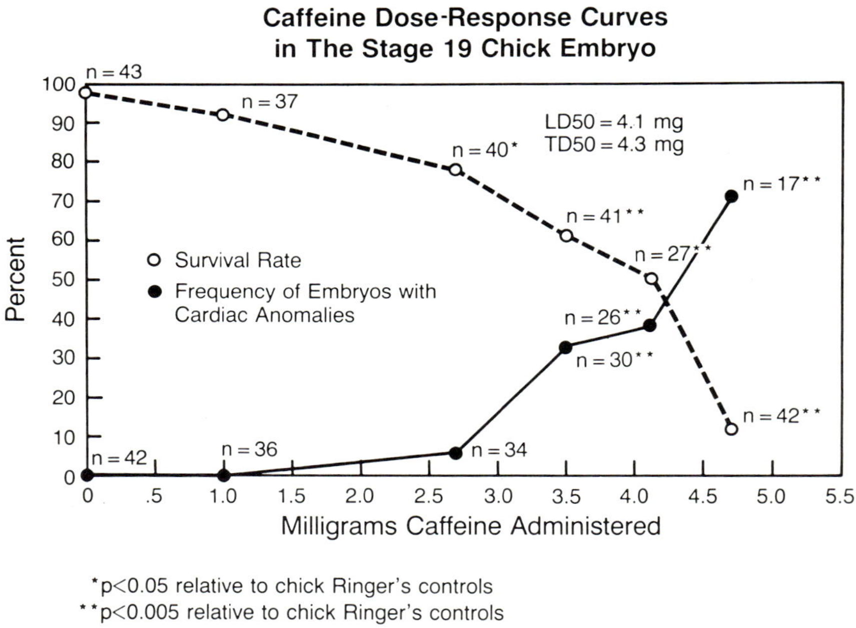

Fig. 1. Dose-response data derived from administration of caffeine to 3-day chick embryos (stage 19). Survival rates were computed as the fraction of embryos that survived to day 14 of incubation based on total number of embryos treated. Malformation frequencies were computed as the fraction of embryos with a heart malformation based on number of embryos that survived to day 11 of incubation. Sample numbers (n) in each group are shown.

TABLE I. Distribution of Specific Caffeine-Induced Cardiac Malformations in the Chick Embryo

	Frequency of embryos with					
	Ventricular septal defect and overriding aorta		Common aortico-pulmonary trunk		Pulmonary stenosis[1]	
Treatment	n	%	n	%	n	%
Chick Ringer's (C/R) solution, 1.0 ml	0/42	0.0	0/42	0.0	0/42	0.0
1.0 mg caffeine	0/36	0.0	0/36	0.0	0/36	0.0
2.7 mg caffeine	2/34	5.9	0/34	0.0	0/34	0.0
3.5 mg caffeine	4/30	13.3[2]	3/30	10.0	3/30	10.0
4.1 mg caffeine	2/26	7.7	6/26	23.1[3]	2/26	7.7
4.7 mg caffeine	1/17	5.9	6/17	35.3[3]	5/17	29.4[3]

[1]Complexed with ventricular septal defect and overriding aorta.
[2]$p < 0.05$ relative to C/R controls.
[3]$p < 0.005$ relative to C/R controls.

er's solution showed no appreciable changes in cardiac function within 60 minutes. However, exposure of embryos to 3.5 mg caffeine produced several marked changes in cardiac function. These included: dilation of the common ventricle and weak ventricular contractility in all embryos within 60 minutes after exposure to this dose of caffeine. Both end-diastolic and end-systolic volumes were markedly increased following the administration of caffeine (Fig. 3). Alterations in function were seen within 3 minutes after exposure to caffeine and persisted 60 minutes afterward.

These studies have shown that adminstration of caffeine to the 3-day chick embryo causes significant hemodynamic changes and interference with normal developmental rotation of the aorta and aorticopulmonary septation. Cardiac malformations were induced at doses of caffeine that markedly increased embryonic mortality. The teratogenic effect of caffeine on the heart seems to be more likely a result of a toxic effect on the embryo than a direct alteration of cardiac cell function. In addition, it appears that physiologic changes in the cardiovascular system also play an important role in the pathogenesis of caffeine-induced cardiac malformations. Marked cardiac functional changes following caffeine administration included dilation of the common ventricle and weak ventricular contractility. However, dilation of the ventricle may have resulted either from a direct pharmacologic action (as caffeine is a vasodilating agent [4]), or may be a manifestation of heart failure due to toxicity. It is suggested that the anomalies produced by caffeine in this study are secondary to dilation of the embryonic heart. Jaffee [5] has previ-

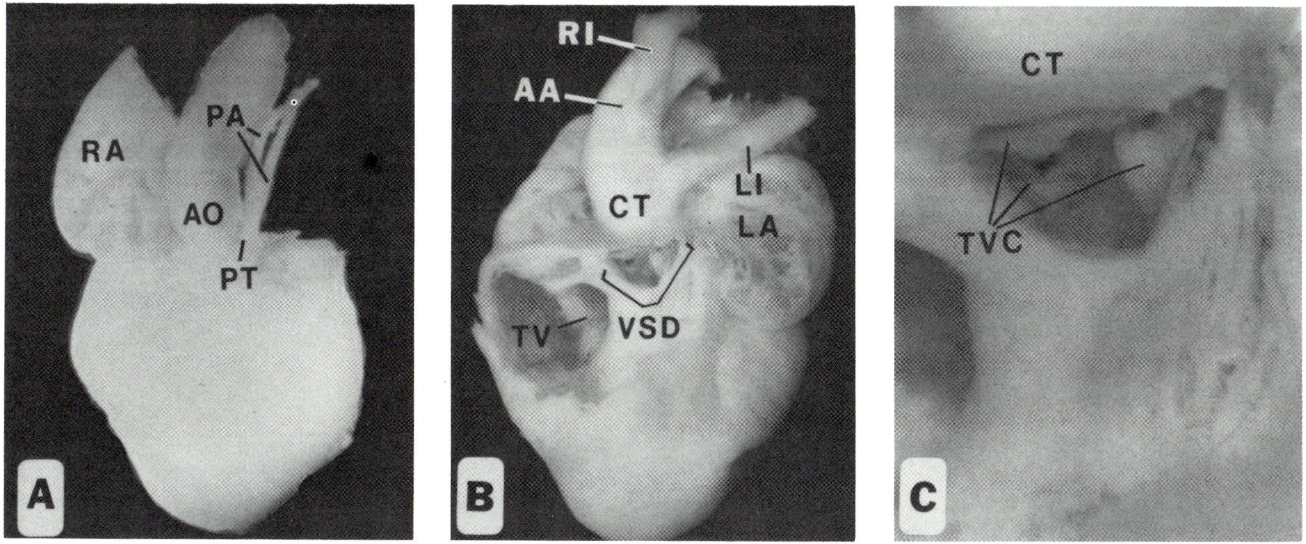

Fig. 2. A) Photograph showing the right ventricular view of the heart from a 13-day chick embryo that was treated with 4.1 mg caffeine on day 3 of incubation. The pulmonary trunk (PT) was markedly stenotic with severely hypoplastic pulmonary arteries (PA). Detailed examination of the heart showed a ventricular septal defect with an overriding aortic valve. The left atrium has been removed for better visualization of the PT and PA. RA, right atrium; AO, aortic root. Magnification ×24. B) Right ventricular view of a 17-day chick embryo exposed to 4.1 mg caffeine on day 3 of incubation. Examination of this heart showed a common aorticopulmonary trunk (CT) with a large ventricular septal defect (VSD). RI, right innominate; LI, left innominate; AA, aortic arch; LA, left atrium; TV, tricuspid valve. Magnification ×19. C) Photograph showing higher magnification of Figure 2B. Note the tricuspid truncal valve. TVC, truncal valve cusp. Magnification ×38.

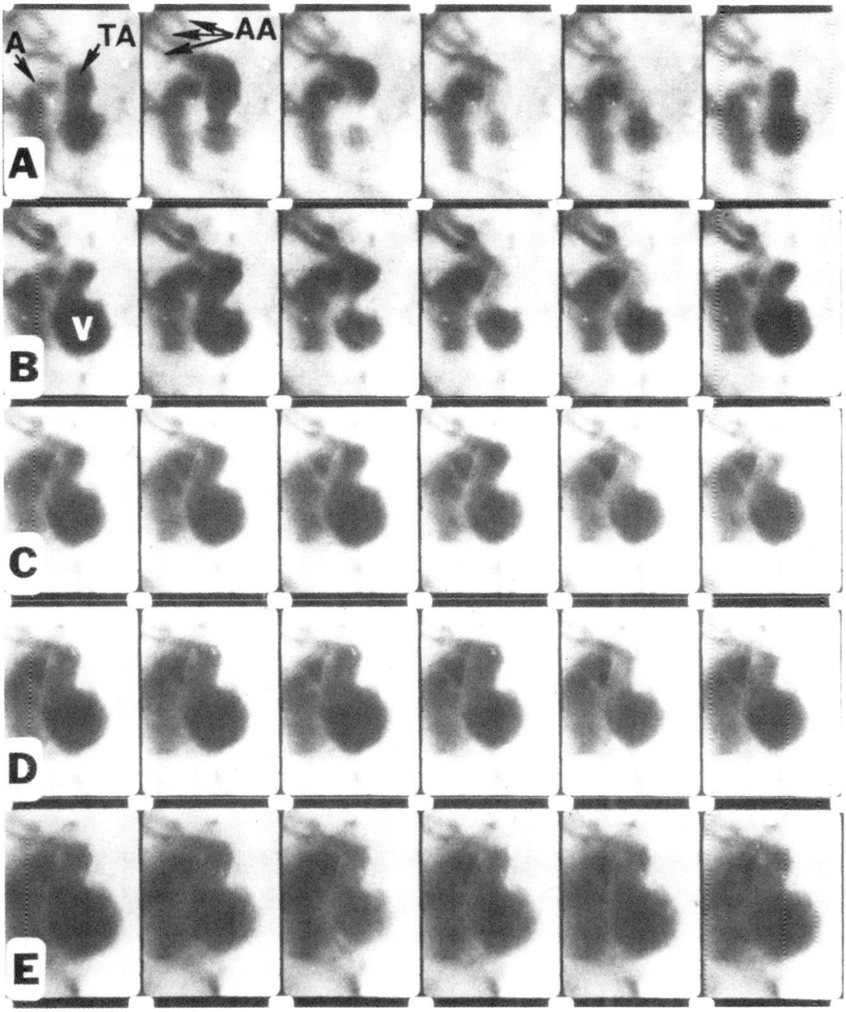

Fig. 3. Microcinegraphs showing cardiac function in a stage 19 chick embryo before treatment with caffeine (A), and at 3 minutes (B), 10 minutes (C), 30 minutes (D), and 60 minutes (E) following administration of a teratogenic dose of caffeine (3.5 mg/egg). It is clear from these microcinegraphs that caffeine induced not only dilation of the common ventricle (V) but also weak ventricular contractility. The transverse dimension of the ventricle decreased only slightly 10–60 minutes after treatment as compared with the pretreatment control (Fig. 3A) sequence (see 3rd and 4th frames in Fig. 3C and 3D and 2nd and 3rd frames in Fig. 3E). It is noteworthy that caffeine markedly reduced blood flow through the third right aortic arch in this embryo. AA, right aortic arch; TA, truncus arteriosus; A, atrium. Magnification ×17.

ously induced VSDs, dextropositional anomalies of the aorta, and CAT by exposing chick embryos to low oxygen environments. Furthermore, Grabowski and Schroeder [6] have demonstrated that exposure of chick embryos to hypoxia may produce dilation of the heart, just as we have observed following caffeine administration.

A comparison of caffeine dosage administered to chick embryos in this study with that to which a human embryo may be exposed during pregnancy is difficult to assess. However, if the assumption is valid that caffeine is distributed throughout the egg and not concentrated exclusively in the embryo itself, then the doses employed in this study are similar to the doses in 7–31 cups of coffee or 3–15 Anacin® tablets. We hope that results will stimulate further testing of caffeine on the development of the heart in mammalian models together with a complete morphologic analyis of the heart defects in the chick.

REFERENCES

1. Fabro S, Brown NA: Caffeine in pregnancy. State of the science. Reprod Toxicol 1:2–3, 1982.
2. Food and Drug Administration: Report on Caffeine, 1980.
3. Fujii T, Nishimura H: Adverse effects of prolonged administration of caffeine on rat fetus. Toxicol Appl Pharmacol 22:449–457, 1972.
4. Rall TW: Central nervous system stimulants. The xanthines. In Gilman AG, Goodman LS, Gilman A (eds.): "The Pharmacological Basis of Therapeutics," 6th ed. New York: Macmillan, 1980, pp 592–607.
5. Jaffee OC: The effects of moderate hypoxia and moderate hypoxia with hypercapnia on cardiac development in chick embryos. Teratology 10:275–282, 1974.
6. Grabowski CT, Schroeder RE: A time-lapse photographic study of chick embryos exposed to teratogenic doses of hypoxia. J Embryol Exp Morphol 19:347–362, 1968.

Experimentally Induced Cardiovascular Malformations in the Chick Embryo. Part II. Teratogenic Effect of Tedral® (Theophylline, Ephedrine, and Phenobarbital) on Cardiac Development in Chick Embryos

Rumiko Matsuoka, MD, Enid F. Gilbert, MD, Harold J. Bruyere, Jr, PhD, Tzann-Tarn Fang, MD, Toshio Nishikawa, MD, and John M. Opitz, MD

Department of Pathology, University of Wisconsin, School of Medicine, Madison, Wisconsin 53792 (RM, EFG, HJB, T-T F, TN) and Department of Medical Genetics, Shodair Children's Hospital, Helena, Montana 59604 (JMO)

We have shown previously that methylxanthine (theophylline and caffeine) administration causes malformations in the cardiovascular system of the chick [1–4]. Aneurysms of the ascending aorta with incomplete rotation of the aorticopulmonary trunk (characterized by malformations such as double outlet right ventricle and overriding aorta) and ventricular septal defect have been produced by the administration of theophylline in the chick embryo.

We have reported a detailed examination [5] of an aborted human embryo whose mother had accidentally taken 4 tablets of Tedral® (Parke-Davis, 1 tablet containing 130 mg theophylline, 25 mg ephedrine, and 8 mg phenobarbital) for an upper respiratory tract infection. Soon after ingestion of the Tedral®, the mother developed acute chest pain and a fast, irregular heart beat. Spontaneous abortion occurred at approximately 80 days of gestation. The embryo had a truncus arteriosus. Therefore, we performed an experimental study of the effect of Tedral® on cardiovascular morphogenesis in chick embryos (Table I).

Tedral® containing 1.0 mg/ml, 2.0 mg/ml, and 2.8 mg/ml theophylline in combination with ephedrine and phenobarbital in a relative dose ratio of theophylline 33: ephedrine 6: phenobarbital 2, was administered to 250 chick

Birth Defects: Original Article Series, Volume 23, Number 1, pages 449–452

TABLE I. Concentrations of Agents in Tedral® Used in These Studies

Group	Agent concentration in Tedral®		
	Theophylline	Ephedrine	Phenobarbital
A	2.8 mg/ml (0.015M)	0.54 mg/ml (0.002M)	0.17 mg/ml (0.0007M)
B	2.0 mg/ml (0.01M)	0.38 mg/ml (0.0015M)	0.12 mg/ml (0.0005M)
C	1.0 mg/ml (0.005M)	0.19 mg/ml (0.00075M)	0.06 mg/ml (0.00025M)

embryos. Tedral® containing larger concentrations of theophylline (2.0–2.8 mg/ml) produced aneurysms of the ascending aorta with associated cardiovascular malformations in 100% of embryos treated. These studies have shown that 1) administration of theophylline alone produces cardiovascular malformations in chick embryos, 2) the effect of theophylline on cardiovascular morphogenesis is amplified when ephedrine and phenobarbital are administered, and 3) the production of specific conotruncal malformations following Tedral® administration depends on the developmental stage at which the drug is given to the embryo. The most frequent anomalies observed following Tedral® administration are double outlet right ventricle with bilateral conus and ventricular septal defect. Aortic aneurysms are larger and cardiovascular malformations more complex in embryos exposed to Tedral® than those treated with theophylline alone (Fig. 1). Complex cardiac defects included transposition of the great arteries, double outlet right ventricle with double inlet left ventricle, and truncus arteriosus communis.

Figure 2 shows comparative effects on cardiovascular morphogenesis of administration of Tedral® and theophylline to 5-day chick embryos (Hamburger-Hamilton stages 24–26). Administration of all Tedral® combinations produced aortic aneurysms and other cardiovascular malformations in significantly higher frequencies ($P < 0.05$) than corresponding doses of theophylline administered alone. Aortic aneurysms with other cardiovascular malformations were seen in 100% of embryos treated with Tedral® combinations A and B. However, parallel doses of theophylline produced aneurysms in only 27.3% (2.8 mg) and 25.0% (2.0 mg) of embryos treated. Aneurysms were not induced by treatment with ephedrine, phenobarbital, or 0.15 M sodium chloride.

Other cardiovascular anomalies induced by Tedral® were also observed among 89 embryos with anomalies: 28 embryos (31.5%) with hypoplastic or atretic right pulmonary artery; 3 embryos with hypoplastic left pulmonary artery; 1 embryo with infundibular and valvular pulmonary atresia, DORV,

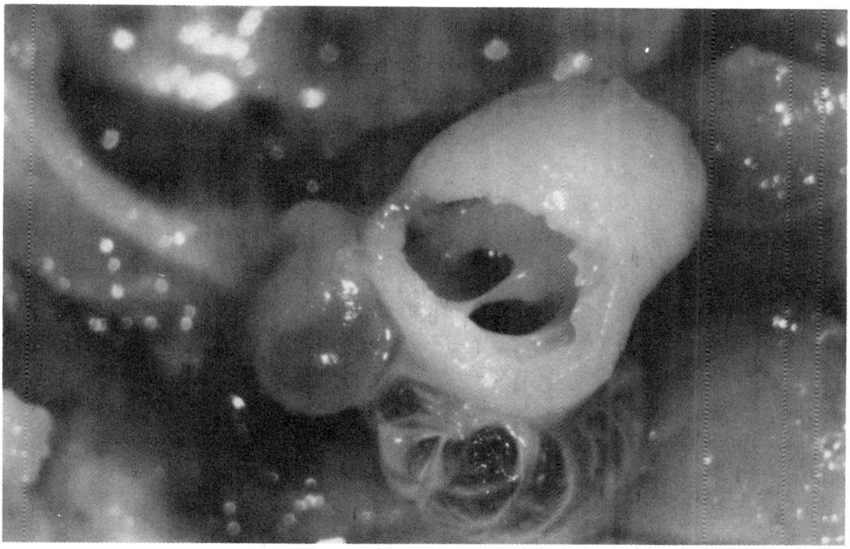

Fig. 1. Right ventricular view of 16-day embryonic chick heart showing large aortic aneurysm and ventricular septal defect induced by administration of Tedral®.

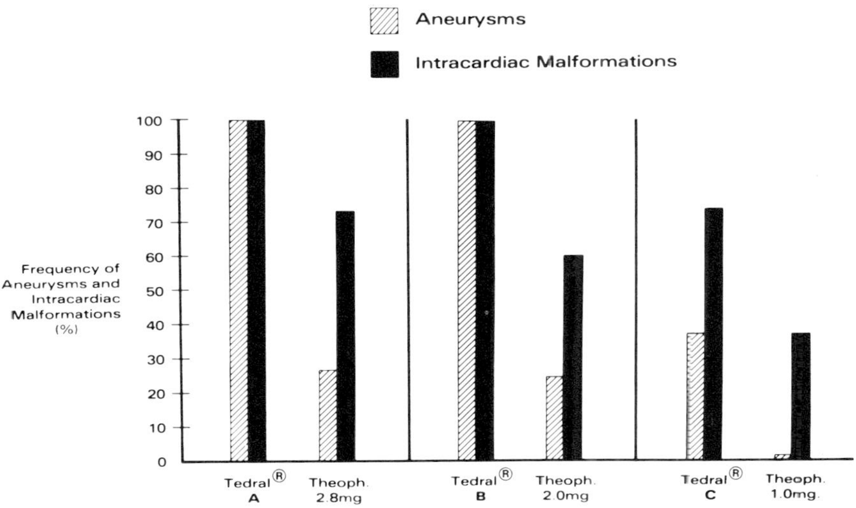

Fig. 2. Histogram showing comparative effects of Tedral® and theophylline with respect to aneurysms and intracardiac malformations.

and bilateral conus; 2 embryos with tricuspid atresia, common atrium due to complete absence of the septum primum and VSD; and 3 embryos with double aortic arch. None of these malformations were observed following exposure of embryos to 2.8 mg theophylline alone.

These data clearly indicate that 1) the combination of drugs in Tedral® is a potent cardiovascular teratogen in the chick embryo; 2) Tedral® administration produces more frequent and more complex (wider spectrum) cardiovascular anomalies in the chick embryo than parallel treatments with corresponding doses of theophylline, ephedrine, or phenobarbital; and 3) theophylline appears to be the major agent contained in Tedral® responsible for cardiovascular malformations and its action is synergistic with ephedrine and/or phenobarbital.

REFERENCES

1. Ishikawa S, Gilbert EF, Bruyere HJ Jr, Cheung MO: Aortic aneurysms subsequent to theophylline administration in chick embryos. Circulation 54:185 (Abstract), 1976.
2. Ishikawa S, Gilbert EF, Bruyere HJ Jr, Cheung MO: Theophylline induced conotruncal malformations in embryonic chick hearts. Teratology 15:27A, 1977.
3. Ishikawa S, Gilbert EF, Bruyere HJ Jr, Cheung MO: Aortic aneurysm associated with cardiac defects in theophylline stimulated chick embryos. Teratology 18:23–30, 1978.
4. Gilbert EF, Bruyere HJ Jr, Ishikawa S, Cheung MO, Hodach RJ: The effects of methylxanthines on catecholamine stimulated and normal chick embryos. Teratology 16:47–52, 1977.
5. Matsuoka R, Gilbert EF, Bruyere HJ Jr, Opitz JM: An aborted human fetus with truncus-arteriosus communis—Possible teratogenic effect of Tedral. Heart and Vessels 1:176–178, 1985.

Experimentally Induced Cardiovascular Malformations in the Chick Embryo. Part III. The Teratogenic Effect of Phenobarbital on the Embryonic Chick Heart

Toshio Nishikawa, MD, Harold J. Bruyere, Jr, PhD, Yasuo Takagi, MD, Rumiko Matsuoka, MD, and Enid F. Gilbert, MD

Department of Pathology, University of Wisconsin, School of Medicine, Madison, Wisconsin 53792

Anticonvulsant drugs have been reported to be teratogenic in humans [1–3]. Numerous clinical studies have demonstrated an increased frequency of congenital malformations in offspring following maternal anticonvulsant therapy during pregnancy [4–8]. In these reports phenobarbital (PB) was often cited as an anticonvulsant drug used alone or in combination with other drugs. The most frequent documented anomalies following maternal anticonvulsant therapy are cleft lip and cleft palate. However, congenital cardiac defects are not uncommon [9]. McColl et al [10], administered PB to pregnant rabbits and observed aortic arch anomalies and small auricles in offspring. However, the mechanism of PB teratogenicity in the cardiovascular (CV) system has not been studied. We have studied the effects of PB administration on morphogenesis of the chick CV system at developmental stages 17–26 [11] (days 3–5 of development), and have established pathophysiologic evidence to support a theory that changes in cardiac function may be related to the pathogenesis of PB-induced CV malformations.

White Leghorn eggs were incubated and prepared using the materials and methods described previously [12]. A single dose of sodium phenobarbital (1.75×10^{-5} mole, Elkins-Sinn Inc., Cherry Hill, N.J.) in 1 ml 0.9% sodium chloride solution was administered topically to chick embryos (Hamburger-

Birth Defects: Original Article Series, Volume 23, Number 1, pages 453–458

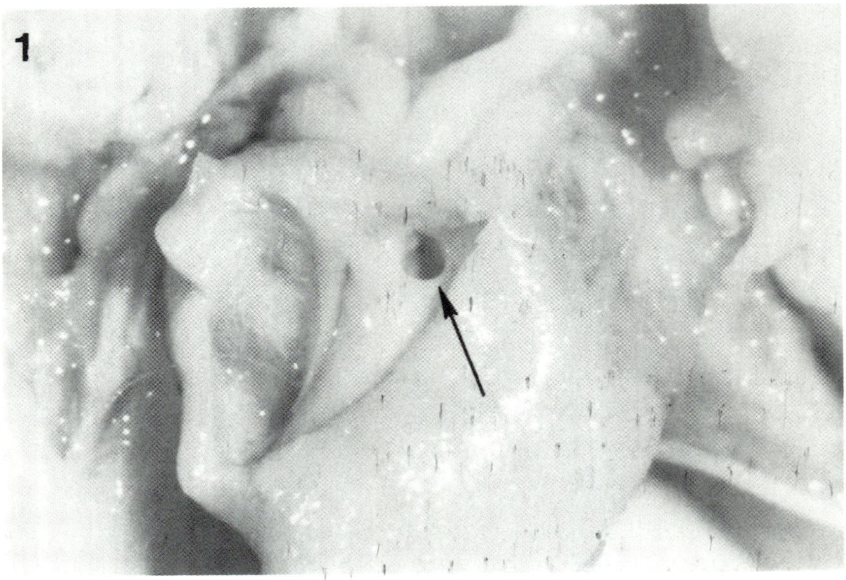
1

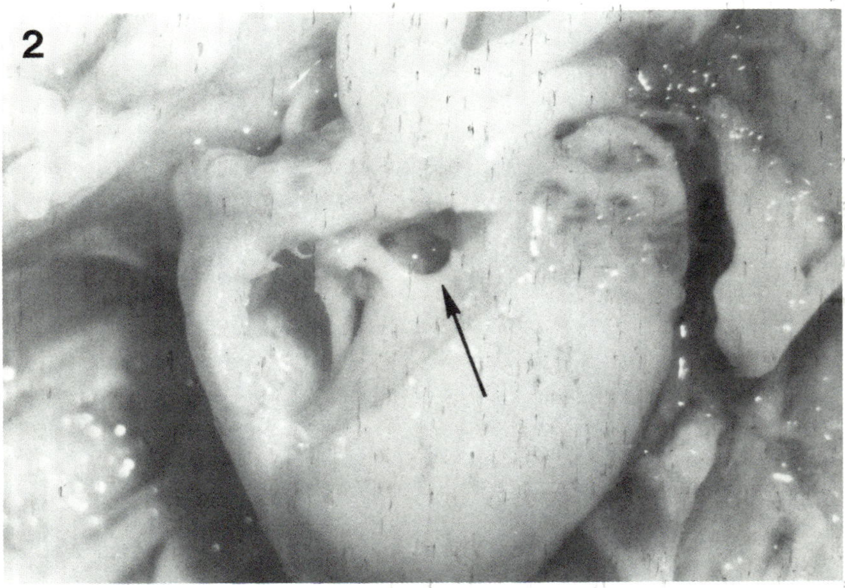
2

Hamilton stages 17–26) through observation windows in the shells. Control embryos received 1 ml of 0.9% sodium chloride solution.

The heart rate was measured in 4-day-old embryos by visually observing with a hand-held lens and counting ventricular contractions for 1 minute.

Ninety-six surviving embryos treated with PB at stages 17–26 had cardiovascular anomalies. Embryos with malformations included 62 specimens with isolated ventricular septal defect (VSD) (Fig. 1), 22 with VSD associated with overriding aorta (Fig. 2), 11 with double outlet right ventricle (DORV) (Fig. 3), and 24 with aortic arch anomalies (AAA). Among the embryos with DORV, the pulmonary artery arose normally, but the aorta originated entirely from the right ventricle. The aortic valve was positioned higher than normal and was located in the same frontal and cross-sectional planes as the pulmonary valve. Ventricular septal defects were located below the crista supraventricularis in a subaortic position. There was no pulmonary stenosis in any of the cases of DORV. Embryos with AAA included 18 specimens with a remnant of the left 4th aortic arch (Fig. 4) and 7 specimens with absence of the right 3rd aortic arch. The frequency of CV defects among control embryos was 8.9%. All anomalies observed were small infundibular VSDs.

Several investigators have investigated the potential teratogenic effects of barbiturates. Skeletal malformations were observed in rats [13, 14], mice [15], and rabbits [16]. Aortic arch anomalies have also been noted [16]; however, to our knowledge, intracardiac malformations have not previously been reported in laboratory animals. In the present study, 99% of phenobarbital (PB) treated chick embryos had cardiac anomalies. These anomalies included isolated ventricular septal defect (VSD), VSD with overriding aorta, and double outlet right ventricle (DORV).

Variations in conotruncal maturation, bulbar rotation, conal absorption, and/or bulbar ostial shift play major roles in the development of slightly different cardiac anomalies. Lev et al [16] suggested that DORV with subaortic VSD and VSD with overriding aorta are similar malformations in that they may belong to one spectrum of cardiac defects. DORV with subaortic VSD and VSD with overriding aorta have been reported previously in the chick embryo [17–21].

Fig. 1. Right ventricular view of a 14-day chick embryo heart with infundibular "simple, punched-out type" ventricular septal defect (arrow).

Fig. 2. Right ventricular view of a 14-day chick embryo heart with an infundibular ventricular septal defect and overriding aorta (arrow).

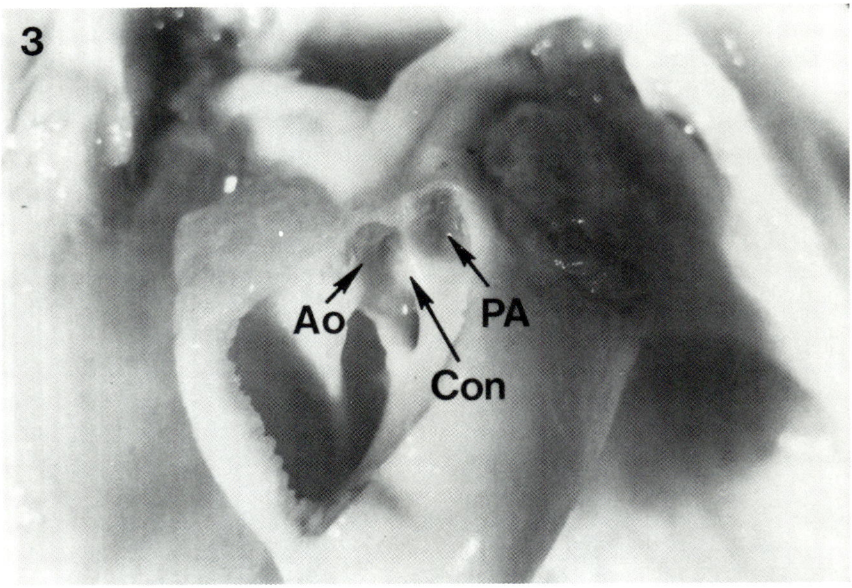
3
Ao
PA
Con

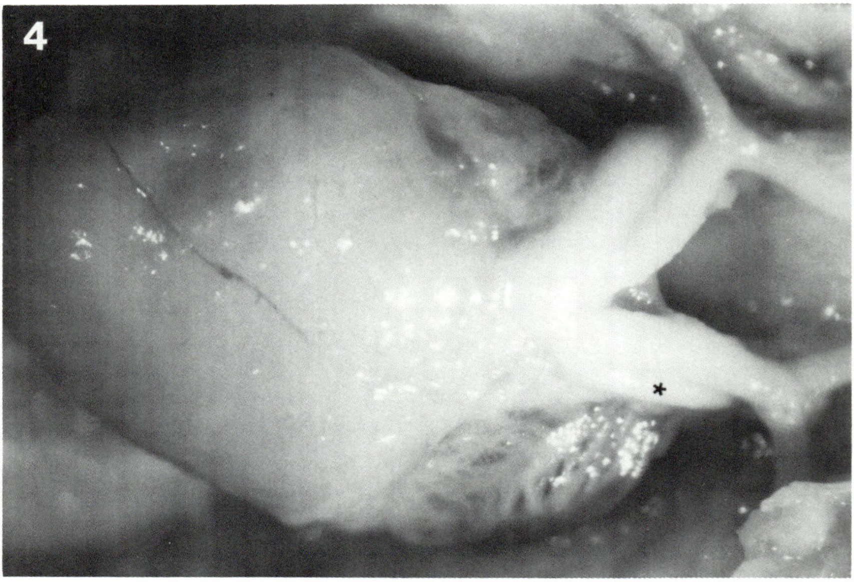
4
*

In this study PB significantly decreased the heart rate in those chick embryos that ultimately developed cardiac malformations. There is good evidence that a negative chronotropic effect during cardiogenesis may predispose to cardiac anomalies. De la Cruz and others [22–24] noted a decreased heart rate in chick embryos exposed to agents that also induced cardiac anomalies.

Arrhythmogenesis may be a more important contributing factor to cardiac teratogenesis. In our study, PB-induced arrhythmia (>30 minute) correlated well with cardiac malformations characterized by dextroposition of the aorta.

REFERENCES

1. Meyer JG: The teratological effects of anticonvulsants and the effects on pregnancy and birth. Eur Neurol 10:179–190, 1973.
2. Smithells RW: Environmental teratogens of man. Br Med Bull 32:27–33, 1976.
3. Paulson GW, Paulson RB: Teratogenic effects of anticonvulsants. Arch Neurol 38:140–143, 1981.
4. Speidel BD, Meadow SR: Maternal epilepsy and abnormalities of the fetus and newborn. Lancet 2:839–843, 1972.
5. Fredric J: Epilepsy and pregnancy: A report from the Oxford record linkage study. Br Med J 2:442–448, 1973.
6. Hill RM: Teratogenesis and antiepileptic drugs. N Engl J Med 289:1089–1090, 1973.
7. Hill RM, Verniaud WM, Horning MG, McCulley LB, Morgan NF: Infants exposed *in utero* to antiepileptic drugs. Am J Dis Child 127:645–653, 1974.
8. Shapiro S, Hartz SC, Siskind V, Mitchell AA, Slone D, Rosenberg L, Monson RR, Heinonen OP: Anticonvulsants and parental epilepsy in the development of birth defects. Lancet 1:272–275, 1976.
9. Anderson RC: Cardiac defects in children of mothers receiving anticonvulsant therapy during pregnancy. J Pediatr 89:318–319, 1976.
10. McColl JD, Robinson S, Globus M: Effect of some therapeutic agents on the rabbit fetus. Toxicol Appl Pharmacol 10:244–252, 1967.
11. Hamburger V, Hamilton HL: A series of normal stages in the development of the chick embryo. J Morphol 88:49–92, 1951.
12. Hodach RJ, Gilbert EF, Fallon JF: Aortic arch anomalies associated with the administration of epinephrine in chick embryos. Teratology 9:203–210, 1974.
13. McColl JD, Globus M, Robinson S: Drug induced skeletal malformations in the rat. Experientia 19:183–185, 1963.

Fig. 3. Right ventricular view of a 14-day chick embryo heart with double outlet right ventricle. Note the side-by-side location of the pulmonic (PA) and aortic (Ao) outlets from the right ventricle with subaortic and subpulmonic conus (Con).

Fig. 4. External view of a 14-day chick embryo heart with a remnant of the 4th aortic arch(*).

14. Persaud TVN: Tierexperimentelle Untersuchungen zur Frage der teratogenen Wirkung von Barbituraten. Acta Biol Med Ger 14:89–90, 1965.
15. Fritz H, Muller D, Hess R: Comparative study of the teratogenicity of phenobarbitone, diphenylhydantoin and carbamazepine in mice. Toxicology 6:323–330, 1976.
16. Lev M, Bharati S, Meng CCL, Liberthson RR, Paul MH, Idriss F: A concept of double-outlet right ventricle. J Thorac Cardiovasc Surg 64:271–281, 1972.
17. Gessner IH: Spectrum of congenital cardiac anomalies produced in chick embryos by mechanical interference with cardiogenesis. Circ Res 18:625–633, 1966.
18. Gessner IH, Van Mierop LHS: Experimental production of cardiac defects: The spectrum of dextroposition of the aorta. Am J Cardiol 25:272–278, 1970.
19. Ishikawa S, Gilbert EF, Bruyere HJ Jr, Cheung MO: Aortic aneurysm associated with cardiac defects in theophylline stimulated chick embryos. Teratology 18:23–30, 1978.
20. Arteaga M, de la Cruz MV, Sanchez C, Diaz GF: Double outlet right ventricle. Experimental morphogenesis in the chick embryo heart. Pediatr Cardiol 3:219–227, 1982.
21. Robertson AC, Foulks JG, Daniel EE: The effects of phenobarbital-induced myocardial depression on cardiac electrolyte distribution. J Pharmacol Exp Ther 122:281–294, 1958.
22. de la Cruz MV, Campillo-Sainz C, Munoz-Armas S: Congenital heart defects in chick embryos subjected to temperature variations. Circ Res 18:257–262, 1966.
23. Grabowski CT, Tsai ENC, Toben HR: The effects of teratogenic doses of hypoxia on the blood pressure of chick embryos. Teratology 2:67–76, 1970.
24. Gilani SH, Silvestri A: The effect of propranolol upon chick embryo cardiogenesis. Exp Cell Biol 45:158–166, 1977.

Experimentally Induced Cardiovascular Malformations in the Chick Embryo. Part IV. Evidence for H2-Receptor Stimulation in the Production of Cardiovascular Malformations by Histamine in Chick Embryos

Yasuo Takagi, MD, **Harold J. Bruyere, Jr**, PhD, **Toshio Nishikawa**, MD, **and Enid F. Gilbert**, MD

Department of Pathology, University of Wisconsin, School of Medicine, Madison, Wisconsin 53792

Hemodynamic flow patterns in the embryonic circulation are important in producing morphologic changes in the cardiac chambers and great vessels [1–4]. Relatively specific cardiovascular malformations have been produced in chicks by mechanically altering these blood flow patterns [5–8]. Administrations of cardioactive chemical substances such as sympathomimetic amines [9–11], acetylcholine [11], and theophylline [12–14] have also resulted in cardiovascular malformations.

Histamine (H) has positive inotropic and chronotropic effects [15–17]. The physiologic actions of H are mediated by at least 2 distinct receptor classes designated H1 and H2 [5,18]. The negative dromotropic effect of H is mediated by the H1-receptor [19–21]. The receptor that mediates the positive chronotropic effect of H has been designated as H2 [5]. The positive inotropic effects of H in the ventricle appear to be due to H2-receptor stimulation [20,22–24], whereas receptors that mediate the positive inotropic effect of H in atria appear to be of the H1 class [25]. Cimetidine, a nonthiourea analog of metiamide, is a specific competitive H2-receptor antagonist [26]. Diphenyhydramine [27] is an H1-receptor antagonist.

Birth Defects: Original Article Series, Volume 23, Number 1, pages 459–464

We investigated the effects of H upon morphology in the rapidly developing embryonic chick cardiovascular system and used H-receptor antagonists in an attempt to prevent the teratogenic effect of H.

Fertile white Leghorn eggs were used. On the fifth day of incubation, at embryonic developmental stages 24–26 Hamburger-Hamilton [28], compounds were administered to the surface of extraembryonic membranes in the vicinity of the embryonic heart.

Four concentrations of H (10^{-7} mole, 2×10^{-6} mole and 5×10^{-6} mole per 0.1 ml) were used to determine the dose response of the drug. A volume of 0.1 ml of H solution was administered every 2 hours for 6 consecutive hours. The concentrations of H and the corresponding anomaly ratios are shown in Figure 1.

Cimetidine (C) (Sigma), an H2-receptor antagonist, and diphenhydramine hydrochloride (D) (Sigma), an H1-receptor antagonist, were used (10^{-6} mole per 0.1 ml). A 0.1 ml volume of these drugs was administered to extraem-

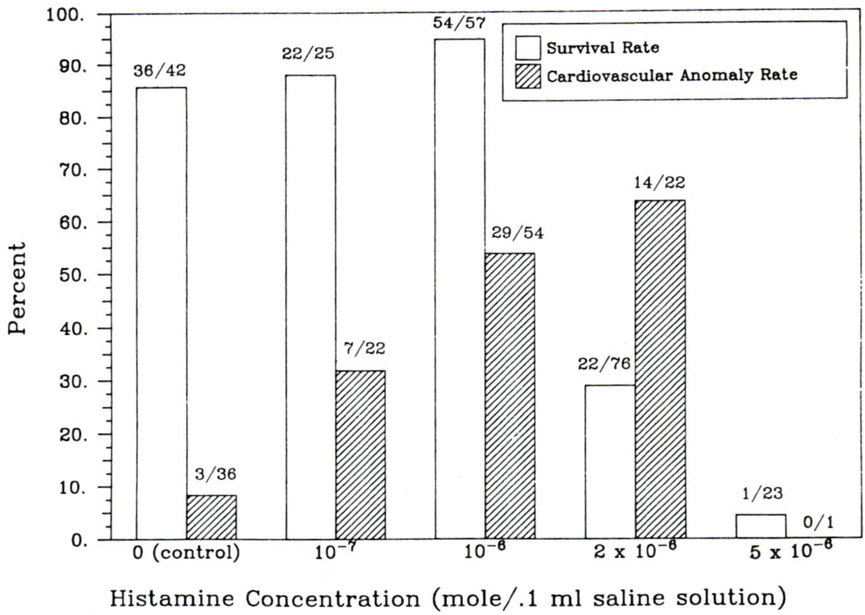

Fig. 1. Histogram showing dose responses to histamine in embryonic chicks. Significant differences in anomaly rate were noted between saline control specimens and embryos treated with 1×10^{-6} or 2×10^{-6} mole histamine ($P < 0.001$). A dose of 1×10^{-6} mole histamine demonstrated a high anomaly rate but did not affect survival.

bryonic membranes 10 minutes before the first administration of H. A 0.1 ml volume of saline was administered to control embryos in the same manner.

From the 14th to 17th day of incubation embryos were sacrificed and hearts of embryos that survived to necropsy were perfused with Carnoy fixative (60% ethanol, 30% chloroform, and 10% acetic acid).

Administrations of 1×10^{-6} mole H demonstrated the highest cardiovascular anomaly rate with no significant change in survival rate relative to controls.

Table I describes specific types of anomalies induced by H with their corresponding frequencies. Isolated ventricular septal defect (VSD) or aortic arch (AA) anomaly in embryos treated with 1×10^{-6} mole H were significantly higher than those seen in the control group. AA anomalies included remnant of the left 4th AA, absence of the right 3rd AA, absence of both 3rd AA, and absence of the right 4th AA. Four cases of double outlet right ventricle (DORV) with a large subaortic VSD were also noted following H administration.

The highest heart rate was attained 10 minutes after each injection of H. Although mean heart rate decreased 10–20 minutes after exposure to H, the mean heart rate 120 minutes after H administration was higher than in corresponding saline-treated control animals.

Pretreatment with 1×10^{-6} mole cimetidine significantly reduced the incidence of total anomalies from 54% to 24% ($P \leqslant 0.025$). An especially significant reduction in AA anomaly incidence was also noted.

TABLE I. Frequencies and Types of Cardiovascular Anomalies Induced by Histamine Administration to Chick Embryos

	Incidence					
	Isolated VSD*		DORV†		Aortic arch anomaly	
Agent, dose	n	%	n	%	n	%
Histamine, 1×10^{-7} mole	6/22	27	0/22	0	2/22	9
Histamine, 1×10^{-6} mole	17/54	31‡	4/54	7	11/54	20**
Histamine, 2×10^{-6} mole	7/22	32††	0/22	0	9/22	41‡‡
0.9% Sodium chloride, 0.1 ml	2/36	6	0/36	0	1/36	3

*Isolated VSD, ventricular septal defect without associated intracardiac anomalies.
†DORV, double outlet right ventricle.
‡Significantly different from control value, $P < 0.01$.
**Significantly different from control value, $P < 0.05$.
††Significantly different from control value, $P < 0.025$.
‡‡Significantly different from control value, $P < 0.001$.

Diphenhydramine hydrochloride (D) pretreatment on total cardiovascular anomaly rate showed no significant differences in frequencies of specific anomalies between D-pretreated embryos and H-treated controls.

These data indicate that histamine (H) induces cardiovascular malformations in 4½–5 day embryonic chicks (stages 24–26).

H is known to have a positive inotropic and chronotropic effect and negative dromotropic effect [15,24]. A possible mechanism of action of H that explains its positive inotropic effects is similar to that established for catecholamines: this physiologic effect of H may be directly related to increased levels of intracellular cyclic adenosine 3′5′-monophosphate (cAMP) [22] as a result of an H-receptor mediated stimulation of cardiac adenyl cyclase [17]. The rise in cAMP leads to a cellular influx of Ca^{++} ions during the cardiac action potential, and this, in turn, results in an increase in contractility. This effect is not through a β-adrenergic mechanism Josephson et al [23], Hodach et al [10], and Bruyere et al [29] demonstrated that agents that stimulate β-adrenoceptors also produce cardiovascular malformations when administered to chick embryos. Gilbert et al [30] suggested that cardiovascular anomalies might be induced in chick embryos via β-1 adrenoreceptor stimulation, activation of adenyl cyclase, and subsequent elevation of cAMP. Significant changes in cardiac function induced by a β-receptor stimulant may have a teratogenic effect on the developing heart [31].

Our studies have shown that 1×10^{-6} mole C protected embryos from the induction of cardiovascular anomalies by H ($P \leqslant 0.025$). D had no appreciable effect in preventing H-induced anomalies at the doses employed. Thus, these blocking studies with C and D suggest that H2-receptor stimulation plays a major role in the production of cardiovascular anomalies by H.

Our studies have shown that H induces cardiovascular anomalies in the chick embryo. These malformations are prevented by pretreatment with an H2-receptor antagonist. Our findings suggest that these anomalies are produced by stimulation of cardiac H2-receptors.

REFERENCES

1. Bremer JL: The presence and influence of two spiral streams in the heart of chick embryo. Am J Anat 49:409–440, 1932.
2. Jaffee OC: Hemodynamics and cardiogenesis. J Morphol 110:217–225, 1962.
3. Jaffee OC: Hemodynamic factors in the development of the chick embryo heart. Anat Rec 151:69–75, 1965.
4. Jaffee OC: The development of the arterial outflow tract in the chick embryo heart. Anat Rec 158:35–42, 1967.
5. Black JW, Duncan WAM, Durant GJ, Ganelline CR, Parson ME: Definition and antagonism of histamine H2-receptor. Nature (London) 236:385–390, 1972.

6. Gessner IH: Spectrum of congenital cardiac anomalies produced in chick embryos by mechanical interference with cardiogenesis. Circ Res 18:625–633, 1966.
7. Gessner IH, Van Mierop LHS: Experimental production of cardiac defects: The spectrum of dextroposition of the aorta. Am J Cardiol 25:272–278, 1970.
8. Harh JY, Paul MH, Gallen WJ, Friedberg DZ, Kaplan S: Experimental production of hypoplastic left heart syndrome in the chick embryo. Am J Cardiol 31:51–56, 1973.
9. Hodach RJ, Gilbert EF, Fallon JF: Aortic arch anomalies associated with the administration of epinephrine in chick embryos. Teratology 9:203–210, 1974.
10. Hodach RJ, Hodach AE, Fallon JF, Folts JD, Bruyere HJ Jr, Gilbert EF: The role of beta-adrenergic activity in the production of cardiac and aortic arch anomalies in chick embryos. Teratology 12:33–45, 1975.
11. Ishikawa S, Kawamura T, Takao A, Ando M, Miwa H, Okai O: Cardiovascular malformations following acetylcholine chloride administration to chick embryos. Teratology 12:198–199 (Abstract), 1975.
12. Ishikawa S, Gilbert EF, Bruyere HJ Jr, Cheung MO: Aortic aneurysms subsequent to theophylline administration in chick embryos. Circulation 54:185 (Abstract), 1976.
13. Gilbert EF, Bruyere HJ Jr, Ishikawa S, Cheung MO, Hodach RJ: The effects of methylxanthines on catecholamine-stimulated and normal chick embryos. Teratology 16:47–52, 1977.
14. Ishikawa S, Gilbert EF, Bruyere HJ Jr, Cheung MO: Aortic aneurysm associated with cardiac defects in theophylline stimulated chick embryos. Teratology 18:23–30, 1978.
15. Bartlet AL: The action of histamine on the isolated heart. Br J Pharmacol 21:450–461, 1963.
16. Dean PM: Investigation into the modes of action of histamine on the isolated rabbit heart. Br J Pharmacol 32:65–77, 1968.
17. McNeill JH, Muschek LD: Histamine effects on cardiac contractility, phosphorylase and adenyl cyclase. J Mol Cell Cardiol 4:611–624, 1972.
18. Ash ASF, Schild HO: Receptors mediating actions of histamine. Br J Pharmacol Chemother 27:427–439, 1966.
19. Levi R, Kuye JO: Pharmacological characterization of cardiac histamine receptors: Sensitivity to H1-receptor antagonists. Eur J Pharmacol 27:330–338, 1974.
20. Levi R, Capurro N, Lee CH: Pharmacological characterization of cardiac histamine receptors: Sensitivity to H1- and H2-receptor agonists and antagonists. Eur J Pharmacol 30:328–335, 1975.
21. Levi R, Ganelline CR, Allan G, Willens HJ: Selective impairment of atrioventricular conduction by 2-(2-pyridyl)-ethylamine and 2-(2-thiazolyl)-ethylamine, two histamine H1-receptor agonists. Eur J Pharmacol 34:237–240, 1975.
22. McNeill JH, Verma SC: Blockade by brimamide of the effects of histamine and histamine analogs on cardiac contractility, phosphorylase activation and cyclase adenosine monophosphate. J Pharmacol Exp Ther 188:180–188, 1974.
23. Josephson I, Renaud JF, Vogel S, McLean M, Sperelakis N: Mechanism of the histamine-induced positive inotropic action in cardiac muscle. Eur J Pharmacol 35:393–398, 1976.
24. Johnson CL, Mizoguchi H: The interaction of histamine and guanyl-nucleotides with cardiac adenylate cyclase and its relationship to cardiac contractility. J Pharmacol Exp Ther 200:174–186, 1977.
25. Steinberg MI, Holland DR: Separate receptors mediating the positive inotropic and chronotropic effect of histamine in guinea pig atria. Eur J Pharmacol 34:95–104, 1975.
26. Brimblecome RW, Duncan WAM, Durant GJ, Emmett JC, Ganelline CR, Parson ME: Cimetidine: A non-thiourea H2-receptor antagonist. J Intern Med Res 3:86–92, 1975.

27. Loew ER, MacMillan R, Katser ME: The antihistamine properties of BENADRYL, beta-dimethyl-aminoethyl benzhydryl ether hydrochloride. J Pharmacol Exp Ther 86:229–238, 1946.
28. Hamburger V, Hamilton HL: A series of normal stages in the development of the chick embryo. J Morphol 88:49–92, 1951.
29. Bruyere HJ Jr, Matsuoka R, Carlsson E, Cheung MO, Dean R, Gilbert EF: Cardiovascular malformations associated with administration of prenalterol to young chick embryos. Teratology 28:75–82, 1983.
30. Gilbert EF, Bruyere HJ Jr, Ishikawa S, Cheung MO, Hodach RJ: The effect of practolol and butoxamine on aortic arch malformation in beta adrenoreceptor stimulated chick embryos. Teratology 15:317–323, 1977.
31. Gilbert EF, Bruyere HJ Jr, Ishikawa S, Foulke LM, Helmann SR: Role of decreased cardiac output in isoproternol-induced cardiovascular teratogenesis in chick embryos. Teratology 21:299–307, 1980.

Index